AF688929

Clinical Oncology: New Paradigms

Clinical Oncology: New Paradigms

Editor: Maria Walters

AMERICAN
MEDICAL PUBLISHERS
www.americanmedicalpublishers.com

AMERICAN
MEDICAL PUBLISHERS
www.americanmedicalpublishers.com

Cataloging-in-Publication Data

Clinical oncology : new paradigms / edited by Maria Walters.
p. cm.
Includes bibliographical references and index.
ISBN 978-1-63927-638-7
1. Oncology. 2. Cancer--Treatment. 3. Cancer--Diagnosis. I. Walters, Maria.
RC254 .C55 2023
616.994--dc23

© American Medical Publishers, 2023

American Medical Publishers,
41 Flatbush Avenue,
1st Floor, New York,
NY 11217, USA

ISBN 978-1-63927-638-7 (Hardback)

This book contains information obtained from authentic and highly regarded sources. Copyright for all individual chapters remain with the respective authors as indicated. All chapters are published with permission under the Creative Commons Attribution License or equivalent. A wide variety of references are listed. Permission and sources are indicated; for detailed attributions, please refer to the permissions page and list of contributors. Reasonable efforts have been made to publish reliable data and information, but the authors, editors and publisher cannot assume any responsibility for the validity of all materials or the consequences of their use.

Trademark Notice: Registered trademark of products or corporate names are used only for explanation and identification without intent to infringe.

Contents

Preface VII

Chapter 1 **Computerized Cytological Features for Papillary Thyroid Cancer Diagnosis—Preliminary Report** 1
Shyang-Rong Shih, I-Shiow Jan, Kuen-Yuan Chen, Wan-Yu Chuang, Chih-Yuan Wang, Yung-Lien Hsiao, Tien-Chun Chang and Argon Chen

Chapter 2 **Cold Atmospheric Plasma Restores Paclitaxel Sensitivity to Paclitaxel-Resistant Breast Cancer Cells by Reversing Expression of Resistance-Related Genes** 13
Sungbin Park, Heejoo Kim, Hwee Won Ji, Hyeon Woo Kim, Sung Hwan Yun, Eun Ha Choi and Sun Jung Kim

Chapter 3 **The Interaction of Selenium with Chemotherapy and Radiation on Normal and Malignant Human Mononuclear Blood Cells** 26
Richard J. Lobb, Gregory M. Jacobson, Ray T. Cursons and Michael B. Jameson

Chapter 4 **Methylseleninic Acid Induces Lipid Peroxidation and Radiation Sensitivity in Head and Neck Cancer Cells** 38
John T. Lafin, Ehab H. Sarsour, Amanda L. Kalen, Brett A. Wagner, Garry R. Buettner and Prabhat C. Goswami

Chapter 5 **Identification of a Novel Quinoxaline-Isoselenourea Targeting the STAT3 Pathway as a Potential Melanoma Therapeutic** 53
Verónica Alcolea, Deepkamal N. Karelia, Manoj K. Pandey, Daniel Plano, Parvesh Singh, Juan Antonio Palop, Shantu Amin, Carmen Sanmartín and Arun K. Sharma

Chapter 6 **Overview of Radiolabeled Somatostatin Analogs for Cancer Imaging and Therapy** 70
Romain Eychenne, Christelle Bouvry, Mickael Bourgeois, Pascal Loyer, Eric Benoist and Nicolas Lepareur

Chapter 7 **Involvement of Differentially Expressed microRNAs in the PEGylated Liposome Encapsulated ^{188}Rhenium-Mediated Suppression of Orthotopic Hypopharyngeal Tumor** 104
Bing-Ze Lin, Shen-Ying Wan, Min-Ying Lin, Chih-Hsien Chang, Ting-Wen Chen, Muh-Hwa Yang and Yi-Jang Lee

Chapter 8 **The Influence of Cell Type and Culture Medium on Determining Cancer Selectivity of Cold Atmospheric Plasma Treatment** 128
Eline Biscop, Abraham Lin, Wilma Van Boxem, Jinthe Van Loenhout, Joey De Backer, Christophe Deben, Sylvia Dewilde, Evelien Smits and Annemie Bogaerts

Chapter 9 **Cold Plasma-Treated Ringer's Saline: A Weapon to Target Osteosarcoma** 142
Miguel Mateu-Sanz, Juan Tornín, Bénédicte Brulin, Anna Khlyustova, Maria-Pau Ginebra, Pierre Layrolle and Cristina Canal

Chapter 10 **Cold-Atmospheric Plasma Induces Tumor Cell Death in Preclinical In Vivo and In Vitro Models of Human Cholangiocarcinoma** 160
Javier Vaquero, Florian Judée, Marie Vallette, Henri Decauchy, Ander Arbelaiz, Lynda Aoudjehane, Olivier Scatton, Ester Gonzalez-Sanchez, Fatiha Merabtene, Jérémy Augustin, Chantal Housset, Thierry Dufour and Laura Fouassier

Chapter 11 **Selenium-Binding Protein 1 in Human Health and Disease** 181
Mostafa Elhodaky and Alan M. Diamond

Chapter 12 **PET Radiotracers for CNS-Adrenergic Receptors: Developments and Perspectives** 195
Santosh Reddy Alluri, Sung Won Kim, Nora D. Volkow and Kun-Eek Kil

Chapter 13 **Pyrazoles as Key Scaffolds for the Development of Fluorine-18 Labeled Radiotracers for Positron Emission Tomography (PET)** 213
Pedro M. O. Gomes, Artur M. S. Silva and Vera L. M. Silva

Permissions

List of Contributors

Index

Preface

I am honored to present to you this unique book which encompasses the most up-to-date data in the field. I was extremely pleased to get this opportunity of editing the work of experts from across the globe. I have also written papers in this field and researched the various aspects revolving around the progress of the discipline. I have tried to unify my knowledge along with that of stalwarts from every corner of the world, to produce a text which not only benefits the readers but also facilitates the growth of the field.

Oncology refers to a branch of medicine concerned with the diagnosis, prevention and treatment of cancer. There are four major divisions of oncology, which includes radiation oncology, medical oncology, clinical oncology and surgical oncology. Clinical oncology encompasses all non-surgical cancer treatments, such as systemic therapies and radiotherapy. The domains of clinical oncology and radiotherapy have undergone fast transformations as a result of technological advancements. Improvement in the imaging quality and computer processing power has enhanced radiotherapy, which allows the treatment to be delivered effectively, safely and efficiently for better patient outcomes. Since a cancer diagnosis may cause anxiety and distress, clinicians can also utilize a variety of interventions to provide emotional support such as SPIKES. This book explores all the important aspects of clinical oncology in the modern day. It is a compilation of chapters that discuss the most vital concepts and emerging trends in this field. This book will serve as a reference to a broad spectrum of readers.

Finally, I would like to thank all the contributing authors for their valuable time and contributions. This book would not have been possible without their efforts. I would also like to thank my friends and family for their constant support.

Editor

1

Computerized Cytological Features for Papillary Thyroid Cancer Diagnosis—Preliminary Report

Shyang-Rong Shih [1,2,3], I-Shiow Jan [4], Kuen-Yuan Chen [5], Wan-Yu Chuang [6], Chih-Yuan Wang [1,2], Yung-Lien Hsiao [2], Tien-Chun Chang [1,3,7,*] and Argon Chen [8,*]

1 National Taiwan University College of Medicine, Taipei 10051, Taiwan; srshih@ntu.edu.tw (S.-R.S.); cyw1965@gmail.com (C.-Y.W.)
2 Department of Internal Medicine, National Taiwan University Hospital, Taipei 10002, Taiwan; hsaio17@yahoo.com.tw
3 Center of Anti-Aging and Health Consultation, National Taiwan University Hospital, Taipei 10002, Taiwan
4 Department of Laboratory Medicine, National Taiwan University Hospital, Taipei 10002, Taiwan; isjan15719@ntu.edu.tw
5 Department of Surgery, National Taiwan University Hospital, Taipei 10002, Taiwan; dtsurg51@gmail.com
6 AmCad BioMed Corporation, Taipei 10547, Taiwan; rachel.chuang@amcad.com.tw
7 Far Eastern Polyclinic, Taipei 10043, Taiwan
8 Institute of Industrial Engineering, National Taiwan University, Taipei 10617, Taiwan
* Correspondence: tienchunchang@ntu.edu.tw (T.-C.C.); achen@ntu.edu.tw (A.C.)

Abstract: Fine needle aspiration cytology (FNAC) is the final diagnosis of thyroid nodules before surgery. It is important to further improve the indeterminate FNAC diagnosis results using computerized cytological features. This retrospective cross-sectional study included 240 cases, of whom 110 had histologic diagnosis of papillary thyroid cancers (PTC), 100 had nodular/adenomatous goiters/hyperplasia (benign goiters), 10 had follicular/Hurthle cell carcinomas, and 20 had follicular adenomas. Morphological and chromatic features of FNAC were quantified and analyzed. The result showed that six quantified cytological features were found significantly different between patients with a histologic diagnosis of PTC and patients with histologic diagnosis of benign goiters in multivariate analysis. These cytological features were used to estimate the malignancy risk in nodules with indeterminate FNAC results. The Area Under the Receiver Operating Characteristics (AUROC) of the diagnostic accuracy with a benign or malignant nature was 81.3% ($p < 0.001$), 78.7% ($p = 0.014$), and 56.8% ($p = 0.52$) for nodules with FNAC results of atypia, which is suspicious for malignancy and follicular neoplasm, respectively. In conclusion, quantification of cytological features could be used to develop a computer-aided tool for diagnosing PTC in thyroid nodules with indeterminate FNAC results.

Keywords: thyroid cytology; diagnosis; computer analysis; morphometry

---

1. Introduction

Thyroid nodules are common. They can be detected in 19%–67% of the normal population using high-resolution sonography, and 5%–15% are malignant [1]. Fine needle aspiration cytology (FNAC) has an essential role in evaluating thyroid nodules before surgery. In samples satisfactory for interpretation, 2%–5% are reported as definitively malignant and 55%–74% as definitively benign [2–5]. The remaining samples have indeterminate cytology, including atypia of undetermined significance or follicular lesion of undetermined significance (AUS/FLUS) (2%–18%), follicular neoplasm or suspicious for a follicular neoplasm (FN/SFN) (2%–25%), and suspicious for malignancy (SUSP) (1%–6%) [6]. Therefore, researchers are seeking methods to further improve preoperative diagnosis or prognostic prediction of thyroid nodules, including genetic evaluation and computerized cytological morphometry [6–8]. Commercial molecular tests for thyroid FNAC include ThyroSeq, Afirma, RosettaGX Reveal, ThyGenX, and ThyraMIR [9]. Their sensitivity for the diagnosis of thyroid cancer ranges from 74% to 91%, with specificity from 49% to 93%, negative predictive value (NPV) from 92% to 97%, and positive predictive value (PPV) from 37% to 83% in tumors with cytological categories of AUS/FLUS and FN. The molecular approach is an ideal "rule-in" test if the PPV for histopathologically-proven malignancy is high. On the other hand, the molecular approach is an ideal "rule out" test if the NPV is high. Most molecular tests listed above have high NPV and lower PPV [6]. The reproducibility of some genetic tests measured in different populations has been questioned [10–12]. Moreover, the molecular tests are expensive and not widely available. Computerized cytomorphometry enables objective quantification of selected morphologic and chromatic parameters in individual cells [13]. It serves as a sequential reader to the conventional cytological evaluation. We aimed to analyze the cytological features of benign and malignant thyroid nodules using computerized cytomorphometry to aid in the differential diagnosis of FNAC. Papillary thyroid cancer (PTC) is the most common thyroid malignancy and constitutes up to 90% of differentiated follicular cell-derived thyroid cancers (FCTC) worldwide [14]. In this preliminary study, we focused on the cytological features of PTC and the other type of FCTC, namely, follicular thyroid cancer (FTC), in comparison with those benign follicular cell-derived lesions.

2. Results

Table 1 shows demographic characteristics, according to categories of cytological diagnoses. Malignant tumors accounted for 13.33%, 57.5%, 31.25%, 94.34%, and 100%, respectively, of the benign, AUS, FN/SFN, SUSP, and malignant categories on cytological diagnosis. Patients' age and sex were not significantly different between the pathologically diagnosed benign and malignant tumors in each of the cytological categories. In patients with pathologic diagnosis of PTC, five cases had follicular variants of PTC (FVPTC). Three of them had non-encapsulated subtype of FVPTC (NFVPTC) and two had mixed classical type of PTC (cPTC) and NFVPTC. The other 105 PTCs were cPTC.

2.1. Diagnosis of Papillary Thyroid Cancer (PTC) and Benign Follicular Lesions Other than Adenoma

In pathologic diagnosis of PTC and benign nodular/adenomatous goiter/hyperplasia, eight cytological features in FNAC specimens were significantly different between pathologically benign and malignant nodules, including mean nuclear size (MNS), standard deviation of nuclear size (SDNS), mean of nuclear elongation (MNElon), coefficient of variation of nuclear elongation, nuclear-cytoplasmic saturation ratio (NCSR), nuclear-cytoplasmic ratio (NCR), nuclear polarity (NP), and inclusion Index (II) (Table 2).

These eight features were then analyzed using stepwise logistic regression with the *p*-value of entering variables set at 0.05 and the *p*-value of removing variables set at 0.1. Six features, i.e., MNS, MNElon, NCSR, NCR, NP, and II, remained significant and were retained in the model. A logistic regression model was then built using these six cytological features as independent variates and pathologic diagnosis as the dependent variate (benign: 0, malignant: 1) (Table 3).

With the logistic regression model, the probability of malignancy could then be estimated using the following. Probability $= \frac{1}{1+e^{-\log it(p)}}$ where $logit(p) = -9.71158 + 0.06557\text{MNS} + 8.94005\text{MNElon} - 1.27953\text{NCSR} + 1.895\text{NCR} + 0.038098\text{NP} + 32.1987\text{II}$.

Table 1. Basic characteristics of the study subjects.

Cytological Diagnosis (Bethesda Category)	Benign			Atypia of Undetermined Significance or Follicular Lesion of Undetermined Significance (AUS)			Follicular Neoplasm or Suspicious for a Follicular Neoplasm (FNSFN)			Suspicious for Malignancy (SUSP)			Malignant
Pathologic Diagnosis	**Benign**	**Malignant (%)**	p	**Benign**	**Malignant (%)**	p	**Benign**	**Malignant (%)**	p	**Benign**	**Malignant (%)**	p	**Malignant (%)**
Number	78	12 (13.33%)		17	23 (57.5%)		22	10 (31.25%)		3	50 (94.34%)		25 (100%)
Age (SD)	52 (12)	50 (19)	0.525	46 (14)	44 (11)	0.564	55 (12)	54 (20)	0.817	50 (29)	52 (11)	0.868	51 (15)
Gender (Female: Male)	69:9	10:2	0.629	13:4	16:7	0.645	18:4	6:4	0.215	3:0	38:12	0.355	22:3

p-values were calculated by independent samples t-test for the age and by Mann-Whitney test for the gender.

Table 2. Cytomorphometry of fine needle aspiration specimens in different pathologic diagnosis.

Pathologic Diagnosis	Papillary Thyroid Cancer and Benign Follicular Lesions other than Follicular Adenoma		Follicular Neoplasm		p *
	Nodular Hyperplasia/Goiter, Adenomatous Hyperplasia/Goiter (Group 1)	**Papillary Thyroid Cancer (Group 2)**	**Follicular Adenoma (Group 3)**	**Follicular Carcinoma Hurthle Cell Carcinoma (Group 4)**	
Number	100	110	20	10	
Age (year)	53 (13)	50 (13)	48 (14)	48 (19)	0.358
Gender (Female: Male)	87:13	85:25	16:4	7:3	0.247
Mean nuclear size (μm^2)	56.03 (43.46–74.93)	75.07 (65.67–87.15)	81.42 (60.69–95.13)	77.60 (58.38–98.14)	<0.001 †,‡,§
Standard deviation of nuclear size (μm^2)	8.02 (5.06–11.23)	10.57 (8.16–14.36)	12.92 (5.90–16.02)	12.71 (8.95–20.16)	0.007 †
Coefficient of variation of nuclear size	0.150 (0.095–0.214)	0.144 (0.114–0.192)	0.161 (0.077–0.292)	0.163 (0.137–0.180)	0.927
Mean nuclear circularity	0.839 (0.819–0.851)	0.832 (0.817–0.840)	0.846 (0.831–0.861)	0.839 (0.811–0.852)	0.062
Standard deviation of nuclear circularity	0.019 (0.014–0.029)	0.021 (0.015–0.031)	0.014 (0.011–0.023)	0.020 (0.015–0.024)	0.632
Coefficient of variation of nuclear circularity	0.023 (0.016–0.036)	0.025 (0.018–0.038)	0.016 (0.013–0.027)	0.024 (0.018–0.030)	0.672
Mean nuclear elongation	0.505 (0.457–0.559)	0.546 (0.503–0.569)	0.478 (0.453–0.541)	0.506 (0.486–0.572)	<0.001 †,‖
Standard deviation of nuclear elongation	0.067 (0.049–0.080)	0.062 (0.051–0.077)	0.066 (0.046–0.098)	0.069 (0.054–0.078)	0.11
Coefficient of variation of nuclear elongation	0.134 (0.099–0.165)	0.115 (0.092–0.141)	0.133 (0.098–0.196)	0.120 (0.108–0.154)	0.012 †
Mean nuclear ellipticity	0.872 (0.852–0.881)	0.871 (0.860–0.879)	0.880 (0.864–0.892)	0.876 (0.861–0.889)	0.017 ‡
Standard deviation of nuclear ellipticity	0.014 (0.010–0.021)	0.015 (0.011–0.020)	0.014 (0.008–0.019)	0.014 (0.012–0.023)	0.528
Coefficient of variation of nuclear ellipticity	0.015 (0.011–0.024)	0.017 (0.012–0.024)	0.015 (0.009–0.022)	0.016 (0.014–0.027)	0.556
Nuclear-to-cytoplasmic hue ratio	1.024 (1.011–1.043)	1.036 (1.016–1.053)	1.015 (0.998–1.026)	1.027 (1.012–1.053)	0.001 ‖
Standard deviation of Nuclear-to-cytoplasmic hue ratio	0.985 (0.864–1.087)	0.983 (0.885–1.116)	0.901 (0.822–0.984)	0.902 (0.830–0.990)	0.082
Nuclear-to-cytoplasmic saturation ratio	1.944 (1.652–2.422)	1.693 (1.570–1.979)	2.232 (1.914–2.347)	2.322 (1.731–2.566)	<0.001 †,‖
Standard deviation of Nuclear-to-cytoplasmic saturation ratio	0.911 (0.797–1.109)	0.908 (0.774–1.013)	0.937 (0.813–1.152)	0.920 (0.848–0.991)	0.105
Nuclear-to-cytoplasmic value ratio	0.833 (0.791–0.872)	0.835 (0.805–0.858)	0.798 (0.756–0.863)	0.864 (0.789–0.869)	0.232
Standard deviation of Nuclear-to-cytoplasmic value ratio	1.086 (0.935–1.194)	1.099 (0.986–1.286)	0.987 (0.933–1.158)	1.133 (0.945–1.227)	0.506
Nuclear-to-cytoplasmic ratio	0.998 (0.740–1.373)	1.230 (1.020–1.556)	1.056 (0.755–1.806)	0.941 (0.806–1.114)	0.025 †
Nuclear polarity	14.02 (5.04–23.49)	22.48 (15.27–32.69)	13.09 (4.19–18.26)	12.75 (7.56–19.01)	<0.001 †,‖
Inclusion index	0 (0.000–0.004)	0.006 (0.002–0.012)	0.004 (0.000–0.007)	0.007 (0.005–0.018)	0.011 †
Overlapping index	0.436 (0.340–0.577)	0.500 (0.432–0.589)	0.473 (0.290–0.581)	0.452 (0.374–0.596)	0.221

Data are presented as mean ± SD if the continuous variable is normally distributed, and as a median (interquartile range) if not normally distributed. * P was obtained using the ANOVA test to compare the difference between the four groups. † The results are significantly different between group 1 and group 2, ‡ significantly different between group 1 and group 3, § significantly different between group 1 and group 4, and ‖ significantly different between group 2 and group 3 when using the Scheffé test for all pairwise comparisons.

Table 3. The relationship between pathologic diagnosis and cytological characteristics in pathologic diagnosis of papillary thyroid cancer and benign follicular lesions other than follicular adenoma. Multivariate logistic regression analysis was performed using pathological diagnosis as the dependent variate (malignant: 1, benign: 0) and six cytological characteristics as independent variates ($n = 210$).

Variable	Coefficient	*p*
Mean nuclear size (μm^2)	0.06557	<0.0001
Mean nuclear elongation	8.94005	0.0239
Nuclear-to-cytoplasmic saturation ratio	−1.27953	0.0008
Nuclear-to-cytoplasmic ratio	1.89500	<0.0001
Nuclear polarity	0.038098	0.0259
Inclusion index	32.19870	0.0473
Constant	−9.71158	0.0001

With the estimated probability of malignancy calculated for each case, the receiver operating characteristic (ROC) curve analysis was performed. In pathologic diagnosis of papillary thyroid cancer and benign follicular lesions other than follicular adenoma, the value for the area under the ROC curve (AUROC) was 87.7% ($p < 0.001$) (Figure 1A). The threshold probability for making diagnosis was then calculated to be 0.535 based on the optimum cut-off point on the ROC curve closest to (0,1). The corresponding diagnosis sensitivity, specificity, PPV, and NPV were 84.5%, 81.0%, 82.3%, and 82.5%, respectively. Figure 2 shows the differentiation performance of the logistic model using box plots for different cytological categories.

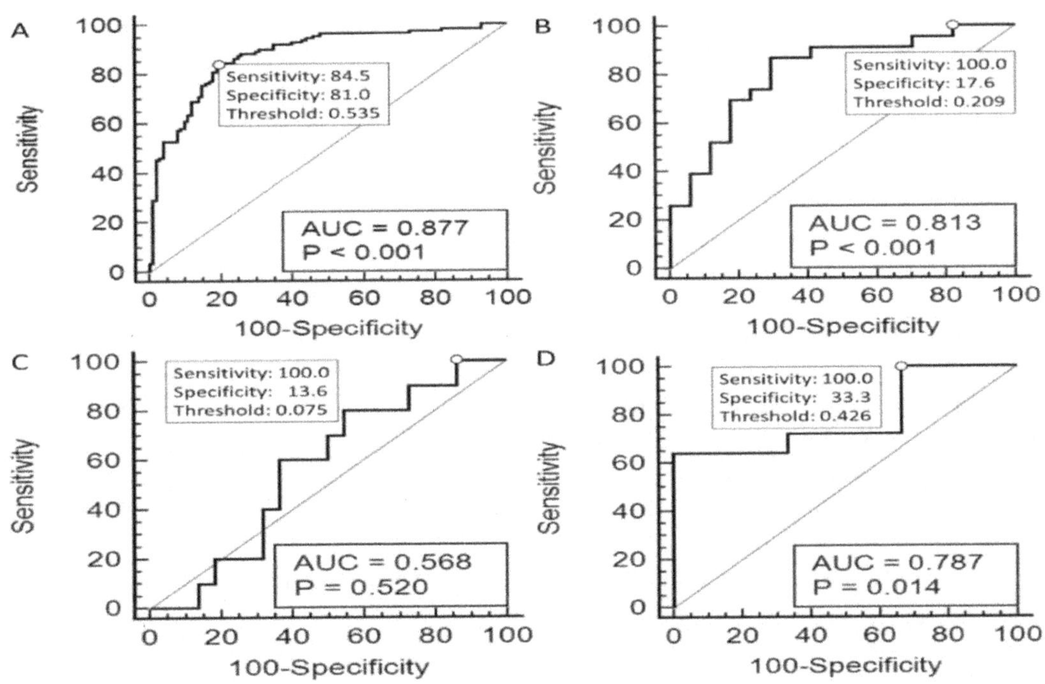

Figure 1. Receiver operating characteristic curves and their area under the curve (AUC), where positive and negative outcomes were defined as malignant and benign, respectively. (**A**) In pathologic diagnosis of papillary thyroid cancer and benign follicular lesions other than follicular adenoma ($n = 210$). (**B**) In Bethesda cytological category of atypia of undetermined significance or follicular lesion of undetermined significance ($n = 40$). (**C**) In Bethesda cytological category of follicular neoplasm or suspicious for a follicular neoplasm ($n = 32$). (**D**) In Bethesda cytological category of suspicious for malignancy ($n = 53$). In panel A, the threshold value was set at the cut-off point that was closest to (0,1). In panel B, C, and D, the threshold value was set at the sensitivity that was 100% aligned with specificity that is as high as possible.

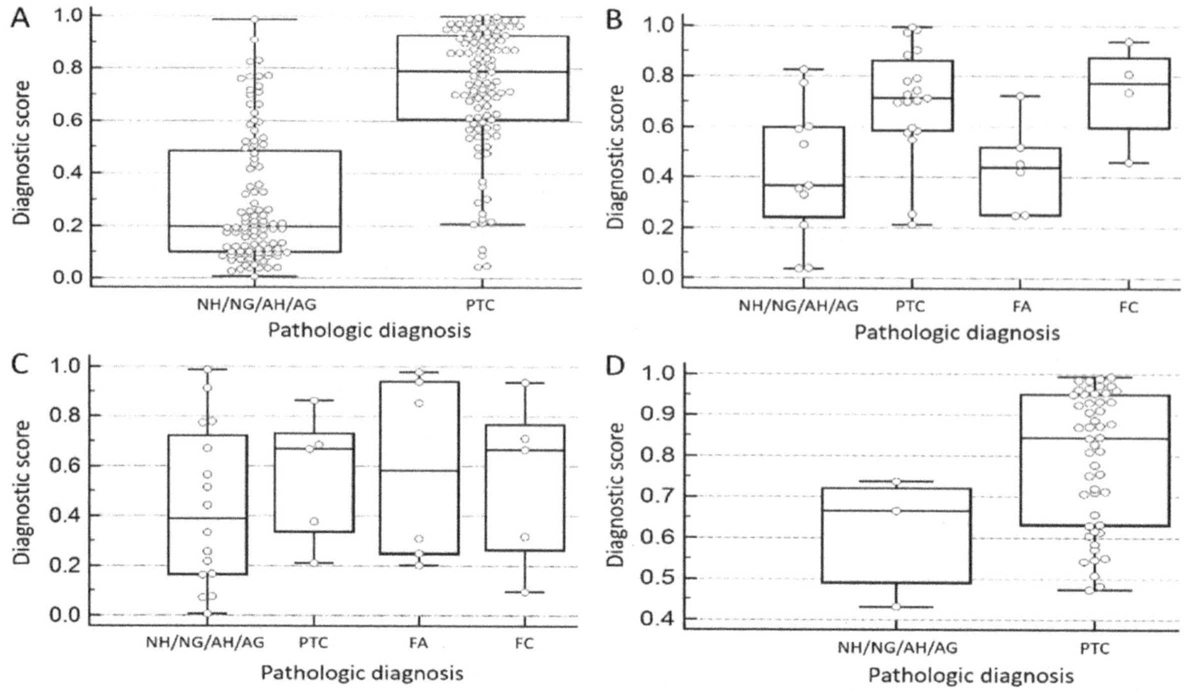

Figure 2. Box plots of the relationship between a diagnostic score and pathologic diagnosis. (**A**) In pathologic diagnosis of papillary thyroid cancer and benign follicular lesions other than follicular adenoma (n = 210). (**B**) In Bethesda cytological category of atypia of undetermined significance or follicular lesion of undetermined significance (n = 40). (**C**) In Bethesda cytological category of follicular neoplasm or suspicious for a follicular neoplasm (n = 32). (**D**) In Bethesda cytological category of suspicions for malignancy (n = 53). NH: Nodular hyperplasia. NG: Nodular goiter. AH: Adenomatous hyperplasia. AG: Adenomatous goiter. PTC: Papillary thyroid cancer. FA: Follicular adenoma. FC: Follicular carcinoma.

2.2. Performance of the Logistic Model in Cytologically Indeterminate Categories

The ROC curve analyses were performed for cases in the indeterminate AUS, FN/SFN, and SUSP cytological categories and their AUROC values were 81.3% ($p < 0.001$), 56.8% ($p = 0.52$), and 78.7% ($p = 0.014$), respectively (Table 4). The optimum threshold probabilities based on the cut-off point closest to (0,1) for the AUS, FN/SFN, and SUSP categories were calculated to be 0.523, 0.304, and 0.733, with (sensitivity percentage, specificity percentage) equal to (87.0, 70.6), (80.0, 45.5), and (64.0, 100.0), respectively (Table 4, model 2). The logistic model was more sensitive for the AUS category and was very specific for the SUSP category, while the model was not as effective for FN/SFN cases.

Table 4. Prediction of pathologic diagnosis of thyroid cancer using a diagnostic score.

Cytological Diagnosis	AUROC (p-Value)	Model 1: Threshold Value was Set at the Sensitivity that was 100% with the Specificity as High as Possible					Model 2: Threshold Value was Set at the Cut-off Point on the ROC Curve that was Closest to (0,1)				
		Sensitivity	Specificity	PPV	NPV	Threshold Value	Sensitivity	Specificity	PPV	NPV	Threshold Value
AUS	0.813 (<0.001)	100.00%	17.60%	62.20%	100.00%	0.209	87.00%	70.60%	80.00%	80.00%	0.523
FN/SFN	0.568 (0.520)	100.00%	13.60%	34.50%	100.00%	0.075	80.00%	45.50%	40.00%	83.30%	0.304
SUSP	0.787 (0.014)	100.00%	33.30%	96.20%	100.00%	0.426	64.00%	100.00%	100.00%	14.30%	0.733

PPV: positive predictive value. NPV: negative predictive value. AUS: atypia of undetermined significance or follicular lesion of undetermined significance. FN/SFN: follicular neoplasm or suspicious for a follicular neoplasm. SUSP: suspicious for malignancy.

To assist the cytologist in further differentiating the benign cases from the indeterminate cases, one may choose the threshold probabilities to ensure a sensitivity of 100%, i.e., no malignant cases missed, with the specificity as high as possible. Table 4 shows the diagnosis results under various threshold probabilities set at different cut-off points of the ROC curves. With the cut-off points ensuring 100% sensitivity, it can be seen that the threshold probability values were 0.209, 0.075, and 0.426 for the AUS, FN/SFN, and SUSP categories and the specificities can reach 17.6%, 13.6%, and 33.3%, respectively (Figure 1 panel B, C, and D, Table 4 and model 1). With the assistance of the logistic model constructed by the computerized cytological features, 3 out of 17 benign AUS cases, 3 out of 22 benign FN/SFN cases, and 1 out of 3 benign SUSP cases might have avoided aggressive treatment, such as surgical thyroidectomy.

3. Discussion

This study proposed several new parameters for computerized morphometry of thyroid FNAC specimens. We can quantify not only morphological but also chromatic features. Our study shows that computerized quantification of cytological characteristics can help to differentiate 17.6%–33.3% of cases as benign rather than malignant, with 100% sensitivity, for the Bethesda categories of AUS and SUSP. Even for the FN/SFN category, 13.6% of cases can be further differentiated as benign with 100% sensitivity, using a model based on PTC cases and benign nodular/adenomatous goiter/hyperplasia. This is because the model is designed to differentiate not only PTC nodules but also benign nodular adenomatous goiter and hyperplasia. Among the three of 22 benign cases of FN/SFN differentiated with the model, one was an adenomatous goiter and two were hyperplastic nodules. The cytological features used in this model for differential diagnosis included mean nuclear size (MNS), mean nuclear elongation (MNElon), nuclear-to-cytoplasmic saturation ratio (NCSR), nuclear-to-cytoplasmic ratio (NCR), nuclear polarity (NP), and inclusion index (II).

Much effort has focused on genetic analysis to aid in diagnosis of indeterminate cytology reports for thyroid nodules. *BRAF*, *NRAS*, *HRAS*, and *KRAS* point mutations, and *RET/PTC1*, *RET/PTC3*, and *PAX8/PPARc* rearrangements were reported to be helpful [6]. Several commercial thyroid FNAC molecular tests are available, including ThyroSeq, Afirma, RosettaGX Reveal, ThyGenX, and ThyraMIR [9]. However, genetic examination is expensive and not widely available. We previously demonstrated that computerized morphometry of FNAC samples helps predict recurrence of PTC [7]. The nucleus-cell ratio and variation of nuclear area showed significant and positive correlations with recurrence ($p = 0.002$ and 0.044, respectively). The present study quantified cytological features and identified differences between benign and malignant thyroid nodules. Larger nuclear size and higher nuclear-to cytoplasmic ratio are related to malignancy. This may be related to cellular duplication activity [8], and was reportedly associated with prognosis for several cancers, including malignant melanoma, rhabdomyosarcoma, and renal cell carcinoma [15–17]. Our study also showed that NCSR is related to diagnosis. PTC cells show less difference in saturation between nuclei and cytoplasm than benign follicular cells. There has been no other description of the association between this chromatic feature and malignancy in the literature. PTC cells had greater mean nuclear elongation than benign follicular cells in our study. This also had not been mentioned in the research. PTC cells are usually found in a papillaroid arrangement. In the cross section of each papilla, the elongated cells are arranged in a spiral shape, which results in a different direction for each cell and greater nuclear polarity in PTC. Inclusion bodies are characteristic features of PTC, and, therefore, the index of inclusion is higher in PTC.

This computerized diagnostic score was developed for the purpose of assisting cytopathologists and clinicians in challenging situations of indeterminate thyroid cytology. According to the American Thyroid Association guideline, in the situation of indeterminate thyroid cytologic results, clinicians should discuss with the patients to decide further management, including repeated FNAC, genetic study, or thyroidectomy [1]. In our dataset of AUS cases, we can set the cut-off point of the diagnostic score at 0.523 to get the best overall diagnostic power (sensitivity: 87%, specificity: 70.6%) for the differentiation of benign and malignant tumors (Table 4). Less aggressive management such as repeated FNAC may be preferred for cases with diagnostic scores less than 0.523. In contrast, more aggressive management such as thyroidectomy may be preferred for patients with diagnostic scores more than 0.523. Or we can set the cut-off point at 0.209 to get the best sensitivity (100%) for the purpose of avoiding unnecessary operation, which, in our dataset, avoids 13.6% (3 out of 22) of benign FN/SFN cases in our dataset from aggressive treatment. This scenario may also be used in the situation with the cytological diagnosis result of suspicions of malignancy (SUSP). We can set the diagnostic score of computerized cytomorphometry at 0.733 to get the best overall diagnostic power (sensitivity: 64%, specificity: 100%) (Table 4). We could set the cut-off point at 0.426 to get the best sensitivity (100%) while avoiding extensive thyroidectomy, i.e., 33% (1 out of 3) of benign SUSP cases in our dataset, could have been exempted from aggressive treatment. In the situation of follicular neoplasm (FN)/suspicious of FN (SFN), the overall diagnostic power for differentiation of follicular adenoma (FA) and follicular thyroid carcinoma (FTC) is poor (Table 4). The comparison of the diagnostic score of FA and FTC was shown in Figure 2C. The ROC curve of the diagnostic score to differentiate benign and malignant lesions in FN/SFN was shown in Figure 1C with the AUC of 0.568 and p value of 0.52. However, if we set the cut-off point of the diagnostic score at 0.075 to get the best sensitivity (100%), we could still avoid 13.6% (3 out of 22) benign FN/SFN cases in our dataset from aggressive treatment.

The cytological features that can differentiate benign from malignant thyroid tumors in AUS/FLUS and SUSP categories of cytological specimens do not perform well for the category of FN/SFN. This indicates that the cytological characteristics of tumors with a follicular growth pattern are different from those of tumors with a papillary growth pattern. This is supported by the fact that the oncogenes associated with these two growth patterns are also different [18]. Since the diagnosis of follicular neoplasm depends on the histologic analysis of vascular and/or capsular invasion, the literature has reported that it is difficult to differentiate benign from malignant follicular neoplasms in cytological specimens [6] and it is not surprising to see that the computerized cytological features proposed by this study have also failed to differentiate the follicular neoplasms effectively.

In our study, the Red-Green-Blue (RGB) color space of image pixels were first converted into the color space of hue (H), saturation (S), and value (V). To the best of our knowledge, this is the first study to evaluate the thyroid FNAC with indeterminate categories using the color space of HSV. In the study conducted by Celik ZE et al., morphological and chromatic variables were used to establish their computerized cytomorphometry system, which included five variables [19]. Among these five variables, only one was chromatic variable and was in grey scale. In another study [20], Gilshtein H et al. applied 50 variables in their computerized cytomorphometry, but the texture of nuclear chromatin was also in gray scale. In addition, our study collected a large dataset of 240 cases. Prior research included 125 cases of indeterminate cytological categories while the previous studies had only 40 and 58 cases, respectively.

The major limitation of this study is the small number of patients in each Bethesda category. In our dataset, more than 95% of PTC (105 out of 110) were cPTC and only five cases were follicular variants of PTC. We have noted that the cPTC constitutes 80% of all PTC in the literature [21] and further study is needed especially for the non-invasive follicular thyroid neoplasm with papillary like nuclear features (NIFTP) because of its different malignant potential [22]. For a more comprehensive clinical use, we should also collect a sufficient sample of other types of thyroid cancers, such as anaplastic thyroid cancer, poorly differentiated thyroid cancer, and medullary thyroid cancers, to be included in the analysis. However, the findings of the current study are still of value in differential diagnosis of PTC, which constitutes most thyroid cancers. Another concern is the use of Riu's stain, which is not widely used in other countries, and the proposed cytological features should be further evaluated using different stains. However, since the Riu's stain, which is also a type of Romanowsky stain [23], has the appearance resembling the Diff-Quik stain [24]. Similar results may be anticipated for the use of the Diff-Quik stain. However, different staining methods may result in different NCHR, NCSR, and NCVR values. We should collect and analyze specimens of other staining methods such as the Papanicolaou stain in the future.

4. Materials and Methods

This study followed the ethical principles of the Declaration of Helsinki and was approved by the Institutional Review Board of the National Taiwan University Hospital (NTUH) (protocol number: 201603064RIPB). The study protocol with the waiver of informed consent has been approved by NTUH's research ethics committee and was registered on ClinicalTrials.gov (protocol number: NCT03105648).

4.1. Study Subjects

We recruited 244 cases who had pathologic diagnoses of benign nodules, PTC, follicular thyroid carcinoma (FTC), or Hurthle cell carcinoma, and had underwent FNAC by endocrinologists in NTUH between 2010 and 2017, which was followed by thyroidectomy. Three cases with a pathologic diagnosis of lymphocytic thyroiditis and 1 with a pathologic diagnosis of Graves' disease were excluded (Figure 3). The analysis of 240 cases included 110 cases with PTC, 100 with nodular/adenomatous goiter/hyperplasia, 10 with follicular/Hurthle cell carcinoma, and 20 with follicular adenoma.

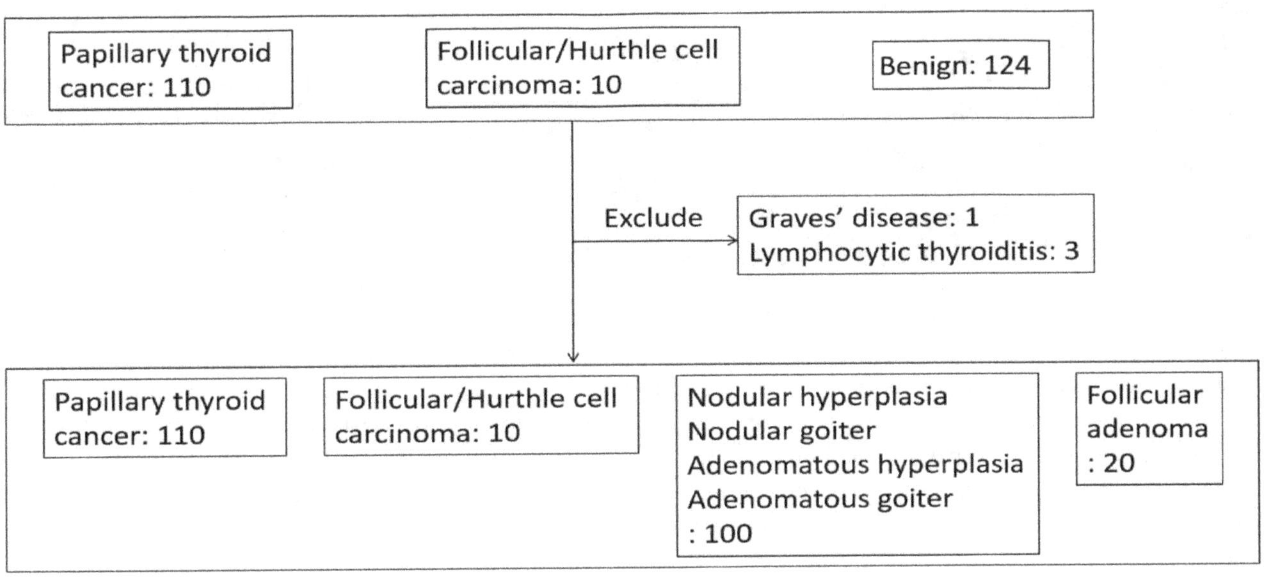

Figure 3. Flowchart of subject recruitment.

FNAC specimens underwent Riu's staining, which is a type of Romanowsky staining [23]. Riu's staining was performed in the following standard procedure. After air drying, the smears were covered with solution A (0.05% methylene blue and 0.17% eosin Y in methanol) for 30 s, which was followed by placement of solution B (0.12% azure I, 0.14% methylene blue, 2.52% $Na_2HPO_4 \cdot 12H_2O$, and 1.25% KH_2PO_4 in distilled water) for 90 s. The stain mixtures were then washed off and the slides were observed under a light microscope. Digital images of these stained FNAC specimens were obtained and analyzed.

4.2. Computerized Analysis of Cytologic Features

Digital cytological images in matrices of color pixels were collected for computerized analysis (Figure 4).

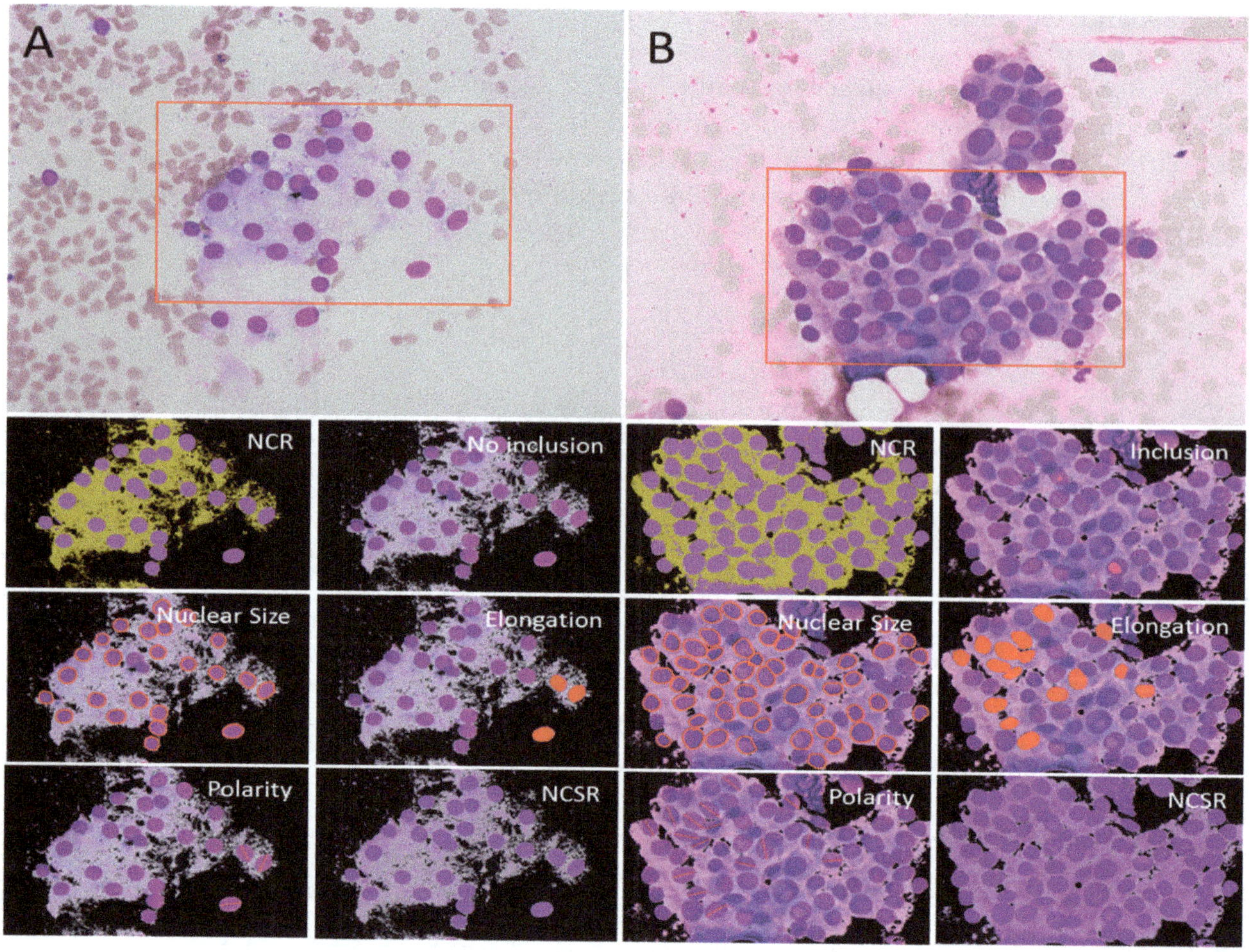

Figure 4. Visual comparison for clinically important features. The images from a case of hyperplasia (**A**) and a case of papillary thyroid carcinoma (**B**) acquired from a thyroid fine-needle aspiration cytology smear (Riu's stain, 400×). The image (red rectangle region of interest) was cropped for computerized analysis. NCR (nuclear-cytoplasmic ratio visualized with nuclei in purple, cytoplasm in yellow), intranuclear inclusion (pink), nuclear size (nuclei segmented by red contours), elongation (elongated nuclei in red), polarity (alignment of red major axes of elongated nuclei), and NCSR (nuclear-cytoplasmic saturation ratio visualized with a saturation contrast between nuclei and cytoplasm).

The image processing and analysis were performed using AmCAD-CA (AmCad BioMed Corp., Taipei, Taiwan). The digital cytological images were segmented into three clusters, including background, cytoplasm, and nucleus, based on the pixel value in hue and saturation with Otsu's method. After segmentation, the background cluster was set to zero, and the Canny edge detection was performed on the remaining image to find the boundary of nuclear area. The detailed algorithm used by the software can be seen in the patent [25] filed by the software company. The pixel values in the Red-Green-Blue (RGB) color space were first converted into the color space of hue (H), saturation (S), and value (V). The H of nuclei and cytoplasm in the same cytologic specimen was compared and the difference was calculated in a nuclear-to-cytoplasmic hue ratio (NCHR) using a formula presented in the Supplementary Material. Nuclear-cytoplasmic saturation ratio (NCSR) and nuclear-cytoplasmic value ratio (NCVR) were generated in similar fashion. Nuclear-cytoplasmic ratio (NCR) was defined as the ratio of the area of the nuclei and cytoplasm. The segmented margin of the nuclei could then be used for statistical values, such as the sample mean (M), the sample standard deviation (SD), and the coefficient of variation (CV = SD/M) of the morphological features including nuclear size, circularity, ellipticity, elongation, nuclear polarity, inclusion, and overlapping. Circularity indicated roundness of a cell nucleus by considering the nuclear perimeter and area. Ellipticity evaluated nuclear surface smoothness by considering axis lengths, perimeter, and area of the nucleus. Elongation assessed nuclear extension by considering both major and minor axis lengths of the nucleus. The overlapping index was defined as the ratio of overlapped nuclei to the total nuclear area. The index of nuclear polarity (NP) was defined as the variability of nuclear long-axis angles. The above calculating formulae were listed in the Supplementary Material.

4.3. *Statistical Analysis*

A total of 22 quantified cytological features, including 16 morphological and 6 chromatic features, were computed and analyzed. Analysis of variance and the Scheffé test were used to compare the differences in cytological features among 4 types of thyroid nodules based on a pathologic diagnosis. The D'Agostino-Pearson test was used to test for normal distribution of each feature. Multivariate logistic regression analysis was used to investigate the relationship between cytological features and pathologic results. Statistical analysis was performed using MedCalc Version 17.6 (MedCalc Software, Mariakerke, Belgium) and Stata/SE 14.0 for Windows (StataCorp LP, TX, USA). A p value less than 0.05 was considered statistically significant.

5. Conclusions

Our study showed that quantification of cytological morphological and chromatic features could be used to develop a computer-aided tool for diagnosing thyroid nodules. We will recruit more cases and other types of thyroid cancer to improve the diagnostic scoring system and examine the cytological features of specimens prepared with other staining methods.

Author Contributions: Conceptualization, S.-R.S., A.C., I.-S.J., and T.-C.C. Methodology, A.C. and I.-S.J. Software, W.-Y.C. Validation, W.-Y.C. and A.C. Formal Analysis, W.-Y.C. and A.C. Investigation, S.-R.S. and A.C. Resources, S.-R.S. and I.-S.J. Data Curation, C.-Y.W., I.-S.J., T.-C.C., K.-Y.C., W.-Y.C., and Y.-L.H. Writing—Original Draft Preparation, S.-R.S., W.-Y.C., and A.C. Writing—Review & Editing, S.-R.S., C.-Y.W., and A.C. Visualization, W.-Y.C. and A.C. Supervision, T.-C.C. Project Administration, S.-R.S. and A.C. Funding Acquisition, S.-R.S. and A.C.

Acknowledgments: We thank the staff of the Eighth Core Lab, Department of Medical Research, National Taiwan University Hospital, Liver Disease Prevention and Treatment Research Foundation, Taiwan, and Wong-Yuan Endocrine Fund, Taiwan, for their support during the study.

References

1. Cooper, D.S.; Doherty, G.M.; Haugen, B.R.; Kloos, R.T.; Lee, S.L.; Mandel, S.J.; Mazzaferri, E.L.; McIver, B.; Pacini, F.; Schlumberger, M.; et al. Revised American Thyroid Association Management Guidelines for Patients with Thyroid Nodules and Differentiated Thyroid Cancer. *Thyroid* **2009**, *19*, 1167–1214. [CrossRef] [PubMed]
2. Bongiovanni, M.; Spitale, A.; Faquin, W.C.; Mazzucchelli, L.; Baloch, Z.W. The Bethesda System for Reporting Thyroid Cytopathology: A Meta-Analysis. *Acta Cytol.* **2012**, *56*, 333–339. [CrossRef] [PubMed]
3. Luu, M.H.; Fischer, A.H.; Pisharodi, L.; Owens, C.L. Improved preoperative definitive diagnosis of papillary thyroid carcinoma in FNAs prepared with both ThinPrep and conventional smears compared with FNAs prepared with ThinPrep alone. *Cancer Cytopathol.* **2011**, *119*, 68–73. [CrossRef] [PubMed]
4. Nayar, R.; Ivanovic, M. The indeterminate thyroid fine-needle aspiration: Experience from an academic center using terminology similar to that proposed in the 2007 National Cancer Institute Thyroid Fine Needle Aspiration State of the Science Conference. *Cancer* **2009**, *117*, 195–202. [CrossRef] [PubMed]
5. Theoharis, C.G.; Schofield, K.M.; Hammers, L.; Udelsman, R.; Chhieng, D.C. The Bethesda Thyroid Fine-Needle Aspiration Classification System: Year 1 at an Academic Institution. *Thyroid* **2009**, *19*, 1215–1223. [CrossRef] [PubMed]
6. Haugen, B.R.; Alexander, E.K.; Bible, K.C.; Doherty, G.M.; Mandel, S.J.; Nikiforov, Y.E.; Pacini, F.; Randolph, G.W.; Sawka, A.M.; Schlumberger, M.; et al. 2015 American Thyroid Association Management

Guidelines for Adult Patients with Thyroid Nodules and Differentiated Thyroid Cancer: The American Thyroid Association Guidelines Task Force on Thyroid Nodules and Differentiated Thyroid Cancer. *Thyroid* **2016**, *26*, 1–133. [CrossRef] [PubMed]

7. Shih, S.R.; Chang, Y.C.; Li, H.Y.; Liau, J.Y.; Lee, C.Y.; Chen, C.M.; Chang, T.C. Preoperative prediction of papillary thyroid carcinoma prognosis with the assistance of computerized morphometry of cytology samples obtained by fine-needle aspiration: Preliminary report. *Head Neck* **2013**, *35*, 28–34. [CrossRef]
8. Shih, S.-R.; Li, H.-Y.; Hsiao, Y.-L.; Chang, T.-C. Prognostic Significance of Cytologic Features in Fine-Needle Aspiration Cytology Samples of Papillary Thyroid Carcinoma: Preliminary Report. *Thyroid* **2006**, *16*, 775–780. [CrossRef]
9. Nikiforov, Y.E. Role of molecular markers in thyroid nodule management: Then and now. *Endocr. Pract.* **2017**, *23*, 979–988. [CrossRef]
10. Harrell, R.M.; Bimston, D.N. Surgical utility of Afirma: Effects of high cancer prevalence and oncocytic cell types in patients with indeterminate thyroid cytology. *Endocr. Pract.* **2014**, *20*, 364–369. [CrossRef]
11. Marti, J.L.; Avadhani, V.; Donatelli, L.A.; Niyogi, S.; Wang, B.; Wong, R.J.; Shaha, A.R.; Ghossein, R.A.; Lin, O.; Morris, L.G.T.; et al. Wide Inter-institutional Variation in Performance of a Molecular Classifier for Indeterminate Thyroid Nodules. *Ann. Surg. Oncol.* **2015**, *22*, 3996–4001. [CrossRef] [PubMed]
12. McIver, B.; Castro, M.R.; Morris, J.C.; Bernet, V.; Smallridge, R.; Henry, M.; Kosok, L.; Reddi, H. An Independent Study of a Gene Expression Classifier (Afirma) in the Evaluation of Cytologically Indeterminate Thyroid Nodules. *J. Clin. Endocrinol. Metab.* **2014**, *99*, 4069–4077. [CrossRef] [PubMed]
13. Wang, S.-L.; Wu, M.-T.; Yang, S.-F.; Chan, H.-M.; Chai, C.-Y. Computerized nuclear morphometry in thyroid follicular neoplasms. *Pathol. Int.* **2005**, *55*, 703–706. [CrossRef] [PubMed]
14. Schlumberger, M.-J.; Filetti, S.; Alexander, E.K.; Hay, I.D. Nontoxic diffuse goiter, nodular thyroid disorders, and thyroid malignancies. In *Williams Textbook of Endocrinology*; Elsevier: Amsterdam, The Netherlands, 2016; pp. 449–488.
15. Karbowniczek, M.; Chosia, M.; Domagała, W. Nuclear morphometry of MIB-1 positive and negative tumor cells in primary and metastatic malignant melanoma of the skin. *Pol. J. Pathol.* **1999**, *50*, 235–241.
16. Kazanowska, B.; Jelen, M.; Reich, A.; Tarnawski, W.; Chybicka, A. The role of nuclear morphometry in prediction of prognosis for rhabdomyosarcoma in children. *Histopathology* **2004**, *45*, 352–359. [CrossRef]
17. Paraskevakou, E.; Kavantzas, N.; Pavlopoulos, P.M.; Delibasis, A.; Yova, D.; Davaris, P. Computerized nuclear morphometry of renal cell carcinomas. *Gen. Diagn. Pathol.* **1996**, *142*, 101–104.
18. Nikiforov, Y.E.; Seethala, R.R.; Tallini, G.; Baloch, Z.W.; Basolo, F.; Thompson, L.D.R.; Barletta, J.A.; Wenig, B.M.; Al Ghuzlan, A.; Kakudo, K.; et al. Nomenclature Revision for Encapsulated Follicular Variant of Papillary Thyroid Carcinoma: A Paradigm Shift to Reduce Overtreatment of Indolent Tumors. *JAMA Oncol.* **2016**, *2*, 1023–1029. [CrossRef]
19. Celik, Z.E.; Altinay, S.; Kilinc, F.; Arslan, N.; Yilmaz, B.S.; Karabagli, P.; Ugurluoglu, C. Using Computerized Cytomorphometry to Distinguish between Benign and Malignant Cases in Thyroid Fine-Needle Aspiration Cytology. *Diagn. Cytopathol.* **2016**, *44*, 902–911. [CrossRef]
20. Gilshtein, H.; Mekel, M.; Malkin, L.; Ben-Izhak, O.; Sabo, E. Computerized cytometry and wavelet analysis of follicular lesions for detecting malignancy: A pilot study in thyroid cytology. *Surgery* **2017**, *161*, 212–219. [CrossRef]
21. Gupta, S.; Ajise, O.; Dultz, L.; Wang, B.; Nonaka, D.; Ogilvie, J.; Heller, K.S.; Patel, K.N. Follicular variant of papillary thyroid cancer: Encapsulated, nonencapsulated, and diffuse: Distinct biologic and clinical entities. *Arch. Otolaryngol. Head Neck Surg.* **2012**, *138*, 227–233. [CrossRef]
22. Bongiovanni, M.; Faquin, W.; Giovanella, L.; Durante, C.; Kopp, P.; Trimboli, P. Impact of non-invasive follicular thyroid neoplasms with papillary-like nuclear features (NIFTP) on risk of malignancy in patients undergoing lobectomy/thyroidectomy for suspicious for malignancy or malignant fine-needle aspiration cytology findings: A systematic review and meta-analysis. *Eur. J. Endocrinol.* **2019**. [CrossRef]
23. Riu, C.H. A new rapid method of staining thin blood film: First report. *Taiwan I Hsueh Hui Tsa Chih.* **1953**, *52*, 348–352.
24. Wright, J.H. A Rapid Method for the Differential Staining of Blood Films and Malarial Parasites. *J. Med. Res.* **1902**, *7*, 138–144. [PubMed]
25. Chen, A.; Hsiao, Y.H.; Chang, T.C.; Jan, I.S.; Shih, S.R.; Wang, H.M. Cytological Image Processing Device, and Method for Quantifying Characteristics of Cytological Image. Patent Number TWI630581B, 21 July 2018.

2

Cold Atmospheric Plasma Restores Paclitaxel Sensitivity to Paclitaxel-Resistant Breast Cancer Cells by Reversing Expression of Resistance-Related Genes

Sungbin Park [1,†], Heejoo Kim [1,†], Hwee Won Ji [1], Hyeon Woo Kim [1], Sung Hwan Yun [1], Eun Ha Choi [2] and Sun Jung Kim [1,*]

1 Department of Life Science, Dongguk University-Seoul, Goyang 10326, Korea; do31100@dongguk.edu (S.P.); heejoo0923@dongguk.edu (H.K.); hweewon96@dongguk.edu (H.W.J.); opopr5@dongguk.edu (H.W.K.); skskbby@dongguk.edu (S.H.Y.)

2 Plasma Bioscience Research Center, Kwangwoon University, Seoul 01897, Korea; ehchoi@kw.ac.kr

* Correspondence: sunjungk@dongguk.edu

† These authors contributed equally to this paper.

Abstract: Paclitaxel (Tx) is a widely used therapeutic chemical for breast cancer treatment; however, cancer recurrence remains an obstacle for improved prognosis of cancer patients. In this study, cold atmospheric plasma (CAP) was tested for its potential to overcome the drug resistance. After developing Tx-resistant MCF-7 (MCF-7/TxR) breast cancer cells, CAP was applied to the cells, and its effect on the recovery of drug sensitivity was assessed in both cellular and molecular aspects. Sensitivity to Tx in the MCF-7/TxR cells was restored up to 73% by CAP. A comparison of genome-wide expression profiles between the TxR cells and the CAP-treated cells identified 49 genes that commonly appeared with significant changes. Notably, 20 genes, such as KIF13B, GOLM1, and TLE4, showed opposite expression profiles. The protein expression levels of selected genes, DAGLA and CEACAM1, were recovered to those of their parental cells by CAP. Taken together, CAP inhibited the growth of MCF-7/TxR cancer cells and recovered Tx sensitivity by resetting the expression of multiple drug resistance–related genes. These findings may contribute to extending the application of CAP to the treatment of TxR cancer.

Keywords: apoptosis; cold atmospheric plasma; breast cancer; genome-wide expression; reactive oxygen species

---

1. Introduction

Recurrence of cancer due to the acquisition of resistance to chemotherapy remains a serious obstacle for the clinical treatment of cancer patients [1]. A high ratio of cancer patients who receive chemotherapy acquire drug resistance [2,3]. Among breast cancer patients, an estimated one in three will eventually develop recurrent or metastatic disease, causing poor prognosis with a median 5-year survival of <25% [4]. Paclitaxel (Tx) has been widely used to treat a variety of cancer types, including breast cancer [5]. Tx binds to β-tubulin subunits of the microtubule, preventing them from undergoing the depolymerization process, which is crucial during the course of mitosis [6]. Subsequently, the dissociation of the spindle is inhibited, and therefore, the cell cycle is blocked in the G2/M phase and apoptosis [7].

A few molecular mechanisms have explained Tx resistance (TxR). Altered microtubule physiology is a major dominator escaping the cytotoxicity of the drug [8]. Moreover, the HER2 signaling cascade influences several routes of resistance, such as drug efflux and drug metabolism [9]. HER2 overexpression was found not only in cultured TxR cells [10] but also in TxR cancer patients [11]. A cascade of protein kinases involving ERK1/2 is activated by HER2 via phosphorylation, and then target genes such as cyclin A, cyclin B, and CD44 are induced to enhance cell proliferation and stemness [12]. TxR can also be conferred by the upregulation of drug efflux pumps, such as ABCB1 [13] and MRP3 [14], which are often overexpressed in HER2-overexpressing tumors. Strategies to circumvent TxR include blockades of ABCB1 and MRP efflux and the development of systemic agents with low susceptibility to common resistance mechanisms, such as HER2 overexpression [15]. Despite these works to eradicate TxR cancer, a high percentage of TxR cancers still remain aggressive and threaten the prognosis of cancer patients [16].

Cold atmospheric plasma (CAP) has received attention from basic biological science, as well as medical researchers, due to its ability to specifically induce the death of cancer cells over normal cells [17,18]. A wide spectrum of cancer cells, including breast, ovary, liver, lung, brain, and skin cancer cells, underwent apoptosis, suggesting the potential of CAP as an alternative cancer treatment option [19,20]. Given the heterogeneity of cancer cells, including drug-resistant cancer cells, it is hoped that CAP is also able to induce apoptosis of these cells and even to help recover sensitivity to the therapeutic chemicals. In previous studies, CAP returned the temozolomide-resistant glioblastoma cells [21] and cisplatin-resistant ovarian cancer cells [22] to a drug-sensitive state, in addition to inducing apoptosis. However, little is known about the molecular mechanism by which CAP resets the protein expression levels of resistant cancer cells to those of their parental cancer cells. A study identified the "cell death/survival and cancer" network as the pivotal pathway that was deregulated by CAP for the tamoxifen-resistant MCF-7 breast cancer cells [23]. In particular, MX1 and HOXC6 genes were identified to be directly involved during the acquisition of tamoxifen resistance and recovery of sensitivity by CAP. With this limited information, however, it is premature to conclude that CAP recovers sensitivity to diverse therapeutics in drug-resistant cancers.

In this study, we explored the potential of CAP to inhibit the proliferation of cancer cells carrying a more extended range of drug resistance using MCF-7/TxR. Next, the gene signature responsible for the resistance and sensitivity to Tx was identified at the genome-wide level. The expression of selected genes that were deregulated by Tx and CAP was further examined at the protein level.

2. Results

2.1. *CAP Recovered Tx Sensitivity in MCF-7/TxR Cells*

MCF-7/TxR cells were developed by continually exposing the MCF-7 cells to Tx of step-wise increased concentrations up to 60 ng/ml in the culture media. The MCF-7/TxR cells produced slightly higher levels of reactive oxygen species (ROS) compared to the parental MCF-7 cells, while both cell types responded to CAP with increased ROS levels (Figure 1). To determine whether the recovery of sensitivity by CAP comes from any decreased pumping-out activity of the cell for chemicals, fluorescence-tagged Tx and doxorubicin, which itself emits fluorescence, were used, and then the fluorescence was measured by Fluorescence Activated Cell Sorter (FACS). As a result, no significant difference was found for either chemical in the CAP-treated MCF-7/TxR cells compared to the non-treated control cells, indicating that the sensitivity recovery is not from any change in the drug transport rate across the plasma membrane (Figure 2).

The potential of CAP to recover the MCF-7/TxR cells' sensitivity to Tx was monitored by two experimental approaches. First, the cells were treated with CAP followed by Tx in amounts of 30 and 60 ng/mL. Then, the survival of cells was examined by a colony formation assay (Figure 3A and Figure S1). MCF-7/TxR cells proliferated more quickly than MCF-7, but the proliferation was suppressed by CAP. Notably, CAP treatment reset the resistant cells' sensitivity to Tx in a dose-dependent manner. When the CAP-treated MCF-7/TxR cells were treated with Tx of 60 ng/mL, their growth decreased by 73%, while that of the non-treated cells decreased by only 50%. Second, the effect of CAP on sensitivity recovery was examined by tracking the growth of the cells for 5 days using a dye-based assay. The result also indicated a higher growth rate for the MCF-7/TxR cells (Figure 3B) and recovery of drug sensitivity when the cells were treated with CAP (Figure 3C). All these data support the fact that CAP sets the state of drug resistance back to the sensitive state, enabling Tx to induce the death of the chemo-resistant cancer cells.

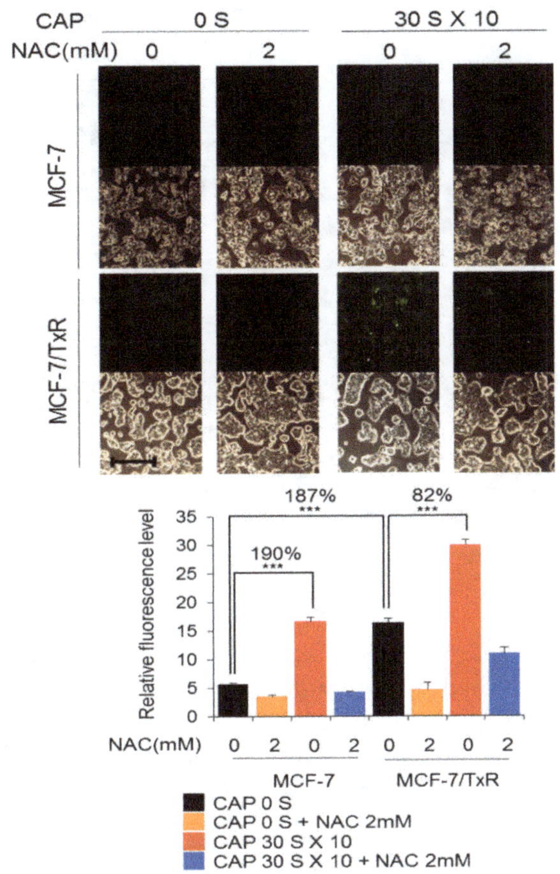

Figure 1. CAP increases ROS in MCF-7/TxR cells. Fluorescence microscope images were taken of MCF-7 and MCF-7/TxR cells by treating the cells with a fluorescent dye DCFH-DA after CAP treatment. N-acetylcysteine (NAC) was used to quench intracellular ROS. Monochrome images were obtained with a bright field microscope. Scale bar, 400 μm. *** $p < 0.001$.

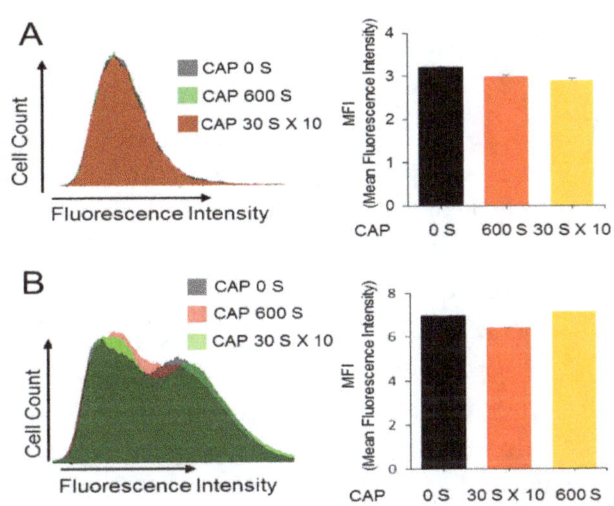

Figure 2. CAP does not affect uptake of Tx into MCF-7/TxR cells. MCF-7 and MCF-7/TxR cells were cultured in drug-containing media and treated with CAP. The uptake rate of doxorubicin (**A**) or Flutax-1 (**B**) in the MCF-7/TxR cells was examined by FACS, and the results are represented by bar graphs. All assays were performed in triplicate, and the results are expressed as mean ± SE.

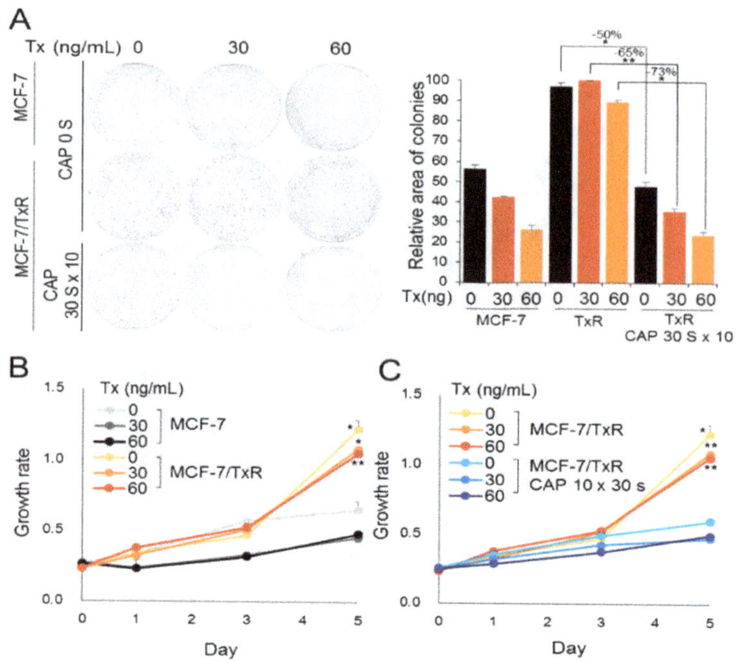

Figure 3. CAP sensitizes MCF-7/TxR cells to Tx. (**A**) The effect of CAP on the sensitivity of MCF-7 and MCF-7/TxR to Tx was examined by colony formation. The area of colonies is represented by a bar graph. (**B**) Effect of Tx on the growth rate of MCF-7/TxR vs. MCF-7. Cell growth was examined by CCK-8 assay. (**C**) Effect of CAP on growth rate of MCF-7/TxR in presence of Tx. All assays were performed in triplicate, and the results are expressed as mean ± SE. * $p < 0.05$, ** $p < 0.01$.

2.2. Expression of a Set of Genes Is Reversed from MCF-7 via MCF-7/TxR to CAP-Treated MCF-7/TxR Cells

To investigate the molecular mechanism of CAP for the sensitivity recovery, a genome-wide expression array analysis was performed. The array covering 58,201 human genes was analyzed in duplicate for each set of MCF-7 vs. MCF-7/TxR and MCF-7/TxR vs. CAP-treated MCF-7/TxR. With the cut ratio higher than 1.3 fold, 1335 genes showed expression differences in the MCF-7 vs. MCF-7/TxR and 367 genes in the MCF-7/TxR and MCF-7/TxR vs. CAP-treated MCF-7/TxR, representing 49 genes that appeared in both sets (Figure 4A). Finally, 20 genes showed the opposite alteration during the course from MCF-7 via MCF-7/TxR to CAP-treated MCF-7/TxR (Table S1). The expression of genes from the array data was re-examined by qPCR for six genes that were selected from the 20 genes in Figure 4A, and the result confirmed the same alteration by Tx and CAP (Figure 4B).

With the 1335 genes from the MCF-7 vs. MCF-7/TxR, the Ingenuity Pathway Analysis (IPA) network analysis was performed, and this represented "Nutritional Disease, Organismal Injury and Abnormalities, Carbohydrate Metabolism" as the top network (Figure 5A). Notably, TGF-β1 comprises a hub of the network through interacting with many genes regulated by TGF-β1, such as TLE4, PLEK2, and CPQ. Meanwhile, the network of the 367 genes from MCF-7/TxR vs. CAP-treated MCF-7/TxR represented "Embryonic Development, Nervous System Development and Function, Organ Development" as the top network (Figure 5B). In the network, the ERK1/2 hub was notable, showing interaction with multiple genes, including DLK1, SPRY4, and APH1A.

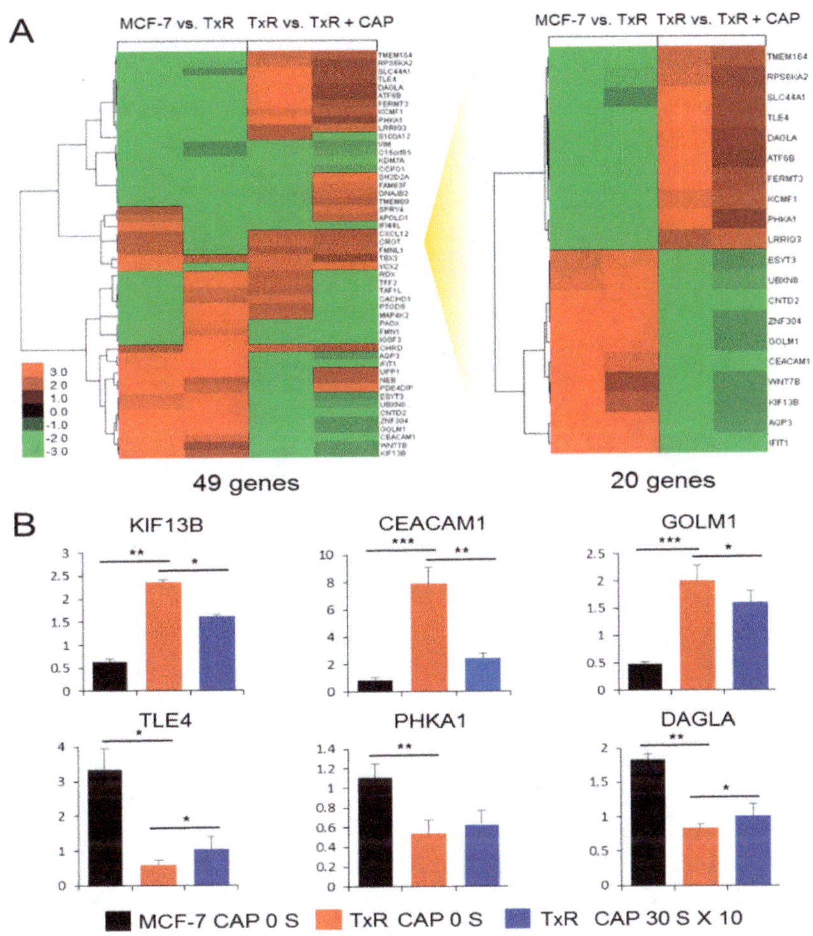

Figure 4. Clustering of genes affected by Tx and CAP in MCF-7 and MCF-7/TxR. (**A**) Heatmap analysis of 49 genes that exhibited expression changes (|fold change| ≥ 1.3) both in MCF-7 vs. MCF-7/TxR and MCF-7/TxR vs. CAP-treated MCF-7/TxR. Twenty genes showed opposite expression profiles at the two comparisons. Data are from expression arrays in duplicate. (**B**) qPCR of six genes that were selected from (**A**) showing upregulation in MCF-7 vs. MCF-7/TxR and downregulation in MCF-7/TxR vs. CAP-treated MCF-7/TxR (upper graphs), or vice versa (lower graphs). All assays were performed in triplicate, and the results are depicted as mean ± SE. * $p < 0.05$, ** $p < 0.01$, *** $p < 0.001$.

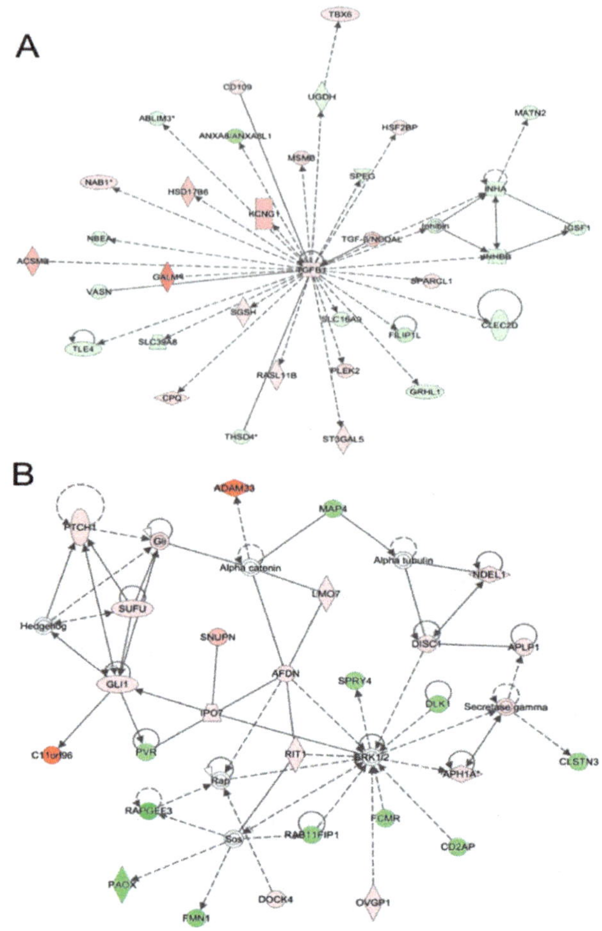

Figure 5. Highest confidence network of genes displaying altered expression levels by acquisition of TxR or by CAP. Most reliable IPA network of genes showing altered expression in MCF-7/TxR vs. MCF-7 (**A**) and CAP-treated MCF-7/TxR vs. MCF-7/TxR (**B**). The top networks are "Nutritional Disease, Organismal Injury and Abnormalities, and Carbohydrate Metabolism" (**A**) and "Embryonic Development, Nervous System Development and Function, and Organ Development" (**B**). Up- and downregulated genes are green and red, respectively, with the color intensity of the expression change. Dashed and solid lines denote direct and indirect interactions, respectively.

2.3. CEACAM1 and DAGLA Are Regulated during the Restoration of Sensitivity to Tx by CAP

Even though 20 genes were deregulated during the acquisition of drug resistance and recovery, their contribution to these processes had to be determined. To address this, we selected and focused on two genes: CEACAM1 from the downregulated group and DAGLA from the upregulated group in the CAP-treated MCF-7/TxR cells. After having confirmed the deregulation of gene expression found in the microarray for the two genes by qPCR, their expression was further examined by Western blot analysis. As a result, the profile of protein expression was similar to that of RNA expression (Figure 6A,B). In detail, expression of DAGLA was decreased in the MCF-7/TxR compared to MCF-7 but increased by CAP. In the case of CEACAM1, the expression profile was the opposite (i.e., increased in the MCF-7/TxR but decreased by CAP). Notably, the effect of CAP on the protein expression of the two genes was deteriorated by NAC, an ROS inhibitor (Figure 6C,D).

Next, the effect of the two genes on drug sensitivity was monitored at their dysregulated conditions through colony formation assay. When DAGLA was downregulated by siRNA, MCF-7/TxR proliferated at a higher rate up to 40% than the control siRNA-treated cells (Figure 7A and Figure S2A). Meanwhile, lower cell growth up to 8% compared to control was observed when CEACAM1 was downregulated (Figure 7B and Figure S2B). However, all the siRNA-treated cells did not show significant change of sensitivity to Tx, even though a few samples such as 30 ng/mL of Tx- and siRNA-treated cells for DAGLA and CEACAM1 showed difference up to 1.5 fold compared to control.

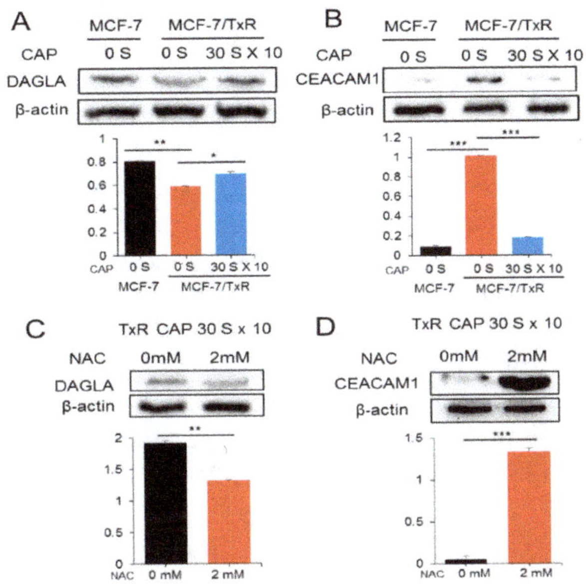

Figure 6. Protein expression of DAGLA and CEACMA1 in CAP-treated MCF-7/TxR cells. The protein expression of DAGLA (**A**) and CEACAM1 (**B**) in CAP-exposed MCF-7/TxR cells was examined by Western blot analysis. The protein expression of DAGLA and CEACAM1 showed a similar profile to that of microarray and qPCR. (**C**,**D**) The effect of CAP on the expression of DAGLA and CEACAM1 was examined after NAC treatment. NAC deteriorated the effect of CAP on the two proteins. The protein band in the Western blot was measured by a gel document system, and the levels are represented by bar graphs. All assays were performed in triplicate, and the results are depicted as mean ± SE. * $p < 0.05$, ** $p < 0.01$, *** $p < 0.001$.

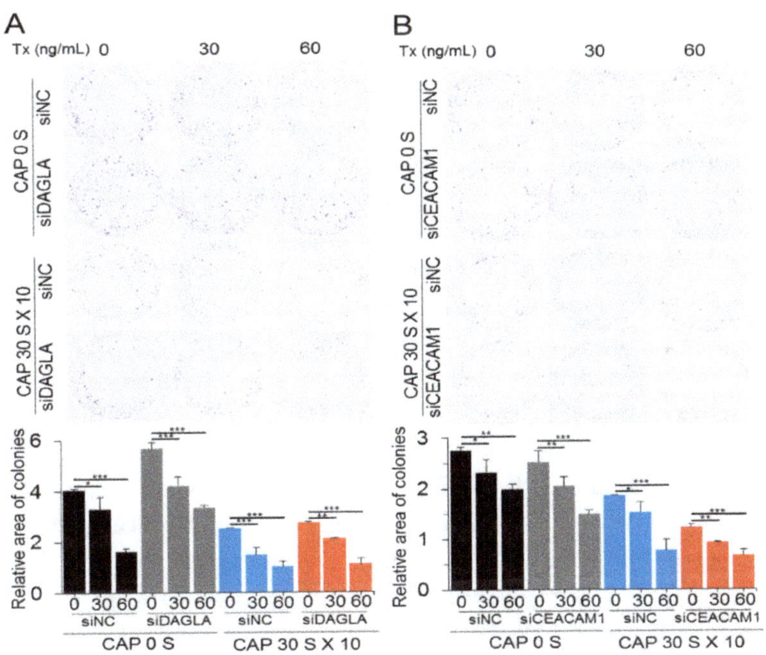

Figure 7. DAGLA and CEACAM1 are involved in the CAP-mediated recovery of sensitivity to Tx. Effect of DAGLA (**A**) and CEACAM1 (**B**) on the recovery of Tx sensitivity was determined by downregulating the genes using siRNA in MCF-7/TxR cells. The sensitivity to Tx was examined by colony formation assay after treating cells with CAP and Tx. siNC, negative-control siRNA. All assays were performed in triplicate, and the results are depicted as mean ± SE. * $p < 0.05$, ** $p < 0.01$, *** $p < 0.001$.

3. Discussion

This study aimed to evaluate the potential of CAP to overcome TxR and thereby prevent cancer recurrence in a cell model system. The underlying molecular mechanism of sensitivity recovery was investigated through tracking the change of genome-wide expression during the acquisition of TxR and during the recovery of sensitivity by CAP. Notably, the level of ROS in the MCF-7/TxR cells was higher than in MCF-7, and the difference became more significant when the cells were exposed to CAP. This is reminiscent of the fact that drug-resistant cancer cells in general produce higher levels of ROS than their parental cancer cells [24]. An increase of ROS in cells can contribute to a higher growth rate, but levels higher than a threshold can induce cell death or apoptosis [25]. Therefore, the increased ROS levels in the drug-resistant cells may serve as a double-edged sword: they may increase the cells' proliferation rate but make them more vulnerable to CAP. In fact, the MCF-7/TxR cells showed a higher growth rate than MCF-7 and a higher level of death induction by CAP.

In this study, CAP did not affect the net intracellular level of Tx (i.e., transport of Tx across the plasma membrane after CAP treatment was not changed significantly). In contrast, the expression of genes previously known to be responsible for drug resistance, such as Bcl2L13 (1.86-fold decrease) [26,27] and HOXA9 (2.14-fold increase) [28], was changed by CAP. This discrepancy explains the complication of drug transport in the MCF-7/TxR cells. Thus, genes in pathways associated with processes other than transport may have been affected during the acquisition of TxR. In fact, among the gene signatures identified in MCF-7 vs. MCF-7/TxR and MCF-7/TxR vs. CAP-treated MCF-7/TxR, only a portion shared common pathways and genes. Elucidation of the molecular mechanism of the differentially expressed genes could contribute to constructing the scenario of how TxR emerges and to establishing how to manipulate the TxR cancer. Notably, TGF-β took part in the central hub of the IPA network constructed with deregulated genes in the MCF-7/TxR cells. In addition, canonical pathway analysis identified the "interferon signaling", "Wnt/β-catenin", and "iNOS signaling" pathways as the most significant pathways. All these are pivotal to drive cellular differentiation and cancer development [29–31].

CEACAM1 is a glycoprotein belonging to the carcinoembryonic antigen (CEA) family that is expressed in a wide variety of cells [32]. The prognostic value of CEACAM1 in cancer is controversial: CEACAM1 expression correlates with good prognosis in mammary carcinomas, whereas in melanomas, upregulation of CEACAM1 is accompanied by poor overall survival [33,34]. It is notable that CEACAM1 was upregulated in the MCF-7/TxR cells and downregulated by CAP. Meanwhile, DAGLA was downregulated in the MCF-7/TxR cells but upregulated by CAP. DAGLA catalyzes the hydrolysis of diacylglycerol to 2-arachidonoylglycerol and free fatty acids [35]. So far, little has been found regarding its possible role in human tumorigenesis. A study indicated the upregulation of DAGLA in oral cancer [36]. However, no information is available on other cancers, including breast cancer. Database analysis identified the downregulation of DAGLA in breast cancer tissue compared to normal tissues (Figure S3A). In addition, breast cancer patients with higher expression of DAGLA showed better prognosis than those with lower expression, suggesting DAGLA as a tumor suppressor in breast cancer. In the case of CEACAM1, no significance was found in either expression or prognosis between normal and cancer tissues (Figure S3B). CAP has previously shown to recover sensitivity to tamoxifen, however, remarkably different gene and network signature for Tx resistance was identified by genome-wide expression analysis, suggesting a differential molecular mechanism of CAP acting on the Tx-resistant cancer cells from the tamoxifen-resistant cancer. It should be mentioned that DAGLA and CEACAM1 were deregulated while the sensitivity was recovered by CAP, however, they are not directly responsible for the sensitivity recovery because downregulation with siRNA did not induce significant change of sensitivity to Tx. Validating other genes from the microarray data (Figure 4A) is needed to identify genes which are pivotal to the recovery of sensitivity. Altogether, these data indicate that CAP recovers Tx sensitivity at least in part by modulating the expression of oncogenes or tumor suppressors.

A limitation of this study is the lack of verification of the in vitro data on in vivo platforms, such as an animal model. Applying CAP treatment in combination with Tx to tumor tissues formed from xenografted MCF-7/TxR cells and tracking the molecular change could clearly demonstrate the potential of CAP to recover Tx sensitivity. Also, using only the ROS inhibitor obscures defining the specific casts in CAP that regulate the identified genes. Further study should include finely tuning the CAP treatment conditions, including power strength and duration, to overcome obstacles while applying it to in vivo systems.

4. Materials and Methods

4.1. Cell Culture and CAP Treatment

The MCF-7 human breast cancer cell line was purchased from the American Type Culture Collection (ATCC) (Manassas, VA, USA) and cultured in RPMI-1640 medium (Gibco, Los Angeles, CA, USA) supplemented with 10% fetal bovine serum (Capricorn, Ebsdorfergrund, Germany) and 2% penicillin/streptomycin (Capricorn) at 37 °C in a humidified incubator containing 5% CO_2. The MCF-7/TxR cell line was generated by sequential exposure to increasing doses of Tx (Sigma-Aldrich, St. Louis, MO, USA) up to 60 ng/mL The mesh-dielectric barrier discharge (DBD) type of CAP device was produced at the Plasma Bioscience Research Center (Kwangwoon University, Seoul, Korea). The surface of culture media was treated with CAP from a 4 mm distance 10 times each for 30 s 1 h apart (10×30 s) with the energy of 0.3 kV and 12.9 kHz at an argon gas flow of 1.8 L/min.

4.2. Colony Formation and Cell Proliferation Analysis

For the colony formation assay, 3×10^3 cells of MCF-7 and MCF-7/TxR were seeded in 60 mm culture dishes with 2 mL medium and treated with CAP followed by exposure to either Tx (Sigma-Aldrich) or DMSO as a vehicle control 24 h later. siRNAs were transfected 24 h before CAP treatment. After incubating the cells for 14–21 days, colonies were fixed with methanol/acetic acid (7:1) and stained with 0.2% crystal violet solution (Sigma-Aldrich). The colony area was analyzed using the ImageJ software program [37]. For the cell proliferation assay, 3×10^3 cells were seeded per well of a 96-well plate with 100 μL medium and 24 h later treated with CAP and Tx. The cell growth rate was monitored at specific time points using CCK-8 solution (Enzo, New York, NY, USA) following the supplier's protocol.

4.3. Reactive Oxygen Species (ROS) Detection

For ROS detection, 5×10^5 cells seeded in a well of a 6-well plate were treated with CAP by the 10×30 s scheme. The cells were treated with 20 μM of DCFH-DA (Sigma-Aldrich) for 30 min in a humidified incubator at 37 °C 24 h later. The ROS level was calculated by measuring fluorescence using an Infinite 200 Pro fluorescence plate reader (Tecan, Mannedorf, Switzerland). To inhibit ROS synthesis, N-acetylcysteine (NAC) (Sigma-Aldrich) was added in a final concentration of 2 mM 2 h before CAP treatment.

4.4. Microarray Analysis

For the microarray analysis, 3×10^5 cells of MCF-7, MCF-7/TxR, and CAP-treated MCF-7/TxR were seeded in 60 mm culture dishes and cultured for 24 h before harvest. Total RNA was extracted using a ZR-Duet DNA/RNA MiniPrep kit (Zymo Research, Irvine, CA, USA). Labeled cRNA was synthesized from 600 ng of RNA and hybridized on SurePrint G3 Custom Gene Expression Microarrays, 8 × 60K (Agilent, Santa Clara, CA, USA) following the Agilent One-Color Microarray-Based Gene Expression Analysis protocol (Agilent, V 6.5, 2010). The hybridized array was analyzed using an Agilent SureScan Microarray Scanner. All array data were uploaded to the Gene Expression Omnibus (GEO) database, and they can be accessed via their website (http://www.ncbi.nlm.nih.gov/geo/; Series accession number GSE131480).

4.5. Pathway and Clustering Analysis

Pathway analysis was performed using the Ingenuity Pathway Analysis (IPA) software (Qiagen, Redwood City, CA, USA) by submitting gene pools comprised of genes showing expression change ≥ 1.3 and p-value < 0.05. Clustering analysis was performed using the Clustering 3.0 software (http://bonsai.hgc.jp/~mdehoon/software/cluster/) and then visualized using the TreeView program (http://jtreeview.sourceforge.net/).

4.6. Quantitative RT-PCR (qPCR)

Total RNA was extracted from cells 24 h after CAP treatment using the ZR-Duet DNA/RNA MiniPrep kit (Zymo Research) and reverse transcribed to cDNA using ReverTra Ace qPCR RT Master Mix with gDNA Remover (Toyobo, Osaka, Japan). DNA was amplified using KAPA SYBR FAST qPCR Kit Master Mix ABI Prism (Kapa Biosystems, Wilmington, MA, USA) on an ABI 7300 instrument (Applied Biosystems, Foster City, CA, USA). The relative gene expression level was calculated using the $2^{-\Delta\Delta Ct}$ method with glyceraldehyde-3-phosphate dehydrogenase (GAPDH) as an internal control. The PCR condition was as follows: denaturation at 95 °C for 3 min, 40 cycles of denaturation at 95 °C for 3 s, and annealing/extension at 60 °C for 40 s. Primer sequences used for qPCR are listed in Table S2.

4.7. Western Blot Analysis

To extract total proteins from cultured cells, the cells were collected and suspended in ice-cold RIPA lysis buffer with a protease inhibitor cocktail (Thermo Fisher Scientific, Waltham, MA, USA). After determining protein concentration by BCA assay (Thermo Fisher Scientific), 50 μg of the protein was subjected to SDS-PAGE. After electrophoresis, the proteins were transferred onto PVDF membranes (Whatman, Maidstone, UK), and then the membranes were soaked in blocking solution (5% non-fat milk diluted in 0.1% Tween-20 TBS) for 1 h at room temperature. The blots were incubated overnight at 4 °C with anti-CEACAM1 (1:500, Bioss, Woburn, MA, USA) and anti-DAGLA (1:500, Bioss) antibodies. The blots were additionally probed with an anti-β-actin antibody (1:800, Bioss) as an internal reference. After incubation with HRP-conjugated goat/rabbit anti-rabbit secondary antibodies (1:1000, GeneTex, Irvine, CA, USA) for 1 h, protein bands were visualized with ECL reagent (AbFrontier, Seoul, Korea) and quantified with Image Lab software (Bio-Rad, Hercules, CA, USA). The whole blot figures can be accessed in Supplementary Materials (Figure S4).

4.8. Fluorescene Activated Cell Sorter (FACS) Analysis

Apoptosis and drug transport were evaluated by FACS. For the apoptosis analysis, 1×10^6 cells were seeded in a 60 mm dish, treated with CAP, and cultured for 24 h. 1×10^5 washed cells were treated with 5 μL of FITC Annexin V and 5 μL of propidium iodide (PI) using an FITC Annexin Apoptosis Detection Kit (BD Technologies, Franklin Lakes, NJ, USA). Samples were analyzed using a FACS Canto II flow cytometer (BD Technologies). To monitor drug uptake by cells, 1×10^6 cells seeded in a 60 mm dish were treated with Flutax (Santa Cruz Biotechnology, Santa Cruz, CA, USA, sc-203958) for 4 h or doxorubicin (Cayman Chemical, Ann Arbor, MI, USA, 15007) for 24 h, respectively, at final concentration of 10 μM. Fluorescene was detected with FACSAria III (BD Technologies) and analyzed with BD FACSDiva software.

4.9. Statistical Analysis

Student's t-test was applied to compare gene expression levels between CAP-exposed MCF-7/TxR and control cells. For the statistical analysis, SPSS for Windows, version 23.0 (SPSS, Chicago, IL, USA), was used. All experimental data were obtained by independently performing experiments at least three times and considered statistically significant when the p-value was lower than 0.05. Gene expression data of normal and cancer tissues were obtained from The Cancer Genome Atlas database (TCGA, https://cancergenome.nih.gov). The association between gene expression levels and the overall survival rate of breast cancer patients was evaluated using the Kaplan–Meier Plotter (http://kmplot.com/analysis).

5. Conclusions

CAP was shown to set the MCF-7/TxR cells back to the Tx-sensitive state, offering the potential application of CAP for the treatment of TxR cancer. At the molecular level, CAP recovered the expression of a set of genes that had been deregulated in the course of TxR. Among the genes, tumor related DAGLA and CEACAM1 were proven essential for the acquisition of resistance and for the recovery of sensitivity. These genes could be developed as diagnostic markers and could be molecular targets for the clinical treatment of TxR breast cancer.

Author Contributions: Conceptualization, S.J.K.; methodology, S.P. and H.K.; validation, H.W.J. and H.W.K.; data curation, S.H.Y.; writing—original draft preparation, S.P. and H.K.; writing—review and editing, S.J.K. and E.H.C.; funding acquisition, S.J.K. and E.H.C.

References

1. Baguley, B.C. Multiple Drug Resistance Mechanisms in Cancer. *Mol. Biotechnol.* **2010**, *46*, 308–316. [CrossRef] [PubMed]
2. Gottesman, M.M. Mechanisms of Cancer Drug Resistance. *Annu. Rev. Med.* **2002**, *53*, 615–627. [CrossRef] [PubMed]
3. Driscoll, L.O.; Clynes, M. Biomarkers and Multiple Drug Resistance in Breast Cancer. *Curr. Cancer Drug Targets* **2006**, *6*, 365–384. [CrossRef] [PubMed]
4. Giordano, S.H.; Buzdar, A.U.; Smith, T.L.; Kau, S.-W.; Yang, Y.; Hortobagyi, G.N. Is breast cancer survival improving? *Cancer* **2004**, *100*, 44–52. [CrossRef] [PubMed]
5. Wang, F.; Porter, M.; Konstantopoulos, A.; Zhang, P.; Cui, H. Preclinical development of drug delivery systems for paclitaxel-based cancer chemotherapy. *J. Control. Release* **2017**, *267*, 100–118. [CrossRef] [PubMed]
6. Shao, Z.; Zhao, H. Manipulating Natural Product Biosynthetic Pathways via DNA Assembler. *Curr. Protoc. Chem. Biol.* **2014**, *6*, 65–100. [CrossRef]
7. Woods, C.M.; Zhu, J.; McQueney, P.A.; Bollag, D.; Lazarides, E. Taxol-induced mitotic block triggers rapid onset of a p53-independent apoptotic pathway. *Mol. Med.* **1995**, *1*, 506–526. [CrossRef]
8. Froidevaux-Klipfel, L.; Targa, B.; Cantaloube, I.; Ahmed-Zaïd, H.; Poüs, C.; Baillet, A. Septin cooperation with tubulin polyglutamylation contributes to cancer cell adaptation to taxanes. *Oncotarget* **2015**, *6*, 36063–36080. [CrossRef]
9. De Hoon, J.P.J.; Veeck, J.; Vriens, B.E.P.J.; Calon, T.G.A.; van Engeland, M.; Tjan-Heijnen, V.C.G. Taxane resistance in breast cancer: A closed HER2 circuit? *Biochim. et Biophys. Acta (BBA) Rev. Cancer* **2012**, *1825*, 197–206. [CrossRef]
10. Nemoto, K.; Matsushita, H.; Ogawa, Y.; Takeda, K.; Takahashi, C.; Britton, K.R.; Takai, Y.; Miyazaki, S.; Miyata, T.; Yamada, S. Radiation Therapy Combined with Cis-Diammine-Glycolatoplatinum (Nedaplatin) and 5-Fluorouracil for Untreated and Recurrent Esophageal Cancer. *Am. J. Clin. Oncol.* **2003**, *26*, 46–49. [CrossRef]
11. Modi, S.; DiGiovanna, M.P.; Lu, Z.; Moskowitz, C.; Panageas, K.S.; Van Poznak, C.; Hudis, C.A.; Norton, L.; Tan, L.; Stern, D.F.; et al. Phosphorylated/Activated HER2 as a Marker of Clinical Resistance to Single Agent Taxane Chemotherapy for Metastatic Breast Cancer. *Cancer Investig.* **2005**, *23*, 483–487. [CrossRef] [PubMed]
12. To, K.; Fotovati, A.; Reipas, K.M.; Law, J.H.; Hu, K.; Wang, J.; Astanehe, A.; Davies, A.H.; Lee, L.; Stratford, A.L.; et al. Y-Box Binding Protein-1 Induces the Expression of *CD44* and *CD49f* Leading to Enhanced Self-Renewal, Mammosphere Growth, and Drug Resistance. *Cancer Res.* **2010**, *70*, 2840. [CrossRef] [PubMed]
13. Ro, J.; Sahin, A.; Ro, J.Y.; Fritsche, H.; Hortobagyi, G.; Blick, M. Immunohistochemical analysis of P-glycoprotein expression correlated with chemotherapy resistance in locally advanced breast cancer. *Hum. Pathol.* **1990**, *21*, 787–791. [CrossRef]
14. Proffered papers and posters. *Target. Oncol.* **2007**, *2*, S20–S63. [CrossRef]
15. Zelnak, A. Overcoming Taxane and Anthracycline Resistance. *Breast J.* **2010**, *16*, 309–312. [CrossRef] [PubMed]

16. Murray, S.; Briasoulis, E.; Linardou, H.; Bafaloukos, D.; Papadimitriou, C. Taxane resistance in breast cancer: Mechanisms, predictive biomarkers and circumvention strategies. *Cancer Treat. Rev.* **2012**, *38*, 890–903. [CrossRef] [PubMed]
17. Biscop, E.; Lin, A.; Van Boxem, W.; Van Loenhout, J.; De Backer, J.; Deben, C.; Dewilde, S.; Smits, E.; Bogaerts, A. The Influence of Cell Type and Culture Medium on Determining Cancer Selectivity of Cold Atmospheric Plasma Treatment. *Cancers* **2019**, *11*, 1287. [CrossRef]
18. Babington, P.; Rajjoub, K.; Canady, J.; Siu, A.; Keidar, M.; Sherman, J.H. Use of cold atmospheric plasma in the treatment of cancer. *Biointerphases* **2015**, *10*, 029403. [CrossRef]
19. Keidar, M.; Yan, D.; Beilis, I.I.; Trink, B.; Sherman, J.H. Plasmas for Treating Cancer: Opportunities for Adaptive and Self-Adaptive Approaches. *Trends Biotechnol.* **2018**, *36*, 586–593. [CrossRef]
20. Von Woedtke, T.; Schmidt, A.; Bekeschus, S.; Wende, K.; Weltmann, K.-D. Plasma Medicine: A Field of Applied Redox Biology. *In Vivo* **2019**, *33*, 1011–1026. [CrossRef]
21. Köritzer, J.; Boxhammer, V.; Schäfer, A.; Shimizu, T.; Klämpfl, T.G.; Li, Y.-F.; Welz, C.; Schwenk-Zieger, S.; Morfill, G.E.; Zimmermann, J.L.; et al. Restoration of sensitivity in chemo-resistant glioma cells by cold atmospheric plasma. *PLoS ONE* **2013**, *8*, e64498. [CrossRef] [PubMed]
22. Utsumi, F.; Kajiyama, H.; Nakamura, K.; Tanaka, H.; Mizuno, M.; Ishikawa, K.; Kondo, H.; Kano, H.; Hori, M.; Kikkawa, F. Effect of indirect nonequilibrium atmospheric pressure plasma on anti-proliferative activity against chronic chemo-resistant ovarian cancer cells in vitro and in vivo. *PLoS ONE* **2013**, *8*, e81576. [CrossRef] [PubMed]
23. Lee, S.; Lee, H.; Jeong, D.; Ham, J.; Park, S.; Choi, E.H.; Kim, S.J. Cold atmospheric plasma restores tamoxifen sensitivity in resistant MCF-7 breast cancer cell. *Free Radic. Biol. Med.* **2017**, *110*, 280–290. [CrossRef] [PubMed]
24. Cui, Q.; Wang, J.-Q.; Assaraf, Y.G.; Ren, L.; Gupta, P.; Wei, L.; Ashby, C.R.; Yang, D.-H.; Chen, Z.-S. Modulating ROS to overcome multidrug resistance in cancer. *Drug Resist. Updates* **2018**, *41*, 1–25. [CrossRef] [PubMed]
25. Galadari, S.; Rahman, A.; Pallichankandy, S.; Thayyullathil, F. Reactive oxygen species and cancer paradox: To promote or to suppress? *Free Radic. Biol. Med.* **2017**, *104*, 144–164. [CrossRef]
26. Panayotopoulou, E.G.; Müller, A.-K.; Börries, M.; Busch, H.; Hu, G.; Lev, S. Targeting of apoptotic pathways by SMAC or BH3 mimetics distinctly sensitizes paclitaxel-resistant triple negative breast cancer cells. *Oncotarget* **2017**, *8*, 45088–45104. [CrossRef]
27. Jensen, S.A.; Calvert, A.E.; Volpert, G.; Kouri, F.M.; Hurley, L.A.; Luciano, J.P.; Wu, Y.; Chalastanis, A.; Futerman, A.H.; Stegh, A.H. Bcl2L13 is a ceramide synthase inhibitor in glioblastoma. *Proc. Natl. Acad. Sci. USA* **2014**, *111*, 5682–5687. [CrossRef]
28. Pontikakis, S.; Papadaki, C.; Tzardi, M.; Trypaki, M.; Sfakianaki, M.; Koinis, F.; Lagoudaki, E.; Giannikaki, L.; Kalykaki, A.; Kontopodis, E.; et al. Predictive value of ATP7b, BRCA1, BRCA2, PARP1, UIMC1 (RAP80), HOXA9, DAXX, TXN (TRX1), THBS1 (TSP1) and PRR13 (TXR1) genes in patients with epithelial ovarian cancer who received platinum-taxane first-line therapy. *Pharm. J.* **2017**, *17*, 506–514. [CrossRef]
29. Pickup, M.; Novitskiy, S.; Moses, H.L. The roles of TGFβ in the tumour microenvironment. *Nat. Rev. Cancer* **2013**, *13*, 788–799. [CrossRef]
30. Yin, P.; Wang, W.; Zhang, Z.; Bai, Y.; Gao, J.; Zhao, C. Wnt signaling in human and mouse breast cancer: Focusing on Wnt ligands, receptors and antagonists. *Cancer Sci.* **2018**, *109*, 3368–3375. [CrossRef]
31. Cheng, H.; Wang, L.; Mollica, M.; Re, A.T.; Wu, S.; Zuo, L. Nitric oxide in cancer metastasis. *Cancer Lett.* **2014**, *353*, 1–7. [CrossRef] [PubMed]
32. Calinescu, A.; Turcu, G.; Nedelcu, R.I.; Brinzea, A.; Hodorogea, A.; Antohe, M.; Diaconu, C.; Bleotu, C.; Pirici, D.; Jilaveanu, L.B.; et al. On the Dual Role of Carcinoembryonic Antigen-Related Cell Adhesion Molecule 1 (CEACAM1) in Human Malignancies. *J. Immunol. Res.* **2018**, *2018*, 7169081. [CrossRef] [PubMed]
33. Ortenberg, R.; Galore-Haskel, G.; Greenberg, I.; Zamlin, B.; Sapoznik, S.; Greenberg, E.; Barshack, I.; Avivi, C.; Feiler, Y.; Zan-Bar, I.; et al. CEACAM1 promotes melanoma cell growth through Sox-2. *Neoplasia* **2014**, *16*, 451–460. [CrossRef] [PubMed]
34. Helfrich, I.; Singer, B.B. Size Matters: The Functional Role of the CEACAM1 Isoform Signature and Its Impact for NK Cell-Mediated Killing in Melanoma. *Cancers* **2019**, *11*, 356. [CrossRef]
35. Powell, D.R.; Gay, J.P.; Wilganowski, N.; Doree, D.; Savelieva, K.V.; Lanthorn, T.H.; Read, R.; Vogel, P.; Hansen, G.M.; Brommage, R.; et al. Diacylglycerol Lipase α Knockout Mice Demonstrate Metabolic and Behavioral Phenotypes Similar to Those of Cannabinoid Receptor 1 Knockout Mice. *Front. Endocrinol. (Lausanne)* **2015**, *6*, 86. [CrossRef]

36. Okubo, Y.; Kasamatsu, A.; Yamatoji, M.; Fushimi, K.; Ishigami, T.; Shimizu, T.; Kasama, H.; Shiiba, M.; Tanzawa, H.; Uzawa, K. Diacylglycerol lipase alpha promotes tumorigenesis in oral cancer by cell-cycle progression. *Exp. Cell Res.* **2018**, *367*, 112–118. [CrossRef]
37. Guzmán, C.; Bagga, M.; Kaur, A.; Westermarck, J.; Abankwa, D. ColonyArea: An ImageJ Plugin to Automatically Quantify Colony Formation in Clonogenic Assays. *PLoS ONE* **2014**, *9*, e92444. [CrossRef]

3

The Interaction of Selenium with Chemotherapy and Radiation on Normal and Malignant Human Mononuclear Blood Cells

Richard J. Lobb [1], Gregory M. Jacobson [2], Ray T. Cursons [2] and Michael B. Jameson [3,4,*]

1 Tumour Microenvironment Laboratory, QIMR Berghofer Medical Research Institute, Herston, QLD 4006, Australia; Richard.Lobb@qimrberghofer.edu.au
2 Department of Biological Sciences, University of Waikato, Hamilton 3216, New Zealand; greg.jacobson@waikato.ac.nz (G.M.J.); ray.cursons@waikato.ac.nz (R.T.C.)
3 Oncology Department, Waikato Hospital, Hamilton 3204, New Zealand
4 Waikato Clinical Campus, Faculty of Medical and Health Sciences, University of Auckland, Hamilton 3204, New Zealand
* Correspondence: michael.jameson@waikatodhb.health.nz

Abstract: Selenium, a trace element with anticancer properties, can reduce harmful toxicities of chemotherapy and radiotherapy without compromising efficacy. However, the dose-response relationship in normal versus malignant human cells is unclear. We evaluated how methylseleninic acid (MSA) modulates the toxicity and efficacy of chemotherapy and radiation on malignant and non-malignant human mononuclear blood cells in vitro. We specifically investigated its effects on endoplasmic reticulum stress induction, intracellular glutathione concentration, DNA damage and viability of peripheral blood mononuclear cells and THP1 monocytic leukaemia cells in response to radiation, cytosine arabinoside or doxorubicin chemotherapy. MSA, at lower concentrations, induced protective responses in normal cells but cytotoxic effects in malignant cells, alone and in conjunction with chemotherapy or radiation. However, in normal cells higher concentrations of MSA were directly toxic and increased the cytotoxicity of radiation but not chemotherapy. In malignant cells higher MSA concentrations were generally more effective in combination with cancer treatments. Thus, optimal MSA concentrations differed between normal and malignant cells and treatments. This work supports clinical reports that selenium can significantly reduce dose-limiting toxicities of anticancer therapies and potentially improve efficacy of anticancer treatments. The optimal selenium compound and dose is not yet determined.

Keywords: selenium; glutathione; malignant; viability; DNA damage; ER stress

---

1. Introduction

Selenium (Se) is an essential trace element that is extensively studied in the prevention of numerous malignancies [1], although the majority of research on Se has focused on providing adequate nutritional intake in populations that have inherently low Se intake [2]. However, substantial preclinical data suggests that Se compounds, in supranutritional doses, have direct anticancer effects, mediated by various mechanisms including oxidative capability and modulation of immunological responses, angiogenesis, protein confirmation and DNA repair pathways [3,4]. These same mechanisms allow selenium compounds to act in synergy with cancer therapies and increase the efficacy of these treatments while reducing their normal tissue toxicities, as reviewed by Evans et al. [4]. Se compounds, when added to chemotherapy, resulted in improved tumour response rates and cures in human tumour xenograft animal models and reduced organ-specific toxicity [5–7]. Some aspects of these findings have been replicated in clinical trials, with various Se compounds ameliorating the toxicity of chemotherapy or radiotherapy [8–17], although the trials were not powered to evaluate overall treatment efficacy. These promising results argue for the initiation of larger clinical trials that can definitively assess the contributions of Se compounds to modulating both efficacy and toxicity of chemotherapy and radiation [4,18].

There is unquestionably a major unmet need in this regard. Despite many advances in supportive care, the toxicities of chemotherapy and radiotherapy still limit their efficacy, utility and acceptability to patients and clinicians, and result in poor quality of life for patients, treatment-related deaths and inadequate outcomes [19]. Apart from antiemetics and haemopoietic growth factors, few agents substantially prevent these toxicities, many are poorly-tolerated, and some reduce toxicities while compromising anticancer efficacy [20–22]. In contrast, Se compounds offer the potential, at optimum doses, of being well-tolerated agents that can improve both cancer outcomes and treatment toxicities.

In one study, Se-methyl-selenocysteine was more effective and dose-potent than seleno-l-methionine or sodium selenite in reducing cytotoxic chemotherapy-related mortality and augmenting its anticancer activity [6]. This may relate to the in vivo ability of Se-methyl-selenocysteine to directly generate methylselenol, a compound that is considered the active moiety for the observed effects of Se compounds in cancer cells [23–27]. In preclinical models Se-methyl-selenocysteine dosed at 0.2 mg/mouse/day optimises the mechanisms that mediate protection of normal tissues while enhancing tumour cytotoxicity [5,6,28]. In humans, however, this dose-response relationship has not been well-characterised, and thus the optimal type and dose of Se for use in clinical trials has not yet been determined [4]. Therefore, there is a need to provide a framework for characterising the divergent biological effects of Se in normal and malignant cells in humans, to inform future trials evaluating Se compounds in conjunction with anticancer treatments.

This investigation was undertaken to evaluate whether peripheral blood mononuclear cells (PBMCs) from healthy blood donors and a comparable malignant human cell line, THP1 monocytic leukaemia, could serve as an in vitro model to investigate the differential effects of Se on normal and malignant human mononuclear cells. Se has been previously shown to enhance apoptosis through the induction of endoplasmic reticulum (ER) stress in cancer cells [29], therefore we evaluated the induction of ER stress in both normal and malignant cells in response to Se treatment. Given that ER stress signalling can be induced in response to oxidative triggers, we also investigated the impact of Se on intracellular glutathione levels [30–32], a key component in maintaining redox homeostasis in the cell, and how this influences DNA damage and viability of normal and malignant cells to cytotoxic chemotherapy or radiation [33–35].

Instead of Se-methyl-selenocysteine, which does not generate methylselenol in vitro, we used methylseleninic acid (MSA), which directly provides methylselenol through non-enzymatic reduction, and enabled us to directly evaluate the impact of this active metabolite of Se compounds [25,27]. We used MSA at Se concentrations (2.5, 5 and 15 μM) that could be achieved in plasma in subsequent clinical trials, and were comparable to plasma levels in mice at effective doses [6]. MSA was used alone or in combination with cytotoxic chemotherapy drugs or gamma radiation to evaluate their interactions in normal and malignant cells.

We demonstrate that Se has divergent effects in normal and malignant human mononuclear cells, protecting normal cells from chemotherapy and radiation toxicity while enhancing their therapeutic effects against malignant cells. In this model we were also able to use analytical methods to demonstrate changes in biological pathways that mediate these effects of Se compounds, which could be incorporated into future clinical trials.

2. Results

2.1. Methylseleninic Acid (MSA) Induces Endoplasmic Reticulum (ER) Stress in Normal and Malignant Cells But Differentially Modulates Apoptosis

To investigate the induction of ER stress in normal and malignant cells we measured the cellular expression of 78 kDa glucose-regulated protein (GRP78) and phosphorylated eukaryotic initiation factor 2-alpha (phospho-EIF2α), and splicing of X-box binding protein 1 (XBP1), in response to exposure to increasing concentrations of MSA for 6 h. MSA induced ER stress in both normal and malignant cells, which was seen through an increase in the expression of GRP78, as well as an increase in the splicing of XBP1 (spliced: S-XBP1; unspliced: U-XBP1) and phosphorylation of EIF2α (Figure 1). Interestingly, when we assessed the effect of MSA on the apoptotic response induced by ER stress we found different patterns between normal and cancer cells (Figure 1). Caspase-8 was down-regulated by MSA in a concentration-dependent manner in normal PBMCs yet was upregulated in malignant THP1 cells at the same concentrations, with the maximal differential impact between normal and malignant cells at 5 μM MSA (Figure 1).

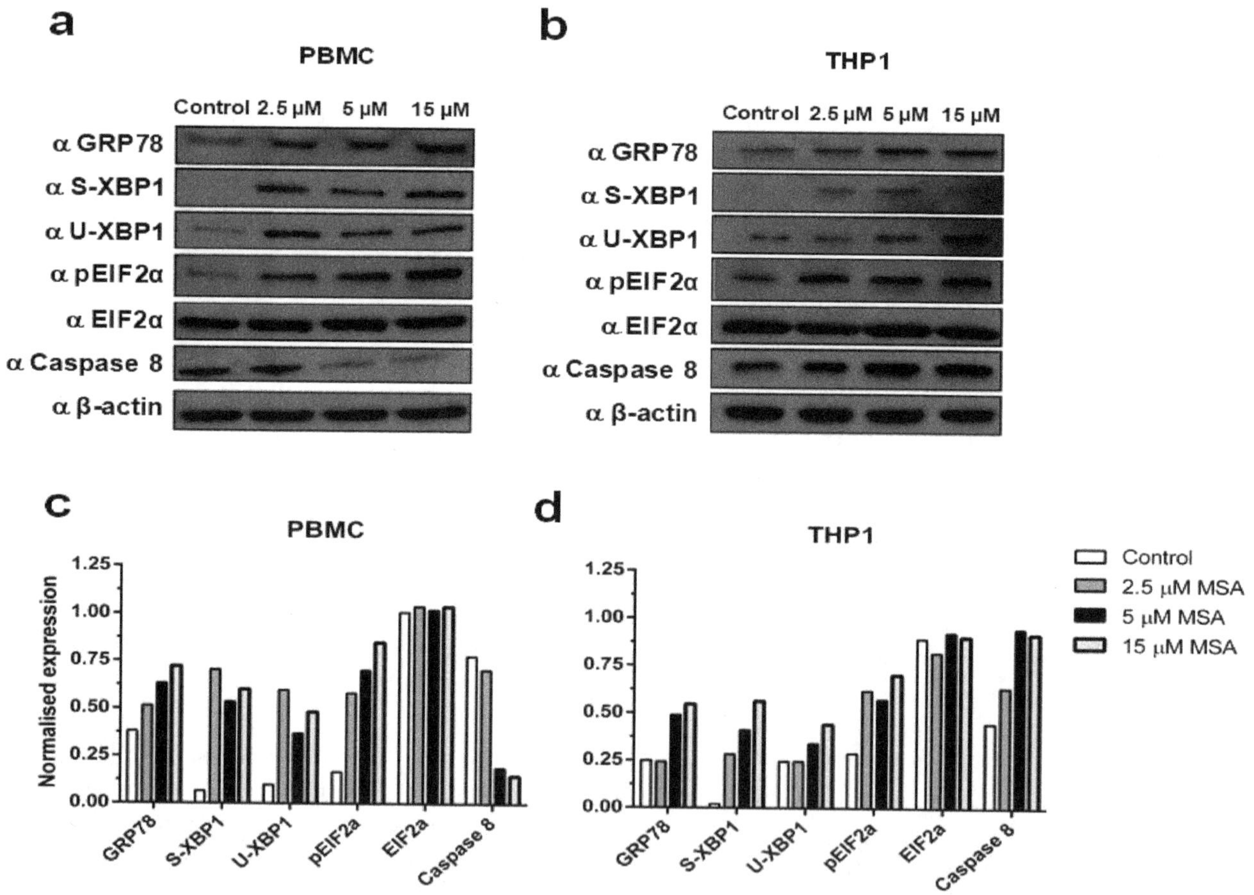

Figure 1. Selenium induces endoplasmic reticulum (ER) stress response in normal and malignant cells. (**a**) Concentration-dependent increase in ER stress proteins and decrease in caspase-8 in peripheral blood mononuclear cells (PBMCs) with 2.5, 5 and 15 μM methylseleninic acid (MSA) at 6 h; (**b**) Concentration-dependent increase in both ER stress proteins and caspase-8 in THP1 cells; (**c**,**d**) Quantification of protein expression in PBMC and THP1 cells.

2.2. MSA Has a Divergent Impact on Glutathione (GSH) Levels in Normal and Malignant Cells

To investigate the link between ER stress and generated oxidative stress we measured intracellular total GSH levels in normal and malignant cells. At 6 h we observed differential effects of MSA in normal and malignant cells (Figure 2a). MSA significantly increased total GSH levels in PBMC (Figure 2a) after 6 h in a concentration-dependent manner (a protective response). Conversely, THP1 cells had a baseline GSH level approximately 40-fold higher than PBMCs that was significantly reduced by MSA in a concentration-dependent manner after 6 h (Figure 2b).

We then tested the duration of the MSA-induced alteration on GSH levels in normal and malignant cells. The increase in GSH observed in PBMCs after 6 h of MSA treatment at 2.5 and 5 μM was maintained at 24 h but returned to baseline levels at 48 h (Figure 2c). However, at 15 μM MSA, the GSH concentration was less elevated at 24 h than at 6 h and also returned to baseline levels at 48 h. In THP1 cells, the depletion of GSH at 24 h was still significant but not concentration-dependent, whereas at 48 h the return of GSH levels towards baseline values was greater with 2.5 and 5 μM compared with 15 μM MSA (Figure 2d).

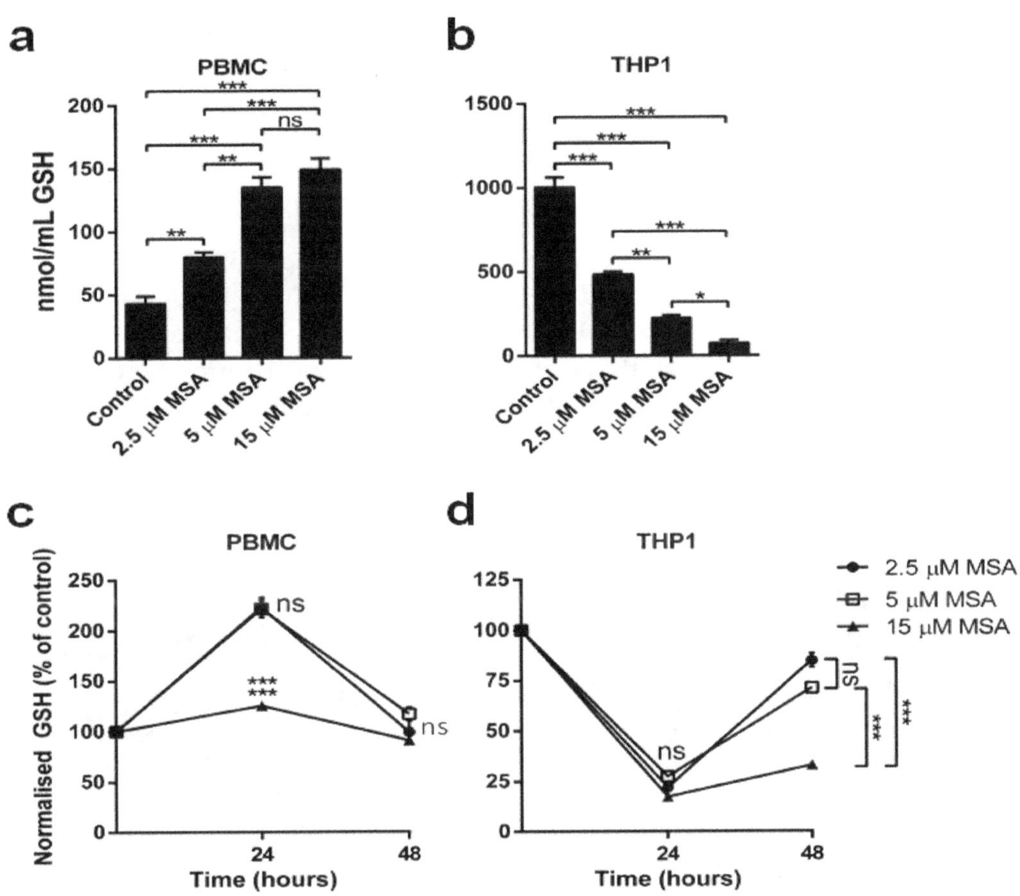

Figure 2. MSA has divergent impact on glutathione (GSH) levels in normal and malignant cells. (**a**,**b**) GSH quantification in PBMC and THP1 cells demonstrates that MSA significantly reduces GSH levels in THP1 cells and significantly increases GSH levels in PBMCs after 6 h ($n = 5$, ± SEM); (**c**,**d**) Timeline of GSH levels in PBMCs and THP1 cells after MSA treatments demonstrates GSH alterations are maintained for up to 24 h. $n = 3$, ± SEM, * $p < 0.05$, ** $p < 0.01$, *** $p < 0.001$, ns, not significant.

Next, we investigated if the MSA-induced GSH response in cells was maintained at 24 h after radiation and chemotherapy treatment. The GSH increase in normal PBMCs was maintained at 24 h when cells were also treated with 2 Gy radiation, cytosine arabinoside (AraC) or doxorubicin (Dox), though the maximum benefit was achieved with 2.5 μM MSA (Figure 3a–c). Furthermore, the depletion of GSH by MSA in malignant THP1 cells was still significantly reduced at 24 h after radiation and chemotherapy treatment, again without the advantage of higher MSA concentrations (Figure 3a–c).

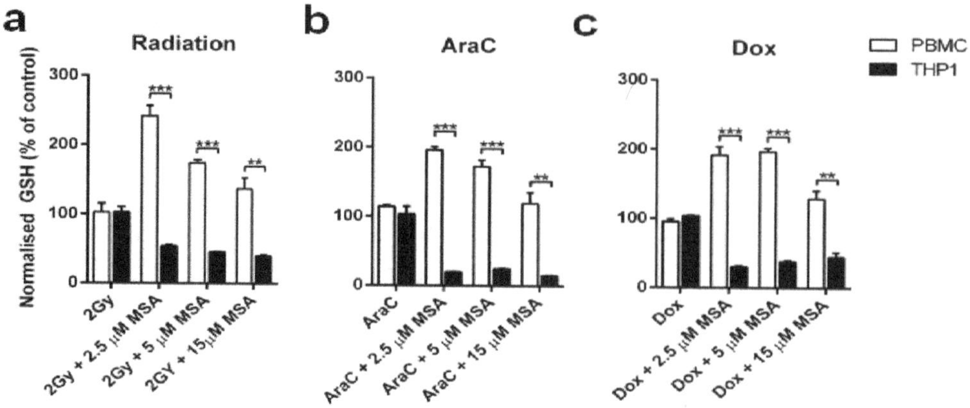

Figure 3. MSA-induced GSH alterations are maintained in the presence of therapeutic treatments. (**a–c**) GSH levels are significantly elevated in PBMCs at 24 h after radiation, AraC or Dox treatment, whereas GSH levels are significantly reduced in THP1 cells 24 h after treatment. $n = 3$, $\pm$ SEM, ** $p < 0.01$, *** $p < 0.001$.

2.3. MSA Reduces DNA Damage in Normal Cells While Increasing DNA Damage in Malignant Cells

Given the divergent effects of MSA on apoptosis induction and GSH expression in normal and malignant cells, we investigated if MSA would protect normal cells from DNA damage due to radiation or chemotherapy, while potentiating the DNA-damaging efficacy of these treatments in malignant cells. Using the comet assay (Figure 4a), this differential effect was pronounced with chemotherapy but not radiation. Treatment with MSA alone at the highest concentration, 15 μM, slightly increased DNA damage levels in normal cells but not in malignant cells, though the lower concentrations had no such effect (Figure 4b).

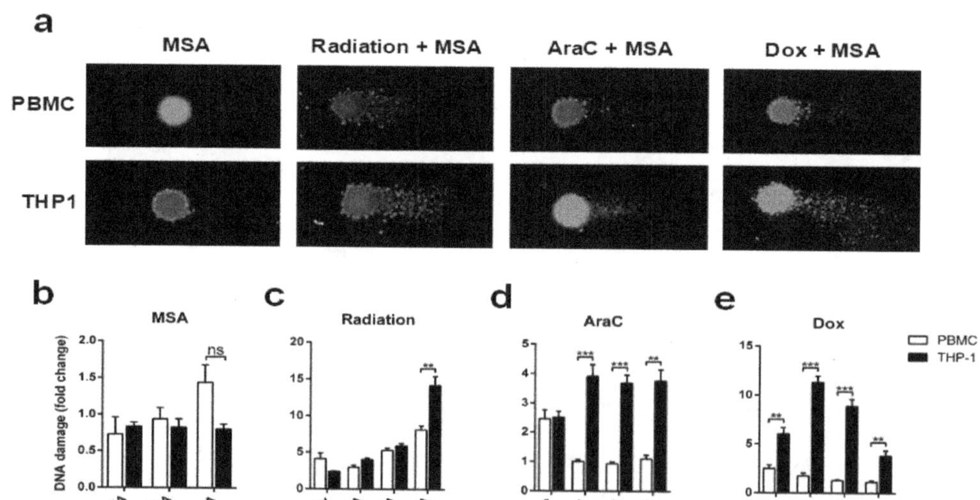

Figure 4. Selenium protects normal cells from DNA damage while enhancing DNA damage in malignant cells. (**a**) Representative image of comet assay (400× magnification) in PBMCs and THP1 cells treated with MSA alone or MSA in combination with radiation, AraC or Dox; (**b**) Quantification of DNA damage in PBMCs and THP1 cells: treatment with MSA 15 μM, but not lower concentrations, slightly increased DNA damage levels in normal but not in malignant cells; (**c**) DNA damage is increased in both PBMCs and THP1 cells exposed to 2 Gy radiation; (**d**,**e**) MSA is significantly protective against DNA damage in PBMCs while significantly increasing DNA damage in THP1 cells treated with AraC or Dox. $n = 3$, $\pm$ SEM, ** $p < 0.01$, *** $p < 0.001$, ns, not significant.

As expected, when PBMCs and THP1 cells were exposed to 2 Gy radiation DNA damage was elevated compared to controls (Figure 4c). While MSA at 2.5 μM reduced radiation-induced DNA damage in PBMC but not THP1 cells, higher concentrations of MSA progressively increased radiation-induced DNA damage in both normal and malignant cells (Figure 4c). DNA damage was significantly increased in PBMCs and THP1 cells when treated with AraC, however adding MSA protected the normal cells while increasing DNA damage in the malignant cells, without a clear concentration dependency (Figure 4d). Dox-induced DNA damage in PBMCs was not potentiated by MSA, while in contrast MSA increased Dox-induced DNA damage in THP1 cells (Figure 4e). However, this effect on THP1 cells was maximal at 2.5 μM MSA, and diminished at higher concentrations (Figure 4e).

2.4. *MSA Treatment Protects Normal Cells While Potentiating Cell Death in Malignant Cells*

We next investigated if the differences in DNA damage culminated in differences in cell viability. MSA alone significantly reduced the viability of THP1 cells with increasing MSA concentrations compared to PBMCs (Figure 5a). Although 2 Gy radiation alone did not affect viability of THP1 cells, adding MSA to radiation significantly reduced THP1 cell viability (Figure 5b). In agreement with the DNA damage induced by radiation, the addition of MSA to this treatment further reduced the viability of PBMCs (Figure 5b). However, when we assessed the combination of MSA with AraC or Dox we found significant differences (Figure 5c,d). Treatment with MSA at all concentrations provided significant protection of PBMCs while progressively increasing toxicity in THP1 cells in response to AraC or Dox treatment (Figure 5c,d).

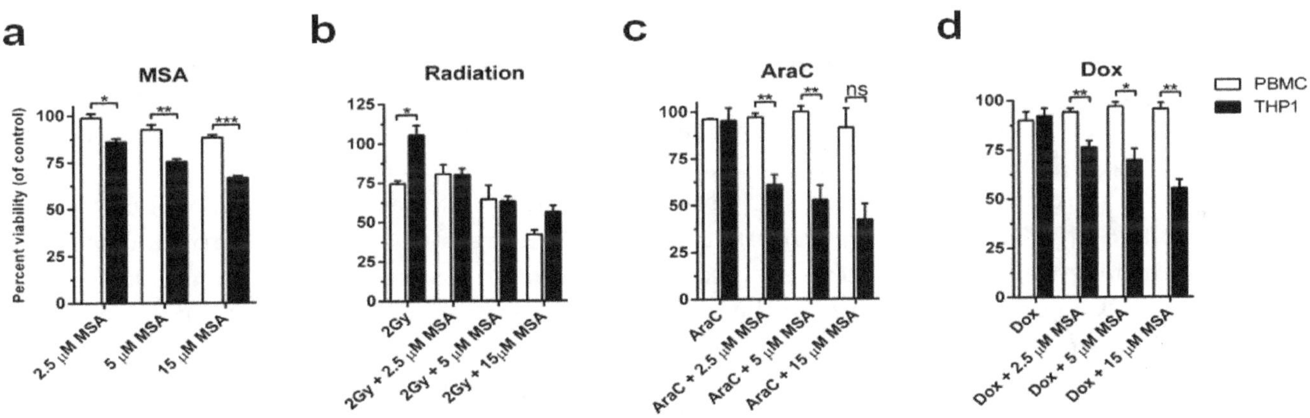

Figure 5. MSA protects normal cells and results in elevated cell killing of malignant cells after 48 h. (**a**) MSA treatment alone significantly reduces cell viability of malignant THP1 cells compared to normal PBMCs; (**b**) MSA does not significantly alter cell viability of PBMCs compared to THP1 cells in response to radiation; (**c**,**d**) MSA significantly protects normal PBMCs from cell death while enhancing the therapeutic activity of AraC or Dox in THP1 cells. $n = 3 \pm$ SEM, * $p < 0.05$, ** $p < 0.01$, *** $p < 0.001$, ns, not significant.

3. Discussion

The toxicity of anticancer therapies is a major ongoing clinical issue and developing agents that usefully modulate the toxicity and efficacy of chemotherapy and radiotherapy without compromising their efficacy is important. Preclinical work and some clinical trials suggest that Se compounds can achieve this, though the Se compounds and doses used have varied widely [4,6]. In the present study, we used an in vitro model of normal and malignant human mononuclear blood cells to investigate the dose-response relationship of Se in modulating the efficacy and toxicity of cancer treatments. We have shown important differences between normal and malignant cells in the dose-response relationship of Se to biological mechanisms that mediate cell survival and response to cancer treatments.

Se compounds have previously been shown to induce ER stress in a concentration- and time-dependent manner in prostate cancer cell lines, which leads to apoptosis in malignant cells [29]. In this study, we found that MSA induced apoptosis through caspase-8 expression in THP1 cells while reducing caspase-8 in PBMCs, in agreement with previous studies that have shown Se compounds induce apoptosis through caspase-8 activation [36]. Moreover, caspase-8-mediated apoptosis has been demonstrated to mediate the therapeutic synergy of Se compounds and chemotherapy treatment in various cancer settings [37,38]. The reduction in caspase-8 induced by MSA in PBMC in this study is consistent with the clinical data that Se compounds, at tested doses, are protective of normal tissues [10,16].

ER stress has been demonstrated to induce reactive oxygen species generation [39]. This results in the depletion of intracellular GSH, causing the cellular environment to become more oxidized, which is associated with increased apoptosis and necrosis [40–42]. GSH contributes to cellular resistance to anticancer treatments through covalent binding and inactivation of drugs [43–47]. Thus the 40-fold higher initial concentration of GSH present in THP-1 cells compared to PBMCs would protect the malignant cells against cytotoxic therapies, whereas the MSA-induced severe depletion of GSH in malignant cells shown in this study may contribute to the increased sensitivity to these treatments with MSA. These results are consistent with work showing that Se compounds inhibit the cisplatin-induced increase in GSH in ovarian cancer cells, thereby preventing chemoresistance [32]. These malignant cells may also have been sensitised to the effects of MSA due to their high concentrations of GSH, as GSH is a cofactor in the metabolic reduction of MSA to methylselenol [31]. This may not be relevant to Se compounds that generate methylselenol through other mechanisms.

Contrary to the effect of MSA seen in malignant cells, it induced a significant increase in GSH in normal cells, which is expected to protect them against cancer therapies. The simultaneous increase in GSH in normal cells and depletion of GSH in malignant cells may contribute to improving the therapeutic ratio of cancer treatment by reducing normal tissue toxicities while increasing the anticancer efficacy. This effect on GSH may mediate, at least in part, the observed ability of Se compounds to reduce the toxicity of chemotherapy and radiation in normal tissues [10,16].

Previous in vitro and in vivo studies have shown that DNA damage and inducible DNA damage is reduced with Se [33,34]. While we demonstrated that MSA reduced chemotherapy-induced DNA damage in normal cells, it was ineffective in protecting them against radiation-induced DNA damage and cytotoxicity. Of particular concern, at the highest concentration tested (15 μM), MSA significantly increased DNA damage from radiation in PBMC. In contrast, all concentrations of MSA increased the DNA damage and cytotoxicity of radiation and chemotherapy in the malignant cells.

This study supports previous work that demonstrated the potential therapeutic benefit of using Se in conjunction with cancer therapeutics, due to its differential effects on chemotherapy- or radiation-treated normal cells relative to malignant cells [48]. It is encouraging in this study that MSA generally protected normal cells while sensitising malignant cells to cytotoxic therapies, and that it informs about mechanisms that plausibly contribute to the reduction of clinically-significant toxicities seen in clinical trials with Se supplementation during cancer treatments [10–12,14].

A very important concern, however, has been raised by this study: in PBMCs the highest concentration of MSA proved toxic, and increased the cytotoxicity and DNA damage from radiation. This could increase the potential for second malignancies and other late complications of radiation, especially if using inorganic forms of Se that are associated with increased genotoxicity compared to several organic forms [49]. These outcomes have not been mentioned in clinical trials to date but the numbers evaluated have been small and follow-up is limited.

There is always a tension in cancer treatment between maximising efficacy while managing toxicities [19]. While Se has considerable and important potential to widen this usually narrow therapeutic window, data from this study strongly suggests that following the traditional cytotoxic therapy paradigm of using the maximum tolerated dose [50,51] may be inappropriate with Se compounds. However, our data also suggests that these interactions are treatment-specific, with greater vulnerability of normal cells when using the highest concentrations of MSA with radiation, but continued protection of normal cells from chemotherapy by MSA at all concentrations. Furthermore, there were marked differences in the concentration-dependence of the improved anticancer effects of chemotherapy or radiation with MSA on malignant THP1 cells. More modest concentrations of MSA proved equally effective to the highest one in terms of inducing ER stress and reducing GSH levels from radiation or chemotherapy, and at inducing DNA damage with chemotherapy drugs. The highest MSA concentration, however, was most effective at inducing DNA damage with radiation and at augmenting the cytotoxicity of radiation or chemotherapy.

4. Materials and Methods

4.1. Mononuclear Cell Isolation

PBMCs were isolated from buffy coats obtained from blood donations given by healthy individuals, and supplied by the New Zealand Blood Service at Waikato Hospital, Hamilton, New Zealand. Ethical approval for their use was granted by the Northern Y Health and Disability Ethics Committee (reference NTY/10/08/065/AM01, 16 August 2011). The mononuclear cell fraction was isolated via density gradient centrifugation using Histopaque® (St. Louis, MO, USA).

4.2. Cell Culture

PBMCs and THP1 cells were cultured in RPMI-1640 medium supplemented with 10% FBS, 1% penicillin (10,000 units/mL) and streptomycin (10,000 μg/mL) at 37 °C in 5% CO_2. Both cell lines were incubated either in the presence of MSA (2.5, 5 and 15 μM), cytosine arabinoside (AraC; 5 ng/mL), or doxorubicin (Dox; 20 nM) alone, as well as the combination of MSA and AraC or Dox. To assess the response to radiation, cells were irradiated with a total of 2 Gy with or without MSA. Cells were incubated with MSA for 6 h prior to treatment with chemotherapy or radiation.

4.3. Western Blot Analysis

Western blotting was carried out as previously described [52]. Briefly, total cell protein was isolated using radioimmunoprecipitation assay (RIPA) buffer (50 mM Tris pH 7.4, 150 mM NaCl, 1% Triton-X-100, 1% Na-deoxycholate, 0.1% sodium dodecyl sulfate (SDS), 1 mM ethylenediaminetetraacetic acid (EDTA), phosphatase inhibitors and protease cocktail inhibitors (Sigma Aldrich, St. Louis, MO, USA), and 1 mM phenylmethanesulfonylfluoride). Proteins were resolved by SDS-polyacriliamide gel (PAGE), transferred to nitrocellulose membranes, blocked in 5% non-fat powdered milk in tris-buffered saline-tween (TBS-T) and probed with antibodies. Protein bands were detected using a FUJIFILM Intelligent dark box II LAS-1000 system.

4.4. Measurement of GSH

Glutathione (GSH) assay kit was purchased from Sigma-Aldrich (St. Louis, MO, USA). The assay was carried out according to the manufacturer's directions. Total GSH was determined using a kinetic assay that measures the reduction of 5,5′-dithiobis-(2-nitrobenzoic) acid (DTNB) to 5-thio-2-nitrobenzoic acid (TNB) at 412 nm.

4.5. Comet Assay

DNA damage was assessed with the comet assay as previously described [53]. Preparation of slides was carried out by coating a pre-agarose-coated slide (1% normal melting point in PBS), with approximately 1000 cells in 0.5% low melting point agarose in PBS. Slides were lysed at 4 °C in a solution containing 1% Triton X-100, 2.5 M NaCl, 100 mM EDTA, and 10 mM Tris pH 10.0 for two hours. Slides were incubated for 20 min in an alkaline buffer (300 mM NaOH and 1 mM EDTA (pH > 13)) and electrophoresed for 20 min at 20 V and 300 mA at 4 °C in the same buffer. Slides were then neutralized and dried in 70% ethanol before being stained with SYBR Gold (Thermo Fisher Scientific, Waltham, MA, USA) and scored using the tail moment [53].

4.6. MTT Assay

Viability was measured with a tetrazolium salt as previously described [52]. The MTT (methyl-thiazol-tetrazolium) assay was used to assess the impact of treatments on cell viability in THP1 cells and PBMCs after 48 h. Cells were incubated with MTT for two hours, lysed in 20% SDS (w/v), 50% dimethylformamide (v/v) pH 4.7, and the absorbance was measured at 570 nm.

4.7. Statistical Analysis

GraphPad Prism version 6.0 (La Jolla, CA, USA) was used for all calculations. Multiple comparisons were controlled for using the Sidak-Bonferroni method. All experiments were performed at a minimum of 3 independent repeats. Differences with p-values less than 0.05 were considered significant.

5. Conclusions

Overall this study suggests that doses of Se compounds that achieve plasma Se concentrations in the range of 2.5–5 μM might achieve the optimal balance between enhancing efficacy and reducing the toxicity of radiation. It is possible that higher doses of Se might safely be used with some chemotherapy drugs. It is noteworthy that dosing to achieve plasma Se levels determined by this in vitro study would not apply to seleno-l-methionine, as it is non-specifically incorporated into the general protein pool, especially albumin, which gives disproportionately high plasma Se levels compared to dosing with equivalent elemental Se doses of sodium selenite or Se-methylselenocysteine [54,55].

The potential of Se to improve the efficacy and reduce toxicities of cancer treatments is important and deserves careful examination in clinical trials. However, when designing these trials, we need to be cognizant of the genotoxicity dose-dependence of the Se compounds to be used, with the potential for increased serious late toxicities of cancer treatments such as secondary malignancies, and evaluate this in our trials. Importantly, this study has demonstrated several laboratory methods that can be incorporated into clinical trials to enable investigators to evaluate the pharmacokinetic-pharmacodynamic relationship of the Se compounds being used in cancer patients. This will assist us in rationally determining the optimal dose and form of Se for use in combination with various cancer treatments in clinical trials; such trials are already underway [4,28].

Author Contributions: Study conception and design, R.J.L., R.T.C. and M.B.J.; methodology, R.J.L., G.M.J., R.T.C. and M.B.J.; acquisition of data: R.J.L. and G.M.J.; analysis and interpretation of data: R.J.L., G.M.J. and M.B.J.; writing—original draft preparation, R.J.L. and M.B.J.; writing—review and editing, R.J.L., G.M.J., R.T.C. and M.B.J.; funding acquisition, M.B.J.

Acknowledgments: We are grateful to blood donors and the New Zealand Blood Service for provision of the buffy coats.

Abbreviations

AraC	Cytosine arabinoside
Dox	Doxorubicin
GSH	Glutathione
MSA	Methylseleninic acid
PBMC	Peripheral blood mononuclear cell

References

1. Rayman, M.P. Selenium in cancer prevention: A review of the evidence and mechanism of action. *Proc. Nutr. Soc.* **2005**, *64*, 527–542. [CrossRef] [PubMed]
2. Rayman, M.P. Selenium and human health. *Lancet* **2012**, *379*, 1256–1268. [CrossRef]

3. Lipinski, B. Sodium Selenite as an Anticancer Agent. *Anticancer Agents Med. Chem.* **2017**, *17*, 658–661. [CrossRef] [PubMed]
4. Evans, S.O.; Khairuddin, P.F.; Jameson, M.B. Optimising Selenium for Modulation of Cancer Treatments. *Anticancer Res.* **2017**, *37*, 6497–6509. [PubMed]
5. Cao, S.; Durrani, F.A.; Rustum, Y.M. Selective Modulation of the Therapeutic Efficacy of Anticancer Drugs by Selenium Containing Compounds against Human Tumor Xenografts. *Clin. Cancer Res.* **2004**, *10*, 2561–2569. [CrossRef] [PubMed]
6. Fakih, M.; Cao, S.; Durrani, F.A.; Rustum, Y.M. Selenium protects against toxicity induced by anticancer drugs and augments antitumor activity: A highly selective, new, and novel approach for the treatment of solid tumors. *Clin. Colorectal Cancer* **2005**, *5*, 132–135. [CrossRef] [PubMed]
7. Francescato, H.D.; Costa, R.S.; Camargo, S.M.R.; Zanetti, M.A.; Lavrador, M.A.; Bianchi, M.D. Effect of oral selenium administration on cisplatin-induced nephrotoxicity in rats. *Pharmacol. Res.* **2001**, *43*, 77–82. [CrossRef] [PubMed]
8. Song, M.; Kumaran, M.N.; Gounder, M.; Gibbon, D.G.; Nieves-Neira, W.; Vaidya, A.; Hellmann, M.; Kane, M.P.; Buckley, B.; Shih, W.; et al. Phase I trial of selenium plus chemotherapy in gynecologic cancers. *Gynecol. Oncol.* **2018**. [CrossRef] [PubMed]
9. Puspitasari, I.M.; Abdulah, R.; Yamazaki, C.; Kameo, S.; Nakano, T.; Koyama, H. Updates on clinical studies of selenium supplementation in radiotherapy. *Radiat. Oncol.* **2014**, *9*, 125. [CrossRef] [PubMed]
10. Sieja, K.; Talerczyk, M. Selenium as an element in the treatment of ovarian cancer in women receiving chemotherapy. *Gynecol. Oncol.* **2004**, *93*, 320–327. [CrossRef] [PubMed]
11. Asfour, I.A.; El Tehewi, M.M.; Ahmed, M.H.; Abdel-Sattar, M.A.; Moustafa, N.N.; Hegab, H.M.; Fathey, O.M. High-dose sodium selenite can induce apoptosis of lymphoma cells in adult patients with non-Hodgkin's lymphoma. *Biol. Trace Elem. Res.* **2009**, *127*, 200–210. [CrossRef] [PubMed]
12. Asfour, I.A.; Fayek, M.; Raouf, S.; Soliman, M.; Hegab, H.M.; El Desoky, H.; Saleh, R.; Moussa, M.A. The impact of high-dose sodium selenite therapy on Bcl-2 expression in adult non-Hodgkin's lymphoma patients: Correlation with response and survival. *Biol. Trace Elem. Res.* **2007**, *120*, 1–10. [CrossRef] [PubMed]
13. Asfour, I.A.; El Shazly, S.; Fayek, M.H.; Hegab, H.M.; Raouf, S.; Moussa, M.A. Effect of high-dose sodium selenite therapy on polymorphonuclear leukocyte apoptosis in non-Hodgkin's lymphoma patients. *Biol. Trace Elem. Res.* **2006**, *110*, 19–32. [CrossRef]
14. Hu, Y.J.; Chen, Y.; Zhang, Y.Q.; Zhou, M.Z.; Song, X.M.; Zhang, B.Z.; Luo, L.; Xu, P.M.; Zhao, Y.N.; Zhao, Y.B.; et al. The protective role of selenium on the toxicity of cisplatin-contained chemotherapy regimen in cancer patients. *Biol. Trace Elem. Res.* **1997**, *56*, 331–341. [CrossRef] [PubMed]
15. Jahangard-Rafsanjani, Z.; Gholami, K.; Hadjibabaie, M.; Shamshiri, A.R.; Alimoghadam, K.; Sarayani, A.; Mojtahedzadeh, M.; Ostadali-Dehaghi, M.; Ghavamzadeh, A. The efficacy of selenium in prevention of oral mucositis in patients undergoing hematopoietic SCT: A randomized clinical trial. *Bone Marrow Transplant.* **2013**, *48*, 832–836. [CrossRef] [PubMed]
16. Muecke, R.; Schomburg, L.; Glatzel, M.; Berndt-Skorka, R.; Baaske, D.; Reichl, B.; Buentzel, J.; Kundt, G.; Prott, F.J.; Devries, A.; et al. Multicenter, phase 3 trial comparing selenium supplementation with observation in gynecologic radiation oncology. *Int. J. Radiat. Oncol. Biol. Phys.* **2010**, *78*, 828–835. [CrossRef] [PubMed]
17. Buntzel, J.; Riesenbeck, D.; Glatzel, M.; Berndt-Skorka, R.; Riedel, T.; Mucke, R.; Kisters, K.; Schonekaes, K.G.; Schafer, U.; Bruns, F.; et al. Limited effects of selenium substitution in the prevention of radiation-associated toxicities. Results of a randomized study in head and neck cancer patients. *Anticancer Res.* **2010**, *30*, 1829–1832. [PubMed]
18. Muecke, R.; Micke, O.; Schomburg, L.; Buentzel, J.; Kisters, K.; Adamietz, I.A. Selenium in Radiation Oncology-15 Years of Experiences in Germany. *Nutrients* **2018**, *10*. [CrossRef] [PubMed]
19. Perry, M.C.; Doll, D.C.; Freter, C.E. *Perry's The Chemotherapy Souce Book*, 5th ed.; Lippincott, Williams & Wilkins: New York, NY, USA, 2012.
20. Mishra, K.; Alsbeih, G. Appraisal of biochemical classes of radioprotectors: Evidence, current status and guidelines for future development. *3Biotech* **2017**, *7*, 292. [CrossRef] [PubMed]
21. Devine, A.; Marignol, L. Potential of Amifostine for Chemoradiotherapy and Radiotherapy-associated Toxicity Reduction in Advanced NSCLC: A Meta-Analysis. *Anticancer Res.* **2016**, *36*, 5–12. [PubMed]
22. Freyer, D.R.; Chen, L.; Krailo, M.D.; Knight, K.; Villaluna, D.; Bliss, B.; Pollock, B.H.; Ramdas, J.; Lange, B.; Van, H.D.; et al. Effects of sodium thiosulfate versus observation on development of cisplatin-induced

hearing loss in children with cancer (ACCL0431): A multicentre, randomised, controlled, open-label, phase 3 trial. *Lancet Oncol.* **2017**, *18*, 63–74. [CrossRef]

23. Liu, M.; Hu, C.; Xu, Q.; Chen, L.; Ma, K.; Xu, N.; Zhu, H. Methylseleninic acid activates Keap1/Nrf2 pathway via up-regulating miR-200a in human oesophageal squamous cell carcinoma cells. *Biosci. Rep.* **2015**, *35*. [CrossRef] [PubMed]
24. Lennicke, C.; Rahn, J.; Bukur, J.; Hochgrafe, F.; Wessjohann, L.A.; Lichtenfels, R.; Seliger, B. Modulation of MHC class I surface expression in B16F10 melanoma cells by methylseleninic acid. *Oncoimmunology* **2017**, *6*, e1259049. [CrossRef] [PubMed]
25. Kassam, S.; Goenaga-Infante, H.; Maharaj, L.; Hiley, C.T.; Juliger, S.; Joel, S.P. Methylseleninic acid inhibits HDAC activity in diffuse large B-cell lymphoma cell lines. *Cancer Chemother. Pharmacol.* **2011**, *68*, 815–821. [CrossRef] [PubMed]
26. Ip, C.; Dong, Y.; Ganther, H.E. New concepts in selenium chemoprevention. *Cancer Metastasis Rev.* **2002**, *21*, 281–289. [CrossRef] [PubMed]
27. Ip, C.; Thompson, H.J.; Zhu, Z.; Ganther, H.E. In vitro and in vivo studies of methylseleninic acid: Evidence that a monomethylated selenium metabolite is critical for cancer chemoprevention. *Cancer Res.* **2000**, *60*, 2882–2886. [PubMed]
28. Zakharia, Y.; Bhattacharya, A.; Rustum, Y.M. Selenium targets resistance biomarkers enhancing efficacy while reducing toxicity of anti-cancer drugs: Preclinical and clinical development. *Oncotarget* **2018**, *9*, 10765–10783. [CrossRef] [PubMed]
29. Wu, Y.; Zhang, H.; Dong, Y.; Park, Y.M.; Ip, C. Endoplasmic reticulum stress signal mediators are targets of selenium action. *Cancer Res.* **2005**, *65*, 9073–9079. [CrossRef] [PubMed]
30. Liu, C.; Liu, H.; Li, Y.; Wu, Z.; Zhu, Y.; Wang, T.; Gao, A.C.; Chen, J.; Zhou, Q. Intracellular glutathione content influences the sensitivity of lung cancer cell lines to methylseleninic acid. *Mol. Carcinog.* **2012**, *51*, 303–314. [CrossRef] [PubMed]
31. Shen, H.M.; Ding, W.X.; Ong, C.N. Intracellular glutathione is a cofactor in methylseleninic acid-induced apoptotic cell death of human hepatoma HEPG(2) cells. *Free Radic. Biol. Med.* **2002**, *33*, 552–561. [CrossRef]
32. Caffrey, P.B.; Frenkel, G.D. Selenium compounds prevent the induction of drug resistance by cisplatin in human ovarian tumor xenografts in vivo. *Cancer Chemother. Pharmacol.* **2000**, *46*, 74–78. [CrossRef] [PubMed]
33. Fischer, J.L.; Mihelc, E.M.; Pollok, K.E.; Smith, M.L. Chemotherapeutic selectivity conferred by selenium: A role for p53-dependent DNA repair. *Mol. Cancer Ther.* **2007**, *6*, 355–361. [CrossRef] [PubMed]
34. Seo, Y.R.; Sweeney, C.; Smith, M.L. Selenomethionine induction of DNA repair response in human fibroblasts. *Oncogene* **2002**, *21*, 3663–3669. [CrossRef] [PubMed]
35. Shin, S.H.; Yoon, M.J.; Kim, M.; Kim, J.I.; Lee, S.J.; Lee, Y.S.; Bae, S. Enhanced lung cancer cell killing by the combination of selenium and ionizing radiation. *Oncol. Rep.* **2007**, *17*, 209–216. [CrossRef] [PubMed]
36. Li, Z.; Carrier, L.; Rowan, B.G. Methylseleninic acid synergizes with tamoxifen to induce caspase-mediated apoptosis in breast cancer cells. *Mol. Cancer Ther.* **2008**, *7*, 3056–3063. [CrossRef] [PubMed]
37. Jiang, C.; Wang, Z.; Ganther, H.; Lu, J. Caspases as key executors of methyl selenium-induced apoptosis (anoikis) of DU-145 prostate cancer cells. *Cancer Res.* **2001**, *61*, 3062–3070. [PubMed]
38. Li, S.; Zhou, Y.; Wang, R.; Zhang, H.; Dong, Y.; Ip, C. Selenium sensitizes MCF-7 breast cancer cells to doxorubicin-induced apoptosis through modulation of phospho-Akt and its downstream substrates. *Mol. Cancer Ther.* **2007**, *6*, 1031–1038. [CrossRef] [PubMed]
39. Malhotra, J.D.; Kaufman, R.J. Endoplasmic reticulum stress and oxidative stress: A vicious cycle or a double-edged sword? *Antioxid. Redox Signal.* **2007**, *9*, 2277–2293. [CrossRef] [PubMed]
40. Cai, J.; Jones, D.P. Superoxide in apoptosis. Mitochondrial generation triggered by cytochrome c loss. *J. Biol. Chem.* **1998**, *273*, 11401–11404. [CrossRef] [PubMed]
41. Engel, R.H.; Evens, A.M. Oxidative stress and apoptosis: A new treatment paradigm in cancer. *Front. Biosci.* **2006**, *11*, 300–312. [CrossRef] [PubMed]
42. Voehringer, D.W.; Meyn, R.E. Redox aspects of Bcl-2 function. *Antioxid. Redox Signal.* **2000**, *2*, 537–550. [CrossRef] [PubMed]
43. Biaglow, J.E.; Varnes, M.E.; Epp, E.R.; Clark, E.P.; Tuttle, S.W.; Held, K.D. Role of glutathione and other thiols in cellular response to radiation and drugs. *Drug Metab. Rev.* **1989**, *20*, 1–12. [CrossRef] [PubMed]
44. Bump, E.A.; Brown, J.M. Role of glutathione in the radiation response of mammalian cells in vitro and in vivo. *Pharmacol. Ther.* **1990**, *47*, 117–136. [CrossRef]

45. Coleman, C.N.; Bump, E.A.; Kramer, R.A. Chemical modifiers of cancer treatment. *J. Clin. Oncol.* **1988**, *6*, 709–733. [CrossRef] [PubMed]
46. Mitchell, J.B.; Russo, A. The role of glutathione in radiation and drug induced cytotoxicity. *Br. J. Cancer Suppl.* **1987**, *8*, 96–104. [PubMed]
47. Tew, K.D. Glutathione-associated enzymes in anticancer drug resistance. *Cancer Res.* **1994**, *54*, 4313–4320. [CrossRef] [PubMed]
48. Vadgama, J.V.; Wu, Y.; Shen, D.; Hsia, S.; Block, J. Effect of selenium in combination with Adriamycin or Taxol on several different cancer cells. *Anticancer Res.* **2000**, *20*, 1391–1414. [PubMed]
49. Valdiglesias, V.; Pasaro, E.; Mendez, J.; Laffon, B. In vitro evaluation of selenium genotoxic, cytotoxic, and protective effects: A review. *Arch. Toxicol.* **2010**, *84*, 337–351. [CrossRef] [PubMed]
50. Brodin, O.; Eksborg, S.; Wallenberg, M.; Asker-Hagelberg, C.; Larsen, E.H.; Mohlkert, D.; Lenneby-Helleday, C.; Jacobsson, H.; Linder, S.; Misra, S.; et al. Pharmacokinetics and Toxicity of Sodium Selenite in the Treatment of Patients with Carcinoma in a Phase I Clinical Trial: The SECAR Study. *Nutrients* **2015**, *7*, 4978–4994. [CrossRef] [PubMed]
51. Corcoran, N.M.; Hovens, C.M.; Michael, M.; Rosenthal, M.A.; Costello, A.J. Open-label, phase I dose-escalation study of sodium selenate, a novel activator of PP2A, in patients with castration-resistant prostate cancer. *Br. J. Cancer* **2010**, *103*, 462–468. [CrossRef] [PubMed]
52. Lobb, R.J.; van, A.R.; Wiegmans, A.; Ham, S.; Larsen, J.E.; Moller, A. Exosomes derived from mesenchymal non-small cell lung cancer cells promote chemoresistance. *Int. J. Cancer* **2017**, *141*, 614–620. [CrossRef] [PubMed]
53. Collins, A.R. The comet assay for DNA damage and repair: Principles, applications, and limitations. *Mol. Biotechnol.* **2004**, *26*, 249–261. [CrossRef]
54. Evans, S.O.; Jacobson, G.M.; Goodman, H.J.B.; Bird, S.; Jameson, M.B. Comparative safety and pharmacokinetic evaluation of three oral selenium compounds in cancer patients. *Biol. Trace Elem. Res.* **2018**. [CrossRef] [PubMed]
55. Marshall, J.R.; Burk, R.F.; Payne, O.R.; Hill, K.E.; Perloff, M.; Davis, W.; Pili, R.; George, S.; Bergan, R. Selenomethionine and methyl selenocysteine: Multiple-dose pharmacokinetics in selenium-replete men. *Oncotarget* **2017**, *8*, 26312–26322. [CrossRef] [PubMed]

4

Methylseleninic Acid Induces Lipid Peroxidation and Radiation Sensitivity in Head and Neck Cancer Cells

John T. Lafin [1], Ehab H. Sarsour [2], Amanda L. Kalen [2], Brett A. Wagner [2], Garry R. Buettner [2] and Prabhat C. Goswami [2,*]

1 Department of Urology, University of Texas Southwestern Medical Center, Dallas, TX 75235, USA; john.lafin@utsouthwestern.edu

2 The University of Iowa Free Radical and Radiation Biology Program, Department of Radiation Oncology, University of Iowa, Iowa City, IA 52242, USA; ehab-sarsour@uiowa.edu (E.H.S.); amanda-kalen@uiowa.edu (A.L.K.); brett-wagner@uiowa.edu (B.A.W.); garry-buettner@uiowa.edu (G.R.B.)

* Correspondence: prabhat-goswami@uiowa.edu

Abstract: Combination radiation and chemotherapy are commonly used to treat locoregionally advanced head and neck squamous cell carcinoma (HNSCC). Aggressive dosing of these therapies is significantly hampered by side effects due to normal tissue toxicity. Selenium represents an adjuvant that selectively sensitizes cancer cells to these treatments modalities, potentially by inducing lipid peroxidation (LPO). This study investigated whether one such selenium compound, methylseleninic acid (MSA), induces LPO and radiation sensitivity in HNSCC cells. Results from 4,4-difluoro-4-bora-3a,4a-diaza-*S*-indacene (BODIPY) C11 oxidation and ferric thiocyanate assays revealed that MSA induced LPO in cells rapidly and persistently. Propidium iodide (PI) exclusion assay found that MSA was more toxic to cancer cells than other related selenium compounds; this toxicity was abrogated by treatment with α-tocopherol, an LPO inhibitor. MSA exhibited no toxicity to normal fibroblasts at similar doses. MSA also sensitized HNSCC cells to radiation as determined by clonogenic assay. Intracellular glutathione in cancer cells was depleted following MSA treatment, and supplementation of the intracellular glutathione pool with *N*-acetylcysteine sensitized cells to MSA. The addition of MSA to a cell-free solution of glutathione resulted in an increase in oxygen consumption, which was abrogated by catalase, suggesting the formation of H_2O_2. Results from this study identify MSA as an inducer of LPO, and reveal its capability to sensitize HNSCC to radiation. MSA may represent a potent adjuvant to radiation therapy in HNSCC.

Keywords: head and neck cancer; selenium; methylseleninic acid; radiation; lipid peroxidation; glutathione; tocopherol

---

1. Introduction

Head and neck squamous cell carcinoma (HNSCC) is a diverse group of cancers that originate from the mouth, nose, throat, or other nearby areas. Over 50,000 new cases of HNSCC are anticipated to arise in the US in 2018; the five-year survival rate is ~64% [1]. Locoregionally advanced HNSCC is often treated with combination radio- and chemotherapy. However, side effects from primary therapy can be debilitating. Radiation and chemotherapy can result in oral mucositis, which can significantly reduce tolerable doses [2]. Even with these aggressive therapy options, about 40% of HNSCC deaths will occur due to the development of therapy resistance [3]. Additional options to sensitize HNSCC cells to current therapies are sorely needed.

Selenium administration shows great promise as a sensitizer to radio- and chemotherapy. Sodium selenite, an inorganic selenium derivative, induces toxicity and radiation sensitization in various cancer cell types with limited effects on normal fibroblasts [4–6]. A recent metastudy reported that selenite supplementation in patients receiving radiation therapy reduced deleterious side effects with no protective effects noted in tumors, supporting the use of selenium as an adjuvant to therapy [7]. These studies and others suggest that selenium may sensitize tumors to intervention, while potentially protecting normal tissue. Unfortunately, sodium selenite exhibits toxicity at relatively low doses, with a reported maximum tolerable dose of 10.2 mg m^{-2} [8]. Organoselenium derivatives, such as selenomethionine (SLM) and methylselenocysteine (MSC), are much less toxic than their inorganic counterparts while maintaining the selective effects noted with selenite [9,10]. Organoselenium derivatives exert their anticancer activities through the formation of a common active metabolite, methylselenol [11,12]. SLM and MSC require the action of specific lyase enzymes, such as methionine gamma-lyase (MGL), to release methylselenol [13]. MGL expression is reported to decline in a number of cancer types, suggesting that the formation of methylselenol in tumor tissue by SLM may be slow, limiting its efficacy [14–17].

Methylseleninic acid (MSA) is an organoselenium derivative that generates methylselenol through its spontaneous reaction with free thiols, such as glutathione [18]. Because the activity of MSA is not reliant upon the expression of lyases, such as MGL, it may represent a more effective antitumor agent than other organoselenium compounds. Previous studies have reported that MSA more effectively reduces TM2H and TM12 hyperplastic mammary cell accumulation than MSC, even at 10-fold lower doses [12]. Additionally, oral administration of MSA reduced the size of PC-3 xenografts in mice by approximately 40%, while administration of SLM, MSC, or sodium selenite exhibited no effects, indicating that MSA is more effective both in vitro and in vivo than other selenium compounds [19]. A combination of MSA and paclitaxel reduced the size of MDA-MB-231 xenografts in mice by about 50%, compared to paclitaxel alone, suggesting that MSA may be an effective adjuvant to current therapies [20]. In these studies, no change in body weight was observed, suggesting that MSA was well tolerated.

Although methylselenol has been identified as the active antitumor metabolite of organoselenium compounds, the mechanism of action following its generation is poorly understood. The combination of MSA and glutathione has been demonstrated to increase lucigenin-based chemiluminescence, which was abrogated by the presence of superoxide dismutase, suggesting the generation of superoxide ($O_2^{\bullet-}$) [18]. Superoxide may be protonated to form hydroperoxyl radical ($HO_2^{\bullet}$) or dismutated to form hydrogen peroxide (H_2O_2), both of which may contribute to the initiation of lipid peroxidation (LPO) [21,22]. Selenium administration has been associated with elevated markers of LPO, suggesting that these initiating effects occur in vivo [23–25]. Because end products of LPO can be highly toxic, MSA-generated methylselenol could, therefore, exhibit toxicity through the superoxide-mediated initiation of LPO. Furthermore, HNSCC patients exhibit higher levels of plasma markers of LPO than matched healthy subjects, suggesting that HNSCC may be particularly susceptible to LPO [26,27].

Results presented herein reveal that MSA exhibits toxicity and radiation sensitization of Cal27 and SCC25 HNSCC cells. Cal27 cells were found to be much more sensitive to MSA compared to SLM or MSC, while normal human fibroblasts were resistant to MSA-induced toxicity. Initiation of oxidative distress via lipid peroxidation appears to be the underlying mechanism for toxicity. Our data suggest that the toxic effects of MSA are mediated by a glutathione-dependent formation of an initiator of LPO. MSA may be a useful adjuvant to radiation therapy.

2. Results

2.1. MSA is More Toxic to HNSCC Cells than Other Organoselenium Derivatives, and Causes Cell Death in a Dose- and Time-Dependent Manner

Organoselenium derivatives SLM and MSC require enzymatic action to generate methylselenol, the common active metabolite. Therefore, methylselenol generation from SLM and MSC will be less in situations where these enzymes are poorly expressed. MSA requires no enzymatic activity to generate methylselenol [18]. To determine if MSA exhibits greater toxicity than other organoselenium compounds, Cal27 cells were treated with MSA, MSC, or SLM for 72 h, and viability was assessed with propidium iodide (PI) exclusion assay. MSC and SLM exhibited no toxicity at doses up to 10 μM, Figure 1A. Treatment with 1 μM MSA resulted in a small but significant increase in PI positive cells, while 10 μM MSA resulted in about 30% PI-positive cells. To ensure that MSA toxicity was not cell-line dependent, the effects of MSA treatment on SCC25 cells were also examined. A dose-dependent increase in PI positive SCC25 cells was observed with MSA treatment, with approximately 30% of the cells staining positive at 10 μM, Figure 1B. These results indicate that Cal27 cells are more sensitive to MSA than other organoselenium derivatives and that MSA-induced toxicity is dose-dependent in both Cal27 and SCC25 cell lines.

The sensitizing effects of organoselenium compounds on cancer cells have been reported to occur as early as 24 h following the beginning of treatment [28]. To determine the temporal aspects of the toxicity resulting from exposure to MSA, Cal27 and SCC25 cells were treated with MSA for varying durations and the toxicity was examined by measuring changes in cell numbers as well as flow cytometry measurements of the percentage of PI-positive (non-viable) and PI-negative (viable) cell populations. SCC25 and Cal27 cells both showed a marked decline in cell number as early as 24 h after initiation of treatment with MSA, with a reduction in cell number of about 75% and 95% in Cal27 and SCC25, respectively, Figure 1C. Cal27 cell numbers continued to decline up to 72 h, while SCC25 cell number appeared to begin to recover at 72 h. The rapid onset of a reduction in cell number correlated with an increase in the percentage of PI-positive Cal 27 cells at 48 h of treatment, Figure 1D. SCC25 cells exhibited significant toxicity as early as 24 h. SCC25 maximal toxicity (45% PI-positive cells) was reached by 48 h in the period examined, while Cal27 reached similar levels at 72 h. Together, these results indicate that the MSA treatment exhibits greater toxicity to HNSCC than treatments with MSC and SLM and that this toxicity is dose- and time-dependent. Furthermore, treatment with MSA appears to be more toxic to SCC25 compared to Cal27 cells.

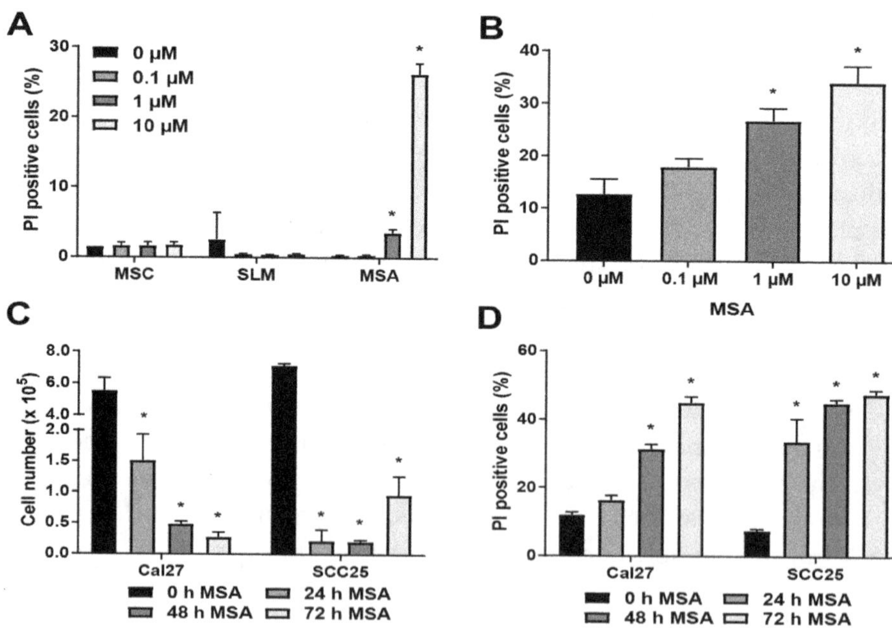

Figure 1. Methylseleninic acid (MSA) is toxic to Cal27 and SCC25 HNSCC cells in a dose- and time-dependent manner. (**A**) PI exclusion assay of Cal27 cells treated with the shown concentrations of Se-methylselenocysteine (MSC), seleno-L-methionine (SLM), or MSA for 72 h. (**B**) Propidium iodide (PI) exclusion assay of SCC25 cells treated with 0 to 10 μM MSA for 72 h. (**C**) Cell counts of Cal27 and SCC25 cells following treatment with 10 μM MSA for 0 to 72 h. (**D**) PI exclusion assay of Cal27 and SCC25 cells after treatment with 10 μM MSA for 0 to 72 h. *, statistical significance relative to 0 μM MSA controls; $p < 0.05$, $n = 3$.

2.2. MSA Treatment Sensitizes HNSCC Cells to Radiation

Selenium compounds, such as sodium selenite and seleno-L-methionine, sensitize cancer cells to radiation [4,5,10,29]. Furthermore, this sensitization is frequently noted to be selective for cancer cells [29]. Fibroblasts are often thought to make up the majority of the non-cancer cellular fraction in the tumor stroma [30,31]. To determine if normal human fibroblasts (NHF) were resistant to MSA toxicity, a PI exclusion assay was utilized. PI-positive (non-viable) NHF population did not increase following MSA treatment, Figure 2A. MSA (1 μM) treatment more than doubled non-viable Cal27 and SCC25 populations, Figure 1A,B, demonstrating the selective effects of MSA to HNSCC over NHF. To determine if MSA sensitizes HNSCC to radiation, Cal27 cells were treated with MSA for 48 h before 2 or 4 Gy irradiation, and toxicity was analyzed by using a clonogenic assay. Irradiated cells without MSA treatment showed a surviving fraction of 0.75 and 0.28 at 2 and 4 Gy, respectively, Figure 2B. Treatment with 0.1 μM MSA did not significantly alter surviving fraction of Cal27 cells: 0.66 and 0.22 at 2 and 4 Gy, respectively. Interestingly, prior treatment with 1 μM MSA significantly reduced the surviving fraction to 0.3 and 0.03 at 2 and 4 Gy compared to a surviving fraction of 0.75 and 0.28 without MSA treatment.

Radiation response is frequently dependent upon the support of the tumor stroma. To determine if the tumor stroma impacts the ability of MSA to sensitize Cal27 cells to radiation, a co-culture clonogenic assay was utilized. Cal27 cells were plated on lawns of quiescent normal human fibroblasts (NHF), and co-cultures were treated with 1 μM MSA for 48 h before irradiation. Even with NHF present, MSA treatment resulted in a 40% decline of surviving fraction following 2 Gy radiation, Figure 2D. Additionally, the lawn of NHF was not disturbed by MSA, further indicating that MSA was not toxic to NHF even in combination with radiation, Figure 2C. These results indicate that MSA treatment potently and selectively sensitizes Cal27 cells to radiation in co-cultures of NHF.

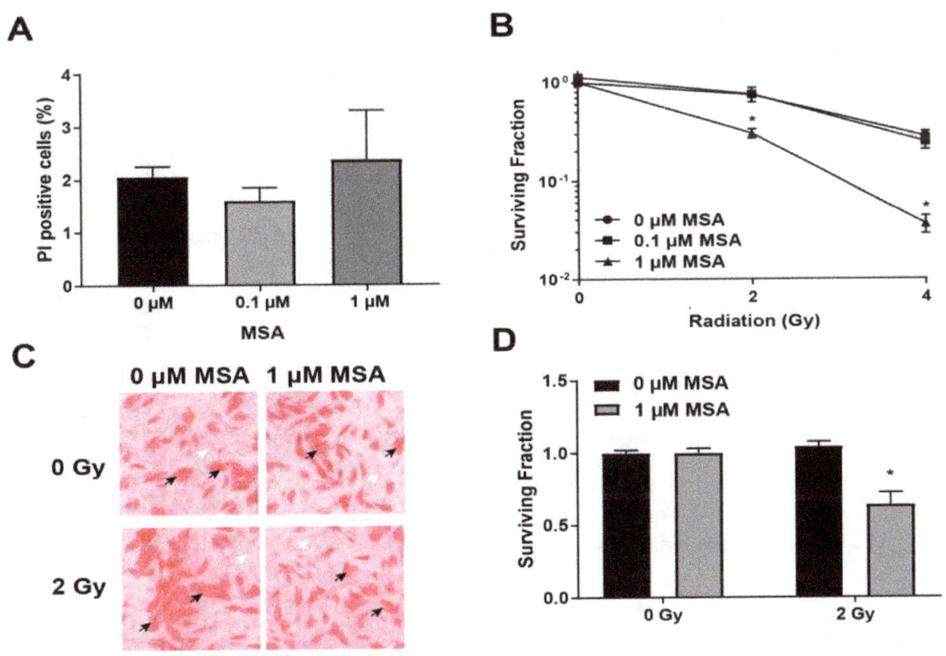

Figure 2. MSA selectively sensitizes head and neck squamous cell carcinoma (HNSCC) cells to radiation. (**A**) PI exclusion assay of normal human fibroblasts (NHF) treated with MSA 24 h. (**B**) Clonogenic assay of Cal27 cells treated with MSA 48 h before irradiation with γ-rays. (**C**) Representative images of Cal27 cells in co-cultures with NHF that were treated with MSA 48 h before irradiation with γ-rays. Black arrows: Cal27 colonies; white arrows: quiescent NHF. (**D**) Quantitation of Cal27 clonogenic survival in co-cultures of Cal27 and NHF that were treated with MSA 48 h before irradiation with γ-rays. *, statistical significance relative to 0 μM MSA controls; $p < 0.05$, $n = 3$.

2.3. MSA Treatment Induces Lipid Peroxidation in HNSCC Cells

Organoselenium compounds are theorized to be metabolized through a multitude of pathways to a central active metabolite, methylselenol, which exerts toxicity. Due to the highly reactive nature of methylselenol, studies concerning its mechanism of toxicity are sorely lacking. However, markers of lipid peroxidation have been found to rise in patients treated with selenium [24], suggesting that high dose selenium may induce lipid peroxidation. To determine if MSA treatment induces lipid peroxidation in HNSCC cells, MSA-treated Cal27 cells were labeled with the dye BODIPY C-11. This dye integrates into membranes and emits maximally at 590 nm. Upon oxidation by an initiator or propagator of lipid peroxidation, the maximal emission shifts to 510 nm. By reading both channels simultaneously, a ratio of oxidized to reduced dye can be calculated, providing a snapshot of lipid peroxidation initiation and propagation. Lipid peroxidation was found to be up to 30% elevated in Cal27 cells treated with MSA for 72 h, Figure 3A. An elevation was noted at a dose as low as 0.1 μM MSA, suggesting a powerful potential for initiation. Examination of lipid peroxidation at very early time intervals indicated that lipid peroxidation was initiated as early as 2 h, and maintained at a relatively stable level up to 72 h, Figure 3B. To determine if these increases in initiation and propagation events resulted in elevated lipid hydroperoxides, the Cayman Lipid Hydroperoxide Assay kit was utilized. Cal27 cells treated with 10 μM MSA for 72 h were found to have 1.16 fmol lipid hydroperoxide per cell, nearly 40 times as much as untreated cells, Figure 3C. These data indicate that treatment with MSA induces lipid peroxidation potently and persistently and that this induction results in a significant accumulation of lipid hydroperoxides.

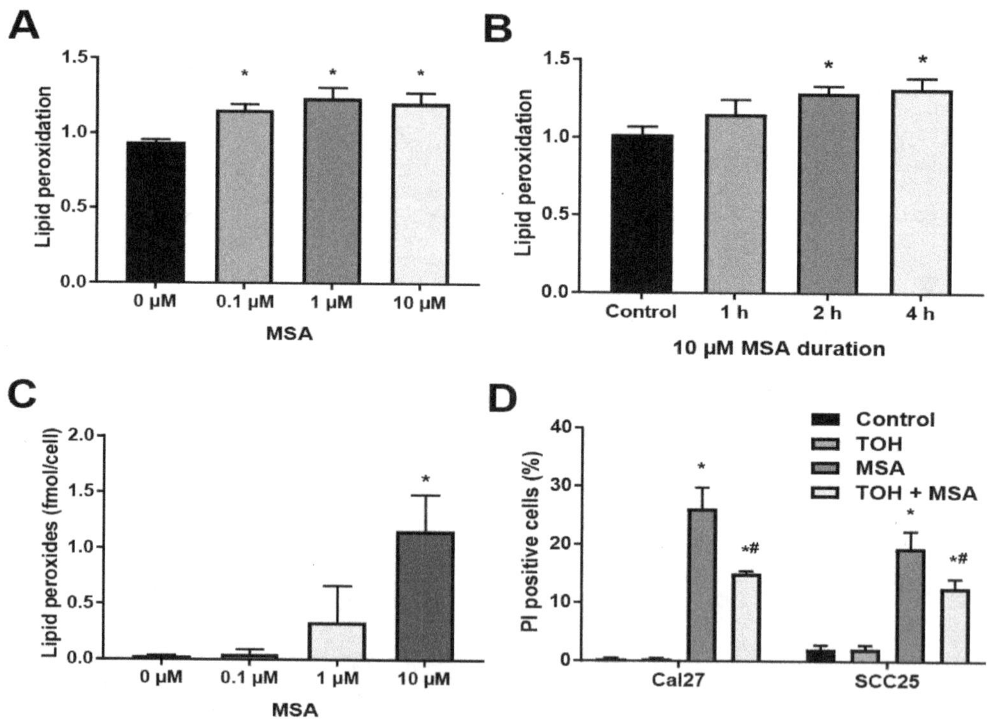

Figure 3. MSA induces lipid peroxidation in HNSCC cells. (**A**) Lipid peroxidation in Cal27 cells assessed by 4,4-difluoro-4-bora-3a,4a-diaza-*S*-indacene (BODIPY) C-11 staining following 72 h treatment with 0 to 10 μM MSA. (**B**) Lipid peroxidation in Cal27 cells following treatment with 10 μM MSA. (**C**) Lipid peroxides in Cal27 cells as assessed by the Cayman Chemical LPO Kit following treatment with 0 to 10 μM MSA for 72 h. (**D**) PI exclusion assay of Cal27 and SCC25 cells treated with 20 μM α-tocopherol acetate (TOH) for 24 h, 10 μM MSA for 72 h, or pre-treatment with TOH for 24 h followed by treatment with MSA. *, statistical significance relative to 0 μM MSA controls; #, statistical significance relative to MSA alone; $p < 0.05$, $n = 3$.

Lipid peroxidation is a deleterious oxidative chain reaction that can form toxic products, such as MDA or 4-HNE. Induction of uncontrolled lipid peroxidation can damage critical biomolecules resulting in cell death. To determine if MSA-induced toxicity is caused by lipid peroxidation, Cal27 and SCC25 cells were pre-treated with a lipid peroxidation chain terminator, α-tocopherol acetate (TOH), before MSA treatment. Treatment with TOH alone did not impact the percentage of PI-positive cell populations in either cell line, Figure 3D. However, treatment with TOH before MSA treatment reduced the percentage of the PI-positive cell population in Cal27 from 26% to 15%, and in SCC25 from 20% to 12%, an approximate 40% decline in the PI-positive populations. These results show that lipid peroxidation is an essential step in MSA-induced toxicity of HNSCC cells.

2.4. *N-Acetyl-L-Cysteine Exacerbates MSA Toxicity in HNSCC*

MSA spontaneously reacts with glutathione (GSH) to form its active metabolite, methylselenol, and GSH disulfide (GSSG), see below [18]. As the principal intracellular redox buffer, GSH is critical to normal cellular function. GSSG may be cytotoxic; it can be recycled to GSH by glutathione reductase, exported from the cell, or form mixed protein disulfides. To determine if MSA treatment influences GSH levels in HNSCC cells, the intracellular GSH content was measured in MSA-treated Cal27 cells using a biochemical assay [32]. Results indicate a dose-dependent decrease of total GSH in MSA-treated Cal27 cells, Figure 4A. Untreated Cal27 cells exhibited a total GSH concentration of about 17 nmol (mg protein)$^{-1}$. Treatment with MSA lowered this to below 10 nmol (mg protein)$^{-1}$, a 40% decline. Despite this marked decline, intracellular GSSG was not found to increase following MSA treatment, but rather also declined, Figure 4B. The decline in GSH levels suggests that GSH may have a significant role in the MSA-induced toxicity of HNSCC. This premise is further supported by results showing *N*-Acetyl-L-Cysteine (NAC) treatments exacerbating MSA-induced toxicity in Cal27 cells, Figure 4C. NAC is a membrane permeable precursor to GSH, stimulating its production; its effects are detectable within 4 h [33,34]. Cal27 cells were treated with 5 mM NAC for 24 h, washed, and treated with 10 μM MSA for 72 h. Cell number declined from 3×10^5 in cultures treated with MSA alone, to 0.5×10^5 cells, Figure 4C. A PI exclusion assay revealed that the combination of NAC and MSA resulted in a 30% non-viable cell population, while MSA alone resulted in only 25%, Figure 4D. Although NAC alone reduced cell number from 11×10^5 to 0.6×10^5, it had no effect on viability. This is consistent with prior reports from our lab that NAC treatment induces a cell cycle arrest [33,34]. These results indicate that GSH facilitates MSA-induced free radical chemistry (see below), leading to lipid peroxidation and HNSCC cytotoxicity.

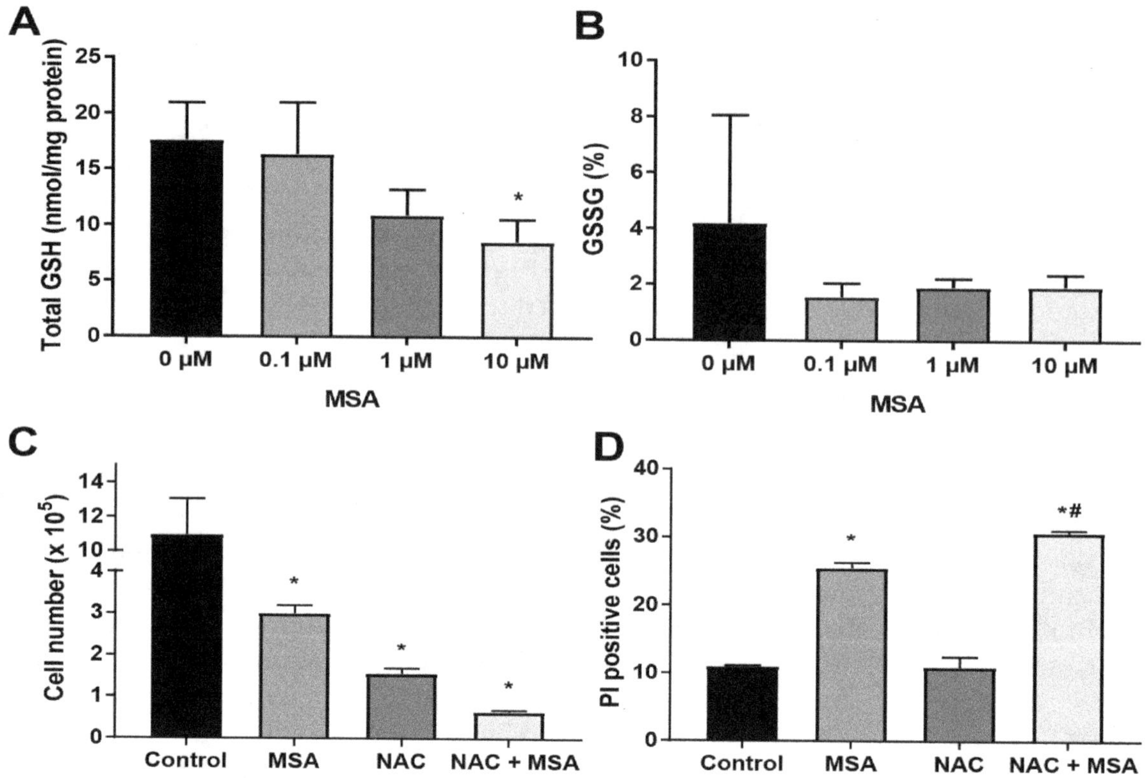

Figure 4. MSA exhibits toxicity in a glutathione (GSH)-dependent manner. (**A**) Total GSH in Cal27 cells treated with 0 to 10 µM MSA for 72 h. (**B**) Percent of GSH existing as glutathione disulfide (GSSG) in Cal27 cells treated with 0 to 10 µM MSA for 72 h. (**C**) Cell counts of Cal27 cells following treatment with 5 mM *N*-Acetyl-L-Cysteine (NAC) for 24 h, and/or 10 µM MSA for 72 h. The NAC + MSA group received 5 mM NAC for 24 h before treatment with MSA. (**D**) PI exclusion assay of Cal27 cells treated with 5 mM NAC for 24 h, and/or 10 µM MSA for 72 h. The NAC + MSA group received 5 mM NAC for 24 h before treatment with MSA. *, statistical significance relative to 0 µM MSA controls; #, statistical significance relative to NAC alone; $p < 0.05$, $n = 3$.

2.5. MSA Treatment Enhances GSH-Dependent O_2 Consumption

MSA can be reduced by free thiols, such as GSH, to form its active metabolite, methylselenol, Figure 5C. Because the pK_a of the selenohydryl group is 5.2, it primarily exists in biological systems as its conjugate base, the highly reactive methylselenolate anion ($MeSe^-$) [35]. This reactive species may initiate a cyclic reaction with molecular oxygen and GSH to cycle between a methylselenyl radical intermediate and methylselenolate anion, forming $O_2^{\bullet-}$ (which is rapidly dismuted to H_2O_2) and GSH to GSSG as products. This cyclic reaction is anticipated to account for the toxicity of organoselenium compounds [18,36]. In support of this chemistry, a previous study demonstrated the involvement of oxygen to the cyclic reaction between a related compound, selenocystamine, and GSH [36]. To determine if MSA may also undergo a similar reaction, O_2 consumption was monitored in a cell-free system containing MSA and GSH, Figure 5A. This system was held at pH 9.2, as this is the reported optimum pH for selenium-catalyzed $O_2^{\bullet-}$ generation [18]. O_2 was observed to disappear from the buffer at a rate of approximately 3 nM s^{-1}. Addition of MSA to buffer did not change the rate of consumption of O_2 (data not shown). Addition of GSH in the absence of MSA resulted in the disappearance of O_2 at a rate of approximately 15 nM s^{-1}, Figure 5B. Interestingly, the addition of MSA (250 µM) following GSH doubled the rate of O_2 consumption to approximately 32 nM s^{-1}. Furthermore, the addition of 500 IU catalase caused the rate of O_2 consumption to return to 13 nM s^{-1}, approximately the same as GSH alone. These results indicate an O_2-dependent reaction occurring between MSA and GSH that may result in the formation, but not accumulation, of H_2O_2. H_2O_2

may also contribute to another O_2-dependent reaction between GSH and MSA. The resulting flux of H_2O_2 may facilitate lipid peroxidation through the iron-dependent generation of $HO^•$, resulting in MSA-induced toxicity of HNSCC. Previous reports indicate elevated markers of LPO in HNSCC patients [26,27], suggesting that MSA-induced selective cytotoxicity may be due to higher baseline levels of LPO in HNSCC compared to normal cells.

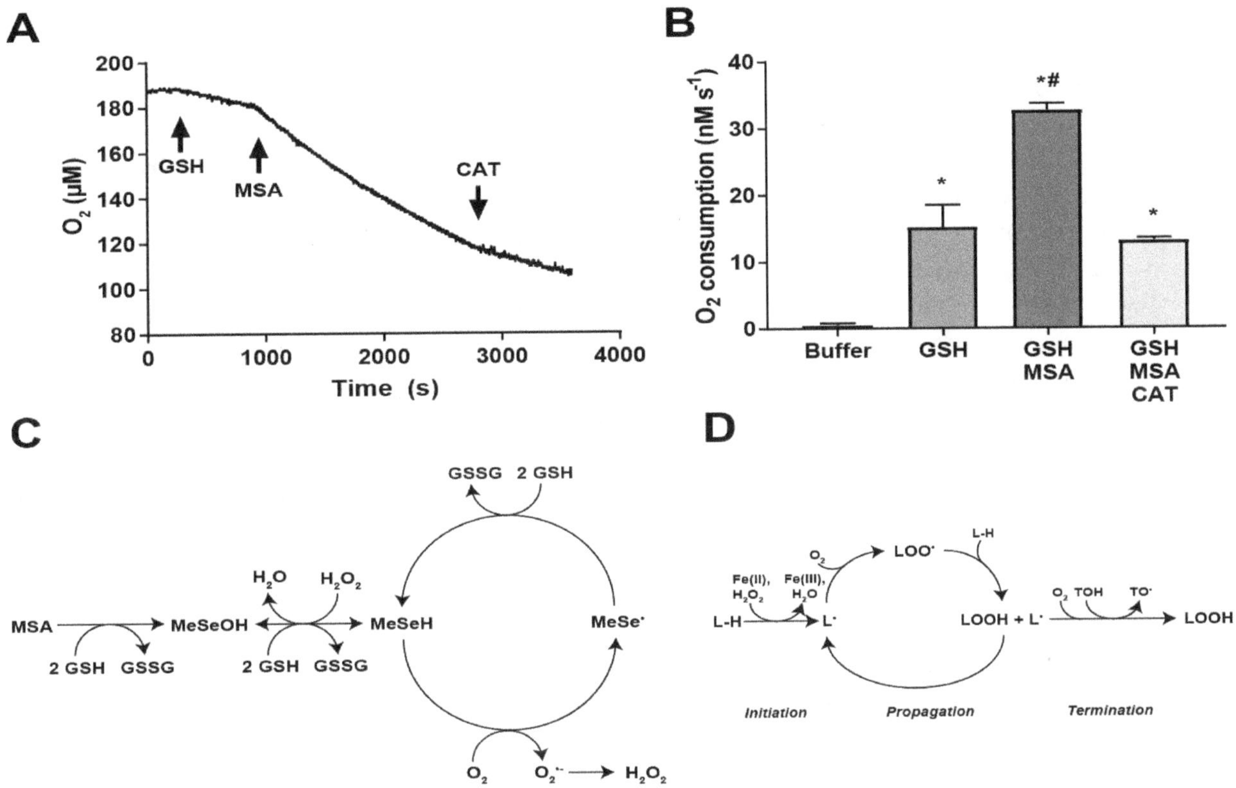

Figure 5. MSA enhances the consumption of O_2 by glutathione. (**A**) Representative trace of O_2 concentration in 3.00 mL pH 9.2 50 mM borate buffer at 37 °C. GSH and MSA added to a final concentration of 2 mM and 250 μM, respectively, at indicated time points. (**B**) Rate of O_2 consumption in 3.00 mL pH 9.2, 50 mM borate buffer at 37 °C. (**C**) Schematic of metabolism of MSA. MSA is reduced by GSH to methylselenol (MeSeH) through a methylselenenic acid (MeSeOH) intermediate. MeSeH may cycle with O_2 and GSH through a methylselenyl radical intermediate (MeSe$^•$) to generate H_2O_2, potentially through an $O_2^{•-}$ intermediate. MeSeH may also exhibit peroxidase activity, consuming H_2O_2. (**D**) Schematic of the process of lipid peroxidation. The process is initiated by abstraction of a hydrogen atom from a lipid, forming a carbon-centered lipid radical (L$^•$). The reaction is propagated by the addition of O_2, followed by abstraction of another hydrogen atom from a neighboring lipid, forming LOOH and a new L$^•$. The chain can be terminated by a donor antioxidant, such as tocopherol (TOH). The resulting tocopheroxyl radical (TO$^•$) radical does not efficiently further oxidize lipids. *, statistical significance relative to buffer alone; #, statistical significance to GSH alone; $p < 0.05$, $n = 3$.

3. Discussion

Results presented here show that MSA treatment results in toxicity and enhanced radiation sensitivity in HNSCC cells and that this toxicity may be facilitated by glutathione and oxygen-mediated reactions resulting in toxicity. BODIPY C-11 oxidation data indicate that lipid peroxidation is associated with this oxidative process, can be detected within 2 h of the initiation of MSA treatment, and persists for at least 72 h. Lipid hydroperoxides were detected in a dose-dependent manner following treatment with MSA, consistent with a role for lipid peroxidation and corroborating BODIPY C-11 oxidation experiments. In a cell-free system, MSA doubled the rate of GSH-dependent O_2 consumption.

Consistent with results from the cell-free experiments, intracellular GSH levels decline in Cal27 cells following exposure to MSA. Supplementation of the intracellular GSH pool by pre-treatment with NAC further sensitized, rather than protected, the cells from MSA-induced toxicity. These results suggest that MSA reacts with intracellular GSH, yielding reactive oxygen species capable of inducing lipid peroxidation and cell death.

MSA exhibited significant toxicity to Cal27 and SCC25 HNSCC cells, Figure 1. Similar organoselenium compounds SLM and MSC did not show any toxicity at doses up to 10 μM, while 10 μM MSA resulted in a nearly 30% PI-positive (non-viable) population of cells, Figure 1A. The active metabolite of all three of the examined compounds is methylselenol [11,12]. SLM and MSC release methylselenol following processing by lyase enzymes, such as MGL [13]. Several reports have identified MGL as a tumor suppressor gene, suggesting that its expression is reduced in tumors [14–17]. Overexpression of MGL in ovarian cancer cells resulted in up to 1000-fold sensitization to SLM [37]. Furthermore, hepatoma xenografts treated with the combination of adenovirus-delivered MGL and SLM (1 μmol d^{-1}, IP) exhibited a drastic decline in tumor size compared to SLM alone, indicating the necessity of MGL for SLM to generate methylselenol [37]. MSA generates methylselenol by a direct and spontaneous reaction with GSH, obviating the need for MGL, Figure 5C [13,18]. Previous studies have identified MSA as more effective than MSC at inducing apoptosis and inhibiting cell growth in murine mammary cell cultures [12]. MSA also more effectively reduced prostate cancer xenograft size than SLM or MSC with no change in body weight [19]. Our results indicate that HNSCC is also more sensitive to MSA than SLM or MSC. MSA was also found to render Cal27 HNSCC cells sensitive to radiation, Figure 2B. Although other selenium compounds have been reported to induce sensitivity of cancer cells to radiation, the ability of MSA to do so has not yet been reported [4,10]. The increased toxicity of MSA compared to other selenium compounds suggests that it may also more effectively sensitize cancer cells to radiation. Additionally, the cytotoxic and sensitizing effects appear to be selective to cancer cells, as NHF were relatively resistant to MSA-induced toxicity, Figure 2A, and quiescent lawns of NHF were undisturbed by a combination of MSA and radiation, Figure 2C.

MSA treatment increased BODIPY C11 oxidation in Cal27 cells, Figure 3A,B. BODIPY C11 may be oxidized by LPO initiators, such as hydroperoxyl radical, and propagators, such as lipid peroxyl radical [38]. The dye is insensitive to LOOH and aldehydic end products of LPO, such as malondialdehyde (MDA) or 4-hydroxynonenal (4-HNE). A dose-dependent increase of BODIPY C11 oxidation was not observed at 72 h of MSA treatment. However, MSA treatment did result in a dose-dependent increase in the accumulation of LOOH, as determined by the Cayman LPO Kit, Figure 3C. Additionally, BODIPY C11 dye oxidation was found to stabilize as early as 2 h of MSA treatment, Figure 3B. These results suggest that MSA induces LPO rapidly and persistently and that this results in an accumulation of toxic lipid hydroperoxides. Furthermore, LPO appears essential to the toxicity of MSA, as pre-treatment with α-tocopherol acetate, an inhibitor of LPO, protected the cells from MSA-induced toxicity, Figure 3D. Previous studies have mainly focused on selenium administration as an inhibitor of LPO, presumably due to the induction of the glutathione peroxidase system [39]. However, evidence exists to suggest that selenium may initiate rather than inhibit LPO. Pre-treatment with sodium selenite (single dose 2 mg kg^{-1}, IP) in a murine model of heavy metal poisoning found a 4-fold increase of liver MDA content over metal alone [23]. Administration of ebselen, a synthetic organoselenium compound, increased liver MDA content in rats by approximately 20% [25]. Serum MDA levels were elevated in ovarian cancer patients following the administration of 50 μg of selenium as selenized yeast (4.8 μM compared to 3.9 μM) [24]. These reports and others suggest that in some circumstances, selenium administration may induce LPO, although the mechanisms are yet unclear. Because MSA more effectively generates methylselenol, the active metabolite, than similar selenium compounds, it may also more potently induce LPO.

MSA treatment of Cal27 cells resulted in a depletion of total intracellular GSH content, Figure 4A,B. MSA has been reported to deplete GSH in A549 lung cancer and HepG2 hepatoma cells [40,41]. In HepG2 cells, a biphasic response was noted: A 10 μM treatment of MSA for 24 h caused intracellular

GSH to increase by about 75%, while 25 μM MSA resulted in an approximate 20% decline in GSH, with no change in GSSG. This biphasic response was not noted in Cal27 cells; total GSH content was unchanged or declined at all doses tested, Figure 3A. Furthermore, treatment with MSA (10 μM) for 24 h decreased cell numbers of Cal27 and SCC25; a significant increase in the non-viable population, Figure 1C,D. Apoptosis of HepG2 cells as detected by LDH was not noted at 10 μM MSA for 24 h, suggesting that HepG2 cells are more resistant to MSA than HNSCC [41]. This concentration coincides with elevated GSH in HepG2, which suggests that the biphasic response may play a role in resistance of MSA. Interestingly, despite a decline in intracellular GSH levels following MSA treatment, no change was noted in GSSG, Figure 4B. This may be due to increased GSSG efflux through membrane transporters, such as MRP1 [42]. GSH may also be consumed without GSSG formation through conjugation, suggesting that MSA treatment may induce increased GSH conjugation forming mixed disulfides. Supplementation of the intracellular thiol pool by pre-treatment with NAC sensitized Cal27 cells to MSA, Figure 4C,D. Similar results were reported with MSA treatment of HepG2 cells [41]. These results suggest that a reaction between MSA and a thiol, such as GSH, is essential for MSA-induced cytotoxicity.

Oxygen consumption by GSH was doubled in the presence of MSA in a cell-free system, Figure 5A,B. Furthermore, the addition of catalase to this system returned the rate of O_2 consumption to those similar to GSH alone. These results suggest the formation, but not accumulation, of H_2O_2. Had H_2O_2 accumulated, the addition of catalase would have returned O_2 to the system, i.e., an increase in the concentration of O_2 would have been observed. Selenol species may exhibit peroxidase activity, as evidenced by the active site selenol of selenium-containing glutathione peroxidases [36]. Methylselenol may, therefore, exhibit peroxidase activity, yielding a methylselenenic acid, which may again react with GSH to regenerate methylselenol, Figure 5C. Previous reports indicate the potential for the formation of $O_2^{\bullet-}$ in systems containing selenium and GSH. The addition of MSA to a solution of GSH is reported to increase lucigenin-based chemiluminescence [13,18]. This effect was abrogated by the presence of superoxide dismutase, suggesting the formation of $O_2^{\bullet-}$. Additionally, an examination of the reaction kinetics of GSH and selenocystamine, an organoselenium compound similar to MSA, suggests a cyclic reaction yielding superoxide [36]. Following $O_2^{\bullet-}$ generation, methylselenol may be regenerated by an additional reduction by GSH, yielding a cyclic reaction capable of generating large amounts of $O_2^{\bullet-}$ [18,36]. These reactions are summarized in Figure 5C. Following its formation, $O_2^{\bullet-}$ can dismute to H_2O_2, either spontaneously or through the action of superoxide dismutase [43]. H_2O_2 may contribute to LPO initiation through the generation of hydroxyl radical by iron-mediated Fenton chemistry [44,45]. Superoxide can also be protonated to form hydroperoxyl radical, which is a powerful LPO initiator [21,22]. The contribution of $O_2^{\bullet-}$ to selenium-based cytotoxicity has been further demonstrated by the protective effects of a superoxide dismutase mimetic [46]. Methylselenol may, therefore, initiate lipid peroxidation chain reactions through superoxide-mediated products.

Overall, results from this study indicate that MSA sensitizes HNSCC cell to radiation and exhibits toxicity through a GSH-dependent induction of LPO. LPO occurs more readily in cells with higher polyunsaturated fatty acid content [47]. Many types of cancer exhibit greater lipid content than their respective normal counterparts, including colon, prostate, pancreatic, and clear cell renal carcinoma [48–52]. MSA may, therefore, exhibit selective cytotoxicity in cancer cells on the basis of altered lipid content. A pre-clinical study examining the efficacy of MSA (4 mg kg^{-1} d^{-1}, PO) in treating prostate cancer xenografts found a nearly 40% reduction in tumor size following MSA treatment, with no change in body weight [19]. Similarly, MSA (4.5 mg kg^{-1} d^{-1}, PO) combined with paclitaxel (10 mg kg^{-1} $week^{-1}$, IP) reduced breast cancer xenograft tumor size with no change in body weight [20]. These studies suggest that MSA is selectively toxic to cancer cells. The work presented herein suggests that this selectivity may be in part due to a differential sensitivity to LPO in cancer compared to normal cells.

4. Materials and Methods

4.1. Cell Culture and Reagents

Head and neck squamous carcinoma cell lines Cal27 (tongue origin, CRL-2095) and SCC25 (tongue origin, CRL-1628) were purchased from ATCC (Manassas, VA, USA). Both lines have mutated p53, are epidermal growth factor receptor (EGFR) positive, and human papillomavirus (HPV) negative. Normal human fibroblasts (NHF) were obtained from the Coriell cell repository (AG01522D). Cells were cultured in Dulbecco's Modified Eagle's Medium (DMEM) (Thermo Fisher Scientific, Waltham, MA, USA), supplemented with antibiotics and 10% bovine calf serum (HNSCC cells, Thermo Fisher Scientific, Waltham, MA, USA) or 10% fetal bovine serum (NHF, Sigma-Aldrich, St. Louis, MO, USA). All cells were grown in humidified incubators set to 37 °C, 5% CO_2, and atmospheric oxygen.

Seleno-L-methionine (SLM, S3132), *N*-acetylcysteine (NAC, A9165), glutathione (GSH, G4251), glutathione disulfide (GSSG, G4376), glutathione reductase (GR, G3664), 2-vinylpyridine (2-VP, 132292), 5,5-dithio-bis-(2-nitrobenzoic acid) (DTNB, D8130), and 5-sulfosalicylic acid (SSA, S2130) were purchased from Sigma-Aldrich. Reduced nicotinamide adenine dinucleotide phosphate (NADPH) (481973) was purchased from EMD Millipore (Burlington, MA, USA). Methyl-Se-selenocysteine (MSC) and methylseleninic acid (MSA) were generous gifts of the laboratory of Youcef Rustum (Roswell Park Cancer Institute, Buffalo, NY, USA). BODIPY 581/591 C-11 (D3861) and CellTracker Green CMFDA (C7025) were purchased from Thermo Fisher Scientific (Waltham, MA, USA). Lipid Hydroperoxide (LPO) Assay Kit (705002) was purchased from Cayman Chemical Company (Ann Arbor, MI, USA).

4.2. Irradiation

Exponentially growing cells were irradiated at the Free Radical and Radiation Research Core Facility at The University of Iowa. All irradiated cells received a single dose of γ-rays from a cesium-137 irradiator (JL Shephard, San Fernando, CA, USA) at a dose rate of 0.65 Gy min^{-1}. Cell survival was measured using a clonogenic assay following a previously published method [53].

4.3. Propidium Iodide Exclusion Assay

Following treatment, cultures were trypsinized, washed, and resuspended in cold phosphate buffered saline (PBS). The suspended cultures were filtered and labeled with 1 $\mu g\ mL^{-1}$ propidium iodide for 5 min on ice. Flow cytometry was completed on a Becton-Dickinson FACScan at the University of Iowa Flow Cytometry Core. Data from 10,000 events were collected in list mode. The population of PI-positive (non-viable) and negative (viable) cells were calculated with FlowJo software (FlowJo, LLC, Ashland, Oregon, USA).

4.4. BODIPY C-11 Assay

Following MSA treatment, adherent cells were washed and labeled with 5 μM BODIPY C-11 in DMEM lacking serum and antibiotics for 15 min at 37 °C. Following labeling, cultures were collected by trypsinization, washed, resuspended in cold PBS and filtered. Samples were read on a Becton-Dickinson LSR II flow cytometer using channels for Texas Red (reduced dye) and fluorescein isothiocyanate (FITC, oxidized dye) simultaneously at The University of Iowa Flow Cytometry Core. Populations were gated and analyzed with FlowJo software (version 7.6.5), and ratios of oxidized:reduced dye were calculated.

4.5. Total Lipid Hydroperoxide Determination

A Cayman Lipid Hydroperoxide Assay Kit was used to determine total lipid hydroperoxides in cell samples. Cal27 cells were treated with MSA for 72 h. Following treatment, cells were collected by trypsinization and counted. Total lipid extracts were obtained and analyzed as recommended by the manufacturer in glass cuvettes on a Beckman DU650 spectrophotometer. Lipid hydroperoxides per cell was quantified by construction of an appropriate standard curve and normalized to cell number, as determined by a Z1 Coulter Counter (Beckman-Coulter, Brea, CA, USA).

4.6. Glutathione Determination

Following treatment, cells were collected by trypsinization, washed, and pellets were lysed in ice cold 5% sulfosalicylic acid. Extracts were stored at −80 °C until analysis. Following centrifugation, the supernatant was removed and used for the glutathione assay; protein precipitate was dissolved in 1% SDS, 0.1 M NaOH for protein determination. Total glutathione was determined as described previously on a Beckman DU-650 spectrophotometer [54]. Glutathione disulfide (GSSG) was determined using the method of Griffith and Anderson [32]. Rates of reaction were compared to glutathione or glutathione disulfide standard curves and normalized to protein content as determined by bicinchoninic acid (BCA) (Thermo Fisher Scientific, Manassas, VA, USA).

4.7. Oxygen Consumption

Involvement of oxygen in the reactions of glutathione and MSA was investigated by recording oxygen consumption during reaction progress in a cell-free system with an ESA BioStat Multi Electrode System and YSI Oxygen Probe (Yellow Springs Instrument Co., Yellow Springs, OH, USA) at the Free Radical and Radiation Research Core Facility at The University of Iowa. Measurements were conducted in 3.00 mL of 50 mM pH 9.2 borate buffer at 37 °C. Initial oxygen concentration was assumed to be 188 μM, as reported previously [55]. The reactants glutathione, MSA, and catalase were introduced sequentially to final concentrations of 2 mM, 250 μM, and 167 IU mL^{-1}, respectively.

4.8. Statistical Analysis

Statistical analysis was completed using Prism (GraphPad Software, San Diego, CA, USA). Two-way ANOVA with post-hoc analysis was completed to determine statistical significance. Homogeneity of variance was assumed at a 95% confidence interval. Results from at least three biological replicates with $p < 0.05$ were considered significant.

Author Contributions: Conceptualization, P.C.G., G.R.B., J.T.L., E.H.S., B.A.W.; methodology, J.T.L., E.H.S., B.A.W., G.R.B.; validation, J.T.L. and A.L.K.; formal analysis, J.T.L., B.A.W., E.H.S.; investigation, J.T.L., A.L.K.; resources, P.C.G., G.R.B.; writing—original draft preparation, J.T.L.; writing—review and editing, P.C.G., G.R.B.; visualization, J.T.L.; supervision, P.C.G., G.R.B.; project administration, P.C.G.; funding acquisition, P.C.G.

Acknowledgments: Youcef Rustum provided methylseleninic acid (MSA) and methylselenocysteine (MSC) as a generous gift for the completion of these studies. We thank Justin Fishbaugh and The University of Iowa Flow Cytometry Core for their aid in completing the flow cytometry measurements. We also thank Michael McCormick and The University of Iowa Free Radical and Radiation Research Core Facility for their expertise in biochemical measurements and irradiation services.

References

1. Howlader, N.A.; Krapcho, M.; Miller, D.; Bishop, K.; Altekruse, S.F.; Kosary, C.L.; Yu, M.; Ruhl, J.; Tatalovich, Z.; Mariotto, A.; et al. *SEER Cancer Statistics Review, 1975–2013*; National Cancer Institute: Bethesda, MD, USA, 2016.
2. Orlandi, E.; Iacovelli, N.A.; Rancati, T.; Cicchetti, A.; Bossi, P.; Pignoli, E.; Bergamini, C.; Licitra, L.; Fallai, C.; Valdagni, R.; et al. Multivariable model for predicting acute oral mucositis during combined IMRT and chemotherapy for locally advanced nasopharyngeal cancer patients. *Oral Oncol.* **2018**, *86*, 266–272. [CrossRef]
3. Pulte, D.; Brenner, H. Changes in survival in head and neck cancers in the late 20th and early 21st century: A period analysis. *Oncologist* **2010**, *15*, 994–1001. [CrossRef]
4. Schueller, P.; Puettmann, S.; Micke, O.; Senner, V.; Schaefer, U.; Willich, N. Selenium influences the radiation sensitivity of C6 rat glioma cells. *Anticancer Res.* **2004**, *24*, 2913–2917.

5. Husbeck, B.; Peehl, D.M.; Knox, S.J. Redox modulation of human prostate carcinoma cells by selenite increases radiation-induced cell killing. *Free Radic. Biol. Med.* **2005**, *38*, 50–57. [CrossRef]
6. Eckers, J.C.; Kalen, A.L.; Xiao, W.; Sarsour, E.H.; Goswami, P.C. Selenoprotein P inhibits radiation-induced late reactive oxygen species accumulation and normal cell injury. *Int. J. Radiat. Oncol. Biol. Phys.* **2013**, *87*, 619–625. [CrossRef]
7. Puspitasari, I.M.; Abdulah, R.; Yamazaki, C.; Kameo, S.; Nakano, T.; Koyama, H. Updates on clinical studies of selenium supplementation in radiotherapy. *Radiat. Oncol.* **2014**, *9*, 125. [CrossRef]
8. Brodin, O.; Eksborg, S.; Wallenberg, M.; Asker-Hagelberg, C.; Larsen, E.H.; Mohlkert, D.; Lenneby-Helleday, C.; Jacobsson, H.; Linder, S.; Misra, S.; et al. Pharmacokinetics and Toxicity of Sodium Selenite in the Treatment of Patients with Carcinoma in a Phase I Clinical Trial: The SECAR Study. *Nutrients* **2015**, *7*, 4978–4994. [CrossRef]
9. Ammar, E.M.; Couri, D. Acute toxicity of sodium selenite and selenomethionine in mice after ICV or IV administration. *Neurotoxicology* **1981**, *2*, 383–386.
10. Shin, S.H.; Yoon, M.J.; Kim, M.; Kim, J.I.; Lee, S.J.; Lee, Y.S.; Bae, S. Enhanced lung cancer cell killing by the combination of selenium and ionizing radiation. *Oncol. Rep.* **2007**, *17*, 209–216. [CrossRef]
11. Ip, C. Lessons from basic research in selenium and cancer prevention. *J. Nutr.* **1998**, *128*, 1845–1854. [CrossRef]
12. Ip, C.; Thompson, H.J.; Zhu, Z.; Ganther, H.E. In vitro and in vivo studies of methylseleninic acid: Evidence that a monomethylated selenium metabolite is critical for cancer chemoprevention. *Cancer Res.* **2000**, *60*, 2882–2886.
13. Spallholz, J.E.; Palace, V.P.; Reid, T.W. Methioninase and selenomethionine but not Se-methylselenocysteine generate methylselenol and superoxide in an in vitro chemiluminescent assay: Implications for the nutritional carcinostatic activity of selenoamino acids. *Biochem. Pharmacol.* **2004**, *67*, 547–554. [CrossRef]
14. Tan, Y.; Sun, X.; Xu, M.; Tan, X.; Sasson, A.; Rashidi, B.; Han, Q.; Tan, X.; Wang, X.; An, Z.; et al. Efficacy of recombinant methioninase in combination with cisplatin on human colon tumors in nude mice. *Clin. Cancer Res. Off. J. Am. Assoc. Cancer Res.* **1999**, *5*, 2157–2163.
15. Yoshioka, T.; Wada, T.; Uchida, N.; Maki, H.; Yoshida, H.; Ide, N.; Kasai, H.; Hojo, K.; Shono, K.; Maekawa, R.; et al. Anticancer efficacy in vivo and in vitro, synergy with 5-fluorouracil, and safety of recombinant methioninase. *Cancer Res.* **1998**, *58*, 2583–2587.
16. Kokkinakis, D.M.; Hoffman, R.M.; Frenkel, E.P.; Wick, J.B.; Han, Q.; Xu, M.; Tan, Y.; Schold, S.C. Synergy between methionine stress and chemotherapy in the treatment of brain tumor xenografts in athymic mice. *Cancer Res.* **2001**, *61*, 4017–4023.
17. Hu, J.; Cheung, N.K. Methionine depletion with recombinant methioninase: In vitro and in vivo efficacy against neuroblastoma and its synergism with chemotherapeutic drugs. *Int. J. Cancer* **2009**, *124*, 1700–1706. [CrossRef]
18. Spallholz, J.E.; Shriver, B.J.; Reid, T.W. Dimethyldiselenide and methylseleninic acid generate superoxide in an in vitro chemiluminescence assay in the presence of glutathione: Implications for the anticarcinogenic activity of L-selenomethionine and L-Se-methylselenocysteine. *Nutr. Cancer* **2001**, *40*, 34–41. [CrossRef]
19. Li, G.-X.; Lee, H.-J.; Wang, Z.; Hu, H.; Liao, J.D.; Watts, J.C.; Combs, G.F.; Lü, J. Superior in vivo inhibitory efficacy of methylseleninic acid against human prostate cancer over selenomethionine or selenite. *Carcinogenesis* **2008**, *29*, 1005–1012. [CrossRef]
20. Qi, Y.; Fu, X.; Xiong, Z.; Zhang, H.; Hill, S.M.; Rowan, B.G.; Dong, Y. Methylseleninic acid enhances paclitaxel efficacy for the treatment of triple-negative breast cancer. *PLoS ONE* **2012**, *7*, e31539. [CrossRef]
21. Aikens, J.; Dix, T.A. Perhydroxyl radical (HOO.) initiated lipid peroxidation. The role of fatty acid hydroperoxides. *J. Biol. Chem.* **1991**, *266*, 15091–15098.
22. Bielski, B.H.; Arudi, R.L.; Sutherland, M.W. A study of the reactivity of HO2/O2- with unsaturated fatty acids. *J. Biol. Chem.* **1983**, *258*, 4759–4761.
23. Rungby, J. Silver-induced lipid peroxidation in mice: Interactions with selenium and nickel. *Toxicology* **1987**, *45*, 135–142. [CrossRef]
24. Sieja, K.; Talerczyk, M. Selenium as an element in the treatment of ovarian cancer in women receiving chemotherapy. *Gynecol. Oncol.* **2004**, *93*, 320–327. [CrossRef]
25. Farina, M.; Soares, F.A.; Zeni, G.; Souza, D.O.; Rocha, J.B. Additive pro-oxidative effects of methylmercury and ebselen in liver from suckling rat pups. *Toxicol. Lett.* **2004**, *146*, 227–235. [CrossRef]

26. Rasheed, M.H.; Beevi, S.S.; Geetha, A. Enhanced lipid peroxidation and nitric oxide products with deranged antioxidant status in patients with head and neck squamous cell carcinoma. *Oral Oncol.* **2007**, *43*, 333–338. [CrossRef]
27. Gupta, A.; Bhatt, M.L.; Misra, M.K. Lipid peroxidation and antioxidant status in head and neck squamous cell carcinoma patients. *Oxid. Med. Cell. Longev.* **2009**, *2*, 68–72. [CrossRef]
28. Chintala, S.; Toth, K.; Cao, S.; Durrani, F.A.; Vaughan, M.M.; Jensen, R.L.; Rustum, Y.M. Se-methylselenocysteine sensitizes hypoxic tumor cells to irinotecan by targeting hypoxia-inducible factor 1alpha. *Cancer Chemother. Pharmacol.* **2010**, *66*, 899–911. [CrossRef]
29. Büntzel, J.; Micke, O.; Glatzel, M.; Schafer, U.; Riesenbeck, D.; Kisters, K.; Bruns, F.; Schänekaes, K.G.; Dawczynski, H.; Mücke, R. Selenium substitution during radiotherapy in head and neck cancer. *Trace Elem. Electrolytes* **2010**, *27*, 235–239. [CrossRef]
30. Orimo, A.; Weinberg, R.A. Stromal fibroblasts in cancer: A novel tumor-promoting cell type. *Cell Cycle* **2006**, *5*, 1597–1601. [CrossRef]
31. Arina, A.; Idel, C.; Hyjek, E.M.; Alegre, M.L.; Wang, Y.; Bindokas, V.P.; Weichselbaum, R.R.; Schreiber, H. Tumor-associated fibroblasts predominantly come from local and not circulating precursors. *Proc. Natl. Acad. Sci. USA* **2016**, *113*, 7551–7556. [CrossRef]
32. Griffith, O.W. Determination of glutathione and glutathione disulfide using glutathione reductase and 2-vinylpyridine. *Anal. Biochem.* **1980**, *106*, 207–212. [CrossRef]
33. Menon, S.G.; Sarsour, E.H.; Spitz, D.R.; Higashikubo, R.; Sturm, M.; Zhang, H.; Goswami, P.C. Redox regulation of the G1 to S phase transition in the mouse embryo fibroblast cell cycle. *Cancer Res.* **2003**, *63*, 2109–2117.
34. Menon, S.G.; Sarsour, E.H.; Kalen, A.L.; Venkataraman, S.; Hitchler, M.J.; Domann, F.E.; Oberley, L.W.; Goswami, P.C. Superoxide signaling mediates *N*-acetyl-L-cysteine-induced G_1 arrest: Regulatory role of cyclin D1 and manganese superoxide dismutase. *Cancer Res.* **2007**, *67*, 6392–6399. [CrossRef]
35. Huber, R.E.; Criddle, R.S. Comparison of the chemical properties of selenocysteine and selenocystine with their sulfur analogs. *Arch. Biochem. Biophys.* **1967**, *122*, 164–173. [CrossRef]
36. Chaudiere, J.; Courtin, O.; Leclaire, J. Glutathione oxidase activity of selenocystamine: A mechanistic study. *Arch. Biochem. Biophys.* **1992**, *296*, 328–336. [CrossRef]
37. Miki, K.; Xu, M.; Gupta, A.; Ba, Y.; Tan, Y.; Al-Refaie, W.; Bouvet, M.; Makuuchi, M.; Moossa, A.R.; Hoffman, R.M. Methioninase cancer gene therapy with selenomethionine as suicide prodrug substrate. *Cancer Res.* **2001**, *61*, 6805–6810.
38. Drummen, G.P.; van Liebergen, L.C.; Op den Kamp, J.A.; Post, J.A. C11-BODIPY(581/591), an oxidation-sensitive fluorescent lipid peroxidation probe: (Micro)spectroscopic characterization and validation of methodology. *Free Radic. Biol. Med.* **2002**, *33*, 473–490. [CrossRef]
39. Rotruck, J.T.; Pope, A.L.; Ganther, H.E.; Swanson, A.B.; Hafeman, D.G.; Hoekstra, W.G. Selenium: Biochemical Role as a Component of Glutathione Peroxidase. *Science* **1973**, *179*, 588–590. [CrossRef]
40. Okuno, T.; Honda, E.; Arakawa, T.; Ogino, H.; Ueno, H. Glutathione-dependent cell cycle G1 arrest and apoptosis induction in human lung cancer A549 cells caused by methylseleninic acid: Comparison with sodium selenite. *Biol. Pharm. Bull.* **2014**, *37*, 1831–1837. [CrossRef]
41. Shen, H.M.; Ding, W.X.; Ong, C.N. Intracellular glutathione is a cofactor in methylseleninic acid-induced apoptotic cell death of human hepatoma HEPG(2) cells. *Free Radic. Biol. Med.* **2002**, *33*, 552–561. [CrossRef]
42. Gordillo, G.M.; Biswas, A.; Khanna, S.; Spieldenner, J.M.; Pan, X.; Sen, C.K. Multidrug Resistance-associated Protein-1 (MRP-1)-dependent Glutathione Disulfide (GSSG) Efflux as a Critical Survival Factor for Oxidant-enriched Tumorigenic Endothelial Cells. *J. Biol. Chem.* **2016**, *291*, 10089–10103. [CrossRef]
43. McCord, J.M.; Fridovich, I. Superoxide dismutase. An enzymic function for erythrocuprein (hemocuprein). *J. Biol. Chem.* **1969**, *244*, 6049–6055.
44. Liochev, S.I.; Fridovich, I. The role of $O_2^{\cdot -}$ in the production of HO·: In vitro and in vivo. *Free Radic. Biol. Med.* **1994**, *16*, 29–33. [CrossRef]
45. Agil, A.; Fuller, C.J.; Jialal, I. Susceptibility of plasma to ferrous iron/hydrogen peroxide-mediated oxidation: Demonstration of a possible Fenton reaction. *Clin. Chem.* **1995**, *41*, 220–225.
46. Zhong, W.; Oberley, T.D. Redox-mediated effects of selenium on apoptosis and cell cycle in the LNCaP human prostate cancer cell line. *Cancer Res.* **2001**, *61*, 7071–7078.
47. Wagner, B.A.; Buettner, G.R.; Burns, C.P. Free radical-mediated lipid peroxidation in cells: Oxidizability is a function of cell lipid bis-allylic hydrogen content. *Biochemistry* **1994**, *33*, 4449–4453. [CrossRef]

48. Accioly, M.T.; Pacheco, P.; Maya-Monteiro, C.M.; Carrossini, N.; Robbs, B.K.; Oliveira, S.S.; Kaufmann, C.; Morgado-Diaz, J.A.; Bozza, P.T.; Viola, J.P. Lipid bodies are reservoirs of cyclooxygenase-2 and sites of prostaglandin-E2 synthesis in colon cancer cells. *Cancer Res.* **2008**, *68*, 1732–1740. [CrossRef]
49. Yue, S.; Li, J.; Lee, S.Y.; Lee, H.J.; Shao, T.; Song, B.; Cheng, L.; Masterson, T.A.; Liu, X.; Ratliff, T.L.; et al. Cholesteryl ester accumulation induced by PTEN loss and PI3K/AKT activation underlies human prostate cancer aggressiveness. *Cell Metab.* **2014**, *19*, 393–406. [CrossRef]
50. Guillaumond, F.; Bidaut, G.; Ouaissi, M.; Servais, S.; Gouirand, V.; Olivares, O.; Lac, S.; Borge, L.; Roques, J.; Gayet, O.; et al. Cholesterol uptake disruption, in association with chemotherapy, is a promising combined metabolic therapy for pancreatic adenocarcinoma. *Proc. Natl. Acad. Sci. USA* **2015**, *112*, 2473–2478. [CrossRef]
51. Toth, K.; Peter, I.; Kremmer, T.; Sugar, J. Lipid-rich cell thyroid adenoma: Histopathology with comparative lipid analysis. *Virchows Arch. APathol. Anat. Histopathol.* **1990**, *417*, 273–276. [CrossRef]
52. Ericsson, J.L.E.; Seljelid, R.; Orrenius, S. Comparative light and electron microscopic observations of the cytoplasmic matrix in renal carcinomas. *Virchows Archiv für Pathologische Anatomie und Physiologie und für Klinische Medizin* **1966**, *341*, 204–223. [CrossRef]
53. Kalen, A.L.; Sarsour, E.H.; Venkataraman, S.; Goswami, P.C. Mn-superoxide dismutase overexpression enhances G2 accumulation and radioresistance in human oral squamous carcinoma cells. *Antioxid. Redox Signal.* **2006**, *8*, 1273–1281. [CrossRef]
54. Tietze, F. Enzymic method for quantitative determination of nanogram amounts of total and oxidized glutathione: Applications to mammalian blood and other tissues. *Anal. Biochem.* **1969**, *27*, 502–522. [CrossRef]
55. Wagner, B.A.; Venkataraman, S.; Buettner, G.R. The rate of oxygen utilization by cells. *Free Radic. Biol. Med.* **2011**, *51*, 700–712. [CrossRef]

5

Identification of a Novel Quinoxaline-Isoselenourea Targeting the STAT3 Pathway as a Potential Melanoma Therapeutic

Verónica Alcolea [1,2], Deepkamal N. Karelia [3,4], Manoj K. Pandey [3,4], Daniel Plano [1,2], Parvesh Singh [5], Juan Antonio Palop [1,2], Shantu Amin [3,4], Carmen Sanmartín [1,2] and Arun K. Sharma [3,4,*]

1 Department of Pharmaceutical Technology and Chemistry, School of Pharmacy and Nutrition, University of Navarra, Irunlarrea 1, E-31008 Pamplona, Spain; valcolea@alumni.unav.es (V.A.); dplano@unav.es (D.P.); jpalop@unav.es (J.A.P.); sanmartin@unav.es (C.S.)
2 Instituto de Investigación Sanitaria de Navarra (IdiSNA), Irunlarrea 3, E-31008 Pamplona, Spain
3 Department of Pharmacology, Penn State Cancer Institute, CH72, Penn State College of Medicine, 500 University Drive, Hershey, PA 17033, USA; dkarelia@pennstatehealth.psu.edu (D.N.K.); pandey@rowan.edu (M.K.P.); sga3@psu.edu (S.A.)
4 Department of Biomedical Sciences, Cooper Medical School of Rowan University, Camden, NJ 08103, USA
5 School of Chemistry and Physics, University of Kwa-Zulu Natal (UKZN), Westville Campus, Durban 4000, South Africa; singhp4@ukzn.ac.za
* Correspondence: aks14@psu.edu

Abstract: The prognosis for patients with metastatic melanoma remains very poor. Constitutive signal transducer and activator of transcription 3 (STAT3) activation has been correlated to metastasis, poor patient survival, larger tumor size, and acquired resistance against vemurafenib (PLX-4032), suggesting its potential as a molecular target. We recently designed a series of isoseleno- and isothio-urea derivatives of several biologically active heterocyclic scaffolds. The cytotoxic effects of lead isoseleno- and isothio-urea derivatives (compounds 1 and 3) were studied in a panel of five melanoma cell lines, including B-RAF^{V600E}-mutant and wild-type (WT) cells. Compound 1 (IC_{50} range 0.8–3.8 μM) showed lower IC_{50} values than compound 3 (IC_{50} range 8.1–38.7 μM) and the mutant B-RAF specific inhibitor PLX-4032 (IC_{50} ranging from 0.4 to >50 μM), especially at a short treatment time (24 h). These effects were long-lasting, since melanoma cells did not recover their proliferative potential after 14 days of treatment. In addition, we confirmed that compound 1 induced cell death by apoptosis using Live-and-Dead, Annexin V, and Caspase3/7 apoptosis assays. Furthermore, compound 1 reduced the protein levels of STAT3 and its phosphorylation, as well as decreased the expression of STAT3-regulated genes involved in metastasis and survival, such as survivin and c-myc. Compound 1 also upregulated the cell cycle inhibitor p21. Docking studies further revealed the favorable binding of compound 1 with the SH2 domain of STAT3, suggesting it acts through STAT3 inhibition. Taken together, our results suggest that compound 1 induces apoptosis by means of the inhibition of the STAT3 pathway, non-specifically targeting both B-RAF-mutant and WT melanoma cells, with much higher cytotoxicity than the current therapeutic drug PLX-4032.

Keywords: selenium; isoselenourea; melanoma; STAT3; apoptosis

---

1. Introduction

Melanoma is originated from the malignant transformation of melanocytes. Its incidence has been rapidly increasing, with a 5-fold increase in the last three decades [1]. The American Cancer Society's estimates for melanoma in the United States for 2018 are: About 91,270 new melanomas will be diagnosed (about 55,150 in men and 36,120 in women) and about 9320 people are expected to die of melanoma (about 5990 men and 3330 women). Nearly 1,330,300 new cases of melanoma and about 126,000 deaths are estimated to occur worldwide in 2018. The regions more affected are those with white population, highest incidences being in Australia, New Zealand, Northern America, and Northern and Western Europe [2]. If diagnosed in early stages, melanoma can be easily removed by surgical excision but in metastatic form, it is one of the most aggressive malignancies with low survival rates [3].

The mitogen-activated protein kinase (MAPK) signaling cascade is a key pathway in melanoma survival and proliferation. Constitutive activation of B-RAF kinase due to B-RAF^{V600E} mutation occurs in nearly 50% of cutaneous melanomas [4]. Moreover, constitutive activation of signal transducer and activator of transcription 3 (STAT3) has been implicated in many oncogenic features, as it regulates the transcription of a variety of genes involved in cell proliferation, apoptosis, angiogenesis, and metastasis. The constitutive activation of STAT3 has been reported in melanoma patients [5]. The high expression of STAT3 has been correlated to large tumor diameter and depth, lymph node metastasis, high expression of MMP-2 and -9, and poor patient survival [6–8].

Traditional treatments for melanoma have shown low response rates and are associated with severe adverse effects. The introduction of agents that specifically target the MAPK pathway, such as vemurafenib (PLX-4032), dabrafenib, and trametinib, has significantly improved the overall survival of patients bearing the B-RAF^{V600E} mutation [9]. Although treatment with these inhibitors induces a quick initial response, the effect is not durable because of the rapid development of drug resistance [10]. The acquired resistance against vemurafenib is implicated in the activation of STAT3 and its signaling pathways [11]. Importantly, suppression of STAT3 activity disrupts B-RAF^{V600E}-mediated induction of anti-apoptotic proteins and reduces melanoma cell survival [12]. In addition, these treatments are ineffective in patients without the B-RAF^{V600E} mutation [10]. Therefore, there is an urgent need to develop novel agents for melanoma treatment.

In the last decade, selenium-containing compounds have emerged as promising anticancer agents due to their efficacy and selectivity [13]. Several studies, including those from our laboratories, have reported the role of different selenium-containing compounds in the prevention and treatment of melanoma, including its metastasis [14–20]. Of these, *Se,Se′*-1,4-phenylenebis(1,2-ethanediyl)bisisoselenourea (PBISe), an isoselenourea derivative, has been found to inhibit proliferation and promote apoptosis in melanoma cells in cell culture models [19]. It should be noted that PBISe was over 10-fold more effective than its isosteric sulfur analog *S,S′*-1,4-phenylenebis(1,2-ethanediyl)bisisothiourea (PBIT). Furthermore, the topical application of PBISe significantly delayed xenografted melanoma tumors growth [21].

In continuation of our pursuits towards developing novel organoselenium compounds as anticancer agents, we recently reported the synthesis and screening of a series of novel isoselenourea and corresponding isothiourea analogs [22]. This series consisted of new hybrid compounds containing an isoselenourea or an isothiourea group and different carbo- and hetero-cyclic scaffolds which have been traditionally included in anticancer agents [22]. Considering the encouraging results of PBISe in melanoma, we decided to evaluate the potential of the novel analogs as potential melanoma therapeutics. For this purpose, we selected an isoselenourea and an isothiourea derivative which showed the highest activity against a melanoma cell line (1205Lu) in our previous screening (compounds 1 and 3, respectively) [22]. The corresponding sulfur analog of compound 1, i.e., isothiourea compound 2, was also tested in order to determine if the compound selenium-containing 1 was more active than the sulfur compound 2 against melanoma cells, similar to what observed in the case of PBISe. This study examines the effects of these compounds on various melanoma cell lines and further evaluates the underlying mechanisms of action of compound 1.

2. Results

2.1. Synthesis of Compounds 1, 2, and 3

The structures of quinoxaline-2,3-diylbis(methylene)dicarbamimidoselenoate dihydrobromide (compound 1), its sulfur analog quinoxaline-2,3-diylbis(methylene)dicarbamimidothioate dihydrobromide (compound 2), and (9,10-dioxo-9,10-dihydroanthracen-2-yl)methyl carbamimidothioate hydrochloride (compound 3) are depicted in Figure 1A. These derivatives were synthesized as previously reported [22]. Briefly, compound 1 was synthesized by treating 2,3-bis(bromomethyl)quinoxaline with selenourea (molar ratio 1:1.1) in absolute ethanol at room temperature for 2 h, and compound 2 by treating 2,3-bis(bromomethyl)quinoxaline with thiourea in absolute ethanol for 3.5 h at reflux. Compound 3 was obtained from 2-(chloromethyl)anthraquinone and thiourea (1:1.1 molar ratio) in absolute ethanol, stirring for 3 h at reflux. The purity of compounds was $\geq 99\%$.

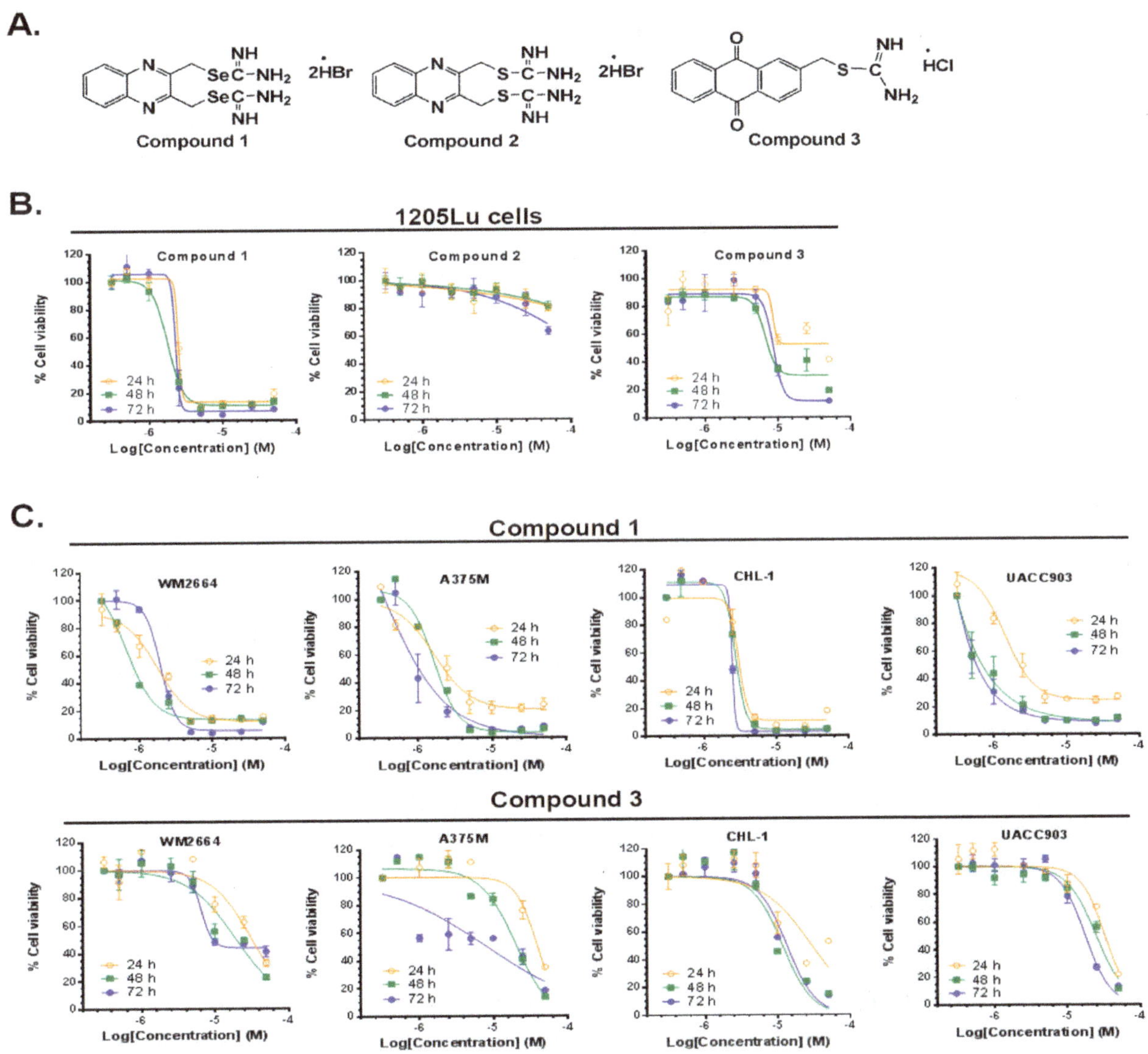

Figure 1. Compounds 1 and 3 were effective at reducing cell viability of different melanoma cancer cell lines. (**A**) Structures of the compounds, (**B**) Screening of the three agents in melanoma cells (1205Lu) for 24, 48, and 72 h using the MTT (cell viability) assay (**C**) Cell viability (MTT) results for compounds 1 and 3 in four different melanoma cancer cell lines at three different time points. Graphs were obtained by performing non-linear regression analysis using variable slope. Error bars represent mean ± SD.

2.2. Compounds 1 and 3 Reduced the Viability of Different Melanoma Cancer Cells

All the compounds were tested against a melanoma cell line (1205Lu) for their effect on cancer cell viability. The MTT (3-(4,5-dimethylthiazol-2-yl)-2,5-diphenyltetrazolium bromide) assay was performed in order to measure cancer cell viability, as previously described [22]. The anti-cancer effect of each agent was tested at seven different concentrations between 0.1 and 50 μM and three time points (24, 48, and 72 h). As shown in Figure 1B, compounds 1 and 3 potently inhibited the cancer cell viability of melanoma cells, while the isosteric sulfur analog (compound 2) of 1 was essentially ineffective up to the maximum concentration (50 μM) used. These results were in accordance with many of our previous reports [14,16,22–24] where isosteric replacement of sulfur by selenium in a small molecule significantly enhanced the anticancer activity. Therefore, compounds 1 and 3 were further screened against a panel of four melanoma cancer cell lines (WM2664, A375M, UACC903, and CHL-1) using the MTT assay. We compared the results with those obtained with PLX-4032, a B-RAF kinase inhibitor used currently in the clinic for melanoma treatment. The results are summarized in Table 1, expressed as IC_{50}, the concentration that produces 50 % of growth inhibition.

Table 1. Effects on cell viability of compounds 1 and 3 and PLX-4032 in five different melanoma cell lines. The results are expressed as mean values for IC_{50} with their respective standard deviation (± SD).

Comp.	Time (h)	Cell Lines				
		WM2664	1205Lu	A375M	UACC903	CHL-1
1	24	1.8 ± 0.4	2.6 ± 0.3	2.6 ± 1.0	3.8 ± 1.6	2.9 ± 0.4
	48	1.1 ± 0.3	1.9 ± 0.3	1.9 ± 0.1	0.8 ± 0.2	3.1 ± 0.4
	72	2.0 ± 0.2	2.0 ± 0.6	1.1 ± 0.2	0.3 ± 0.6	2.5 ± 0.2
3	24	32.7 ± 3.6	33.7 ± 10.1	38.7 ± 1.0	32.6 ± 1.9	29.3 ± 10.6
	48	21.0 ± 2.9	11.3 ± 3.0	21.3 ± 0.8	24.7 ± 2.3	12.3 ± 2.2
	72	22.8 ± 7.0	8.3 ± 0.9	8.1 ± 4.2	22.3 ± 5.6	13.6 ± 1.7
PLX-4032	24	>50.0	>50.0	>50.0	38.5 ± 7.2	>50.0
	48	32.1 ± 14.2	31.4 ± 8.0	3.5 ± 1.1	10.3 ± 2.6	21.2 ± 3.4
	72	3.6 ± 1.5	9.3 ± 3.4	0.4 ± 0.3	17.9 ± 1.3	12.2 ± 1.5

Compound 1 was more cytotoxic across all cell lines compared to compound 3 and PLX-4032 (Figure 1, Table 1). Interestingly, while PLX-4032 was more effective when the B-RAF^{V600E} mutation was present, compounds 1 and 3 also reduced cell viability in the B-RAF wild-type cell line CHL-1, compound 1 being the most potent. It should be noted that PLX-4032 showed no effect at 24 h in four out of the five lines tested, whereas both compounds 1 and 3 produced a reduction of cell viability in the five cell lines at that time point (Figure 1, Table 1). Compound 1 exhibited an IC_{50} lower than 4 μM in all the cell lines tested at 24 h. Furthermore, this compound was more potent than the reference drug in all cell lines at the three time points, with the exception of A375M cell line after 72 h of treatment. Overall, the isoselenourea derivative (compound 1) exhibited much higher potency than the isothiourea analog (compound 3) and, therefore, we selected compound 1 for further in vitro efficacy and mechanism of action elucidation.

2.3. Compound 1 Suppressed the Proliferative Ability of Melanoma Cells (1205Lu and UACC903)

In order to evaluate the long-term effects of compound 1 on melanoma cells, a colony formation assay was employed. For this assay, the cells were treated with either compound 1 or dimethyl sulfoxide (DMSO, control) for 24 h, and then 500 live cells were counted and re-seeded in new plates in the absence of compound 1 or DMSO and allowed to form colonies over a period of 14 days. As shown in Figure 2, compound 1 effectively inhibited the colony formation ability of both 1205Lu and UACC903 melanoma cell lines. At the dose of 1 μM, the ability of melanoma cells to form colonies was reduced to less than 50%, and when cells were treated with 2.5 μM, this percentage was dramatically reduced at levels lower than 20% and 5% for 1205Lu and UACC903 cells, respectively. These studies clearly indicate that the effects of compound 1 on the inhibition of melanoma cells replication are long-lasting.

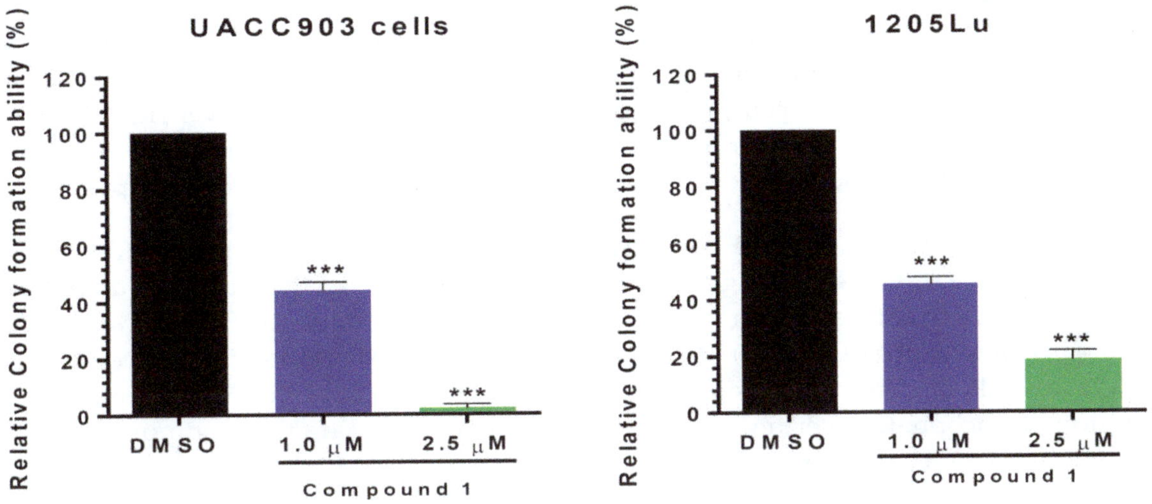

Figure 2. Compound 1 dramatically reduced the colony formation ability of melanoma cells. 1205Lu (**A**) and UACC903 (**B**) cells were treated with 1 or 2.5 μM of compound 1 or dimethyl sulfoxide (DMSO) (control) for 24 h. Subsequently, 500 cells were re-seeded with free compound 1 or DMSO medium for 14 days and stained with 0.5% alcoholic crystal violet. The results are expressed as mean ± SD. *** $p < 0.001$.

2.4. *Compound 1 Increased Melanoma Cell Death in Vitro*

In order to study whether the reduction of cell viability caused by compound 1 was due to cell death and not cell growth inhibition, 1205Lu cells were subjected to the Live-and-Dead assay. As shown in Figure 3, compound 1 increased the number of cells positive for ethidium homodimer staining (dead cells, upper left quadrant) and reduced the cells stained with calcein AM (live cells, lower right quadrant) compared to control cells. After treatment with 1 μM compound 1, no difference was observed between control and treated cells. However, when the dose of compound 1 was increased to 5 μM, the percentage of dead cells increased dramatically up to 25 %. These results suggest that compound 1 was able to induce cell death in vitro in melanoma cells.

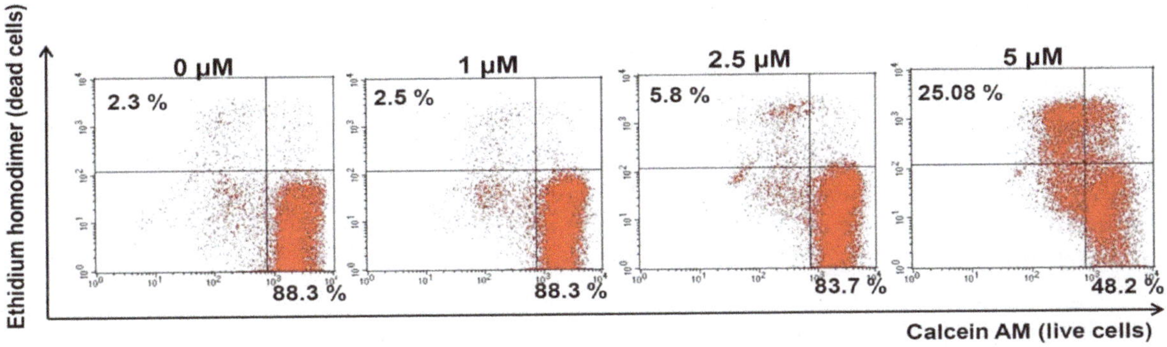

Figure 3. Compound 1 induced cell death in melanoma cells. 1205Lu cells were incubated with 1, 2.5, or 5 μM of compound 1 or DMSO (control) for 24 h and stained with ethidium homodimer and calcein AM. Live and dead cells were quantified by flow cytometry.

2.5. Compound 1 Induced Apoptosis in Melanoma Cells

With the aim of investigating whether the increase in cell death induced by compound 1 was due to apoptosis induction, the Muse™ Annexin V & Dead Cell assay was carried out. Annexin V was employed in this assay to detect the externalization of phosphatidylserine to the cell surface, a process occurring in apoptosis but not in necrosis [25]. A dead cell marker (7-ADD) was also included in the kit as an indicator of cell membrane structural integrity. Therefore, cells negative for both markers (lower left quadrant) were healthy cells, cells positive for Annexin V only (lower right quadrant) were in early apoptosis, and cells positive for both Annexin V and 7-ADD were undergoing apoptotic death (upper right quadrant). Cells positive for 7-ADD only were undergoing necrosis (upper left quadrant).

Compound 1 was tested at three concentrations: 1.75, 2.5, and 5 μM. The dose of 1 μM was not tested because we observed no significant effect at this dose in the previous assay. As shown in Figure 4A, after the treatment with compound 1 at 1.75 μM concentration, 15% of cells were in early apoptosis (lower right quadrant). At 5 μM of compound 1, less than 50% of cells were healthy cells and 25% of cells died by apoptosis (upper right quadrant). Less than 1% of cells died without externalization of phosphatidylserine (upper left quadrant), indicating that compound 1 induced cell death through apoptosis.

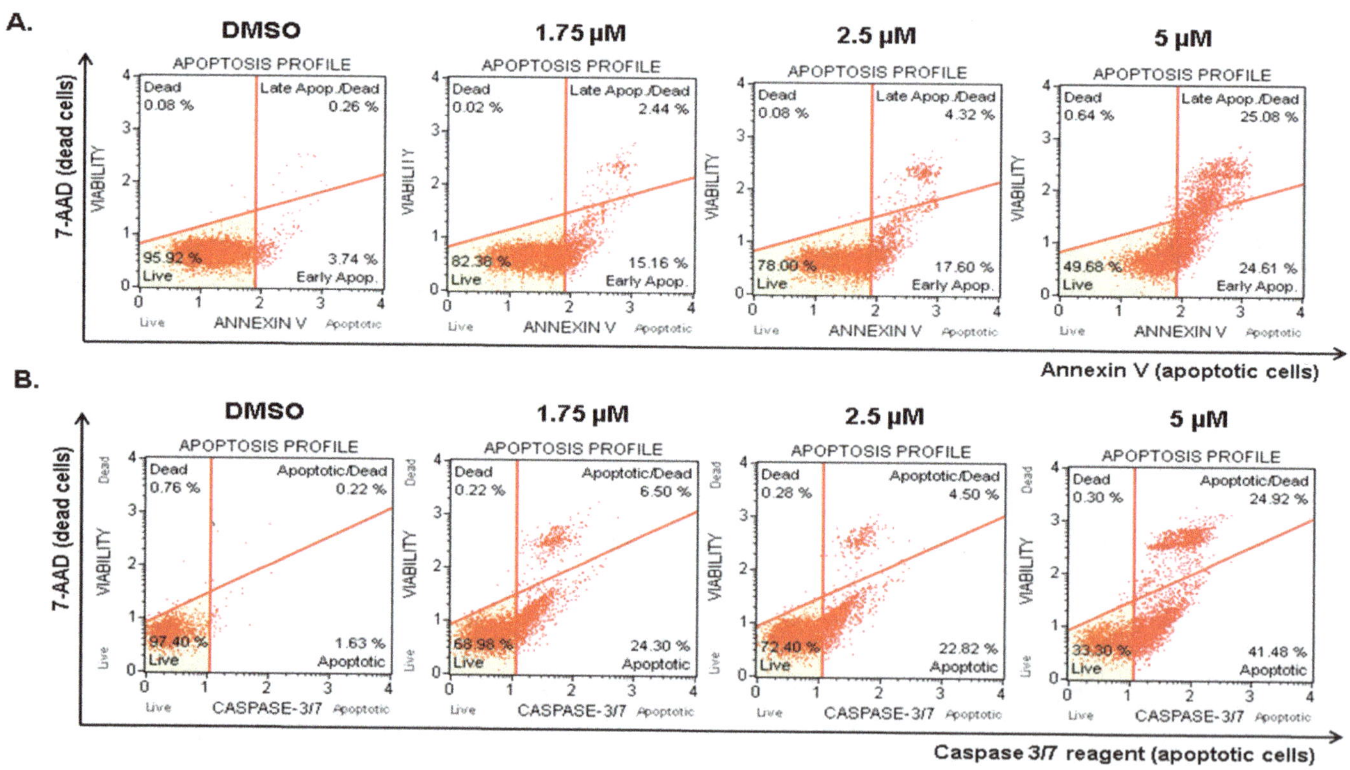

Figure 4. Compound 1 induced apoptotic cell death. After 24 h of incubation with the indicated concentration of compound 1 or DMSO (control), the apoptotic status of 1205Lu cells was analyzed using the Muse™ Annexin V & Dead Cell Kit according to the manufacturer's instructions. (**A**) Analogous independent experiments were analyzed with Muse™ Caspase 3/7 Kit to confirm the results. (**B**) The results of both experiments were analyzed by flow cytometry.

In order to confirm these results, the Muse™ Caspase-3/7 kit was also employed. The kit includes a reagent with a DNA binding dye. In non-apoptotic cells, this reagent is linked to an effector caspase recognition sequence which does not bind to DNA. However, when caspases are active, the dye is released by caspase cleavage and translocated to the nucleus, where it binds to DNA, producing high fluorescence. This kit also includes the dead cell marker 7-ADD. Hence, cells negative for both dyes were healthy cells (lower left quadrant), cells only positive for Caspase 3/7 reagent (lower right quadrant) were supposed to be in early apoptosis, cells positive for both dyes (upper right quadrant) were undergoing apoptotic death, and cells only positive for 7-ADD (upper left quadrant) were undergoing caspase-independent death. The results (Figure 4B) showed the same tendency observed in the Annexin V assay. The doses of 1.75 and 2.5 μM increased the amount of early apoptotic cells (lower right quadrant), and, after treatment with 5 μM compound 1, more than 60% of the cells were positive for caspase 3/7 activity (lower and upper right quadrants). Less than 0.5% of cells died through caspase-independent mechanisms. Overall, our results confirmed that compound 1 is a potent apoptosis inducer.

2.6. Compound 1 did not Inhibit the Phosphorylation of Akt and ERK1/2

The dysregulated expression of Akt and ERK1/2 is associated with cell proliferation and melanoma cell survival [26,27]. Hence, we decided to evaluate whether compound 1 affected the expression and phosphorylation status of these proteins. Interestingly, as shown in Figure 5A, compound 1 did not affect the expression or phosphorylation of Akt or ERK1/2. These observations suggest that the cell inhibitory response to compound 1 is not mediated through the inhibition of Akt and ERK1/2; therefore, other pathways might be implicated.

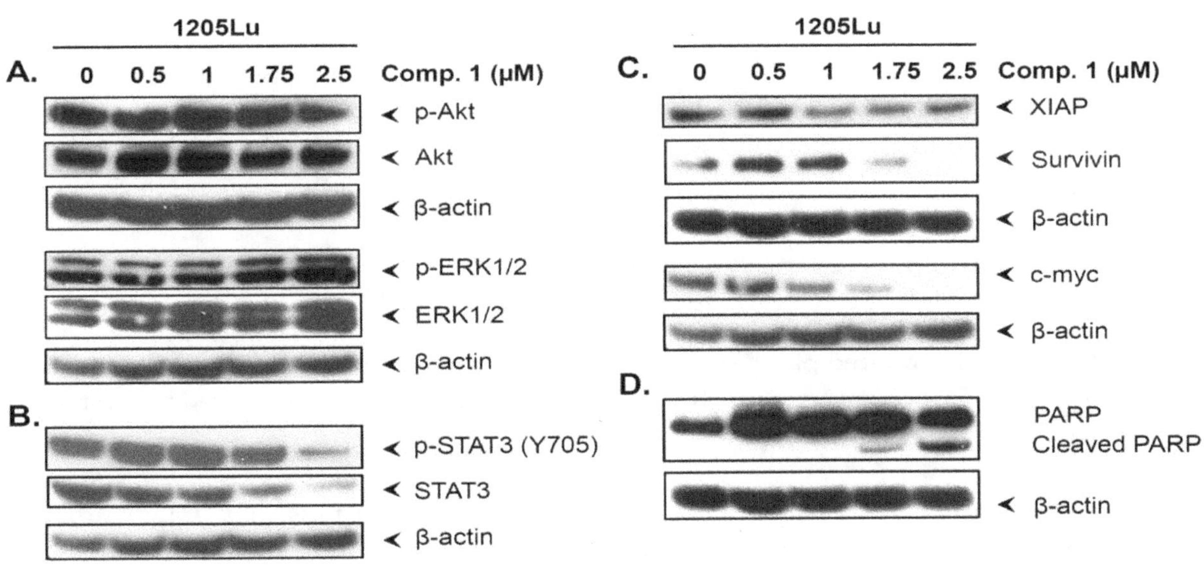

Figure 5. Compound 1 downregulated STAT3 and its downstream target proteins expression. 1205Lu cells were incubated with either DMSO (control) or compound 1 for 24 h. Whole cell lysates were subjected to western blot analysis. Expression of different proteins related to STAT3 and its downstream targets (**A**–**D**) were monitored. ß-actin was used as a loading control.

2.7. Compound 1 Inhibited STAT3 and Related Proteins Expression

To further examine the mechanism of action of compound 1, its effects on proteins implicated in cancer survival and metastasis were studied. STAT3 is highly upregulated in melanoma, and its activation by phosphorylation contributes to cancer progression and survival [12]. Hence, we decided to establish whether compound 1 affected the expression and phosphorylation status of the transcription factor STAT3. As shown in Figure 5B, compound 1 reduced protein levels and phosphorylation of STAT3. At the dose of 2.5 μM, the expression and phosphorylation of STAT3 were dramatically reduced.

STAT3 controls the expression of proteins involved in proliferation, survival, and metastasis formation, such as XIAP, survivin, and c-myc [28–30]. As observed in Figure 5C, compound 1 also downregulated these proteins at the doses at which STAT3 inhibition was observed. In addition, the inhibition of these anti-apoptotic proteins was accompanied by PARP (poly(ADP-ribose) polymerase) cleavage (Figure 5D), which is traditionally employed as a marker of apoptosis [31]. These results suggest that compound 1 has the ability to inhibit STAT3 signaling pathway. Moreover, the induction of apoptosis and cell proliferation inhibitory response of compound 1 may be mediated by STAT3 inhibition.

2.8. Compound 1 Induced the Cell Cycle Inhibitor p21

Recent studies have shown a correlation between the cell cycle inhibitor p21 and transcription factor STAT3 [32]. These studies revealed that p21 is part of a feedback network controlling the down-modulation of STAT activity [32]. Thus, we sought to investigate whether compound 1 activated the expression of this cell cycle inhibitor. As shown in Figure 6, compound 1 induced the expression of p21. These results suggest that the cell inhibitory activities of compound 1 may be mediated by activation of p21.

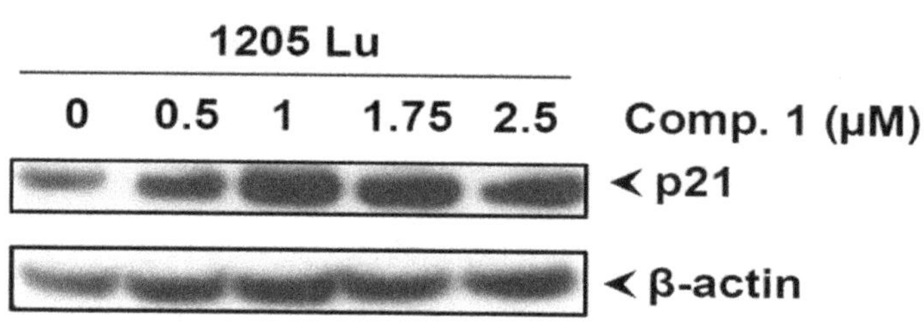

Figure 6. Compound 1 induced p21 expression. After 24 h of treatment with either compound 1 or DMSO (control), 1205Lu cells were collected, and the expression of p21 was analyzed by western blot analysis. ß-actin was used as a loading control.

2.9. Compound 1 Inhibited the Phosphorylation of STAT3, Increased the Expression of p21, and Induced Apoptotic Cell Death in Different Melanoma Cell Lines

The data above demonstrate that compound 1 effectively decreased p-STAT3 levels and increased the expression of p21 and apoptotic cell death in 1205LU cells. However, to rule out cell line-dependent effects of compound 1, we tested all the above biological activities of compound 1 in two additional melanoma cell lines (UACC903 and SK-Mel-8). As shown in Figure 7A, compound 1 inhibited cell proliferation of both melanoma cell lines, with UACC903 cells being more sensitive than SK-Mel-8. As suggested by our Annexin V and Caspase 3/7 activity assay (Figure 7B,C), compound 1 induced apoptotic cell death. Additionally, compound 1 also decreased the phosphorylation of STAT3 (Figure 7D,E) and induced p21 expression similar in both cell lines, to what observed in 1205Lu cells. Hence, the biological activities of compound 1 were consistent across a variety of human melanoma cell lines.

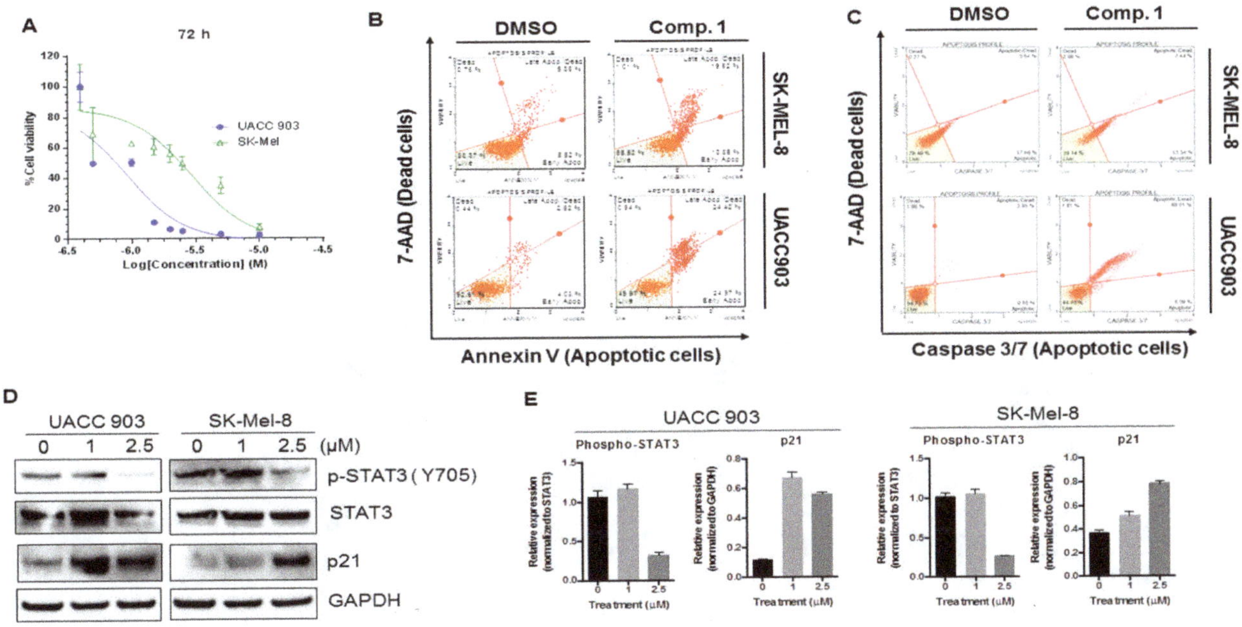

Figure 7. Compound 1 inhibited the phosphorylation of STAT3, increased the expression of p21, and induced apoptotic cell death in UACC 903 and Sk-Mel-8 melanoma cell lines. (**A**) Cell viability (MTT) results for compound 1 in two different melanoma cell lines at 72 h. The graphs were obtained by performing non-linear regression analysis using variable slope. Error bars represent mean ± SD. (**B**,**C**) Human melanoma cells UACC 903 and SK-Mel-8 were treated with compound 1 (2.5 μM) for 24 h, and an apoptotic assay was performed using the Muse^{TM} Annexin V & Dead Cell (**B**) and Caspase 3/7 Kit (**C**) according to the manufacturer's instructions. (**D**) Melanoma cells (UACC 903 and SK-Mel-8) cells were treated with the mentioned concentrations of Compound 1. After 24 h, cells were collected and lysed, and the expression of p-STAT3, STAT3, and p21 was analyzed by western blot. GAPDH was used as a loading control; (**E**) Quantification of protein expression was performed using Image J software, and graphs represent the relative expressions of proteins. The relative expressions were determined using either STAT3 or GAPDH as mentioned.

2.10. Docking

In order to substantiate our experimental findings and to investigate the binding propensities of compound 1 to the SH2 domain of STAT3, docking simulations were employed. The molecular structure [33] of STAT3 (pdb id: 1BG1, resolution 2.25 Å) was retrieved from the protein data bank (www.rcsb.org). CDocker [34], a CHARMm force field-based algorithm embedded in DS version 4.0 (Accelrys; San Diego, CA, USA), was used to flexibly dock compound 1 within the conservative SH2 domain of STAT3. The docking analysis revealed favorable binding of compound 1 with STAT3, based on the computed scoring function (CDocker energy = −23.8 kcal/mol), where the most negative value of CDocker energy indicates good binding affinity of a ligand for a protein. The visualization of the complex (Figure 8A) further revealed that compound 1 penetrated deep inside the STAT3 cavity and settled well by establishing a network of hydrogen bonding and electrostatic forces with the protein. Specifically, compound 1 utilized its nitrogen atom (proton acceptor) of the quinoxaline moiety to form two strong concurrent hydrogen bonds (2.2 Å, 2.8 Å) with the amine (proton donor) functionalities of Arg609 (Figure 8B). This amino acid contributed significantly to STAT3 and SH2 peptide binding, as the mutation of Arg609 has been reported to abolish the peptide-binding ability of this domain [35,36]. Several anticancer agents targeting the same amino acid residue (Arg609) in STAT3 SH2 domain have already been documented in the literature [37,38]. Additionally, a hydrophobic interaction and two electrostatic forces (cation-type) between the –NH_3 group of Lys591 and the aromatic network of compound 1 also facilitated locking its conformation in the binding domain of STAT3. Overall, the docking results revealed compound 1 as a good inhibitor of STAT3 protein and supported our experimental observations.

A

B

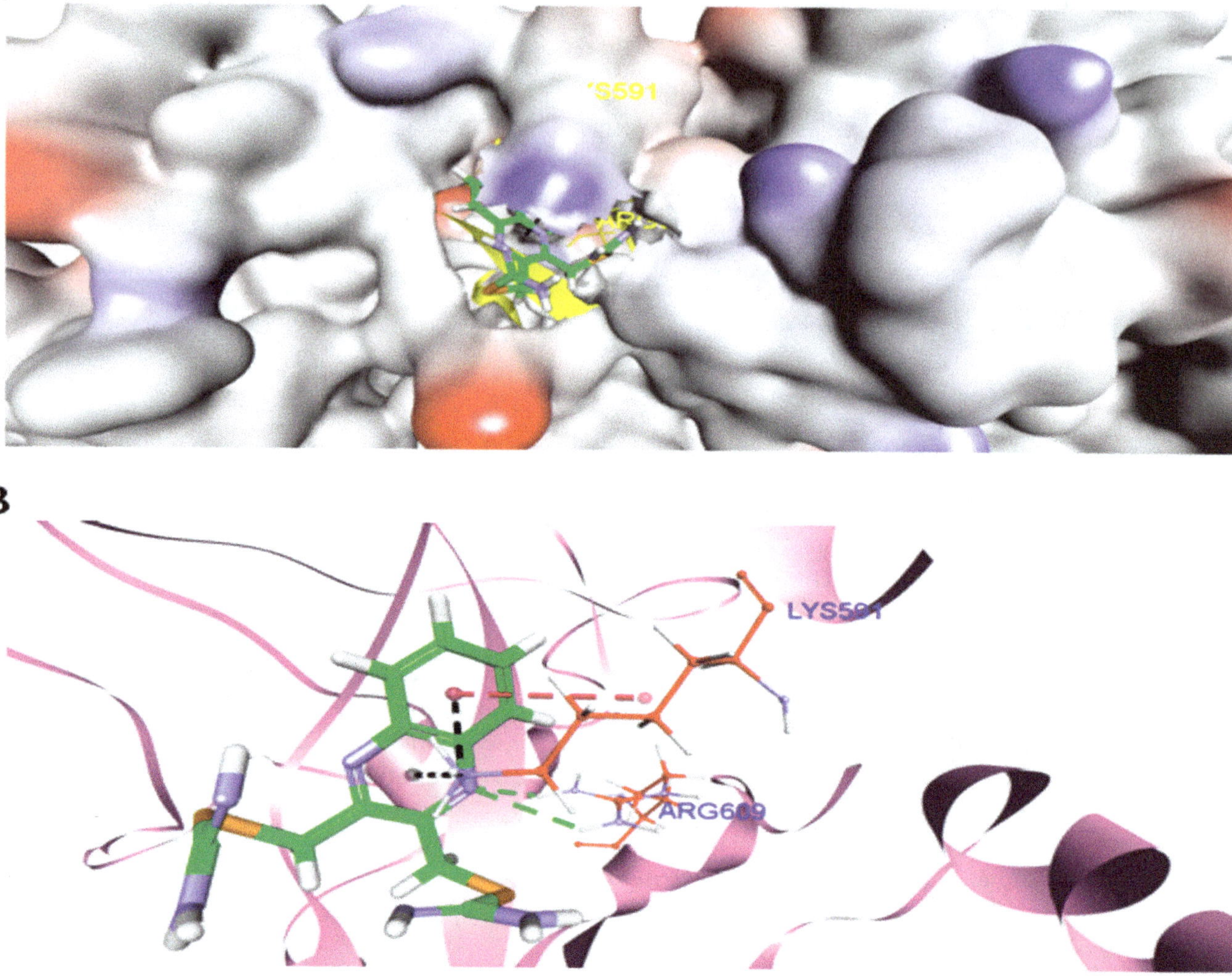

Figure 8. Docked complex of compound 1 with STAT3. (**A**) The surface representation of STAT3 showing deep penetration of compound 1 into the SH2 domain of STAT3 (pdb id: 1BG1), generated by DS (Accelrys). (**B**) Docked conformation of compound 1 in the SH2 domain of STAT3 (pdb id: 1BG1), viewed by DS (Accelrys). Carbon atoms of compound 1 (in sticks format) are colored green. The interacting amino acids of the SH2 domain of STAT3 are colored in red. All other amino acids of STAT3 are depicted in violet (flat ribbon format). Hydrogen bonds are shown in green, electrostatic interactions in black, and hydrophobic interactions are shown as magenta dotted lines.

3. Discussion

In this work, we tested the effects of an isoselenourea derivative and an isothiourea compound on cell viability in a panel of five melanoma cell lines bearing different mutations. The sulfur analog of compound 1 (compound 2) was inactive at the studied doses. This was in accordance with a previous report showing the isoselenourea derivative PBISe, an isosteric selenium analog of PBIT, to be over 10-fold more effective in inhibiting the viability of melanoma cells [19]. However, our recent report [22] also indicates that replacing the isothiourea functionality by an isoselenourea may not always lead to a more potent compound, suggesting that the potency depends on the overall structure of the molecule. For example, the isothiourea analog compound 3 was more effective than its corresponding isoselenourea analog [22]. Compounds 1 and 3 were active against both B-RAF mutant and wild-type

(CHL-1) cells lines, whereas PLX-4032 is only effective against the altered form [39]. In addition, our compounds were also more effective in reducing cell viability at 24 h in all the tested cell lines, compound 1 being at least 10-fold more potent than PLX-4032. In general, as reported in previous works [14,22,23], the selenium-containing derivative was much more active than the isothiourea one in reducing cancer cell growth.

The results from Annexin V and Caspase3/7 assays, as well as the observation of cleaved PARP in western blot, indicated that compound 1 induced apoptotic cell death. Apoptosis is a typical mechanism for selenium compounds to induce cell death [13]. However, the underlying mechanism of apoptosis induction could be remarkably different between distinct selenium-containing small molecules. Activation of caspases, modulation of anti-apoptotic proteins, alteration of oxidative stress-related proteins, cell cycle arrest, or kinases regulation are some of the described mechanisms associated with apoptosis [40]. This fact could explain the different mechanism of action between PBISe and compound 1. Although PBISe inhibited the phosphorylation and total protein levels of Akt in melanoma cells [41], compound 1 did not regulate this protein. We conclude that compound 1 is not effective against either Akt or ERK1/2 and indeed we found that compound 1 inhibits the expression of STAT3. In silico docking simulations conducted on compound 1 using STAT3 as a molecular target also suggested the compound to be a good inhibitor for this target protein. Hydrogen bonding and electrostatic and hydrophobic forces were found to be accountable for their host–guest relationship. Moreover, just like other known STAT3 inhibitors, compound 1 also interacted with Arg609, an essential amino acid for STAT3 function, suggesting its anti-melanoma activity may well be through inhibition of STAT3, in agreement with the experimental results.

STAT3 is a member of the signal-transducer-and-activators-of-transcription family. When phosphorylated, STAT3 dimerizes and translocates to the nucleus, where it modulates the transcription of genes involved in cell survival and proliferation [42]. Constitutive activation of STAT3 has been reported in several tumor types and has been proved to be involved in proliferation, survival, inflammation, invasion, metastasis, and angiogenesis [7]. Several in vitro and in vivo studies have demonstrated that the inhibition of STAT3 leads to tumor growth inhibition [5]. Thus, STAT3 is considered a valid therapeutic target for cancer therapy. STAT3 also has an important role in melanoma development and survival. This protein was found to be constitutively activated in numerous melanoma cell lines and tumor specimens [5]. Furthermore, inhibition of STAT3 signaling led to apoptosis of melanoma cells. Besides, STAT3 upregulation has been associated with acquired resistances to PLX-4032. Melanoma cells resistant to PLX-4032 showed increased STAT3 pathway activity [43], and in vitro silencing of this signaling inhibited the growth of cells resistant to PLX-4032 [11]. Moreover, a combination treatment with WP1066 (a STAT3 inhibitor) and PLX-4032 resulted in more significant growth inhibition of both resistant and sensitive cells to PLX-4032. The downregulation of other proliferative and anti-apoptotic proteins which are under transcriptional regulation of STAT3, such as XIAP, survivin, and c-myc, supports that compound 1 induces apoptosis through STAT3 inhibition. A previous study also reported a relationship between selenium-containing compounds and STAT3 inhibition [44]. The studies by Zuazo et al. demonstrated that imidoselenocarbamate derivatives blocked hypoxia-induced STAT3 phosphorylation [44].

4. Materials and Methods

4.1. Chemistry

All the chemicals were obtained from Sigma Aldrich (Alcobendas, Madrid, Spain) and Acros Organics (Janssen Pharmaceuticalaan, Geel, Belgium). Quinoxaline-2,3-diylbis(methylene)dicarbamimidoselenoate dihydrobromide (compound 1), quinoxaline-2,3-diylbis(methylene)dicarbamimidothioate dihydrobromide (compound 2), and (9,10-dioxo-9,10-dihydroanthracen-2-yl)methyl carbamimidothioate hydrochloride (compound 3) were synthesized and characterized as previously described [22]. Briefly, the corresponding alkyl halide (1 mmol) was added to a mixture of selenourea (2.2 mmol; compound 1) or thiourea (2.2 mmol for compound 2 and 1.1. mmol for 3) in absolute ethanol (20 mL). The mixture was stirred 2 h at r.t. for compound 1 or 3 hat reflux for 2 and 3. The precipitate was filtered and washed with 50 mL of ether (1 and 2) or with dichloromethane and ether (3).

4.2. Reagents and Antibodies

All the chemicals were obtained from Sigma Aldrich (Alcobendas, Madrid, Spain) and Acros Organics (Janssen Pharmaceuticalaan, Geel, Belgium). Quinoxaline-2,3-diylbis(methylene)dicarbamimidoselenoate dihydrobromide (compound 1), quinoxaline-2,3-diylbis(methylene)dicarbamimidothioate dihydrobromide (compound 2) and (9,10-dioxo-9,10-dihydroanthracen-2-yl)methyl carbamimidothioate hydrochloride (compound 3) were synthesized and characterized as previously described [22]. Briefly, the corresponding alkyl halide (1 mmol) was added to a mixture of selenourea (2.2 mmol; compound 1) or thiourea (2.2 mmol for compound 2 and 1.1. mmol for 3) in absolute ethanol (20 mL). The mixture was stirred 2 h at r.t. for compound 1, or 3 h at reflux for compounds 2 and 3. The precipitate was filtered and washed with 50 mL of ether (1 and 2) or with dichloromethane and ether (3). Rabbit anti-phospho-Akt (Cat # 4060), rabbit anti-Akt (Cat # 4685), rabbit anti-phospho-STAT3 (Cat # 9145), rabbit anti-STAT3 (Cat # 12640), rabbit anti-phospho-p44/42 MAPK (Erk1/2) (Cat # 4370), rabbit anti-p44/42 MAPK (Erk1/2) (Cat # 4695), rabbit anti-XIAP (Cat # 14334), rabbit anti-survivin (Cat # 2803), rabbit anti-c-Myc (Cat #9402), rabbit anti-p21waf1/Cip1 (Cat # 2947), and rabbit anti-PARP (Cat # 9542) were obtained from Cell Signaling (Danvers, MA). Antibodies against GAPDH, β-actin, goat anti-rabbit, and goat anti-mouse horseradish peroxidase conjugates, and MTT were purchased from Sigma-Aldrich (St. Louis, MO, USA).

4.3. Cell Culture

Human melanoma cell lines were grown in DMEM medium supplemented with 10 % fetal bovine serum (FBS) and 100 units/mL of penicillin and streptomycin (Corning; Corning, NY, USA). The cells were maintained at 37 °C and 5% CO_2.

4.4. Cell Viability

A total of 3000 cells/well were grown in 96-well plates for 12 h and then treated with either DMSO (control) or increasing concentrations (0.5–50 μM) of compound 1, 3, or PLX-4032 for 24, 48, and 72 h. Three hours before the termination point, 20 μL of MTT were added to measure cellular viability. The resultant formazan crystals were dissolved in 50 μL of DMSO, and absorbance was measured at 570 nm and 630 nm wavelengths. IC_{50} values were calculated using GraphPad Prism version 6.01.

4.5. Colony Formation Assay

Melanoma cells (UACC903 and 1205Lu) were treated with DMSO or compound 1 (1 and 2.5 μM) for 24 h. The cells were then trypsinized and counted, and 500 live cells were seeded in new 10 cm tissue culture plates separated by treatments. The cells were allowed to form colonies for 14 days in DMEM without compound 1 or DMSO in a 5% CO_2 incubator. After 14 days, the medium was removed, and the formed colonies were stained with 0.5% alcoholic crystal violet. The percentage plating efficiency (PE) was calculated by using the following formula:

$$\%PE = \frac{number\ of\ colonies}{number\ of\ cells\ plated} \times 100 \quad (1)$$

The results correspond to the mean ± SD of three independent experiments. Differences between control and treated cells were determined by one-way ANOVA tests, using GraphPad Prism version 6.01.

4.6. Live-and-Dead Assay

The LIVE/DEAD viability/cytotoxicity kit for mammalian cells (Molecular Probes, Invitrogen; Carlsbad, CA, USA) was employed for this experiment. A total of 7.5×10^5 1205Lu cells/well were plated in a 6-well plate and treated with DMSO (control) or increasing amounts of compound 1. After 24 h of incubation, both floating and attached cells were collected and re-suspended in PBS. Further, cells were stained with a calcein AM and ethidium homodimer solution according to the manufacturer's instructions. The number of live and dead cells was determined by flow cytometry (BD FACSCalibur; Heidelberg, Germany).

4.7. Annexin V Assay

1205Lu, UACC903, and SK-Mel-8 (4×10^5 cells/well) were pleated and treated with DMSO (control) or compound 1 at the given concentrations. After 24 h of treatment, both floating and attached cells were collected and stained with the Muse™ Annexin V & Dead Cell Reagent (Millipore; Bedford, MA, USA) for 20 min at room temperature in the dark. The results were collected by Muse™ Cell Analyzer (Millipore).

4.8. Caspase-3/7 Assay

The Muse™ Caspase 3/7 kit (Millipore) was employed for this experiment according to the manufacturer's instructions and our previously published method [22]. 1205Lu, UACC903, and Sk-Mel-8 cells were seeded at a density of 4×10^5 cells/well and treated with DMSO or the indicated amounts of compounds 1 and 3 for 24 h. Next, both floating and attached cells were collected, out of which 50 μL of cells were stained with 5 μL of Muse™ Caspase-3/7 working solution and incubated for 30 min at 37 °C with 5 % CO_2. After incubation, 150 μL of Muse™ Caspase 7-AAD working solution were added to each sample, and the samples were incubated in the dark for 5 min more. The samples were analyzed by Muse™ Cell Analyzer.

4.9. Western Blotting

1205Lu, UACC903, and SK-Mel-8 cells (7×10^5 cells/well) were plated in 6-well plates and treated with compound 1 or DMSO for 24 h. The cells were then collected, and whole cell lysates were prepared in RIPA buffer (Thermo Scientific #89900; Rockford, IL, USA) supplemented with 1% phosphatase inhibitor cocktail 2 (Sigma #P5726-5ML), 1% protease inhibitor (Complete mini, Roche #11836170001; Branchburg, NJ, USA), and 0.5 % of 200 mM phenylmethanesulfonyl fluoride (PMSF) (Sigma #P7626-250 mg). The cell lysates were spun at $15{,}000\times g$ for 10 min to remove any insoluble cell debris. The resultant supernatants were collected and stored at −80 °C until use. The whole cell lysates were resolved by SDS-PAGE. The proteins were transferred to Immobilon®-P PVDF membranes (Millipore # IPVH304F0) and blotted with the indicated antibody overnight at 4 °C. The dilution for primary antibodies was 1:1000, with the exception of p-STAT3 (1:2000), STAT3 (1:200), and β-actin (1:3000). Further, the membranes were incubated with the corresponding peroxidase-linked secondary antibodies (dilution 1:3000) for 1–4 h at room temperature. The antibodies were detected by an enhanced chemiluminescence reagent (Thermo Scientific #1856135 and #1856136).

4.10. Docking Methodology

Different 3D conformations of compound 1 were generated and energetically minimized using the "Generate Conformations" tool in Discovery Studio (DS) 4.0 client (Accelrys). The lowest energetic conformation thus obtained was subjected to the "Prepare Ligands" module to generate its isomers at physiological pH. The CHARMm force field was employed to develop the partial atomic charges on each atom of the isomer. The isomer with the lowest CHARMm energy was used for the docking study.

The X-ray co-ordinates of STAT3 (pdb id: 1BG1, resolution 2.25 Å) were retrieved from the protein data bank (www.rcsb.org). The "Prepare Protein" tool in DS was used to add missing atoms/chains and remove water molecules in the protein structure. The "Prepare Protein" algorithm was employed to protonate amino acid residues according to the physiological conditions. Prior to docking, a binding sphere covering the SH2 domain of STAT3 was generated. CDOCKER [34], a grid-based docking program, was used to dock compound 1 in the SH2 domain, considering the default parameters. The most favorable pose of compound 1 was identified based on the CDOCKER energy (-CDE).

5. Conclusions

In conclusion, compound 1, a quinoxaline-isoselenourea, showed promising efficacy in vitro against melanoma cells. Compound 1 was more effective than the isothiourea derivative 3 and the reference drug PLX-4032, especially at short times of treatment (24 h). As demonstrated by the colony formation assay, the effects of compound 1 in inhibiting cell proliferation were long-lasting. Overall, we demonstrated for the first time that the cell growth inhibitory response of compound 1 may be mediated through the STAT3 pathway as it does not inhibit other pro-survival signaling pathways such as Akt and ERK1/2. On account of the fact that compound 1 inhibits STAT3, it could also be employed in combination therapy with PLX-4032 to overcome acquired resistance to the latter. Interestingly, the response to compound 1 was not dependent on the mutation status of BRAF. Only about half of all melanomas have a mutation in the BRAF gene, and, therefore, compound 1, targeting both BRAF-mutant and WT melanoma cells, may have a broader clinical impact. However, more preclinical studies examining in vivo efficacy, Absorption, Distribution, Metabolism and Excretion (ADME), toxicity, and mechanism of action are required to determine the therapeutic properties and future clinical potential of compound 1.

Author Contributions: Conceptualization, D.P., J.A.P., S.A., C.S., A.K.S.; Methodology, V.A., D.N.K., M.K.P., D.P., P.S.; Writing – Original Draft Preparation, V.A., D.N.K.; Writing – Review & Editing, M.J.P., D.P., J.A.P., S.A., C.S., A.K.S.

Acknowledgments: The authors thank the Department of Pharmacology and Penn State Cancer Institute, Pennsylvania State University College of Medicine for financial support, and the Flow Cytometry Core at of the Pennsylvania State University, College of Medicine. The melanoma cell lines were graciously provided by Gavin Robertson, Penn State College of Medicine, Hershey, PA. V. Alcolea wishes to express her gratitude to the Asociación de Amigos de la Universidad de Navarra for the pre-doctoral fellowship. The Authors are also grateful to the Centre for High-Performance Computing, an initiative supported by the Department of Science and Technology of South Africa for usage of software and cluster support.

Abbreviations

AKT	Protein kinase B
c-myc	Avian myelocytomatosis virus oncogene cellular homolog
ERK1/2	Extracellular signal-regulated kinases 1 and 2
FBS	Fetal bovine serum
MAPK	Mitogen-activated protein kinase
MMP	Matrix metalloproteinase
MTT	3-(4,5-dimethylthiazol-2-yl)-2,5-diphenyltetrazolium bromide
PARP	Poly(ADP-ribose)polymerase
PBISe	*Se,Se'*-1,4-phenylenebis(1,2-ethanediyl)bisisoselenourea
PBIT	*S,S'*-1,4-phenylenebis(1,2-ethanediyl)bisisothiourea
PMSF	Phenylmethanesulfonyl fluoride
STAT3	Signal transducer and activator of transcription 3
XIAP	X-linked inhibitor of apoptosis protein

References

1. Leiter, U.; Eigentler, T.; Garbe, C. Epidemiology of skin cancer. *Adv. Exp. Med. Biol.* **2014**, *810*, 120–140. [PubMed]
2. Bray, F.; Ferlay, J.; Soerjomataram, I.; Siegel, R.L.; Torre, L.A.; Jemal, A. Global cancer statistics 2018:

GLOBOCAN estimates of incidence and mortality worldwide for 36 cancers in 185 countries. *CA Cancer J. Clin.* **2018**, *68*, 394–424. [CrossRef] [PubMed]

3. Di Trolio, R.; Simeone, E.; Di Lorenzo, G.; Buonerba, C.; Ascierto, P.A. The use of interferon in melanoma patients: A systematic review. *Cytokine Growth Factor Rev.* **2015**, *26*, 203–212. [CrossRef] [PubMed]
4. Marzuka, A.; Huang, L.; Theodosakis, N.; Bosenberg, M. Melanoma treatments: Advances and mechanisms. *J. Cell. Physiol.* **2015**, *230*, 2626–2633. [CrossRef] [PubMed]
5. Niu, G.; Bowman, T.; Huang, M.; Shivers, S.; Reintgen, D.; Daud, A.; Chang, A.; Kraker, A.; Jove, R.; Yu, H. Roles of activated Src and Stat3 signaling in melanoma tumor cell growth. *Oncogene* **2002**, *21*, 7001–7010. [CrossRef] [PubMed]
6. Xie, T.X.; Wei, D.; Liu, M.; Gao, A.C.; Ali-Osman, F.; Sawaya, R.; Huang, S. Stat3 activation regulates the expression of matrix metalloproteinase-2 and tumor invasion and metastasis. *Oncogene* **2004**, *23*, 3550–3560. [CrossRef]
7. Siveen, K.S.; Sikka, S.; Surana, R.; Dai, X.; Zhang, J.; Kumar, A.P.; Tan, B.K.; Sethi, G.; Bishayee, A. Targeting the STAT3 signaling pathway in cancer: Role of synthetic and natural inhibitors. *Biochim. Biophys. Acta* **2014**, *1845*, 136–154. [CrossRef]
8. Kusaba, T.; Nakayama, T.; Yamazumi, K.; Yakata, Y.; Yoshizaki, A.; Inoue, K.; Nagayasu, T.; Sekine, I. Activation of STAT3 is a marker of poor prognosis in human colorectal cancer. *Oncol. Rep.* **2006**, *15*, 1445–1451. [CrossRef]
9. Strickland, L.R.; Pal, H.C.; Elmets, C.A.; Afaq, F. Targeting drivers of melanoma with synthetic small molecules and phytochemicals. *Cancer Lett.* **2015**, *359*, 20–35. [CrossRef]
10. Mukherjee, N.; Schwan, J.V.; Fujita, M.; Norris, D.A.; Shellman, Y.G. Alternative treatments for melanoma: Targeting Bcl-2 family members to de-bulk and kill cancer stem cells. *J. Investig. Dermatol.* **2015**, *135*, 2155–2161. [CrossRef]
11. Liu, F.; Cao, J.; Wu, J.; Sullivan, K.; Shen, J.; Ryu, B.; Xu, Z.; Wei, W.; Cui, R. Stat3-targeted therapies overcome the acquired resistance to vemurafenib in melanomas. *J. Investig. Dermatol.* **2013**, *133*, 2041–2049. [CrossRef] [PubMed]
12. Becker, T.M.; Boyd, S.C.; Mijatov, B.; Gowrishankar, K.; Snoyman, S.; Pupo, G.M.; Scolyer, R.A.; Mann, G.J.; Kefford, R.F.; Zhang, X.D.; et al. Mutant B-RAF-Mcl-1 survival signaling depends on the STAT3 transcription factor. *Oncogene* **2014**, *33*, 1158–1166. [CrossRef] [PubMed]
13. Fernandes, A.P.; Gandin, V. Selenium compounds as therapeutic agents in cancer. *Biochim. Biophys. Acta* **2015**, *1850*, 1642–1660. [CrossRef] [PubMed]
14. Sharma, A.K.; Sharma, A.; Desai, D.; Madhunapantula, S.V.; Huh, S.J.; Robertson, G.P.; Amin, S. Synthesis and anticancer activity comparison of phenylalkyl isoselenocyanates with corresponding naturally occurring and synthetic isothiocyanates. *J. Med. Chem.* **2008**, *51*, 7820–7826. [CrossRef] [PubMed]
15. Chen, Y.C.; Prabhu, K.S.; Mastro, A.M. Is selenium a potential treatment for cancer metastasis? *Nutrients* **2013**, *5*, 1149–1168. [CrossRef] [PubMed]
16. Sharma, A.; Sharma, A.K.; Madhunapantula, S.V.; Desai, D.; Huh, S.J.; Mosca, P.; Amin, S.; Robertson, G.P. Targeting Akt3 signaling in malignant melanoma using isoselenocyanates. *Clin. Cancer Res.* **2009**, *15*, 1674–1685. [CrossRef]
17. Nguyen, N.; Sharma, A.; Nguyen, N.; Sharma, A.K.; Desai, D.; Huh, S.J.; Amin, S.; Meyers, C.; Robertson, G.P. Melanoma chemoprevention in skin reconstructs and mouse xenografts using isoselenocyanate-4. *Cancer Prev. Res.* **2011**, *4*, 248–258. [CrossRef]
18. Cassidy, P.B.; Fain, H.D.; Cassidy, J.P., Jr.; Tran, S.M.; Moos, P.J.; Boucher, K.M.; Gerads, R.; Florell, S.R.; Grossman, D.; Leachman, S.A. Selenium for the prevention of cutaneous melanoma. *Nutrients* **2013**, *5*, 725–749. [CrossRef]
19. Madhunapantula, S.V.; Desai, D.; Sharma, A.; Huh, S.J.; Amin, S.; Robertson, G.P. PBISe, a novel selenium-containing drug for the treatment of malignant melanoma. *Mol. Cancer Ther.* **2008**, *7*, 1297–1308. [CrossRef]
20. Karelia, D.N.; Sk, U.H.; Singh, P.; Gowda, A.S.P.; Pandey, M.K.; Ramisetti, S.R.; Amin, S.; Sharma, A.K. Design, synthesis, and identification of a novel napthalamide-isoselenocyanate compound NISC-6 as a dual Topoisomerase-IIalpha and Akt pathway inhibitor, and evaluation of its anti-melanoma activity. *Eur. J. Med. Chem.* **2017**, *135*, 282–295. [CrossRef]
21. Chung, C.Y.; Madhunapantula, S.V.; Desai, D.; Amin, S.; Robertson, G.P. Melanoma prevention using topical PBISe. *Cancer Prev. Res.* **2011** *4*, 935–948. [CrossRef] [PubMed]

22. Alcolea, V.; Plano, D.; Karelia, D.N.; Palop, J.A.; Amin, S.; Sanmartin, C.; Sharma, A.K. Novel seleno- and thio-urea derivatives with potent in vitro activities against several cancer cell lines. *Eur. J. Med. Chem.* **2016**, *113*, 134–144. [CrossRef] [PubMed]

23. Ibanez, E.; Plano, D.; Font, M.; Calvo, A.; Prior, C.; Palop, J.A.; Sanmartin, C. Synthesis and antiproliferative activity of novel symmetrical alkylthio- and alkylseleno-imidocarbamates. *Eur. J. Med. Chem.* **2011**, *46*, 265–274. [CrossRef] [PubMed]

24. Alcolea, V.; Plano, D.; Encio, I.; Palop, J.A.; Sharma, A.K.; Sanmartin, C. Chalcogen containing heterocyclic scaffolds: New hybrids with antitumoral activity. *Eur. J. Med. Chem.* **2016**, *123*, 407–418. [CrossRef] [PubMed]

25. van Engeland, M.; Nieland, L.J.; Ramaekers, F.C.; Schutte, B.; Reutelingsperger, C.P. Annexin V-affinity assay: A review on an apoptosis detection system based on phosphatidylserine exposure. *Cytometry* **1998**, *31*, 1–9. [CrossRef]

26. Stahl, J.M.; Sharma, A.; Cheung, M.; Zimmerman, M.; Cheng, J.Q.; Bosenberg, M.W.; Kester, M.; Sandirasegarane, L.; Robertson, G.P. Deregulated Akt3 activity promotes development of malignant melanoma. *Cancer Res.* **2004**, *64*, 7002–7010. [CrossRef] [PubMed]

27. Zhang, X.D.; Borrow, J.M.; Zhang, X.Y.; Nguyen, T.; Hersey, P. Activation of ERK1/2 protects melanoma cells from TRAIL-induced apoptosis by inhibiting Smac/DIABLO release from mitochondria. *Oncogene* **2003**, *22*, 2869–2881. [CrossRef] [PubMed]

28. Fofaria, N.M.; Srivastava, S.K. Critical role of STAT3 in melanoma metastasis through anoikis resistance. *Oncotarget* **2014**, *5*, 7051–7064. [CrossRef] [PubMed]

29. Kiuchi, N.; Nakajima, K.; Ichiba, M.; Fukada, T.; Narimatsu, M.; Mizuno, K.; Hibi, M.; Hirano, T. STAT3 is required for the gp130-mediated full activation of the c-myc gene. *J. Exp. Med.* **1999**, *189*, 63–73. [CrossRef]

30. Ishdorj, G.; Johnston, J.B.; Gibson, S.B. Inhibition of constitutive activation of STAT3 by curcurbitacin-I (JSI-124) sensitized human B-leukemia cells to apoptosis. *Mol. Cancer Ther.* **2010**, *9*, 3302–3314. [CrossRef]

31. Soldani, C.; Scovassi, A.I. Poly(ADP-ribose) polymerase-1 cleavage during apoptosis: An update. *Apoptosis* **2002**, *7*, 321–328. [CrossRef] [PubMed]

32. Coqueret, O.; Gascan, H. Functional interaction of STAT3 transcription factor with the cell cycle inhibitor p21WAF1/CIP1/SDI1. *J. Biol. Chem.* **2000**, *275*, 18794–18800. [CrossRef] [PubMed]

33. Becker, S.; Groner, B.; Muller, C.W. Three-dimensional structure of the Stat3beta homodimer bound to DNA. *Nature* **1998**, *394*, 145–151. [CrossRef] [PubMed]

34. Wu, G.; Robertson, D.H.; Brooks, C.L., 3rd; Vieth, M. Detailed analysis of grid-based molecular docking: A case study of CDOCKER-A CHARMm-based MD docking algorithm. *J. Comput. Chem.* **2003**, *24*, 1549–1562. [CrossRef] [PubMed]

35. Wang, Y.; Ren, X.; Deng, C.; Yang, L.; Yan, E.; Guo, T.; Li, Y.; Xu, M.X. Mechanism of the inhibition of the STAT3 signaling pathway by EGCG. *Oncol. Rep.* **2013**, *30*, 2691–2696. [CrossRef] [PubMed]

36. Zhang, T.; Kee, W.H.; Seow, K.T.; Fung, W.; Cao, X. The coiled-coil domain of Stat3 is essential for its SH2 domain-mediated receptor binding and subsequent activation induced by epidermal growth factor and interleukin-6. *Mol. Cell. Biol.* **2000**, *20*, 7132–7139. [CrossRef] [PubMed]

37. Yu, W.; Xiao, H.; Lin, J.; Li, C. Discovery of novel STAT3 small molecule inhibitors via in silico site-directed fragment-based drug design. *J. Med. Chem.* **2013**, *56*, 4402–4412. [CrossRef]

38. Bhasin, D.; Cisek, K.; Pandharkar, T.; Regan, N.; Li, C.; Pandit, B.; Lin, J.; Li, P.K. Design, synthesis, and studies of small molecule STAT3 inhibitors. *Bioorg. Med. Chem. Lett.* **2008**, *18*, 391–395. [CrossRef]

39. Tsai, J.; Lee, J.T.; Wang, W.; Zhang, J.; Cho, H.; Mamo, S.; Bremer, R.; Gillette, S.; Kong, J.; Haass, N.K.; et al. Discovery of a selective inhibitor of oncogenic B-Raf kinase with potent antimelanoma activity. *Proc. Natl. Acad. Sci. USA* **2008**, *105*, 3041–3046. [CrossRef]

40. Sanmartin, C.; Plano, D.; Palop, J.A. Selenium compounds and apoptotic modulation: A new perspective in cancer therapy. *Mini Rev. Med. Chem.* **2008**, *8*, 1020–1031. [CrossRef]

41. Tagaram, H.R.; Desai, D.; Li, G.; Liu, D.; Rountree, C.B.; Gowda, K.; Berg, A.; Amin, S.; Staveley-O'Carroll, K.F.; Kimchi, E.T. A Selenium Containing Inhibitor for the Treatment of Hepatocellular Cancer. *Pharmaceuticals* **2016**, *9*, 18. [CrossRef] [PubMed]

42. Thomas, S.J.; Snowden, J.A.; Zeidler, M.P.; Danson, S.J. The role of JAK/STAT signalling in the pathogenesis, prognosis and treatment of solid tumours. *Br. J. Cancer* **2015**, *113*, 365–371. [CrossRef] [PubMed]

43. Girotti, M.R.; Pedersen, M.; Sanchez-Laorden, B.; Viros, A.; Turajlic, S.; Niculescu-Duvaz, D.; Zambon, A.; Sinclair, J.; Hayes, A.; Gore, M.; et al. Inhibiting EGF receptor or SRC family kinase signaling overcomes BRAF inhibitor resistance in melanoma. *Cancer Discov.* **2013**, *3*, 158–167. [CrossRef] [PubMed]
44. Zuazo, A.; Plano, D.; Anso, E.; Lizarraga, E.; Font, M.; Martinez Irujo, J.J. Cytotoxic and proapototic activities of imidoselenocarbamate derivatives are dependent on the release of methylselenol. *Chem. Res. Toxicol.* **2012**, *25*, 2479–2489. [CrossRef] [PubMed]

6

Overview of Radiolabeled Somatostatin Analogs for Cancer Imaging and Therapy

Romain Eychenne [1,2,3], Christelle Bouvry [4,5], Mickael Bourgeois [2,3], Pascal Loyer [6], Eric Benoist [1] and Nicolas Lepareur [4,6,*]

1 UPS, CNRS, SPCMIB (Laboratoire de Synthèse et Physico-Chimie de Molécules d'Intérêt Biologique)—UMR 5068, Université de Toulouse, F-31062 Toulouse, France; eychenne@arronax-nantes.fr (R.E.); benoist@chimie.ups-tlse.fr (E.B.)
2 Groupement d'Intérêt Public ARRONAX, 1 Rue Aronnax, F-44817 Saint Herblain, France; mickael.bourgeois@univ-nantes.fr
3 CNRS, CRCINA (Centre de Recherche en Cancérologie et Immunologie Nantes—Angers)—UMR 1232, ERL 6001, Inserm, Université de Nantes, F-44000 Nantes, France
4 Comprehensive Cancer Center Eugène Marquis, Rennes, F-35000, France; c.bouvry@rennes.unicancer.fr
5 CNRS, ISCR (Institut des Sciences Chimiques de Rennes)—UMR 6226, Univ Rennes, F-35000 Rennes, France
6 INRAE, Institut NUMECAN (Nutrition, Métabolismes et Cancer)—UMR_A 1341, UMR_S 1241, Inserm, Univ Rennes, F-35000 Rennes, France; pascal.loyer@univ-rennes1.fr
* Correspondence: n.lepareur@rennes.unicancer.fr

Abstract: Identified in 1973, somatostatin (SST) is a cyclic hormone peptide with a short biological half-life. Somatostatin receptors (SSTRs) are widely expressed in the whole body, with five subtypes described. The interaction between SST and its receptors leads to the internalization of the ligand–receptor complex and triggers different cellular signaling pathways. Interestingly, the expression of SSTRs is significantly enhanced in many solid tumors, especially gastro-entero-pancreatic neuroendocrine tumors (GEP-NET). Thus, somatostatin analogs (SSAs) have been developed to improve the stability of the endogenous ligand and so extend its half-life. Radiolabeled analogs have been developed with several radioelements such as indium-111, technetium-99 m, and recently gallium-68, fluorine-18, and copper-64, to visualize the distribution of receptor overexpression in tumors. Internal metabolic radiotherapy is also used as a therapeutic strategy (e.g., using yttrium-90, lutetium-177, and actinium-225). With some radiopharmaceuticals now used in clinical practice, somatostatin analogs developed for imaging and therapy are an example of the concept of personalized medicine with a theranostic approach. Here, we review the development of these analogs, from the well-established and authorized ones to the most recently developed radiotracers, which have better pharmacokinetic properties and demonstrate increased efficacy and safety, as well as the search for new clinical indications.

Keywords: somatostatin analogs; radiolabeling; radiopharmaceuticals; radionuclide therapy; imaging

1. Introduction

Somatostatin (SST), also called somatotropin release inhibiting factor (SRIF), is a cyclic peptide hormone, first isolated in 1968 from an ovine hypothalamus, and actually identified in 1973 [1]. It was originally discovered as a growth hormone inhibitor, but is now known to be involved in the inhibition of numerous metabolic processes relating to neurotransmitters, endocrine secretions (e.g., growth hormone, insulin, glucagon, and gastrin) but also modulating exocrine secretions (e.g., gastric acid and pancreatic enzymes). In the body, its synthesis takes place in the form of an inactive precursor of 116 amino acids (AA), preprosomatostatin, which is then converted by the action of proteases into prosomatostatin (96 AA). Depending on where it is produced in the body, enzymes do not cleave the pro-peptide on the same amino acid motif, resulting in two distinct active forms, SRIF-28 and SRIF-14. Although SRIF-14 is predominant in the central nervous system and SRIF-28 in the digestive tract, the distribution of these two biologically active forms is similar.

In the early 1990s, concomitantly to studies on the binding properties and mechanisms of action of somatostatin, five receptor subtypes were discovered (SSTR1 to SSTR5) [2]. These subtypes belong to the family of receptors coupled to G-proteins, and their length varies from 364 to 418 AA. They all exhibit seven α helices with transmembrane domains and most of the differences between subtypes are found in the extracellular (N-terminal) and intracellular (C-terminal) ends. SSTR-1, -3, -4, and -5 have a single subtype, while two variants exist for SSTR2, called SSTR2A and SSTR2B. SSTR1 to 4 link SRIF-14 and -28 with a very high affinity (in the nanomolar order), whereas SSTR5 shows an affinity 5 to 10 times higher, but for SRIF-28 only.

Somatostatin receptors are widely distributed in healthy tissues, with distinct expression throughout the body (Figure 1). It is quite possible to find several subtypes in the same tissue. Each of the SSTRs is involved in the regulation of the various processes: (i) SSTR1 is involved in the antisecretory effects of growth hormone, prolactin (a peptide hormone involved in lactation, reproduction, growth, and immunity) and calcitonin (regulation of calcemia); (ii) SSTR2 also inhibits the secretion of growth hormone and adrenocorticotropin (hormone that stimulates the adrenal glands), glucagon, insulin, interferon-γ (protein produced by immune cells), and stomach acid; (iii) SSTR5 has the same inhibiting effect on growth hormone, adrenocorticotropin, insulin, and inhibits the secretion of amylase (digestive enzyme constituting saliva and pancreatic juice); (iv) SSTR3 reduces cell proliferation and causes cell apoptosis; (v) the functions of SSTR4 are not yet well defined [3].

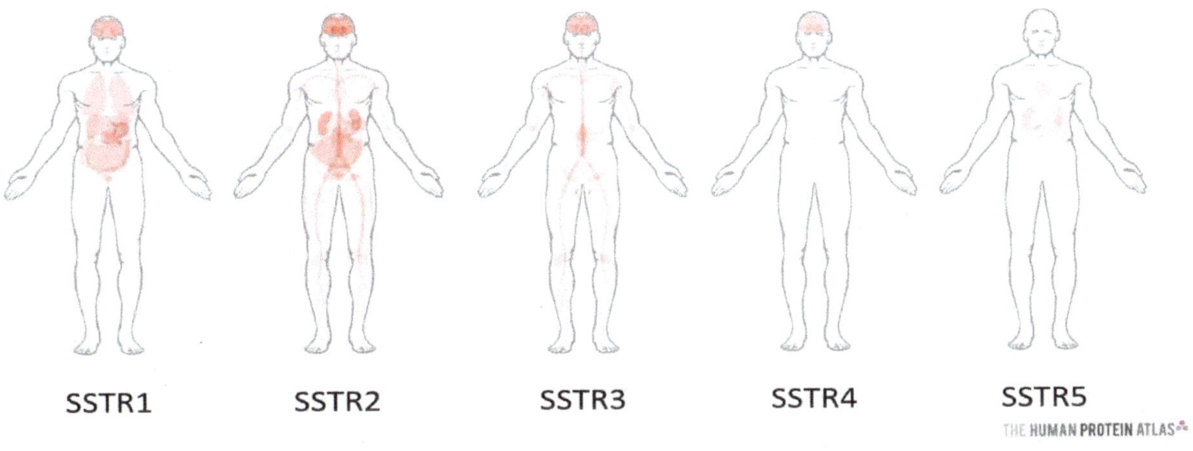

Figure 1. Somatostatin receptors (SSTRs) biodistribution in the body (from The Human Protein Atlas https://www.proteinatlas.org/).

The effects of somatostatin are expressed through different signaling pathways [4,5]. After a cascade of reactions, this leads on the one hand to the inhibition of tumor growth (action on the secretion of hormones) and blocking proliferation via the activation of different tyrosine phosphatases (anti-proliferative and pro-apoptotic action), but also to the inhibition of the secretion of growth factors such as growth hormone or IGF-1 having a major role in the inhibition of tumor growth (anti-angiogenic) (Figure 2) [6,7].

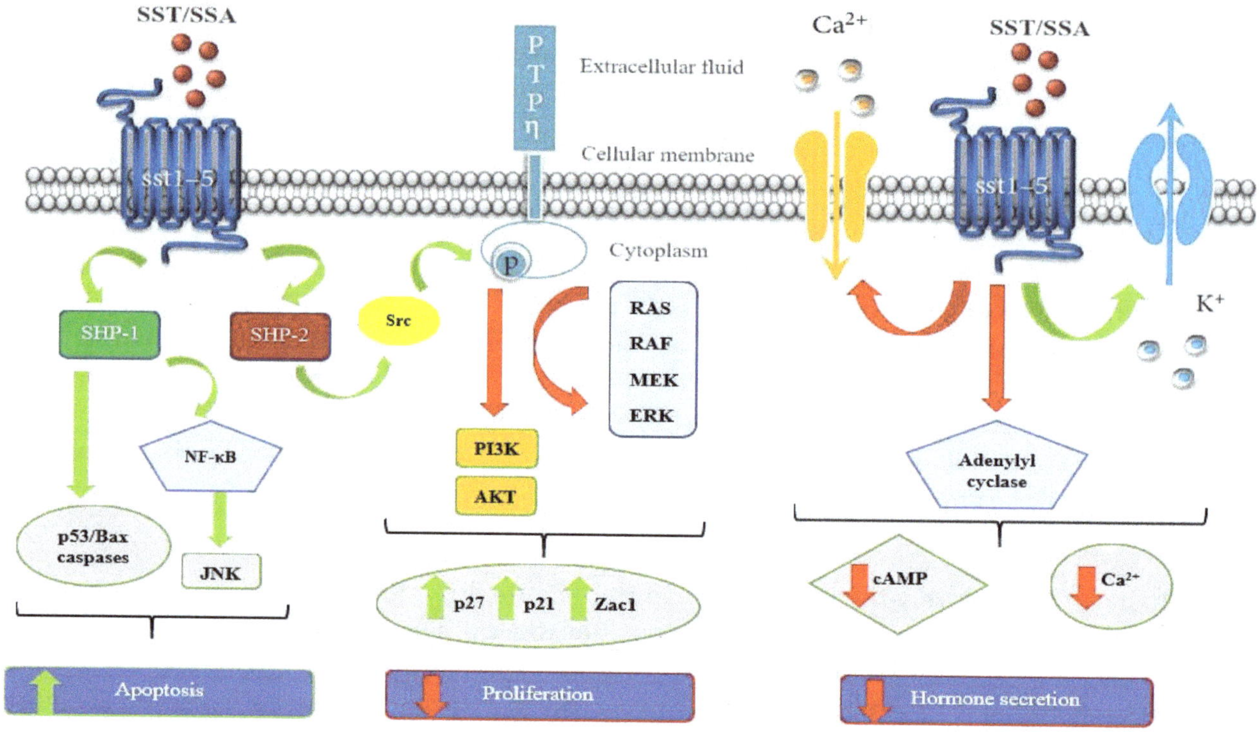

Figure 2. Schematic representation of the signaling pathways induced by somatostatin receptors activation. Green arrows: activated pathways; red arrows: inhibited pathways. Adapted from [8].

Over the past 20 years, our understanding of the phenomena due to the activation of SSTRs has increased thanks to numerous translational and clinical studies, leading to the development of new therapeutic options [3]. The use of SST analogs has demonstrated real effectiveness in the treatment of various pathologies: acromegaly (production of an excess of growth hormone), pancreatitis, complications linked to diabetes and obesity (e.g., retinopathy or nephropathy), action on inflammation and pain in some cases [5,9]. However, SSTRs and SST analogs are mainly known for their presence and role in the detection and treatment of some solid tumors. Tumor cells and peritumoral vessels express receptor subtypes whose density depends on the type of tumors (Table 1) [10–13]. For those overexpressing SSTRs, such as pituitary adenomas, gastroentero-pancreatic neuroendocrine tumors (GEP-NET), or other cancers (e.g., lymphomas, small cell lung cancers, etc.), targeting with SST analogs becomes possible [14]. Many therapeutic protocols based on these analogs (classic octreotide or with a longer release time (octreotide LAR), Lanreotide, Vapreotide, Pasireotide, etc.) have been the subject of phase II and III clinical trials. The majority of results were generally disappointing and did not provide clear evidence of a significant antitumor effect on solid tumors, probably due to the existence of other pathways of tumor progression [15,16].

Table 1. SSTRs expression in different tumor types.

Tumor Type	SSTR Expression	Ref
Astrocytoma	+	[17]
Breast carcinoma	+ (SSTR2)	[11]
Cholangiocarcinoma	+ (SSTR2)	[18]
Colorectal carcinoma	-	[17]
Endometrial carcinoma	-	[17]
Ependymoma	+ (SSTR1, SSTR5)	[11]
Esophageal carcinoma	-	[17]
Ewing sarcoma	-	[17]
Exocrine pancreatic tumor	-	[17]
Gastric carcinoma	+ (SSTR1 > SSTR2, SSTR5)	[11]
Gastrinoma	+ (SSTR2)	[17]
Glioblastoma	-	[17]

Table 1. *Cont.*

Tumor Type	SSTR Expression	Ref
Growth hormone-producing pituitary adenoma	**+** (SSTR2, SSTR5)	[17]
Gut carcinoid	**+** (SSTR2 > SSTR1, SSTR5)	[17]
Hepatocellular carcinoma	+ (SSTR2, SSTR5)	[19]
Insulinoma	+ (SSTR1, SSTR2, SSTR3)	[20]
Leiomyoma	+	[17]
Lymphoma	+ (SSTR2)	[11]
Medullary thyroid carcinoma	+ (SSTR2)	[11]
Medulloblastoma	**+** (SSTR2)	[17]
Meningioma	**+** (SSTR2)	[17]
Neuroblastoma	**+** (SSTR2)	[17]
Non-functioning pituitary adenoma	+ (SSTR3 > SSTR2)	[17]
Non-small cell lung cancer	-	[17]
Ovarian carcinoma	+	[17]
Paraganglioma	**+** (SSTR2)	[17]
Pheochromocytoma	**+** (SSTR1, SSTR2)	[17]
Prostate carcinoma	+ (SSTR1)	[17]
Renal cell carcinoma	+ (SSTR2)	[11]
Small cell lung cancer	+ (SSTR2)	[17]
Urinary bladder carcinoma	-	[17]

Bold +, receptors with particularly high density and incidence. Subtypes preferentially expressed are listed in parentheses, only when compelling evidence is available (immunohistochemistry or autoradiography). Adapted from [11] and [17].

For example, regarding liver tumors, such as hepatocellular carcinoma (HCC), in vitro studies clearly demonstrated (i) the lack of SSTRs expression in healthy liver cells; (ii) overexpression in tumors and metastases of HCC, even though their density is less than in neuroendocrine tumors [21,22]. On the other hand, the results show a heterogeneous expression and strong inter-individual differences. In fact, according to studies, HCCs express high levels of SSTR2 [21,23,24] or SSTR5 [13,19], or even SSTR1 [22] or SSTR3 [25]. In general, around 40% of HCCs studied express somatostatin receptors. These differences could be due to the different methodologies used during the measurements, by studying different stages of the disease or even by heterogeneous behaviors of HCC. Further studies have also found a correlation between the density of SSTRs expression, disease aggressiveness [26], and the rate of tumor recurrence after treatment with octreotide LAR [27]. In a study by Nguyen-Khac et al. [23], 41.2% of extrahepatic metastases express SSTR2. Preclinical tests on HCC cell lines have shown an antiproliferative effect of SST analogs [25,28]. In addition, a real decrease in invasion and cell migration of HCC cells after stimulation of SSTR1 by a specific agonist has also been demonstrated [22]. This action has also been confirmed in vivo [29], with the demonstration of a similar effect on metastatic dissemination [23,30]. These initial results paved the way for clinical trials on patients with HCC, but their conclusions are quite contradictory, [31] showing rather positive effects in the advanced stages [32,33] and others quite negative [34,35]. These outcome discrepancies could come from heterogeneity in the choice of patients, but available data are still insufficient to truly conclude on the effectiveness of analogs of SST alone in the control of HCC tumors [6,31,36]. Cholangiocarcinoma, the other main primary liver tumor, might also be a potential target [18,37].

On the other hand, in certain cases, and in particular for neuroendocrine tumors (a category of tumors where SSTRs are the most expressed), a benefit has been proven via two Phase III studies, which have greatly contributed to the fact that SST analogs are now used in clinical routine [38,39].

2. Somatostatin Analogs

Somatostatin has a short half-life in the body (between one and three minutes), because it is rapidly degraded by peptidases found in plasma and tissues [40]. Therefore, the amount present in the bloodstream is extremely low (between 14 and 32.5 pg/mL). This very short half-life has been considered a limiting factor for possible clinical applications, thus many analogs with better metabolic properties (longer half-life between 1.5 h and 12 h) have been rapidly developed [2,5,9]. These are most often hexapeptide or octapeptide molecules which incorporate the biologically active core of native somatostatin (see some examples in Figure 3). Indeed, studies on the structure–activity correlation have shown that the Phe^7, Trp^8, Lys^9, and Thr^{10} sequence in the form of a β-sheet is necessary for biological activity. The residues Trp^8 and Lys^9 are essential for this activity, whereas Phe^7 and Thr^{10} may undergo some substitutions. Among somatostatin analogs, there are two main categories: the agonists (substances capable of activating somatostatin receptors) and the antagonists (molecules that interact with somatostatin receptors and block or reduce the physiological effect of an agonist). It is also important to note that somatostatin analogs have different affinities for the different receptor subtypes [2].

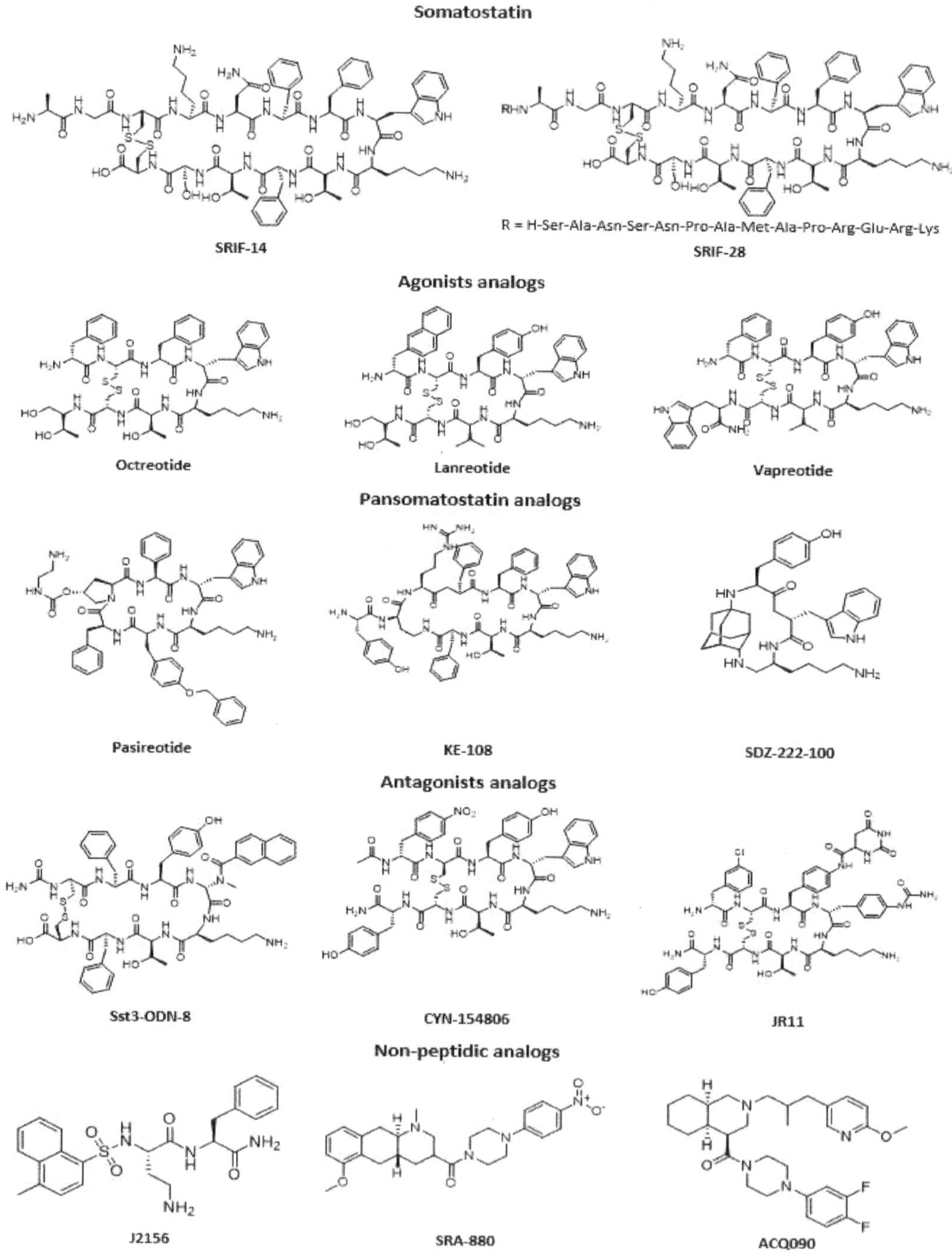

Figure 3. Chemical structures of SRIF-14, SRIF-28, and selected examples of somatostatin analogs.

The first agonist peptide analog to be approved by the FDA was octreotide (SMS 201-995), marketed under the name Sandostatin®. From a structural point of view, it has a D-Trp and a D-Phe, to stabilize the β-sheet and a disulfide bridge closer to the active core, for a better metabolic stability. Its pharmacodynamics is highly similar to native SST, which has made it widely used in clinical trials for the treatment of GEP (gastro-entero-pancreatic) tumors [41,42]. Next, Lanreotide (BIM 23014, tradename Somatuline®), whose structure is similar to that of octreotide (Phe and Thr having been replaced by Tyr and Val respectively), showed comparable characteristics and is also widely used in the treatment of neuroendocrine tumors [43]. In 2005, another analog, Vapreotide (RC160), was marketed under the name Sanvar®, with properties close to those of the two previous analogs, and is also used for the treatment of esophageal varices. More recently, Pasireotide (SOM-230 or Signifor®) was one of the first analogs to show a strong affinity for most of the somatostatin receptor subtypes (pansomatostatin analog). Marketed by Novartis, it is used for the treatment of Cushing's disease [44]. Many other analogs have been developed, from "ultra-short" peptides, such as SDZ 222-100 (an adamantine cyclopeptide), to longer ones, such as KE-108 or CH-275 [5]. Regarding antagonist peptide analogs, the wide variety of compounds that the octapeptide model can offer has allowed the discovery of several structures that can block this kind of receptors. The first antagonist that has been described in the literature is CYN-154806, followed by PRL-2970, sst3-ODN-8 or even non-cyclic models such as BIM-23056 and BIM-23627. New non-peptide compounds have also emerged [45]. These agonists and antagonists (selective or not) constitute a very promising field in the chemistry of somatostatin analogs, in particular because of their pharmacological, pharmacokinetic, and physicochemical properties. This type of compound may have a stronger affinity and/or selectivity for certain subtypes of somatostatin receptors than the majority of peptide analogs. They can thus provide additional information on the exact role of each of these subtypes [5,9].

3. Targeting of Somatostatin Receptors with Radiopharmaceuticals

In the field of medicine, much research is focused on finding methods to achieve earlier detection of pathologies to allow treatment at early stages of the disease, to increase the chances of total recovery. For this purpose, nuclear medicine, through the use of radiopharmaceuticals, is a very powerful tool. Its application can have two different aims: imaging, with the visualization of a radioactive element's distribution in the body, or therapy, with specific irradiation of abnormal cells, thereby reducing damages to nearby healthy tissue. Having a broad range of potential biological targets and desirable pharmacokinetic characteristics—such as high uptake in target tissue and fast blood and non-target tissue clearance—peptides can also be easily chemically modified for incorporation into a radiopharmaceutical, making them a very potent targeting vector for nuclear medicine. Research in that domain has thus gained widespread interest [46–49]. These compounds can be directly labeled with a radionuclide, such as a halogen radioisotope, but they are generally based on a triple structure involving: (i) a radiometal, the radiation of which allows either the localization (γ and β^+ emitters) or the destruction (β^-, α or Auger electron emitters) of the targeted cells; (ii) a bifunctional chelating agent (BFCA), the dual role of which is not only to bind the radiometal in a very stable manner to minimize its dissociation in vivo, but also to allow its conjugation with targeting moiety (or vector) via a functionalized arm; (iii) a targeting moiety (the peptide analog), which aims to convey this set in a specific way to a well-defined target. To limit the influence of the chelating moiety, a linker (or spacer) is usually inserted between the BFCA and the biomolecule (Figure 4).

The choice of the radiometal is crucial, since it deeply influences the design of the chelating structure [50–53]. Several criteria govern the choice of radionuclide: (i) the nature of the radiation emitted, depending on the intended application (diagnosis or therapy); (ii) the half-life, which must be long enough to allow effective fixation of the radiotracer on the target cells, but relatively short to avoid irradiation of the organism (neighboring healthy tissues) and more specifically non-targeted organs; (iii) the isotope decay profile. By emitting its radiation, the nuclide disintegrates into a daughter nuclide, which must be non-radioactive to avoid any additional harmfulness to the organism; (iv) the means of production. Most of the radioelements used in nuclear medicine are artificial. They can be produced in three different ways: from a nuclear reactor, a cyclotron or via a generator. Generator production remains the most convenient way for clinical application, as it can provide in-house radionuclides when a cyclotron is not available nearby, but cyclotron production still remains the cheapest and most used. As an example, Table 2 shows some of the characteristics of radioactive nuclides among the most used today for the radiolabeling of peptides.

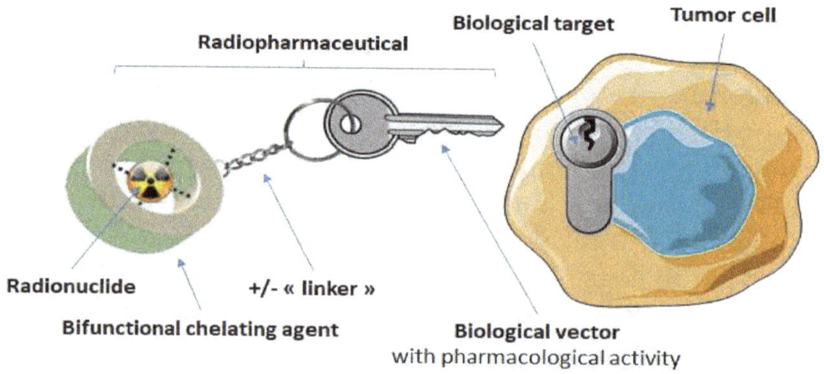

Figure 4. Schematic design of a radiometallated bioconjugate.

Table 2. Some of the main radionuclides studied for imaging and therapy (SPECT—Single-Photon Emission Computed Tomography; PET—Positron Emission Tomography).

Radionuclide	Half-Life (h)	Type of Emission	Energy of Emitted Radiation (keV)	Source	Application
^{99m}Tc	6.01	γ	140	Generator	SPECT imaging
^{111}In	67.4	γ	172, 245	Cyclotron	SPECT imaging
^{18}F	1.83	β^+	634	Cyclotron	PET imaging
^{64}Cu	12.7	$\beta^+/\gamma/\beta^-$	653	Cyclotron	PET imaging
^{68}Ga	1.1	β^+	1190	Generator/Cyclotron	PET imaging
^{90}Y	64.1	β^-	2284	Generator	Therapy
^{177}Lu	160.8	β^-/γ	497	Cyclotron	Therapy
^{188}Re	17	β^-/γ	2118	Generator	Therapy
^{211}At	7.2	α	5870	Cyclotron	Therapy
^{225}Ac	238	α	5830	Generator	Therapy

From a structural point of view, each radiometal has its own properties such as polarizability, degree of oxidation, or coordination number. These features have a direct impact on the choice of the bifunctional chelating agent, in particular in terms of denticity and nature of the donor atoms (most often *O*-, *N*-, or *S*-donors) [54,55]. The BFCA makes it possible to link the biomolecule and the radiometal; its choice is a crucial step in the construction of a radiopharmaceutical. As indicated above, this structure plays a double role: the first is to complex the radioelement in a very stable manner. Several criteria can be evaluated to truly attest to the stability of the complex formed. First of all, the formed radiocomplex must be thermodynamically stable, i.e., the metal-ligand affinity must be as strong as possible. Then it must be kinetically inert. Many metalation reactions take place in the body and the complex formed must be stable enough to avoid any in vivo degradation (e.g., demetallation or transchelation). In addition, radiolabeling conditions with low concentrations are required, ideally with efficient complexation kinetics (high labeling yield) and fast and mild reaction conditions. Beside chemistry considerations, the radiotracer must have: (i) a strong affinity for the target receptor; (ii) a high accumulation for the target and low for the non-target organs; (iii) relatively rapid clearance in the organism; (iv) preferably a mainly renal route of excretion.

Chelating ligands used for the design of radiotracers are usually classified into two categories: macrocyclic and acyclic compounds (Figure 5). Generally, acyclic ligands are less kinetically inert than macrocycles, although some may have shown very good characteristics. On the other hand, these ligands generally have faster metal-chelate binding kinetics compared to macrocyclic analogs, which represents a huge advantage for working with isotopes that have a short lifespan. Despite the coordination properties specific to each metal, some chelating agents—such as polyaminopolycarboxylic acids—are considered to be 'universal' because they can complex different radiometals.

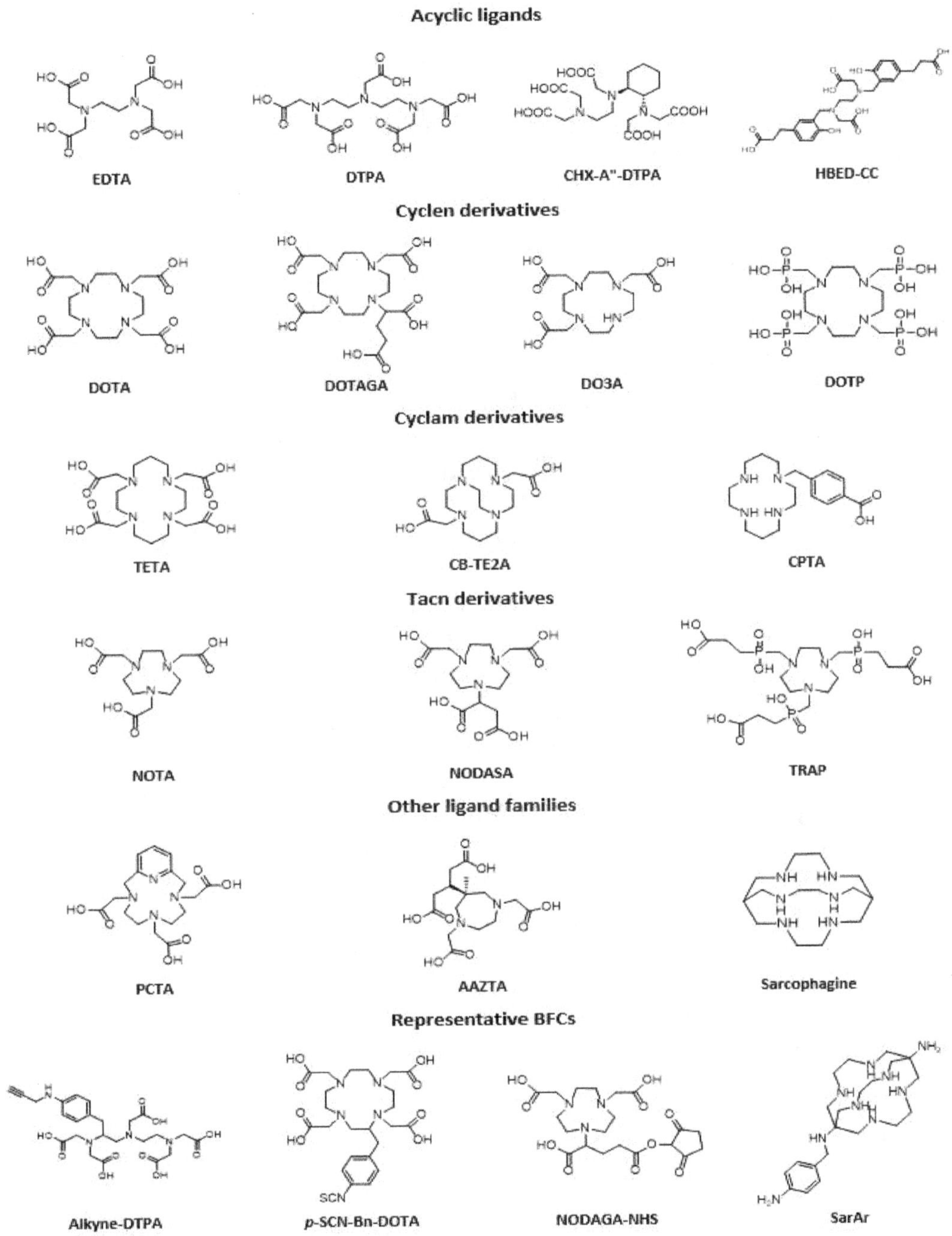

Figure 5. Representative (but not exhaustive) examples of acyclic and macrocyclic polyamino and polyaminocarboxylic chelator families and their derivatives.

Among acyclic ligands, the first BFCAs developed were EDTA (ethylenediaminetetraacetic acid) and DTPA (diethylenetriaminepentaacetic acid). They have been widely used in the chemistry of radiopharmaceuticals, in particular with radioelements such as ^{111}In, ^{90}Y or ^{177}Lu, and even ^{99m}Tc [54]. Later on, DTPA derivatives such as CHX-A''-DTPA with a cyclohexyl moiety bringing more rigidity to the DTPA backbone (allowing a pre-organization of the system) showed better kinetic inertia [56]. Regarding cyclic compounds, cyclen derivatives such as DOTA (1,4,7,10-tetraazacyclododecane-1,4,7,10-tetraacetic acid) and triaza analogs—NOTA (1,4,7-triazacyclononane-1,4,7-triacetic acid)—are among the most studied ligands. NOTA has the smaller chelating cavity of the two, and is generally used for Ga (III) or Cu (II) because it has a particular attraction for these metals, which results in mild radiolabeling conditions and good in vivo stability of the complexes formed. DOTA (which is considered as the gold standard chelator) and its derivatives play an important role in clinical applications because they form very stable complexes with a wide range of trivalent radiometals such as Ga (III), Y (III), In (III), Lu (III), or even divalent such as Cu (II) [57,58]. For DOTA or NOTA, the introduction of a functionalized arm offers the possibility of coupling a biomolecule (NODASA/NODAGA and DOTASA/DOTAGA). Similarly, TETA (1,4,8,11-tetraazacyclotetradecane-1,4,8,11-tetraacetic acid), has mainly been studied with Cu (II) and have shown a stability similar to DOTA [59].

Whether on the side of macrocyclic ligands, derivatives or variations of DOTA (e.g., p-SCN-Bn-DOTA, DOTAGA, CB-DO2A, TCMC …), NOTA (e.g., p-SCN-Bn-NOTA, NETA …), or TETA (e.g., CB-TE2A, p-NH2-Bn-TE3A …), or on the side of acyclic ligands, derivatives or variations of DTPA (e.g., CHX-A′′-DTPA …), a large number of ligands have been developed so far. A wide choice of ligands is available for the design of new agents, and numerous journals have described and carefully classified all the structures that can be used in the design of a radiopharmaceutical, whatever the intended application [46,51,53,54,57,60].

BFCA's second role is to allow the conjugation of the complex with a biomolecule. The nature of this link is very important, because it is essential for it to be stable, and above all, for it to not interfere in any way with the binding to the receiver. The slightest structural modification of the ligand and/or of the biomolecule can have a very marked effect on the affinity to the targeted receptors. To minimize this impact as much as possible, that sometimes a 'spacer' or 'linker' can be used between these two entities. Biomolecules are often functionalized through a primary amine, which provides an ideal conjugation site for a coupling reaction, most often with peptide or thiourea type links. Other links based on thioether, triazole, oxime, or more recently via a copper-free click-chemistry with tetrazine/cyclooctyne may prove to be interesting, in particular, because they have very good stability in vivo [51,54,61].

Many somatostatin analogs have already been labeled with various radioelements, whether for imaging, with probes used today in clinical applications, or for therapy, with many compounds in clinical studies [17,61–63]. These analogs were obtained from modifications in the sequence of amino acids that make up the peptide. For example, replacing Phe^3 in octreotide (OC) with Tyr^3 (TOC) improves the affinity for SSTRs (in particular SSTR2) and introduction of a Thr (TATE) instead of Thr(ol) (TOC) further improves this. By following this procedure, many analogs have been developed and studied, often with the same chelating cavity to be able to compare their properties (Table 3) [64,65].

Table 3. Peptidic sequences of the main somatostatin agonist analogs. Differences towards Octreotide (OC) are highlighted in red.

Peptide	Peptidic Sequence
OC Octreotide	D-Phe^1-cyclo(Cys^2-Phe^3-D-Trp^4-Lys^5-Thr^6-Cys^7)$Thr(ol)^8$
LAN Lanreotide	β-D-Nal^1-cyclo(Cys^2-Tyr^3-D-Trp^4-Lys^5-Val^6-Cys^7)Thr^8-NH_2
VAP Vapreotide	D-Phe^1-cyclo(Cys^2-Phe^3-D-Trp^4-Lys^5-Val^6-Cys^7)Trp^8-NH_2
TOC [Tyr^3]-Octreotide	D-Phe^1-cyclo(Cys^2-Tyr^3-D-Trp^4-Lys^5-Thr^6-Cys^7)$Thr(ol)^8$
TATE [Tyr^3]-Octreotate	D-Phe^1-cyclo(Cys^2-Tyr^3-D-Trp^4-Lys^5-Thr^6-Cys^7)Thr^8
NOC [1-Nal^3]-Octreotide	D-Phe^1-cyclo(Cys^2-1-Nal^3-D-Trp^4-Lys^5-Thr^6-Cys^7)$Thr(ol)^8$
NOC-ATE [1-Nal^3, Thr^8]-Octreotide	D-Phe^1-cyclo(Cys^2-1-Nal^3-D-Trp^4-Lys^5-Thr^6-Cys^7)Thr^8
BOC [$BzThi^3$]-Octreotide	D-Phe^1-cyclo(Cys^2-$BzThi^3$-D-Trp^4-Lys^5-Thr^6-Cys^7)$Thr(ol)^8$
BOC-ATE [$BzThi^3$, Thr^8]-Octreotide	D-Phe^1-cyclo(Cys^2-$BzThi^3$-D-Trp^4-Lys^5-Thr^6-Cys^7)Thr^8

3.1. Radiolabeled Somatostatin Analogs for Imaging

The very first proof of concept for the visualization of tumors expressing SSTRs was carried out with [^{123}I-Tyr^{3}]-octreotide, obtained from an iodination reaction (electrophilic substitution) of tyrosine [66,67]. This compound demonstrated biological activity and an affinity for receptors similar to those of native SST [68]. Despite the obvious interest of this probe, several factors such as the difficult radiolabeling procedure, the significant cost, and particularly, the clearance via the liver and the hepatobiliary system (which makes it difficult to interpret the obtained images) were the main drawbacks of its application [67]. To overcome all of these disadvantages, iodine-123 has been replaced with indium-111, which, through the chelating agent DTPA, has been coupled to octreotide (Figure 6) [69]. In vivo studies of [^{111}In-DTPA^{0}]-octreotide ([^{111}In]-pentetreotide) have shown that it is possible to visualize tumors expressing SSTRs and their metastases, even 24 h after injection. In comparison with the compounds coupled to antibodies, this reveals a relatively rapid clearance via the kidneys, which represents a huge advantage compared to [^{123}I-Tyr^{3}]-octreotide [70,71]. This compound was the first radiopharmaceutical targeting SSTRs to be approved by the FDA (Octreoscan® marketed in 1994). It has been widely used, and has long been considered a 'gold standard' for the visualization of neuroendocrine tumors. It still has a few limits: in fact, it requires a high tumor/noise intensity ratio, shows low spatial resolution, has a moderate affinity for receptors and finally, and possesses a high γ energy which results in a high dose of radioactivity received by the patient. For all these reasons, research in the field of radiopharmaceuticals has focused on other radioelements such as technetium-99m for SPECT and gallium-68 for PET. In addition to having excellent physical properties, these two elements are available from a commercial clinical-grade generator, an important advantage for clinical applications.

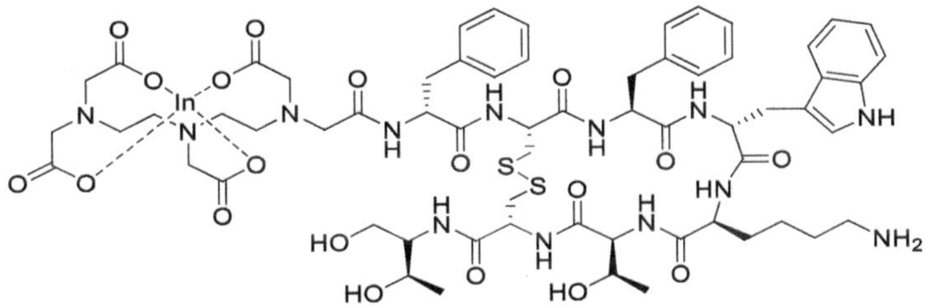

Figure 6. Structure of [^{111}In]-pentetreotide (Octreoscan®).

3.1.1. Gallium-68 and Indium-111

DOTATOC analog was the first to be radiolabeled with indium-111, and its comparative study with Octreoscan® showed similar diagnostic accuracy, but with better biodistribution and clearance [72]. Although DOTATATE alone showed better affinity for SSTRs, the two analogs [^{111}In]-DOTATOC and [^{111}In]-DOTATATE showed relatively similar pharmacokinetic properties [73]. SSTR2 receptors—and to a lesser extent, SSTR5—are most often overexpressed in tumors. Consequently, the majority of the radiotracers described have a strong affinity for these two SSTRs subtypes. Systems such as DOTANOC were designed to develop a probe capable of targeting all subtypes. Compared to DOTATOC and DOTATATE, it has a similar affinity for SSTR2 and SSTR5 subtypes, but a much higher affinity towards SSTR3. Their high internalization rate results in interesting biodistribution data, with a greater accumulation of the probe in the tumor and in the organs or tissues expressing SSTRs (e.g., pancreas and adrenal glands), ending with excretion mainly by kidneys [74].

These three systems, similarly labeled with gallium-68 (Figure 7), have proven to be very good radiotracers, and are currently routinely used in clinical applications [75]. These three radiopharmaceuticals have slightly different pharmacokinetic properties, but their diversity is mainly due to the variation in affinity for certain subtypes. This feature is even more marked depending on the radioelement chosen (^{68}Ga or ^{111}In). This can be explained by the differences in the geometry of the complexes. [^{68}Ga]-DOTATOC is very affine for SSTR2 and more moderate for SSTR5, [^{68}Ga]-DOTATATE is specific to SSTR2 and finally, [^{68}Ga]-DOTANOC binds with great affinity to SSTR2, SSTR3, and SSTR5 [76–78].

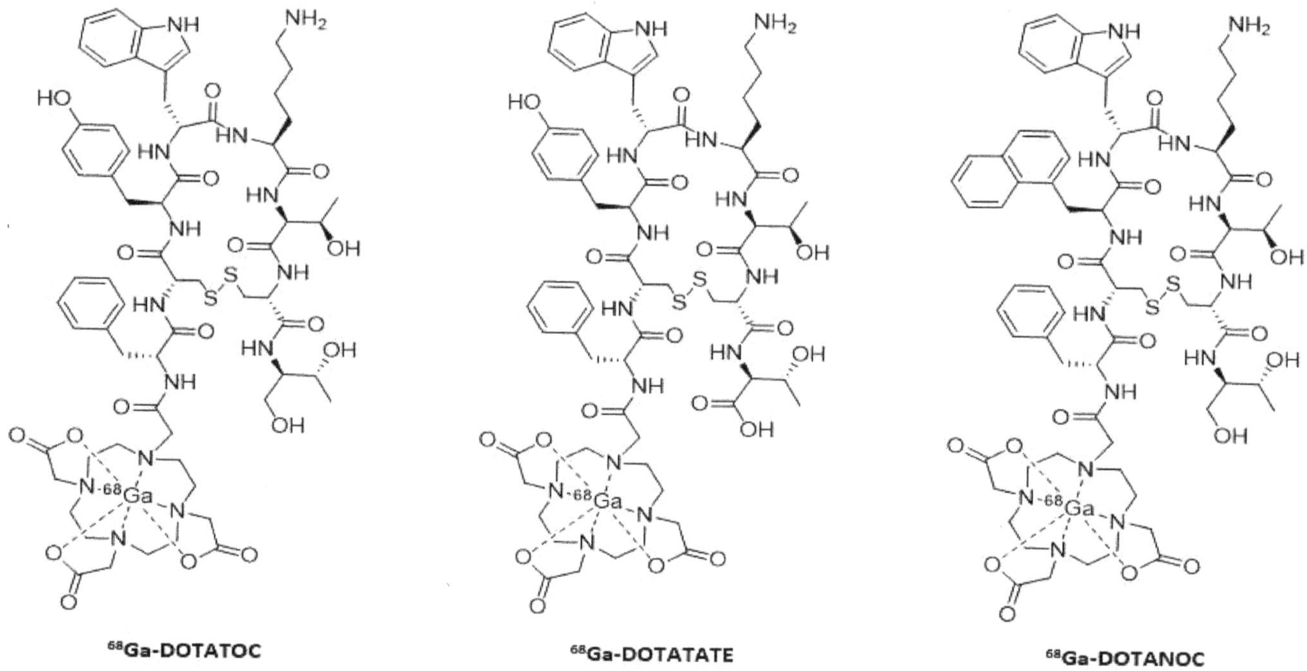

Figure 7. Structures of the three main systems radiolabeled with gallium-68.

A study with DOTANOC aimed at determining the impact of the introduction of a spacer on the pharmacokinetic properties of the formed radiotracer. The aim was to insert polyethyleneglycol (PEG) moieties or sugars between the chelating cavity (DOTA) and the biomolecule (NOC), which resulted in the modification of the lipophilicity or the charge of the final compound. As a result, the hydrophilicity of the system seems to be involved only in the affinity phenomenon towards the receptor, and the overall charge of the compound influences the excretion profile [79].

DOTA is not the only macrocycle to have been coupled to somatostatin analogs. Knowing the attraction of Ga (III) for NOTA, the latter has been the subject of comparative studies. Conjugated with octreotide (NODAGATOC), the compound showed a strong affinity for SSTR2 (similar to that of DOTATOC). Once marked with ^{111}In, affinity was even stronger for SSTR2, with even a gain on SSTR3 and SSTR5 (compared to ^{68}Ga-NODAGATOC), which confirms the influence that the geometry of the complex can have on affinity. In terms of stability, as expected, that of [^{68}Ga]-NODAGATOC was higher than that of [^{111}In]-NODAGATOC. The biodistribution of [^{68}Ga]-NODAGATOC was similar to that of [^{68}Ga]-DOTATOC, but showed a better accumulation in the tumor than [^{111}In]-DOTATOC. This is probably due to the strong agonist character, and the high rate of internalization of the NODAGATOC derivative [80].

A large variety of derivatives have also been investigated, such as DOTALAN, DOTABOC, DOTAGA [81], DOTANOCATE or DOTABOCATE (all derivatives of DOTANOC) [82,83], or THP-TATE (comparison of the overall behavior of the tris chelating system (hydroxypyridinone) with DOTATATE) [84]. New generation analogs with broader affinity profiles or pan-somatostatin analogs have been developed. For instance, AM3 (DOTA-Tyr-cyclo(DAB-Arg-cyclo(Cys-Phe-D-Trp-Lys-Thr-Cys))), a bicyclic somatostatin analog demonstrated affinity to SSTR2, 3, and 5, when labeled with ^{68}Ga. It showed a fast background clearance coupled with a high tumor/non-tumor ratio. [85] KE108 was coupled with DOTA and labeled with ^{111}In and ^{68}Ga, giving [^{111}In/^{68}Ga]-KE88 (DOTA-D-Dab-Arg-Phe-Phe-D-Trp-Lys-Thr-Phe), which bound to all five SSTRs with high affinity. [86] However, in an in vitro study, it had a low SSTR2 uptake, but was very effective for SSTR3-expressing tumors. More recently, a Pasireotide derivative, DOTA-PA1

(DOTA-cyclo-[HyPro-Phe-D-Trp-Lys-Tyr(Bzl)-Phe]) was labeled with ^{68}Ga and was investigated in three human lung cancer models, where it demonstrated superiority compared to [^{68}Ga]-DOTATATE [87]. In parallel, the group from Demokritos Institute, in Athens, developed pansomatostatin radiopeptides based on native somatostatin (SRIF-14 and SRIF-28). Both were derivatized with DOTA chelator and labeled with ^{111}In. Subsequent radiotracers exhibited high affinity and internalization profiles. SRIF-14 derivatives unfortunately demonstrated low in vivo stability. [^{111}In]-DOTA-LTT-SS28, on the contrary, demonstrated a much higher stability and showed more promise [88,89].

3.1.2. Technetium-99m

A wide range of chelating agents have been used to prepare somatostatin analogs labeled with technetium-99m: peptide moieties [90,91], propyleneaminooxime [92], tetraamines [93,94] or a cyclopentadienyl group [95]. Macrocyclic ligands have also been investigated [96]. Three systems stand out for the radiolabeling of somatostatin analogs: HYNIC-TOC and Demotate scaffolds, and P829 (Figure 8).

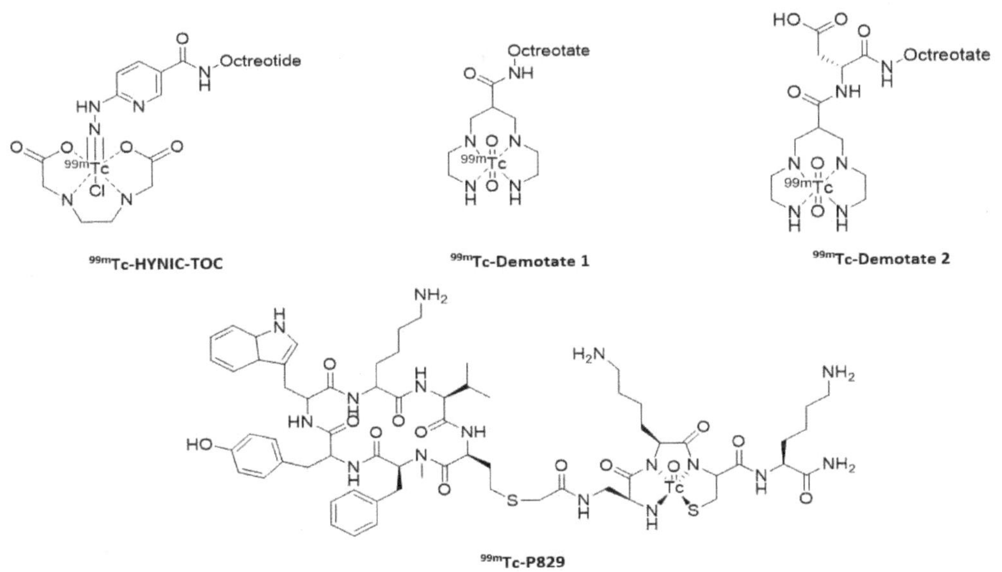

Figure 8. [^{99m}Tc]-labeled somatostatin analogs.

Initially, the HYNIC core (hydrazinonicotinamide) was designed for the radiolabeling of antibodies and proteins with technetium-99m [97], then this was transposed to peptides and more specifically to octreotide. This ligand can complex the metal in a monodentate or bidentate way, therefore, it is necessary to use one or more co-ligands to complete the coordination of the [^{99m}Tc]-HYNIC core. Among the most commonly used co-ligands are tricin, nicotinic acid, or EDDA (ethylenediaminodiacetic acid). Each co-ligand has its own influences on the properties of the complex obtained (e.g., lipophilicity and biodistribution) [98]. The first studies were carried out using tricin as a co-ligand ([^{99m}Tc]-HYNIC-TOC), but quickly EDDA demonstrated a very favorable influence on the pharmacokinetics of the radiotracers [99]. Compared to Octreoscan®, [^{99m}Tc]-EDDA/HYNIC-TOC showed better accumulation in the tumor and a weaker accumulation in the kidneys. The improved spatial resolution, the reduction in the radiation dose received by the patient and the better availability of ^{99m}Tc made it a possible alternative to Octreoscan® [99,100]. Finally, its conjugation with the octreotate analog ([^{99m}Tc]-EDDA/HYNIC-TATE) has shown significantly similar behavior to its octreotide counterpart [101]. [^{99m}Tc]-EDDA/HYNIC-TOC (Tektrotyd®) was granted marketing authorization in Europe in adult patients with gastro-enteropancreatic neuroendocrine tumors (GEP-NET) for localizing primary tumors and their metastases.

The second radiotracer, based on the tetraamine motif 6-R-1,4,8,11-tetraazaundecane, is available in a series with [^{99m}Tc]-Demotate 1 ([^{99m}Tc-N_4^0, Tyr^3]-octreotate) and ^{99m}Tc-Demotate 2 ([^{99m}Tc-N_4^{0-1},

Asp^0, Tyr^3]-octreotate). The first version of this probe demonstrated excellent pharmacokinetic properties, including faster accumulation in the tumor compared to Octreoscan® [102]. The objective of the second version was to improve the qualities of [^{99m}Tc]-Demotate 1, by modifying the overall charge of the complex and adding an Asp residue. In the end, [^{99m}Tc]-Demotate 2 showed overall behavior similar to [^{111}In]-DOTATATE, even if the latter has a faster clearance and a better retention time in the tumor [103]. The last of the main analogs based on technetium-99m is [^{99m}Tc]-P829 (^{99m}Tc-Depreotide), marketed in 2000 by the company CISBio International under the name of NeoSpect®, but recently withdrawn from the market. The P829 peptide (directly radiolabeled with ^{99m}Tc) showed results similar to the other SST analogs [104]. Its use for the detection of neuroendocrine tumors appeared to be less precise than with Octreoscan® [105]. On the other hand, its affinity for SSTR3, subtype which may be the origin of cross-competition from other types of receptors (notably VIP receptors), gave it the ability to bind to a larger number of primary tumors [104]. In particular, it was used clinically for the diagnosis of malignant lung tumors [106–108], for which it got its market authorization [109], and also demonstrated some interest in breast cancer, but it was never confirmed in a larger series of patients [110].

The question that now remains to be answered is that of the clinical interest of a SPECT tracer among the wide choice of PET SSTRs imaging agents [111,112].

3.1.3. Copper-64

Due to the short half-life of ^{68}Ga ($T_{1/2}$ = 67.7 min.) each center willing to perform ^{68}Ga PET imaging must purchase a currently expensive ^{68}Ge/^{68}Ga generator and a specifically shielded hot-cell. For this reason and despite the FDA and EMA market authorizations for [^{68}Ga]-DOTATATE and [^{68}Ga]-DOTATOC and the better diagnostic performances for these two radiopharmaceuticals products, the use of ^{68}Ga appears to be under the dependence of an economic choice for many hospitals and only a few large centers are making the financial investment to perform ^{68}Ga-radiolabeling. In this context, the use of a PET-emitter with a longer half-life such as copper-64 ($T_{1/2}$ = 12.7 h) appears to be an interesting alternative to remove the financial hindrance of gallium-68 [113]. This physical parameter allows for a centralized radiolabeling site with a large multicentric supply of ready-to-use ^{64}Cu-radiolabeled compounds. The chemistry of copper is also well known, which is a real asset in the design of new radiotracers. Many systems already presented before, such as DOTATOC/TATE or NODAGATOC/TATE, or others more copper-specific BFCAs, such as TETA (1,4,8,11-tetraazacyclotetradecane-*N,N',N'',N'''*-tetraacetic acid) [114], and its more stable derivatives such as cross-bridge CB-TE2A (4,11-bis(carboxymethyl)-1,4,8,11-tetraazabicyclo [6.6.2]hexadecane) [115], and CPTA (4-[(1,4,8,11-tetraazacyclotetradec-1-yl)methyl]benzoic acid]) [116] or sarcophagine derivatives [117] have been studied. A review on the development of copper radiolabeled somatostatin analogs was recently published by Marciniak et al. [118].

To validate the clinical interest of [^{64}Cu]-somatostatin analogs, various clinical studies have been conducted around the world. Among the different somatostatin analogs, [^{64}Cu]-DOTATATE was one of the first used. In 2015, [^{64}Cu]-DOTATATE was compared head-to-head to [^{111}In]-DTPA-octreotide in 112 patients and showed that the PET ^{64}Cu-compound was far superior to SPECT ^{111}In compound performances [119]. In 2017, [^{64}Cu]-DOTATATE was challenged to [^{68}Ga]-DOTATOC according to an identical PET/CT imaging modality [120]. The results of this study, where 59 patients were injected with [^{68}Ga]-DOTATOC followed by an injection of [^{64}Cu]-DOTATATE one week later, concluded that the two radiopharmaceuticals had the same sensitivity. Nevertheless, in this cohort of neuroendocrine tumors, [^{64}Cu]-DOTATATE had a substantially better lesion detection rate. The patient follow-up revealed that these additional lesions detected by [^{64}Cu]-DOTATATE were true positives. To evaluate the benefits of this better detection of lesions with [^{64}Cu]-DOTATATE than with [^{68}Ga]-DOTATOC, the correlation between PET image [^{64}Cu]-DOTATATE uptake (expressed in maximal standardized uptake value - SUV_{max}) and overall (OS)/progression free survival (PFS) was studied during 24 months after [^{64}Cu]-DOTATATE PET/CT acquisition. The conclusion of this study claimed a good correlation/prognostic between SUV_{max} and PFS but not with OS [121]. The major drawback of these preliminary human studies consist of the affinities differences for the five SSTRs subtypes between DOTATOC and DOTATATE compounds. To circumvent these discrepancies, an in vitro study in a mouse model was conducted and compared [^{64}Cu]-DOTATATE to [^{68}Ga]-DOTATATE. The results showed a similar pharmacokinetic and absolute uptake between both compounds 1 h post-injection [122]. In Europe, where the PET radiopharmaceutical approved is [^{68}Ga]-DOTATOC, it could be interesting to perform some PET imaging with [^{64}Cu]-DOTATOC to compare the performance of the two tracers. A first-in-human retrospective study was recently conducted and seems to present same results than [^{64}Cu]-DOTATATE with high detection rate of suspected lesion associated to a high target-to-background contrast [123]. A recent first-in-human study also demonstrated potential interest for [^{64}Cu]-SARTATE analog [124].

In conclusion, despite a higher dosimetric impact for copper-64 (only 17.6% of radioactive decay lead to positron emission), copper-64 somatostatin analogs appear to be an advantageous alternative to gallium-68 radiopharmaceuticals. Compared to ^{68}Ga, in addition to economic advantages, ^{64}Cu has a lower positron range which leads to a better PET intrinsic resolution and a higher half-life which allows for a more flexible scanning window. The better patient care management and outcomes remain to be proven and the work is in progress to establish these points [121,125]. In parallel, at present, a radiopharmaceutical industrial company submitted a market authorization from FDA for [^{64}Cu]-DOTATATE and thus confirms the interest of copper-64 in SSTRs imaging.

3.1.4. Other Radiometals

Other radionuclides have also been investigated for SSTRs imaging. Cobalt-55 seems to be a possible alternative to gallium-68 and copper-64 compounds, with similar behavior and lifespan (17.5 h vs. 12.7 h) to the latter, but with a higher positron yield (75.9% vs. 17.6%). Preliminary complexation tests of DOTATOC with the isotope ^{57}Co as a surrogate for ^{55}Co showed a higher affinity for SSTR2 than [^{68}Ga]-DOTATOC, implying a rate of internalization among the highest of all derivatives of SST and thus, a strong accumulation in targeted tissues. Despite similar structures, the analogs of cobalt and gallium have different biological behaviors. This confirms the fact that the physical characteristics of radioactive elements influence the affinity, biodistribution, and pharmacokinetics of radiolabeled peptides [126]. The properties of cobalt-based compounds have been further investigated with the comprehensive evaluation of other octreotide analogs such as DOTANOC and DOTATATE [127]. Furthermore, [^{55}Co]-DOTATATE compared favorably with [^{68}Ga]-DOTATATE and [^{64}Cu]-DOTATATE in an animal model [122]. Associated with the Auger-emitting ^{58m}Co, it could represent a potentially interesting theranostic pair [128].

Scandium and terbium are two metals that recently emerged as possibly useful for theranostic applications, as both possess imaging and therapeutic radionuclides [129]. DOTATOC was radiolabeled with scandium-44 ($T_{1/2}$ = 3.97 h, $E_{\beta+}$ = 632 keV) [130] and terbium-152 ($T_{1/2}$ = 17.5 h, $E_{\beta+}$ = 1140 keV) [131] and rapidly injected in patients in proof-of-concept studies [132,133]. No adverse effects were observed during follow-up periods and images proved suitable for diagnosis. With DOTATATE, it seems the affinity to SSTR2 receptors is lower with scandium than with gallium, thus limiting its interest [134]. In a study comparing the labeling and stability of DOTANOC and NODAGANOC with ^{44}Sc and ^{68}Ga, it was observed that [^{44}Sc]-NODAGANOC labeling was more challenging and less stable than [^{44}Sc]-DOTANOC [135]. The opposite was observed with ^{68}Ga. Recently, a new chelator was proposed, AAZTA (1,4-bis (carboxymethyl)-6-[bis (carboxymethyl)]amino-6-methylperhydro-1,4-diazepine), which enables fast and easy labeling at room temperature. AAZTA-TOC labeled with ^{44}Sc demonstrated high in vitro stability [136]. Affinity tests are now necessary to assess its potential utility. DOTATATE has also been labeled with ^{155}Tb ($T_{1/2}$ = 5.32 days, E_{γ} = 87 keV (32%), 105 keV (25%)) for SPECT imaging [137]. Though a potentially promising radionuclide for theranostic applications, availability of ^{155}Tb is currently the main limitation for further development.

At the turn of the millennium, yttrium-86 ($T_{1/2}$ = 14.74 h, 32% β^+) was thought to be a potential radionuclide of interest, particularly for pretherapeutic dosimetry of ^{90}Y-radiotracers, and notably ^{90}Y-labeled somatostatin analogs [138]. Thus, several octreotide analogs were developed [139,140]. [^{86}Y]-DOTATOC even reached the clinics [139,141]; however, ^{86}Y properties are less than optimal, and availability is limited, so interest soon faded out.

3.1.5. Fluorine-18

Radiometals' production is currently still limited, even for the most advanced ones [142–144]. Fluorine-18, on the contrary, can be mass-produced and distributed daily, thanks to a worldwide network of cyclotrons. Because of this availability, and favorable decay characteristics ($T_{1/2}$ = 110 min, 97% β^+), it thus should be noted that some radiotracers based on fluorine-18 have been described (Figure 9) [145]. The first generations such as 2-[^{18}F]fluoropropionyl-D-Phe^1-octreotide [146] or 4-[^{18}F]fluorobenzoyl-D-Phe^1-octreotide [147] generally showed unfavorable biokinetic properties (low accumulation and low retention in the tumor). The probes developed subsequently contained hydrophilic or charged moieties to reduce the lipophilicity of the radiotracer. In particular, several carbohydrate derivatives of octreotide/octreotate have been developed [148,149]. A disadvantage of fluorine-labeling compared to radiometal labeling is the use of generally long and tedious multi-step procedures. To circumvent this, innovative strategies, enabling fast and purification-less labeling, have been developed, such as the formation of ^{18}F-boron or ^{18}F-silicon bonds, or the use of click-chemistry [150–152]. Another elegant method to label somatostatin analogs is the use of [^{18}F]-aluminum fluoride with radiotracers previously developed for radiometals, such as NOTATOC [153]. These new generation analogs demonstrated general properties (affinity for the targeted receptors, metabolic stability, biodistribution and clearance) which are much more interesting, and some of them have been investigated in patients, where they gave results comparable to [^{68}Ga]-DOTATOC [154,155]. In addition, [^{18}F]F-FET-βAG-TOCA and [^{18}F]-IMP466 ([Al^{18}F]-NOTATOC) are currently being evaluated in phase I clinical trials (EudraCT number 2013-003152-20 and NCT03511768, respectively). Recently published results with [^{18}F]-IMP466 demonstrated it was safe and well-tolerated, with a physiologic uptake pattern similar to [^{68}Ga]-DOTATATE [156]. Besides cost and availability, another advantage of fluorine-18 is its shorter positron range compared with gallium-68, leading to an improved spatial resolution, and thus, better quantification of uptake [157].

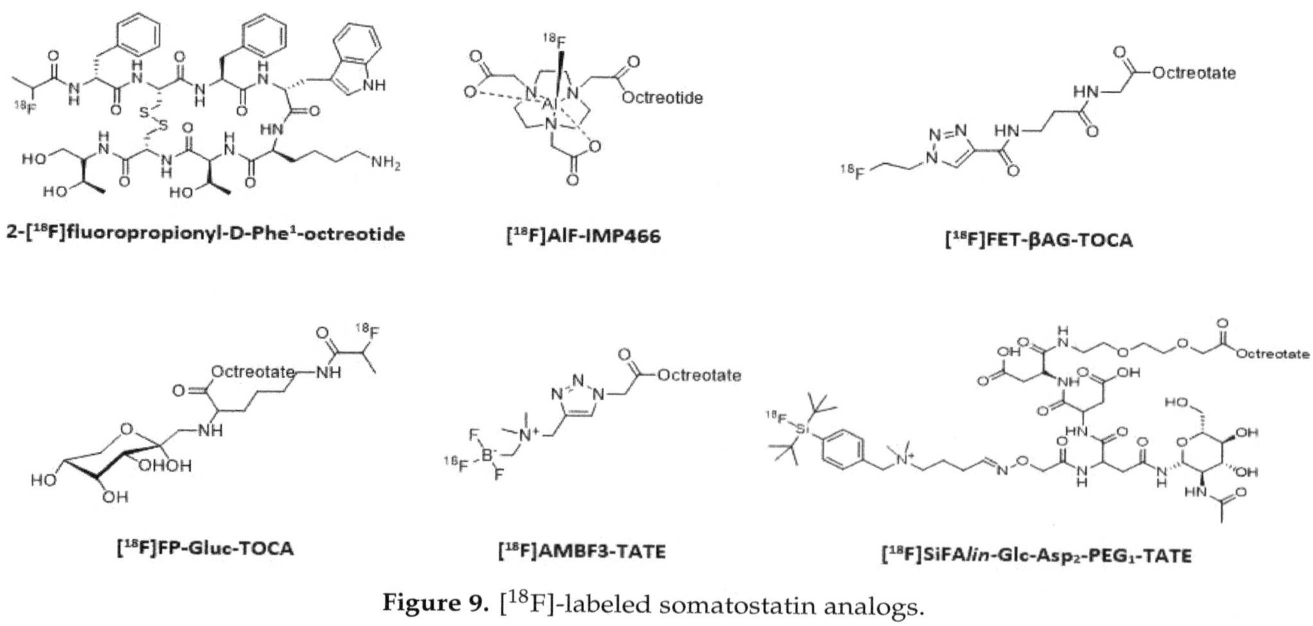

Figure 9. [^{18}F]-labeled somatostatin analogs.

3.2. Radiolabeled Somatostatin Analogs for Therapy

Concerning radionuclide therapy and more particularly peptide receptor radionuclide therapy (PRRT), radioactivity is used to destroy the targeted cells. Radiopharmaceuticals used in therapy are designed in the same way as those used in imaging, only the nature of the radioelement being modified. Contrary to imaging, which uses radioelements having very penetrating but little ionizing radiations, PRRT privileges the use of radionuclides that have little penetrating and more energetic and thus more ionizing radiations. Brought directly to the cancer cell, the radiation emitted by the radioactive decay causes irreversible ionization of the cell's DNA, which induces its apoptosis. The main isotopes used today are iodine-131, yttrium-90, lutetium-177 and, to a lesser extent, rhenium-188 [158]. As mentioned earlier, the purpose of the DOTA-SSA design was to work with a chelating cavity capable of complexing radioelements for imaging or therapy. Consequently, most of the platforms discussed above have been transposed for therapeutic application via the use of β^- emitters [64,74,81,82].

3.2.1. Yttrium-90 and Lutetium-177

Yttrium-90, a pure high energy β^- emitter ($T_{1/2}$ = 64 h, $E_{\beta max}$ = 2.28 MeV), and lutetium-177, a medium energy β^- emitter ($T_{1/2}$ = 6.7 d, $E_{\beta max}$ = 0.5 MeV) with a γ component (208 keV), are currently the most used in PRRT. Each of these two elements has its own advantages for targeted therapy. The particles emitted by ^{90}Y are more energetic and more penetrating; they are able to diffuse on a thicker layer of cells, which is an advantage for the treatment of large tumors. However, even if high energy radiation allows a more uniform irradiation of the tumor, the risk of imposing an excessive dose of radiation on the adjacent tissues is very present. For its part, the ^{177}Lu emits less energetic radiation, more suited to small tumors. In addition, the energy of its γ radiation is sufficient to allow detection by scintigraphy and establish dosimetry during the therapy sequences [159].

The first analog to be studied was [^{90}Y]-DOTATOC (Octreother®), and the first treatment sessions quickly showed good results, stopping the progression of the tumor [72,160,161]. Many studies on this long-used treatment have made it possible to observe a good tolerance for this radiotracer, with fairly mild side effects (fatigue) and in very rare cases a little more severe ones (nausea). However, it also showed some toxicity for the kidneys and the bones, these two aspects being the dose-limiting factors for the patient. In vitro, a greater affinity for SSTR2 has been demonstrated for [^{90}Y]-DOTATATE compared to [^{90}Y]-DOTATOC [64]. However, for the diagnosis in humans, a better contrast between the kidneys and the tumor was found for [^{111}In]-DOTATOC compared to [^{111}In]-DOTATATE [73], which may explain the wider use of DOTATOC analog. Despite this, these two analogs have relatively similar properties and have proven to be effective treatment methods that improve survival in some patients with neuroendocrine tumors (approximately 50 months vs. 18 months without treatment) [162]. In a Phase IIA study with [^{90}Y]-DOTALAN (MAURITIUS trial), this one demonstrated lower tumor uptake in neuroendocrine tumors compared to ^{90}Y-DOTATOC, but could be of potential interest for other tumors, such as HCC or lung cancers [163]. With the perspective of several years of clinical use, PRRT with ^{90}Y-labeled somatostatin analogs appears to be well-tolerated with favorable long-term outcome. Unfortunately, Phase III studies are still lacking [164,165].

The same analogs have also been radiolabeled with lutetium-177. Initially, [^{177}Lu]-DOTATOC was used in cases of relapse of neuroendocrine tumors after treatment with [^{90}Y]-DOTATOC. Despite satisfactory results [166], its subsequently developed analog [^{177}Lu]-DOTATATE has shown more promise, mainly due to a more significant retention time in the tumor. For this reason, octreotate analog (TATE) is being preferred to octreotide (TOC) for labeling with lutetium [164,167]. It is also important to note that, unlike ^{90}Y, no cases of nephrotoxicity after treatment with ^{177}Lu have been reported. In 2005, the possibility of combining these two β^- emitters for therapy in cases where tumors of variable sizes are detected, was demonstrated [168]. From there, different treatment combinations between the four main systems ([^{90}Y]-DOTATOC, [^{90}Y]-DOTATATE, [^{177}Lu]-DOTATOC, and [^{177}Lu]-DOTATATE) have proven to be interesting and sometimes even more effective than using a single treatment modality [169,170]. Similarly, combination treatments with non-labeled somatostatin analogs, chemotherapy, targeted therapy, and/or radiosensitizers might further improve the efficacy and/or tolerability [171,172]. [^{177}Lu]-DOTATATE has been investigated in a phase III trial, in well-differentiated, unresectable or metastatic, progressive midgut neuroendocrine tumors (Netter 1 trial). Treatment with [^{177}Lu]-DOTATATE resulted in a significant tumor response rate of 18% compared with 3% in the high-dose octreotide LAR group, coupled with a 79% risk reduction for disease progression or death [173]. Following these positive findings, [^{177}Lu]-DOTATATE was granted marketing authorization in this indication, both in Europe and in the US (Lutathera®) [174]. Coupled with ^{68}Ga-imaging (Figure 10), it represents a powerful theranostic tool for the management of neuroendocrine tumors (NETs) [175]. Current research with [^{177}Lu]-DOTATATE aims to improve the safety and efficacy of this procedure, enlarge possible indication, notably in advanced, poorly-differentiated, GEP-NETs, [176,177] or other NETs, such as pheomochromocytoma or paraganglioma [178,179].

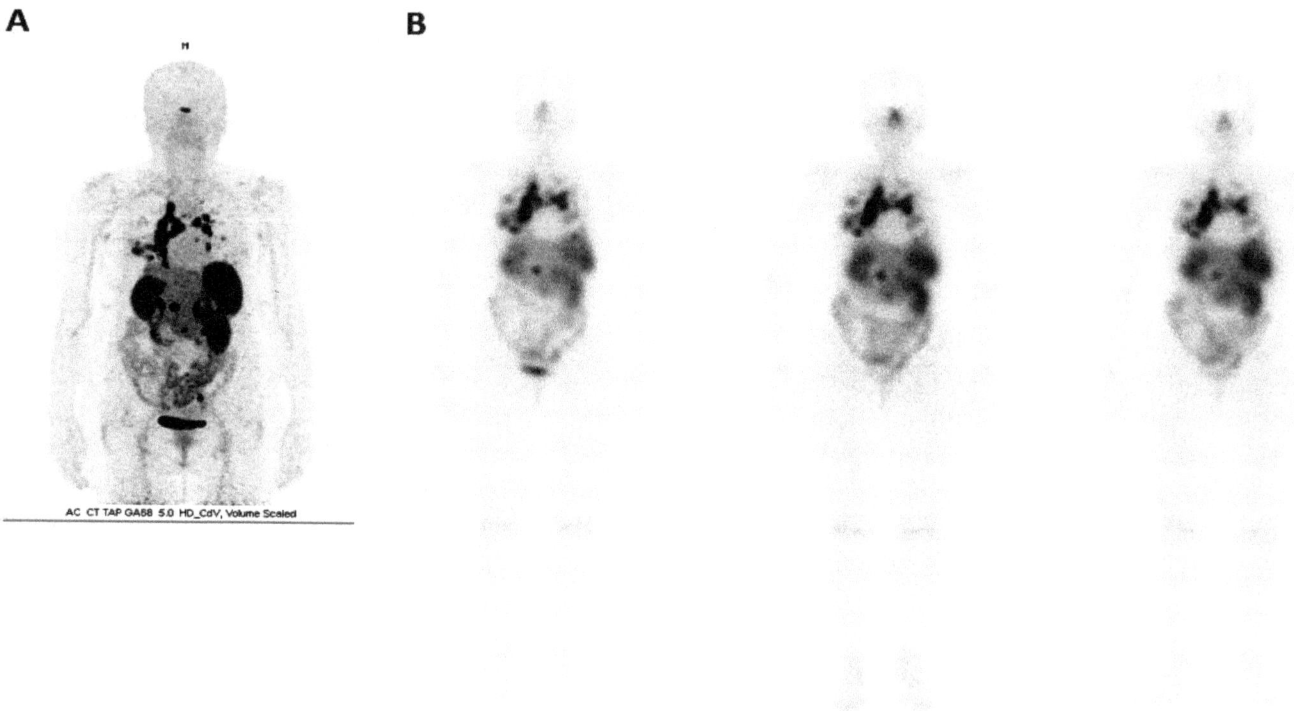

Figure 10. (**A**) [^{68}Ga]-DOTATOC (Somakit®) and (**B**) [^{177}Lu]-DOTATATE (Lutathera®, cures 1, 2, and 3) imaging of a patient treated for progressive metastatic midgut NET (images courtesy of Centre Eugene Marquis, Rennes, France).

3.2.2. Rhenium-188 and Other β-Emitting Radionuclides

Despite equally interesting characteristics, rhenium-188 remains widely less used than ^{90}Y and ^{177}Lu [180]. This is mainly due to more difficult chemistry and the unavailability of a pharmaceutical-grade ^{188}W/^{188}Re generator, as compared to the other two. Vapreotide and Lanreotide analogs have been described in the literature with ^{188}Re. They have been investigated in experimental cancer models (e.g., pancreas, colorectal, lungs and cervical) to reduce tumor growth [181–184]. [^{188}Re]-Lanreotide notably demonstrated favorable pharmacokinetics and distribution profiles (tumor-to-liver ratio) in HCC-bearing rats compared to healthy ones [185]. Another example is an equivalent to Depreotide (P829). After the development of ^{99m}Tc-Depreotide for imaging, the idea was to label this compound with ^{188}Re, to assess its potential in vivo. Although the radiolabeling proceeded successfully, the study showed unacceptable toxicity to non-target organs. To improve its properties, structural modifications of the peptide sequences close to the chelating moiety were tested. This optimization led to P2045, which showed better accumulation in the tumor, weaker retention in the kidneys, and faster urinary excretion than [^{99m}Tc]-depreotide [186]. This new rhenium-based analog of depreotide, [^{188}Re]-P2045 (Figure 11), went up to phase I in therapy for small cell lung cancer [187] and has shown promising in vivo results in the treatment of pancreatic tumors in mice [188]. To the best of our knowledge, no HYNIC-TOC/TATE or demotate derivatives have yet been radiolabeled with rhenium. Recent research with rhenium isotopes has been focusing on tricarbonyl core derivatives for the labeling of NOTA-SSAs [96].

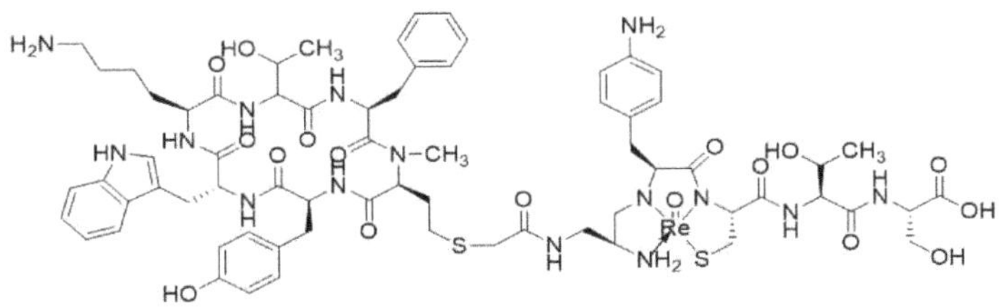

Figure 11. [^{188}Re]-P2045.

In a theranostic perspective, other β-emitting nuclides could have a potential interest—such as ^{47}Sc ($T_{1/2}$ = 3.35 d, $E_{\beta max}$ = 600.8 keV), ^{67}Cu ($T_{1/2}$ = 2.58 d, $E_{\beta max}$ = 577 keV), and ^{161}Tb ($T_{1/2}$ = 6.91 d, $E_{\beta max}$ = 593 keV)—to be coupled with ^{44}Sc, ^{64}Cu, and ^{152}Tb/^{155}Tb respectively [129,158,189]. To date, no ^{67}Cu-labeled somatostatin analogs have been described so far, and only very preliminary studies have been described with [^{161}Tb]-DTPA-Octreotide and [^{47}Sc]-DOTATOC [190,191].

3.2.3. Alpha and Auger Emitters

Recently, alpha emitters have attracted particular attention for radionuclide therapy. Long confined to hematological tumors, they are now being considered for the potential treatment of solid tumors [192]. In vitro, α-labeled somatostatin analogs (DOTATOC and DOTATATE) demonstrated a significantly higher killing effect compared to ^{177}Lu [193–195]. [^{213}Bi]- and [^{225}Ac]-labeled DOTATOC (^{213}Bi: $T_{1/2}$ = 45.6 min, E_α = 5.88 MeV; ^{225}Ac: $T_{1/2}$ = 9.92 d, E_α = 5.83 MeV) have demonstrated promising therapeutic effects in pre-clinical animal studies [196,197]; whereas [^{213}Bi]-DOTATATE, investigated in human small cell lung carcinoma and rat pancreatic tumor models, demonstrated a great therapeutic effect in both small (50 mm^3) and large (200 mm^3) tumors, but with a higher probability for stable disease in small tumors [198]. First, and, to date, the only clinical experience with [^{213}Bi]-DOTATOC, was published by Kratochwil et al., and included seven patients with advanced NETs with liver metastases refractory to treatment with [^{90}Y]-DOTATOC or [^{177}Lu]-DOTATOC [199]. It demonstrated specific tumor binding, lower toxicity than with β-irradiation and partial remission of metastases. Two years after intra-arterial injection of [^{213}Bi]-DOTATOC, all seven patients were still alive. Regarding ^{225}Ac, a first-in-human study included 10 patients with progressive NETs after β-PRRT. As with ^{213}Bi, [^{225}Ac]-DOTATOC was well tolerated and effective [200]. A recent study with [^{225}Ac]-DOTATATE confirmed the potential of these radiotracers as an additional, and valuable, treatment option for patients who are refractory to [^{177}Lu]-DOTATATE therapy. 32 patients with previous [^{177}Lu]-DOTATATE therapy were treated with [^{225}Ac]-DOTATATE (100 kBq/kg body weight). The response was assessed in 24 patients, with 9 stabilized diseases and 15 partial remissions [201].

Though not stricto sensu an α-emitter, lead-212 ($T_{1/2}$ = 10.6 h) eventually decays to stable 2^{08}Pb through a cascade chain with two α-emissions of potential therapeutic interest. A somatostatin analog, DOTAMTATE (Figure 12), has been labeled with ^{212}Pb and investigated in a murine model of neuroendocrine tumor. Results showed a promising safety index with a 3.2-fold increase in median survival and one-third of the animals being tumor-free. A combination with 5-FU (Fluorouracyl) was able to durably cure approximately 80% of the animals. [202] Given these promising outcomes, a Phase I dose-escalation clinical trial has recently been started with [^{212}Pb]-DOTAMTATE (AlphaMedix™) including 50 patients with unresectable or metastatic neuroendocrine tumors (NCT03466216). Preliminary results (nine patients enrolled) demonstrated a favorable safety profile at the tested doses [203].

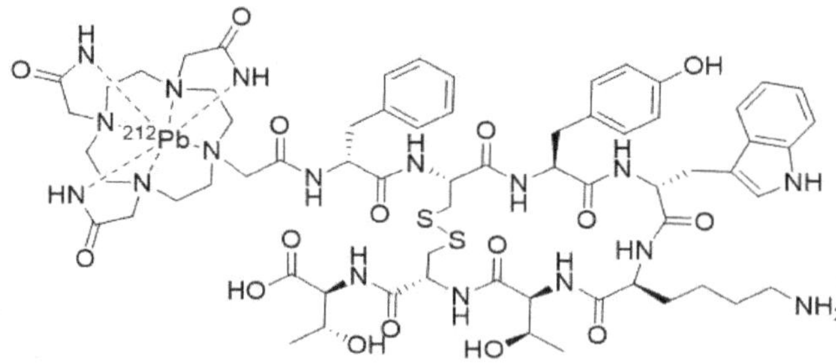

Figure 12. $[^{212}Pb]$-DOTAMTATE.

Cyclotron-produced astatine-211 ($T_{1/2}$ = 7.2 h, E_{α} = 5.87 MeV) is another very promising α-emitting radionuclide. Astatine is the heaviest halogen with a behavior somehow similar to iodine, but, in certain circumstances, it also displays significant metallic characteristics [204]. Direct astatination of somatostatin analogs is feasible, through tyrosine residues, but it led to poor stability of the resulting analogs, therefore different prosthetic groups have been developed [205–207]. Although *N*-(3-$[^{211}At]$astato-4-guanidinomethylbenzoyl)-Phe^{1}-octreotate ($[^{211}At]$-AGMBO) and N^{α}-(1-deoxy-D-fructosyl)-N^{ε}-(3-$[^{211}At]$astatobenzoyl)-Lys^{0}-octreotate ($[^{211}At]$-GABLO) showed disappointing biodistribution results, with poor tumor uptake, $[^{211}At]$-SPC-octreotide displayed a more favorable biodistribution profile, and a dose-dependent apoptosis in an NSCLC murine model.

Auger electron emitters are also very potent for specific tumor cell killing, sparing surrounding cells, with a highly localized energy deposition. Indium-111 emits Auger electrons (E_{Ae-} = 19 keV, 16%), and, as such, has been investigated for therapy. Several clinical trials have been undertaken with high doses of $[^{111}In]$-Pentetreotide. A first study with 20 patients that had neuroendocrine progressive tumors demonstrated stabilization of the disease in 5 patients, and tumor shrinkage in 5 others. All of them had received a cumulated dose higher than 20 GBq [208]. In a study with 50 SSTR-positive patients treated with cumulated doses from 20 to 160 GBq, of which 40 were evaluable, there was a stabilization in 14 patients, minor remission in 6 and partial remission in 1, with mild bone marrow toxicity [209]. However, half of the patients receiving more than 100 GBq developed a myelodysplastic syndrome or leukemia. A dose of 100 GBq was thus considered the maximal tolerated activity. Another study with 27 patients with GEP-NETs found that two doses of 6.6 GBq (180 mCi) were safe and well-tolerated, demonstrating a clinical benefit in 62% of patients [210]. Benefit of ^{111}In-Pentetreotide treatment was shown to last at least 6 months for 70% of patients, while only 31% of them still had sustained benefit after 18 months [211]. Efficacy in large tumors and end-stage patients is limited, mainly because of heterogeneous radiopharmaceutical uptake due to poor tumor vascularity and central necrosis [212]. This has been demonstrated by Capello et al. in a rat tumor model, with different sizes of tumors [213]. Effects were much more pronounced in small ($\leq 1\ cm^2$) tumors than in large ($\geq 8\ cm^2$). They also found a significant increase in tumor receptor density after tumor regrowth, indicating repeated injections would probably be more efficient than single-dose treatment. It could also be worth using PRRT with Auger emitters in an adjuvant setting after surgery, to destroy occult metastases. A final example is $[^{58m}Co]$-DOTATOC. This radiotracer presented for potential use in Auger-based therapy, particularly for disseminated tumor cells and micrometastases, appears to have more beneficial in vitro properties than those of $[^{177}Lu]$-DOTATATE, with a significantly more efficient cell killing effect per cumulated decay, which has to be confirmed in vivo [127].

4. Antagonists vs. Agonists

Pharmacomodulation around the synthetic somatostatin analogs has led to a change of chirality in the first amino-acid (from D to L form) and in cysteine number 2 (from L to D form). These modifications have given a new class of SSTR specific compounds with antagonist effects (Table 4). From a pharmacological point of view, the biological and molecular mechanisms responsible for their targeting effectiveness in vivo are completely different. After binding to an SST receptor, an agonist analog is internalized into the cell as a ligand-receptor complex. This internalization allows it to accumulate in the cell, and to increase the amount of radiation emitted. This very powerful and specific internalization mechanism enables efficient in vivo targeting of receptors. This phenomenon does not occur (or very little) for somatostatin antagonists, and they do not stimulate the G-protein coupled to the SSTR with an associate blockage of the agonist-induced activity. Surprisingly, it has been shown that targeting receptors can also be effective without internalization of the ligand-receptor complex, and some antagonist analogs can sometimes behave better than agonists (e.g., better accumulation in tumor, poor kidney retention, and rapid clearance) [214,215]. This high tumor uptake appears to be a consequence of a greater number of target binding sites for antagonists and a more slowly dissociation than for agonists, which allows for a longer accumulation of radiation [216,217]. The hypothesis of a ligand rebinding mechanism has been put forward, but this still requires some investigation before it can be validated. These first results were confirmed by preclinical studies and by preliminary clinical trials and seems to show superior results for antagonist-based tracers than agonists [218–221]. The first comparative study of antagonists with Octreoscan® confirmed the good characteristics of the [^{111}In]-DOTA-BASS analog, and better accumulation at the level of the tumor and better visualization of metastases. It was truly the first proof of the concept of antagonist SSTRs imaging [222].

Table 4. Main somatostatin antagonist analogs. Differences towards octreotide (OC) are highlighted in red.

Antagonist Peptide	*Peptidic Sequence*
Sst2-ANT (BASS)	p-NO_2-Phe^1-cyclo(D-Cys^2-Tyr^3-D-Trp^4-Lys^5-Thr^6-Cys^7)D-Tyr^8-NH_2
LM3	p-Cl-Phe^1-cyclo(D-Cys^2-Tyr^3-D-Aph^4(Cbm)-Lys^5-Thr^6-Cys^7)D-Tyr^8-NH_2
JR10	p-NO_2-Phe^1-cyclo(D-Cys^2-Tyr^3-D-Aph^4(Cbm)-Lys^5-Thr^6-Cys^7)D-Tyr^8-NH_2
JR11 (Satoreotide)	p-Cl-Phe^1-cyclo(D-Cys^2-Aph^3(Hor)-D-Aph^4(Cbm)-Lys^5-Thr^6-Cys^7)D-Tyr^8-NH_2

Concerning the affinity for each SSTR subtype, it turned out that the nature of the chelator and the radiometal is of great importance for the in vivo pharmacokinetic fate (mainly for the tumor uptake and retention time) [223]. Ultimately, copper-64 based radiotracers seem to be more interesting, especially when comparing their contrast ratio between the tumor and normal tissues which increases over time—a direct consequence of their higher half-life. The influence of radiometals (^{111}In, ^{90}Y, ^{177}Lu, ^{64}Cu, and ^{68}Ga) and chelates (DOTA and NODAGA) on three antagonist families (LM3, JR10, and JR11) were also studied. On the radiometric side, the overall affinity of [^{68}Ga]-DOTA was found to be much lower than for the other elements, which is the opposite of the results obtained with the agonists. For the chelate, the substitution of DOTA by NODAGA seems to greatly improve the affinity of the antagonist analogs. During this study, two particularly promising platforms emerged, DOTA-JR11 and NODAGA-JR11 [224]. Another example highlighting the influence of the chelate is 406-040-15 (cyclo (2–11) H-Cpa-DCys-Asn-Phe-Phe-DTrp-Lys-Thr-Phe-Thr-Cys-2NalNH_2), a pansomatostatin analog, with an SSTR3 antagonist behavior. Chelation to DOTA turned this analog to an agonist [225]. Note that the first antagonist labeled via a [^{99m}Tc]-tricarbonyl core has been described. ^{99m}TcL-sst2-ANT (with L = tridentate ligand type N, S, N) has shown very promising in vivo behavior, but requires some modifications to improve its pharmacokinetics [226].

As for imaging, antagonists are also an interesting alternative for therapy. As discussed above, the first proof of the feasibility of imaging using antagonists was highlighted by comparing Octreoscan® and [^{111}In]-DOTA-BASS. However, this analog has shown only a very modest affinity for the SSTR2 receptor subtype targeted in the therapy of neuroendocrine tumors [214]. To overcome this problem, the second generation of somatostatin antagonists was synthesized to improve affinity for this receptor. DOTA-JR11 showed the highest affinity for SSTR2 and was selected for use in targeted therapy [218]. A pilot study to assess the possibility of treatment with [^{177}Lu]-DOTA-JR11, by comparing it to [^{177}Lu]-DOTATATE, was carried out. This new antagonist has shown favorable properties, such as better accumulation in the tumor and a higher dose received by the tumor, thanks to a longer retention time [227]. Further developments led to a theranostic pair with JR11: one with a NODAGA chelator (satoreotide trizoxetan, OPS-202) and one with DOTA chelator (satoreotide tetraxetan, OPS-201) [228,229]. Satoreotide trizoxetan is currently radiolabeled with ^{68}Ga and used in PET imaging clinical trials (Figure 13) [230,231]. Satoreotide tetraxetan radiolabeled with ^{177}Lu has been evaluated in a therapeutic clinical trial [232]. First clinical results for this somatostatin antagonist theranostic pair seem to be promising with high sensitivity for neuroendocrine tumors and require further studies in larger patient population.

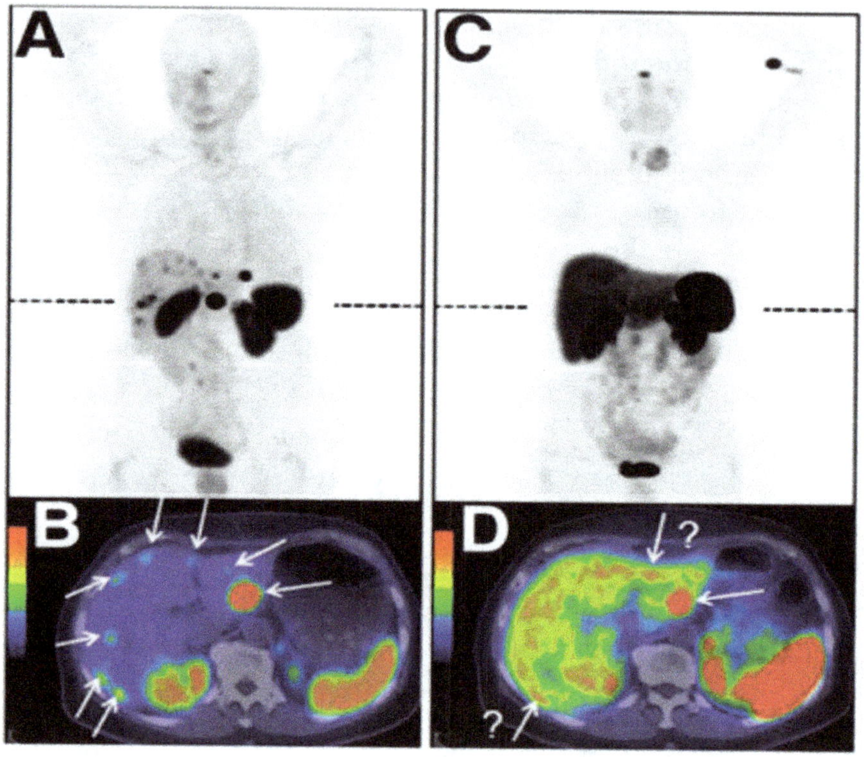

Figure 13. Comparison between [^{68}Ga]-OPS202 (**A**,**B**) and [^{68}Ga]-DOTATOC (**C**,**D**) PET/CT images of the same patient with ileal neuroendocrine tumours, showing bilobar liver metastases (from Rangger et al. [233]).

5. Future Prospects

Regarding clinically established somatostatin analogs, the development of kit-based ^{68}Ga radiotracers, as well as cyclotron production of gallium-68 should improve their availability and worldwide dissemination. Further clinical translation of ^{64}Cu- and ^{18}F-based somatostatin SSAs could also represent an attractive alternative. For therapy, current research focuses on optimizing the dose received by the tumor while sparing healthy tissues. Fractionation, as well as combination of ^{90}Y and ^{177}Lu, have demonstrated their interest [168,234]. The same approach with other treatment modalities, such as external-beam radiotherapy or chemotherapy could enhance treatment response [235,236]. Targeted α-therapy also seems to hold promises and is currently attracting much interest, notably from the industry.

Recent developments showed a switch from agonist to antagonist derivatives, demonstrating higher efficacy. With the advent of new promising radionuclides and somatostatin analogs with better pharmacokinetic properties and binding profiles, the future looks bright for radiolabeled somatostatin analogs, expanding their use for wider indications, than just GEP-NETs. With peptide derivatives with improved targeting, tumors with lower SSTR expression might nonetheless be clinically relevant. In this context, as already demonstrated with some analogs, use of somatostatin-based radiopharmaceuticals might be of interest in pulmonary or hepatic cancers, warranting further studies. The development of bivalent radiotracers to target several receptors concomitantly expressed could be of interest to improve targeting [237]. Similarly, improved detection and sensitivity could be achieved using bimodal agents [238]. Besides, the clinical success for radiolabeled somatostatin analogs both with diagnostic and therapeutic radionuclides paved the way for new promising peptide derivatives, such as bombesin, neurotensin, or CXCR4 ligands, and, in a similar way, PSMA ligands, for cancer theranostics [49,233,239,240].

Author Contributions: All authors contributed to the writing of the manuscript. All authors have read and agreed to the published version of the manuscript.

Acknowledgments: The authors thank Sophie Laffont for providing the [^{68}Ga]-DOTATOC and [^{177}Lu]-DOTATATE pictures.

References

1. Brazeau, P.; Vale, W.; Burgus, R.; Ling, N.; Butcher, M.; Rivier, J.; Guillemin, R. Hypothalamic polypeptide that inhibits the secretion of immunoreactive pituitary growth hormone. *Science* **1973**, *179*, 77–79. [CrossRef] [PubMed]
2. Patel, Y.C.; Greenwood, M.T.; Panetta, R.; Demchyshyn, L.; Niznik, H.; Srikant, C.B. The somatostatin receptor family. *Life Sci.* **1995**, *57*, 1249–1265. [CrossRef]
3. Günther, T.; Tulipano, G.; Dournaud, P.; Bousquet, C.; Csaba, Z.; Kreienkamp, H.J.; Lupp, A.; Korbonits, M.; Castaño, J.P.; Wester, H.J.; et al. International Union of Basic and Clinical Pharmacology. CV. Somatostatin Receptors: Structure, Function, Ligands, and New Nomenclature. *Pharmacol. Rev.* **2018**, *70*, 763–835. [CrossRef]
4. Patel, Y.C. Somatostatin and Its Receptor Family. *Front. Neuroendocrinol.* **1999**, *20*, 157–198. [CrossRef] [PubMed]
5. Weckbecker, G.; Lewis, I.; Albert, R.; Schmid, H.A.; Hoyer, D.; Bruns, C. Opportunities in somatostatin research: Biological, chemical and therapeutic aspects. *Nat. Rev. Drug Discov.* **2003**, *2*, 999–1017. [CrossRef] [PubMed]
6. Abdel-Rahman, O.; Lamarca, A.; Valle, J.W.; Hubner, R.A. Somatostatin receptor expression in hepatocellular carcinoma: Prognostic and therapeutic considerations. *Endocr. Relat. Cancer* **2014**, *21*, R485–R493. [CrossRef]
7. Pyronnet, S.; Bousquet, C.; Najib, S.; Azar, R.; Laklai, H.; Susini, C. Antitumor effects of somatostatin. *Mol. Cell. Endocrinol.* **2008**, *286*, 230–237. [CrossRef]
8. Barbieri, F.; Bajetto, A.; Pattarozzi, A.; Gatti, M.; Würth, R.; Thellung, S.; Corsaro, A.; Villa, V.; Nizzari, M.; Florio, T. Peptide receptor targeting in cancer: The somatostatin paradigm. *Int. J. Pept.* **2013**, *2013*, 926295. [CrossRef]
9. Rai, U.; Thrimawithana, T.R.; Valery, C.; Young, S.A. Therapeutic uses of somatostatin and its analogues: Current view and potential applications. *Pharmacol. Ther.* **2015**, *152*, 98–110. [CrossRef]
10. Reubi, J.C.; Schaer, J.C.; Laissue, J.A.; Waser, B. Somatostatin receptors and their subtypes in human tumors and in peritumoral vessels. *Metabolism* **1996**, *45*, 39–41. [CrossRef]
11. Reubi, J.C.; Waser, B.; Schaer, J.C.; Laissue, J.A. Somatostatin receptor sst1-sst5 expression in normal and neoplastic human tissues using receptor autoradiography with subtype-selective ligands. *Eur. J. Nucl. Med.* **2001**, *28*, 836–846. [CrossRef] [PubMed]
12. Guillermet-Guibert, J.; Lahlou, H.; Pyronnet, S.; Bousquet, C.; Susini, C. Somatostatin receptors as tools for diagnosis and therapy: Molecular aspects. *Best Pract. Res. Clin. Gastroenterol.* **2005**, *19*, 535551. [CrossRef]
13. Hasskarl, J.; Kaufmann, M.; Schmid, H.A. Somatostatin receptors in non-neuroendocrine malignancies: The potential role of somatostatin analogs in solid tumors. *Future Oncol.* **2011**, *7*, 895–913. [CrossRef]
14. Gomes-Porras, M.; Cárdenas-Salas, J.; Álvarez-Escolá, C. Somatostatin Analogs in Clinical Practice: A Review. *Int. J. Mol. Sci.* **2020**, *21*, 1682. [CrossRef]
15. Hejna, M.; Schmidinger, M.; Raderer, M. The clinical role of somatostatin analogues as antineoplastic agents: Much ado about nothing? *Ann. Oncol.* **2002**, *13*, 653–668. [CrossRef]
16. Keskin, O.; Yalcin, S. A review of the use of somatostatin analogs in oncology. *OncoTargets Ther.* **2013**, *6*, 471–483. [CrossRef]
17. Reubi, J.C. Peptide receptors as molecular targets for cancer diagnosis and therapy. *Endocr. Rev.* **2003**, *24*, 389–427. [CrossRef]

18. Zhao, B.; Zhao, H.; Zhao, N.; Zhu, X.G. Cholangiocarcinoma cells express somatostatin receptor subtype 2 and respond to octreotide treatment. *J. Hepatobiliary Pancreat. Surg.* **2002**, *9*, 497–502. [CrossRef]
19. Bläker, M.; Schmitz, M.; Gocht, A.; Burghardt, S.; Schulz, M.; Bröring, D.C.; Pace, A.; Greten, H.; De Weerth, A. Differential expression of somatostatin receptor subtypes in hepatocellular carcinomas. *J. Hepatol.* **2004**, *41*, 112–118. [CrossRef]
20. Reubi, J.C.; Waser, B. Concomitant expression of several peptide receptors in neuroendocrine tumours: Molecular basis for in vivo multireceptor tumour targeting. *Eur. J. Nucl. Med. Mol. Imaging* **2003**, *30*, 781–793. [CrossRef]
21. Reubi, J.C.; Zimmermann, A.; Jonas, S.; Waser, B.; Neuhaus, P.; Läderach, U.; Wiedenmann, B. Regulatory peptide receptors in human hepatocellular carcinomas. *Gut* **1999**, *45*, 766–774. [CrossRef] [PubMed]
22. Reynaert, H.; Rombouts, K.; Vandermonde, A.; Urbain, D.; Kumar, U.; Bioulac-Sage, P.; Pinzani, M.; Rosenbaum, J.; Geerts, A. Expression of somatostatin receptors in normal and cirrhotic human liver and in hepatocellular carcinoma. *Gut* **2004**, *53*, 1180–1189. [CrossRef] [PubMed]
23. Nguyen-Khac, E.; Ollivier, I.; Aparicio, T.; Moullart, V.; Hugentobler, A.; Lebtahi, R.; Lobry, C.; Susini, C.; Duhamel, C.; Hommel, S.; et al. Somatostatin receptor scintigraphy screening in advanced hepatocarcinoma: A multi-center French study. *Cancer Biol. Ther.* **2009**, *8*, 2033–2039. [CrossRef] [PubMed]
24. Verhoef, C.; van Dekken, H.; Hofland, L.J.; Zondervan, P.E.; de Wilt, J.H.; van Marion, R.; de Man, R.A.; IJzermans, J.N.; van Eijck, C.H. Somatostatin receptors in human hepatocellular carcinomas: Biological, patient and tumor characteristics. *Dig. Surg.* **2008**, *25*, 21–26. [CrossRef] [PubMed]
25. Liu, H.L.; Huo, L.; Wang, L. Octreotide inhibits proliferation and induces apoptosis of hepatocellular carcinoma cells. *Acta Pharmacol. Sin.* **2004**, *25*, 1380–1386.
26. Li, S.; Liu, Y.; Shen, Z. Characterization of somatostatin receptor 2 and 5 expression in operable hepatocellular carcinomas. *Hepatogastroenterology* **2012**, *59*, 2054–2058. [CrossRef]
27. Liu, Y.; Jiang, L.; Mu, Y. Somatostatin receptor subtypes 2 and 5 are associated with better survival in operable hepatitis B-related hepatocellular carcinoma following octreotide long-acting release treatment. *Oncol. Lett.* **2013**, *6*, 821–828. [CrossRef]
28. Huang, C.Z.; Huang, A.M.; Liu, J.F.; Wang, B.; Lin, K.C.; Ye, Y.B. Somatostatin Octapeptide Inhibits Cell Invasion and Metastasis in Hepatocellular Carcinoma Through PEBP1. *Cell Physiol. Biochem.* **2018**, *47*, 2340–2349. [CrossRef]
29. Hua, Y.P.; Huang, J.F.; Liang, L.J.; Li, S.Q.; Lai, J.M.; Liang, H.Z. The study of inhibition effect of octreotide on the growth of hepatocellular carcinoma xenografts in situ in nude mice. *Chin. J. Surg.* **2005**, *43*, 721–725.
30. Jia, W.D.; Xu, G.L.; Wang, W.; Wang, Z.H.; Li, J.S.; Ma, J.L.; Ren, W.H.; Ge, Y.S.; Yu, J.H.; Liu, W.B. A somatostatin analogue, octreotide, inhibits the occurrence of second primary tumors and lung metastasis after resection of hepatocellular carcinoma in mice. *Tohoku J. Exp. Med.* **2009**, *218*, 155160. [CrossRef]
31. Reynaert, H.; Colle, I. Treatment of Advanced Hepatocellular Carcinoma with Somatostatin Analogues: A Review of the Literature. *Int. J. Mol. Sci.* **2019**, *20*, 4811. [CrossRef] [PubMed]
32. Kouroumalis, E.; Skordilis, P.; Thermos, K.; Vasilaki, A.; Moschandrea, J.; Manousos, O.N. Treatment of hepatocellular carcinoma with octreotide: A randomised controlled study. *Gut* **1998**, *42*, 442–447. [CrossRef] [PubMed]
33. Dimitroulopoulos, D.; Xinopoulos, D.; Tsamakidis, K.; Zisimopoulos, A.; Andriotis, E.; Panagiotakos, D.; Fotopoulou, A.; Chrysohoou, C.; Bazinis, A.; Daskalopoulou, D.; et al. Long acting octreotide in the treatment of advanced hepatocellular cancer and overexpression of somatostatin receptors: Randomized placebo-controlled trial. *World J. Gastroenterol.* **2007**, *13*, 3164–3170. [CrossRef] [PubMed]
34. Becker, G.; Allgaier, H.P.; Olschewski, M.; Zähringer, A.; Blum, H.E.; HECTOR Study Group. Long-acting octreotide versus placebo for treatment of advanced HCC: A randomized controlled double-blind study. *Hepatology* **2007**, *45*, 9–15. [CrossRef]
35. Barbare, J.C.; Bouché, O.; Bonnetain, F.; Dahan, L.; Lombard-Bohas, C.; Faroux, R.; Raoul, J.L.; Cattan, S.; Lemoine, A.; Blanc, J.F.; et al. Treatment of advanced hepatocellular carcinoma with long-acting octreotide: A phase III multicenter, randomised, double blind placebo-controlled study. *Eur. J. Cancer* **2009**, *45*, 1788–1797. [CrossRef]
36. Samonakis, D.N.; Notas, G.; Christodoulakis, N.; Kouroumalis, E.A. Mechanisms of action and resistance of somatostatin analogues for the treatment of hepatocellular carcinoma: A message not well taken. *Dig. Dis. Sci.* **2008**, *53*, 2359–2365. [CrossRef]

37. Kaemmerer, D.; Schindler, R.; Mußbach, F.; Dahmen, U.; Altendorf-Hofmann, A.; Dirsch, O.; Sänger, J.; Schulz, S.; Lupp, A. Somatostatin and CXCR4 chemokine receptor expression in hepatocellular and cholangiocellular carcinomas: Tumor capillaries as promising targets. *BMC Cancer* **2017**, *17*, 896. [CrossRef]
38. Rinke, A.; Müller, H.H.; Schade-Brittinger, C.; Klose, K.J.; Barth, P.; Wied, M.; Mayer, C.; Aminossadati, B.; Pape, U.F.; Bläker, M.; et al. Placebo-controlled, double-blind, prospective, randomized study on the effect of octreotide LAR in the control of tumor growth in patients with metastatic neuroendocrine midgut tumors: A report from the PROMID study group. *J. Clin. Oncol.* **2009**, *27*, 4656–4663. [CrossRef]
39. Caplin, M.E.; Pavel, M.; Ćwikła, J.B.; Phan, A.T.; Raderer, M.; Sedláčková, E.; Cadiot, G.; Wolin, E.M.; Capdevila, J.; Wall, L.; et al. Anti-tumour effects of lanreotide for pancreatic and intestinal neuroendocrine tumours: The CLARINET open-label extension study. *Endocr. Relat. Cancer* **2016**, *23*, 191–199. [CrossRef]
40. Sheppard, M.; Shapiro, B.; Pimstone, B.; Kronheim, S.; Berelowitz, M.; Gregory, M. Metabolic clearance and plasma half-disappearance time of exogenous somatostatin in man. *J. Clin. Endocrinol. Metab.* **1979**, *48*, 50–53. [CrossRef]
41. Lowell, A.; Freda, P.U. From somatostatin to octreotide LAR: Evolution of a somatostatin analogue. *Curr. Med. Res. Opin.* **2009**, *25*, 2989–2999. [CrossRef]
42. Öberg, K.; Lamberts, S.W.J. Somatostatin analogues in acromegaly and gastroenteropancreatic neuroendocrine tumours: Past, present and future. *Endocr. Relat. Cancer* **2016**, *23*, R551–R566. [CrossRef] [PubMed]
43. Ryan, P.; McBride, A.; Ray, D.; Pulgar, S.; Ramirez, R.A.; Elquza, E.; Favaro, J.P.; Dranitsaris, G. Lanreotide vs. octreotide LAR for patients with advanced gastroenteropancreatic neuroendocrine tumors: An observational time and motion analysis. *J. Oncol. Pharm. Pract.* **2019**, *25*, 1425–1433. [CrossRef] [PubMed]
44. Feelders, R.A.; Yasothan, U.; Kirkpatrick, P. Pasireotide. *Nat. Rev. Drug Discov.* **2012**, *11*, 597–598. [CrossRef]
45. Crider, A.M. Recent Advances in the Development of Nonpeptide Somatostatin Receptor Ligands. *Mini Rev. Med. Chem.* **2002**, *2*, 507–517. [CrossRef]
46. Correia, J.D.; Paulo, A.; Raposinho, P.D.; Santos, I. Radiometallated peptides for molecular imaging and targeted therapy. *Dalton Trans.* **2011**, *40*, 6144–6167. [CrossRef]
47. Jamous, M.; Haberkorn, U.; Mier, W. Synthesis of Peptide Radiopharmaceuticals for the Therapy and Diagnosis of Tumor Diseases. *Molecules* **2013**, *18*, 3379–3409. [CrossRef]
48. Tornesello, A.L.; Buonaguro, L.; Tornesello, M.L.; Buonaguro, F.M. New Insights in the Design of Bioactive Peptides and Chelating Agents for Imaging and Therapy in Oncology. *Molecules* **2017**, *22*, 1282. [CrossRef]
49. Tornesello, A.L.; Tornesello, M.L.; Buonaguro, F.M. An Overview of Bioactive Peptides for in vivo Imaging and Therapy in Human Diseases. *Mini Rev. Med. Chem.* **2017**, *17*, 758–770. [CrossRef]
50. Cutler, C.S.; Hennkens, H.M.; Sisay, N.; Huclier-Markai, S.; Jurisson, S.S. Radiometals for Combined Imaging and Therapy. *Chem. Rev.* **2013**, *113*, 858–883. [CrossRef]
51. Ramogida, C.F.; Orvig, C. Tumour Targeting with Radiometals for Diagnosis and Therapy. *Chem. Commun.* **2013**, *49*, 4720–4739. [CrossRef] [PubMed]
52. Blower, P.J. A nuclear chocolate box: The periodic table of nuclear medicine. *Dalton Trans.* **2015**, *44*, 4819–4844. [CrossRef] [PubMed]
53. Kostelnik, T.I.; Orvig, C. Radioactive Main Group and Rare Earth Metals for Imaging and Therapy. *Chem. Rev.* **2019**, *119*, 902–956. [CrossRef] [PubMed]
54. Price, E.W.; Orvig, C. Matching Chelators to Radiometals for Radiopharmaceuticals. *Chem. Soc. Rev.* **2014**, *43*, 260–290. [CrossRef] [PubMed]
55. Boros, E.; Packard, A.B. Radioactive Transition Metals for Imaging and Therapy. *Chem. Rev.* **2019**, *119*, 870–901. [CrossRef]
56. Hancock, R.D.; Martell, A.E. Ligand design for selective complexation of metal ions in aqueous solution. *Chem. Rev.* **1989**, *89*, 1875–1914. [CrossRef]
57. Stasiuk, G.J.; Long, N.J. The ubiquitous DOTA and its derivatives: The impact of 1,4,7,10-tetraazacyclododecane-1,4,7,10-tetraacetic acid on biomedical imaging. *Chem. Commun.* **2013**, *49*, 2732–2746. [CrossRef]
58. Baranyai, Z.; Tircsó, G.; Rösch, F. The Use of the Macrocyclic Chelator DOTA in Radiochemical Separations. *Eur. J. Inorg. Chem.* **2020**, 36–56. [CrossRef]
59. Sun, X.; Wuest, M.; Weisman, G.R.; Wong, E.H.; Reed, D.P.; Boswell, C.A.; Motekaitis, R.; Martell, A.E.; Welch, M.J.; Anderson, C.J. Radiolabeling and in vivo behavior of copper-64-labeled cross-bridged cyclam ligands. *J. Med. Chem.* **2002**, *45*, 469–477. [CrossRef]
60. Bhattacharyya, S.; Dixit, M. Metallic radionuclides in the development of diagnostic and therapeutic radiopharmaceuticals. *Dalton Trans.* **2011**, *40*, 6112–6128. [CrossRef]

61. Mushtaq, S.; Yun, S.J.; Jeon, J. Recent Advances in Bioorthogonal Click Chemistry for Efficient Synthesis of Radiotracers and Radiopharmaceuticals. *Molecules* **2019**, *24*, 3567. [CrossRef] [PubMed]
62. Reubi, J.C.; Maecke, H.R. Peptide-based probes for cancer imaging. *J. Nucl. Med.* **2008**, *49*, 1735–1738. [CrossRef] [PubMed]
63. Maecke, H.R.; Reubi, J.C. Somatostatin receptors as targets for nuclear medicine imaging and radionuclide treatment. *J. Nucl. Med.* **2011**, *52*, 841–844. [CrossRef] [PubMed]
64. Reubi, J.C.; Schär, J.C.; Waser, B.; Wenger, S.; Heppeler, A.; Schmitt, J.S.; Mäcke, H.R. Affinity profiles for human somatostatin receptor subtypes SST1-SST5 of somatostatin radiotracers selected for scintigraphic and radiotherapeutic use. *Eur. J. Nucl. Med.* **2000**, *27*, 273–282. [CrossRef]
65. Fani, M.; Maecke, H.R. Radiopharmaceutical development of radiolabeled peptides. *Eur. J. Nucl. Med. Mol. Imaging* **2012**, *39*, S11–S30. [CrossRef]
66. Lamberts, S.W.; Bakker, W.H.; Reubi, J.C.; Krenning, E.P. Somatostatin-receptor imaging in the localization of endocrine tumors. *N. Engl. J. Med.* **1990**, *323*, 1246–1249. [CrossRef]
67. Bakker, W.H.; Krenning, E.P.; Breeman, W.A.; Kooij, P.P.; Reubi, J.C.; Koper, J.W.; de Jong, M.; Laméris, J.S.; Visser, T.J.; Lamberts, S.W. In vivo use of a radioiodinated somatostatin analogue: Dynamics, metabolism, and binding to somatostatin receptor-positive tumors in man. *J. Nucl. Med.* **1991**, *32*, 1184–1189.
68. Bakker, W.H.; Krenning, E.P.; Breeman, W.A.; Koper, J.W.; Kooij, P.P.; Reubi, J.C.; Klijn, J.G.; Visser, T.J.; Docter, R.; Lamberts, S.W. Receptor scintigraphy with a radioiodinated somatostatin analogue: Radiolabeling, purification, biologic activity, and in vivo application in animals. *J. Nucl. Med.* **1990**, *31*, 1501–1509.
69. Bakker, W.H.; Albert, R.; Bruns, C.; Breeman, W.A.; Hofland, L.J.; Marbach, P.; Pless, J.; Pralet, D.; Stolz, B.; Koper, J.W.; et al. [^{111}In-DTPA-D-Phe^{1}]-octreotide, a potential radiopharmaceutical for imaging of somatostatin receptor-positive tumors: Synthesis, radiolabeling and in vitro validation. *Life Sci.* **1991**, *49*, 1583–1591. [CrossRef]
70. Bakker, W.H.; Krenning, E.P.; Reubi, J.C.; Breeman, W.A.; Setyono-Han, B.; de Jong, M.; Kooij, P.P.; Bruns, C.; van Hagen, P.M.; Marbach, P.; et al. In vivo application of [^{111}In-DTPA-D-Phe^{1}]-octreotide for detection of somatostatin receptor-positive tumors in rats. *Life Sci.* **1991**, *49*, 1593–1601. [CrossRef]
71. Krenning, E.P.; Bakker, W.H.; Kooij, P.P.; Breeman, W.A.; Oei, H.Y.; de Jong, M.; Reubi, J.C.; Visser, T.J.; Bruns, C.; Kwekkeboom, D.J.; et al. Somatostatin receptor scintigraphy with indium-111-DTPA-D-Phe-1-octreotide in man: Metabolism, dosimetry and comparison with iodine-123-Tyr-3-octreotide. *J. Nucl. Med.* **1992**, *33*, 652–658. [PubMed]
72. Otte, A.; Jermann, E.; Behe, M.; Goetze, M.; Bucher, H.C.; Roser, H.W.; Heppeler, A.; Mueller-Brand, J.; Maecke, H.R. DOTATOC: A powerful new tool for receptor-mediated radionuclide therapy. *Eur. J. Nucl. Med.* **1997**, *24*, 792–795. [CrossRef] [PubMed]
73. Forrer, F.; Uusijärvi, H.; Waldherr, C.; Cremonesi, M.; Bernhardt, P.; Mueller-Brand, J.; Maecke, H.R. A comparison of ^{111}In-DOTATOC and ^{111}In-DOTATATE: Biodistribution and dosimetry in the same patients with metastatic neuroendocrine tumours. *Eur. J. Nucl. Med. Mol. Imaging* **2004**, *31*, 1257–1262. [CrossRef] [PubMed]
74. Wild, D.; Schmitt, J.S.; Ginj, M.; Mäcke, H.R.; Bernard, B.F.; Krenning, E.; De Jong, M.; Wenger, S.; Reubi, J.C. DOTA-NOC, a high-affinity ligand of somatostatin receptor subtypes 2, 3 and 5 for labeling with various radiometals. *Eur. J. Nucl. Med. Mol. Imaging* **2003**, *30*, 1338–1347. [CrossRef]
75. Virgolini, I.; Ambrosini, V.; Bomanji, J.B.; Baum, R.P.; Fanti, S.; Gabriel, M.; Papathanasiou, N.D.; Pepe, G.; Oyen, W.; De Cristoforo, C.; et al. Procedure guidelines for PET/CT tumour imaging with ^{68}Ga-DOTA-conjugated peptides: ^{68}Ga-DOTA-TOC, ^{68}Ga-DOTA-NOC, ^{68}Ga-DOTA-TATE. *Eur. J. Nucl. Med. Mol. Imaging* **2010**, *37*, 2004–2010. [CrossRef]
76. Hofmann, M.; Maecke, H.; Börner, R.; Weckesser, E.; Schöffski, P.; Oei, L.; Schumacher, J.; Henze, M.; Heppeler, A.; Meyer, J.; et al. Biokinetics and imaging with the somatostatin receptor PET radioligand ^{68}Ga-DOTATOC: Preliminary data. *Eur. J. Nucl. Med.* **2001**, *28*, 1751–1757. [CrossRef]
77. Hofman, M.S.; Lau, W.F.; Hicks, R.J. Somatostatin receptor imaging with ^{68}Ga DOTATATE PET/CT: Clinical utility, normal patterns, pearls, and pitfalls in interpretation. *Radiographics* **2015**, *35*, 500–516. [CrossRef]
78. Wild, D.; Mäcke, H.R.; Waser, B.; Reubi, J.C.; Ginj, M.; Rasch, H.; Müller-Brand, J.; Hofmann, M. ^{68}Ga-DOTANOC: A first compound for PET imaging with high affinity for somatostatin receptor subtypes 2 and 5. *Eur. J. Nucl. Med. Mol. Imaging* **2005**, *32*, 724. [CrossRef]

79. Antunes, P.; Ginj, M.; Walter, M.A.; Chen, J.; Reubi, J.C.; Maecke, H.R. Influence of different spacers on the biological profile of a DOTA-Somatostatin analogue. *Bioconjugate Chem.* **2007**, *18*, 84–92. [CrossRef]
80. Eisenwiener, K.P.; Prata, M.I.; Buschmann, I.; Zhang, H.W.; Santos, A.C.; Wenger, S.; Reubi, J.C.; Mäcke, H.R. NODAGATOC, a new chelator-coupled somatostatin analogue labeled with [$^{67/68}$Ga] and [^{111}In] for SPECT, PET, and targeted therapeutic applications of somatostatin receptor (hsst2) expressing tumors. *Bioconjugate Chem.* **2002**, *13*, 530–541. [CrossRef]
81. Laznickova, A.; Laznicek, M.; Trejtnar, F.; Maecke, H.R.; Eisenwiener, K.P.; Reubi, J.C. Biodistribution of two octreotate analogs radiolabeled with indium and yttrium in rats. *Anticancer Res.* **2010**, *30*, 2177–2184. [PubMed]
82. Ginj, M.; Chen, J.; Walter, M.A.; Eltschinger, V.; Reubi, J.C.; Maecke, H.R. Preclinical evaluation of new and highly potent analogues of octreotide for predictive imaging and targeted radiotherapy. *Clin. Cancer Res.* **2005**, *11*, 1136–1145. [PubMed]
83. Boubaker, A.; Prior, J.O.; Willi, J.P.; Champendal, M.; Kosinski, M.; Bischof-Delaloye, A.; Maecke, H.R.; Ginj, M.; Baechler, S.; Buchegger, F. Biokinetics and dosimetry of ^{111}In-DOTA-NOC-ATE compared with ^{111}In-DTPA-octreotide. *Eur. J. Nucl. Med. Mol. Imaging* **2012**, *39*, 1868–1875. [CrossRef] [PubMed]
84. Ma, M.T.; Cullinane, C.; Waldeck, K.; Roselt, P.; Hicks, R.J.; Blower, P.J. Rapid kit-based ^{68}Ga-labeling and PET imaging with THP-Tyr^3-octreotate: A preliminary comparison with DOTA-Tyr3octreotate. *EJNMMI Res.* **2015**, *5*, 52. [CrossRef] [PubMed]
85. Fani, M.; Mueller, A.; Tamma, M.L.; Nicolas, G.; Rink, H.R.; Cescato, R.; Reubi, J.C.; Maecke, H.R. Radiolabeled bicyclic somatostatin-based analogs: A novel class of potential radiotracers for SPECT/PET of neuroendocrine tumors. *J. Nucl. Med.* **2010**, *51*, 1771–1779. [CrossRef]
86. Ginj, M.; Zhang, H.; Eisenwiener, K.P.; Wild, D.; Schulz, S.; Rink, H.; Cescato, R.; Reubi, J.C.; Maecke, H.R. New pansomatostatin ligands and their chelated versions: Affinity profile, agonist activity, internalization, and tumor targeting. *Clin. Cancer Res.* **2008**, *14*, 2019–2027. [CrossRef]
87. Liu, F.; Liu, T.; Xu, X.; Guo, X.; Li, N.; Xiong, C.; Li, C.; Zhu, H.; Yang, Z. Design, Synthesis, and Biological Evaluation of ^{68}Ga-DOTA-PA1 for Lung Cancer: A Novel PET Tracer for Multiple Somatostatin Receptor Imaging. *Mol. Pharm.* **2018**, *15*, 619–628. [CrossRef]
88. Tatsi, A.; Maina, T.; Cescato, R.; Waser, B.; Krenning, E.P.; de Jong, M.; Cordopatis, P.; Reubi, J.C.; Nock, B.A. [^{111}In-DOTA]Somatostatin-14 analogs as potential pansomatostatin-like radiotracers—First results of a preclinical study. *EJNMMI Res.* **2012**, *2*, 25. [CrossRef]
89. Maina, T.; Cescato, R.; Waser, B.; Tatsi, A.; Kaloudi, A.; Krenning, E.P.; de Jong, M.; Nock, B.A.; Reubi, J.C. [^{111}In-DOTA]LTT-SS28, a first pansomatostatin radioligand for in vivo targeting of somatostatin receptor-positive tumors. *J. Med. Chem.* **2014**, *57*, 6564–6571. [CrossRef]
90. Pearson, D.A.; Lister-James, J.; McBride, W.J.; Wilson, D.M.; Martel, L.J.; Civitello, E.R.; Taylor, J.E.; Moyer, B.R.; Dean, R.T. Somatostatin receptor-binding peptides labeled with technetium-99m: Chemistry and initial biological studies. *J. Med. Chem.* **1996**, *39*, 1361–1371. [CrossRef]
91. Decristoforo, C.; Mather, S.J. Preparation, ^{99m}Tc-labeling and in vitro characterization of HYNIC and N3S modified RC-160 and [Tyr^3]octreotide. *Bioconjugate Chem.* **1999**, *10*, 431–438. [CrossRef] [PubMed]
92. Maina, T.; Stolz, B.; Albert, R.; Bruns, C.; Koch, P.; Mäcke, H. Synthesis, radiochemistry and biological evaluation of a new somatostatin analogue (SDZ 219-387) labeled with technetium-99m. *Eur. J. Nucl. Med.* **1994**, *21*, 437–444. [CrossRef] [PubMed]
93. Thakur, M.L.; Kolan, H.; Li, J.; Wiaderkiewicz, R.; Pallela, V.R.; Duggaraju, R.; Schally, A.V. Radiolabeled somatostatin analogues in prostate cancer. *Nucl. Med. Biol.* **1997**, *24*, 105–113. [CrossRef]
94. Abiraj, K.; Ursillo, S.; Tamma, M.L.; Rylova, S.N.; Waser, B.; Constable, E.C.; Fani, M.; Nicolas, G.P.; Reubi, J.C.; Maecke, H.R. The tetraamine chelator outperforms HYNIC in a new technetium-99m-labeled somatostatin receptor 2 antagonist. *EJNMMI Res.* **2018**, *8*, 75. [CrossRef]
95. Spradau, T.W.; Edwards, W.B.; Anderson, C.J.; Welch, M.J.; Katzenellenbogen, J.A. Synthesis and biological evaluation of Tc-99m-cyclopentadienyltricarbonyltechnetium-labeled octreotide. *Nucl. Med. Biol.* **1999**, *26*, 1–7. [CrossRef]
96. Makris, G.; Kuchuk, M.; Gallazzi, F.; Jurisson, S.S.; Smith, C.J.; Hennkens, H.M. Somatostatin receptor targeting with hydrophilic [^{99m}Tc/^{186}Re]Tc/Re-tricarbonyl NODAGA and NOTA complexes. *Nucl. Med. Biol.* **2019**, *71*, 39–46. [CrossRef]
97. Abrams, M.J.; Juweid, M.; tenKate, C.I.; Schwartz, D.A.; Hauser, M.M.; Gaul, F.E.; Fuccello, A.J.; Rubin, R.H.;

Strauss, H.W.; Fischman, A.J. Technetium-99m-human polyclonal IgG radiolabeled via the hydrazino nicotinamide derivative for imaging focal sites of infection in rats. *J. Nucl. Med.* **1990**, *31*, 2022–2028.
98. Mikolajczak, R.; Maecke, H.R. Radiopharmaceuticals for somatostatin receptor imaging. *Nucl. Med. Rev. Cent. East Eur.* **2016**, *19*, 126–132. [CrossRef]
99. Decristoforo, C.; Melendez-Alafort, L.; Sosabowski, J.K.; Mather, S.J. ^{99m}Tc-HYNIC-[Tyr^3]octreotide for imaging somatostatin receptor positive tumors: Preclinical evaluation and comparison with ^{111}In-octreotide. *J. Nucl. Med.* **2000**, *41*, 1114–1119.
100. Gabriel, M.; Decristoforo, C.; Donnemiller, E.; Ulmer, H.; Watfah Rychlinski, C.; Mather, S.J.; Moncayo, R. An intrapatient comparison of ^{99m}Tc-EDDA/HYNIC-TOC with ^{111}In-DTPA-Octreotide for diagnosis of somatostatin receptor expressing tumors. *J. Nucl. Med.* **2003**, *44*, 708–716.
101. Cwikla, J.B.; Mikolajczak, R.; Pawlak, D.; Buscombe, J.R.; Nasierowska-Guttmejer, A.; Bator, A.; Maecke, H.R.; Walecki, J. Initial direct comparison of ^{99m}Tc-TOC and ^{99m}Tc-TATE in identifying sites of disease in patients with proven GEP NETs. *J. Nucl. Med.* **2008**, *49*, 1060–1065. [CrossRef] [PubMed]
102. Decristoforo, C.; Maina, T.; Nock, B.; Gabriel, M.; Cordopatis, P.; Moncayo, R. ^{99m}Tc-Demotate 1: First data in tumour patients-results of a pilot/phase I study. *Eur. J. Nucl. Med. Mol. Imaging* **2003**, *30*, 1211–1219. [CrossRef] [PubMed]
103. Maina, T.; Nock, B.A.; Cordopatis, P.; Bernard, B.F.; Breeman, W.A.; van Gameren, A.; van den Berg, R.; Reubi, J.C.; Krenning, E.P.; de Jong, M. [^{99m}Tc]Demotate 2 in the detection of sst2-positive tumours: A preclinical comparison with [^{111}In]DOTA-tate. *Eur. J. Nucl. Med. Mol. Imaging* **2006**, *33*, 831–840. [CrossRef] [PubMed]
104. Virgolini, I.; Leimer, M.; Handmaker, H.; Lastoria, S.; Bischof, C.; Muto, P.; Pangerl, T.; Gludovacz, D.; Peck-Radosavljevic, M.; Lister-James, J.; et al. Somatostatin receptor subtype specificity and in vivo binding of a novel tumor tracer, ^{99m}Tc-P829. *Cancer Res.* **1998**, *58*, 1850–1859.
105. Lebtahi, R.; Le Cloirec, J.; Houzard, C.; Daou, D.; Sobhani, I.; Sassolas, G.; Mignon, M.; Bourguet, P.; Le Guludec, D. Detection of neuroendocrine tumors: ^{99m}Tc-P829 scintigraphy compared with ^{111}In-pentetreotide scintigraphy. *J. Nucl. Med.* **2002**, *43*, 889–895.
106. Blum, J.E.; Handmaker, H.; Rinne, N.A. The utility of a somatostatin-type receptor binding peptide radiopharmaceutical (P829) in the evaluation of solitary pulmonary nodules. *Chest* **1999**, *115*, 224–232. [CrossRef]
107. Bååth, M.; Kolbeck, K.G.; Danielsson, R. Somatostatin receptor scintigraphy with ^{99m}Tc-Depreotide (NeoSpect) in discriminating between malignant and benign lesions in the diagnosis of lung cancer: A pilot study. *Acta Radiol.* **2004**, *45*, 833–839. [CrossRef]
108. Axelsson, R.; Herlin, G.; Bååth, M.; Aspelin, P.; Kolbeck, K.G. Role of scintigraphy with technetium-99m depreotide in the diagnosis and management of patients with suspected lung cancer. *Acta Radiol.* **2008**, *49*, 295–302. [CrossRef]
109. Menda, Y.; Kahn, D. Somatostatin receptor imaging of non-small cell lung cancer with ^{99m}Tc depreotide. *Semin. Nucl. Med.* **2002**, *32*, 92–96. [CrossRef]
110. Van Den Bossche, B.; D'haeninck, E.; Bacher, K.; Thierens, H.; Van Belle, S.; Dierckx, R.A.; Van de Wiele, C. Biodistribution and dosimetry of ^{99m}Tc-depreotide (P829) in patients suffering from breast carcinoma. *Cancer Biother. Radiopharm.* **2004**, *19*, 776–783. [CrossRef]
111. Briganti, V.; Cuccurullo, V.; Di Stasio, G.D.; Mansi, L. Gamma Emitters in Pancreatic Endocrine Tumors Imaging in the PET Era: Is there a Clinical Space for ^{99m}Tc-peptides? *Curr. Radiopharm.* **2019**, *12*, 156–170. [CrossRef] [PubMed]
112. Boschi, A.; Uccelli, L.; Martini, P. A Picture of Modern Tc-99m Radiopharmaceuticals: Production, Chemistry, and Applications in Molecular Imaging. *Appl. Sci.* **2019**, *9*, 2526. [CrossRef]
113. Boschi, A.; Martini, P.; Janevik-Ivanovska, E.; Duatti, A. The emerging role of copper-64 radiopharmaceuticals as cancer theranostics. *Drug Discov. Today* **2018**, *23*, 1489–1501. [CrossRef] [PubMed]
114. Anderson, C.J.; Dehdashti, F.; Cutler, P.D.; Schwarz, S.W.; Laforest, R.; Bass, L.A.; Lewis, J.S.; McCarthy, D.W. ^{64}Cu-TETA-octreotide as a PET imaging agent for patients with neuroendocrine tumors. *J. Nucl. Med.* **2001**, *42*, 213–221.
115. Sprague, J.E.; Peng, Y.; Sun, X.; Weisman, G.R.; Wong, E.H.; Achilefu, S.; Anderson, C.J. Preparation and biological evaluation of copper-64-labeled Tyr^3-octreotate using a cross-bridged macrocyclic chelator. *Clin. Cancer Res.* **2004**, *10*, 8674–8682. [CrossRef]

116. Edwards, W.B.; Fields, C.G.; Anderson, C.J.; Pajeau, T.S.; Welch, M.J.; Fields, G.B. Generally Applicable, Convenient Solid-Phase Synthesis and Receptor Affinities of Octreotide Analogs. *J. Med. Chem.* **1994**, *37*, 3749–3757. [CrossRef]

117. Paterson, B.M.; Roselt, P.; Denoyer, D.; Cullinane, C.; Binns, D.; Noonan, W.; Jeffery, C.M.; Price, R.I.; White, J.M.; Hicks, R.J.; et al. PET imaging of tumours with a ^{64}Cu labeled macrobicyclic cage amine ligand tethered to Tyr^{3}-octreotate. *Dalton Trans.* **2014**, *43*, 1386–1396. [CrossRef]

118. Marciniak, A.; Brasuń, J. Somatostatin analogues labeled with copper radioisotopes: Currrent status. *J. Radioanal. Nucl. Chem.* **2017**, *313*, 279–289. [CrossRef]

119. Pfeifer, A.; Knigge, U.; Binderup, T.; Mortensen, J.; Oturai, P.; Loft, A.; Berthelsen, A.K.; Langer, S.W.; Rasmussen, P.; Elema, D.; et al. ^{64}Cu-DOTATATE PET for Neuroendocrine Tumors: A Prospective Head-to-Head Comparison with ^{111}In-DTPA-Octreotide in 112 Patients. *J. Nucl. Med.* **2015**, *56*, 847–854. [CrossRef]

120. Johnbeck, C.B.; Knigge, U.; Loft, A.; Berthelsen, A.K.; Mortensen, J.; Oturai, P.; Langer, S.W.; Elema, D.R.; Kjaer, A. Head-to-head comparison of ^{64}Cu-DOTATATE and ^{68}Ga-DOTATOC PET/CT: A prospective study of 59 patients with neuroendocrine tumors. *J. Nucl. Med.* **2017**, *58*, 451–458. [CrossRef]

121. Carlsen, E.A.; Johnbeck, C.B.; Binderup, T.; Loft, M.; Pfeifer, A.; Mortensen, J.; Oturai, P.; Loft, A.; Berthelsen, A.K.; Langer, S.W.; et al. ^{64}Cu-DOTATATE PET/CT and prediction of overall and progression-free survival in patients with neuroendocrine neoplasms. *J. Nucl. Med.* **2020**. [CrossRef]

122. Andersen, T.L.; Baun, C.; Olsen, B.B.; Dam, J.H.; Thisgaard, H. Improving Contrast and Detectability: Imaging with [^{55}Co]Co-DOTATATE in Comparison with [^{64}Cu]Cu-DOTATATE and [^{68}Ga]Ga-DOTATATE. *J. Nucl. Med.* **2020**, *61*, 228–233. [CrossRef] [PubMed]

123. Mirzaei, S.; Revheim, M.; Raynor, W.; Zehetner, W.; Knoll, P.; Zandieh, S.; Alavi, A. ^{64}Cu-DOTATOC PET-CT in Patients with Neuroendocrine Tumors. *Oncol. Ther.* **2019**, *8*, 125–131. [CrossRef]

124. Hicks, R.J.; Jackson, P.; Kong, G.; Ware, R.E.; Hofman, M.S.; Pattison, D.A.; Akhurst, T.A.; Drummond, E.; Roselt, P.; Callahan, J.; et al. ^{64}Cu-SARTATE PET Imaging of Patients with Neuroendocrine Tumors Demonstrates High Tumor Uptake and Retention, Potentially Allowing Prospective Dosimetry for Peptide Receptor Radionuclide Therapy. *J. Nucl. Med.* **2019**, *60*, 777–785. [CrossRef] [PubMed]

125. Delpassand, E.S.; Ranganathan, D.; Wagh, N.; Shafie, A.; Gaber, A.; Abbasi, A.; Kjaer, A.; Tworowska, I.; Núñez, R. ^{64}Cu-DOTATATE PET/CT for Imaging Patients with Known or Suspected Somatostatin Receptor-Positive Neuroendocrine Tumors: Results of the First US Prospective, Reader-Blinded Clinical Trial. *J. Nucl. Med.* **2020**, *61*, 890–896. [CrossRef] [PubMed]

126. Heppeler, A.; André, J.P.; Buschmann, I.; Wang, X.; Reubi, J.C.; Hennig, M.; Kaden, T.A.; Maecke, H.R. Metal-ion-dependent biological properties of a chelator-derived somatostatin analogue for tumour targeting. *Chem. Eur. J.* **2008**, *14*, 3026–3034. [CrossRef] [PubMed]

127. Thisgaard, H.; Olsen, B.B.; Dam, J.H.; Bollen, P.; Mollenhauer, J.; Høilund-Carlsen, P.F. Evaluation of cobalt-labeled octreotide analogs for molecular imaging and Auger electron-based radionuclide therapy. *J. Nucl. Med.* **2014**, *55*, 1311–1316. [CrossRef]

128. Thisgaard, H.; Olesen, M.; Dam, J.H. Radiosynthesis of Co-55- and Co-58m-labeled DOTATOC for positron emission tomography imaging and targeted radionuclide therapy. *J. Label. Compd. Radiopharm.* **2011**, *54*, 758–762. [CrossRef]

129. Müller, C.; Domnanich, K.A.; Umbricht, C.A.; van der Meulen, N.P. Scandium and terbium radionuclides for radiotheranostics: Current state of development towards clinical application. *Br. J. Radiol.* **2018**, *91*, 20180074. [CrossRef]

130. Pruszyński, M.; Majkowska-Pilip, A.; Loktionova, N.S.; Eppard, E.; Roesch, F. Radiolabeling of DOTATOC with the long-lived positron emitter ^{44}Sc. *Appl. Radiat. Isot.* **2012**, *70*, 974–979. [CrossRef]

131. Müller, C.; Vermeulen, C.; Johnston, K.; Köster, U.; Schmid, R.; Türler, A.; van der Meulen, N.P. Preclinical in vivo application of ^{152}Tb-DOTANOC: A radiolanthanide for PET imaging. *EJNMMI Res.* **2016**, *6*, 35. [CrossRef] [PubMed]

132. Singh, A.; van der Meulen, N.P.; Muller, C.; Klette, I.; Kulkarni, H.R.; Türler, A.; Schibli, R.; Baum, R.P. First-in-human PET/CT imaging of metastatic neuroendocrine neoplasms with cyclotron-produced ^{44}Sc-DOTATOC: A proof-of-concept study. *Cancer Biother. Radiopharm.* **2017**, *32*, 124–132. [CrossRef] [PubMed]

133. Baum, R.P.; Singh, A.; Benešová, M.; Vermeulen, C.; Gnesin, S.; Köster, U.; Johnston, K.; Müller, D.;

Senftleben, S.; Kulkarni, H.R.; et al. Clinical evaluation of the radiolanthanide terbium-152: First-in-human PET/CT with ^{152}Tb-DOTATOC. *Dalton Trans.* **2017**, *46*, 14638–14646. [CrossRef] [PubMed]

134. Koumarianou, E.; Pawlak, D.; Korsak, A.; Mikolajczak, R. Comparison of receptor affinity of ^{nat}Sc-DOTA-TATE versus ^{nat}Ga-DOTA-TATE. *Nucl. Med. Rev. Cent. East Eur.* **2011**, *14*, 85–89. [CrossRef]
135. Domnanich, K.A.; Müller, C.; Farkas, R.; Schmid, R.M.; Ponsard, B.; Schibli, R.; Türler, A.; van der Meulen, N.P. ^{44}Sc for labeling of DOTA- and NODAGA-functionalized peptides: Preclinical in vitro and in vivo investigations. *EJNMMI Radiopharm. Chem.* **2017**, *1*, 8. [CrossRef]
136. Sinnes, J.P.; Nagel, J.; Rösch, F. AAZTA5/AAZTA5-TOC: Synthesis and radiochemical evaluation with ^{68}Ga, ^{44}Sc and ^{177}Lu. *EJNMMI Radiopharm. Chem.* **2019**, *4*, 18. [CrossRef]
137. Müller, C.; Fischer, E.; Behe, M.; Köster, U.; Dorrer, H.; Reber, J.; Haller, S.; Cohrs, S.; Blanc, A.; Grünberg, J.; et al. Future prospects for SPECT imaging using the radiolanthanide terbium-155—Production and preclinical evaluation in tumor-bearing mice. *Nucl. Med. Biol.* **2014**, *41*, e58–e65. [CrossRef]
138. Walrand, S.; Jamar, F.; Mathieu, I.; De Camps, J.; Lonneux, M.; Sibomana, M.; Labar, D.; Michel, C.; Pauwels, S. Quantitation in PET using isotopes emitting prompt single gammas: Application to yttrium-86. *Eur. J. Nucl. Med. Mol. Imaging* **2003**, *30*, 354–361. [CrossRef]
139. Helisch, A.; Förster, G.J.; Reber, H.; Buchholz, H.G.; Arnold, R.; Göke, B.; Weber, M.M.; Wiedenmann, B.; Pauwels, S.; Haus, U.; et al. Pre-therapeutic dosimetry and biodistribution of ^{86}Y-DOTA-Phe^1-Tyr^3-octreotide versus ^{111}In-pentetreotide in patients with advanced neuroendocrine tumours. *Eur. J. Nucl. Med. Mol. Imaging* **2004**, *31*, 1386–1392. [CrossRef]
140. Clifford, T.; Boswell, C.A.; Biddlecombe, G.B.; Lewis, J.S.; Brechbiel, M.W. Validation of a novel CHX-A "derivative suitable for peptide conjugation: Small animal PET/CT imaging using yttrium-86-CHX-A"-octreotide. *J. Med. Chem.* **2006**, *49*, 4297–4304. [CrossRef]
141. Jamar, F.; Barone, R.; Mathieu, I.; Walrand, S.; Labar, D.; Carlier, P.; de Camps, J.; Schran, H.; Chen, T.; Smith, M.C.; et al. ^{86}Y-DOTA^0-D-Phe^1-Tyr^3-octreotide (SMT487)—A phase 1 clinical study: Pharmacokinetics, biodistribution and renal protective effect of different regimens of amino acid co-infusion. *Eur. J. Nucl. Med. Mol. Imaging* **2003**, *30*, 510–518. [CrossRef] [PubMed]
142. Mikolajczak, R.; van der Meulen, N.P.; Lapi, S.E. Radiometals for imaging and theranostics, current production, and future perspectives. *J. Label. Compd. Radiopharm.* **2019**, *62*, 615–634. [CrossRef] [PubMed]
143. do Carmo, S.J.C.; Scott, P.J.H.; Alves, F. Production of radiometals in liquid targets. *EJNMMI Radiopharm. Chem.* **2020**, *5*, 2. [CrossRef] [PubMed]
144. Talip, Z.; Favaretto, C.; Geistlich, S.; Meulen, N.P.V. A Step-by-Step Guide for the Novel Radiometal Production for Medical Applications: Case Studies with ^{68}Ga, ^{44}Sc, ^{177}Lu and ^{161}Tb. *Molecules* **2020**, *25*, 966. [CrossRef]
145. Waldmann, C.M.; Stuparu, A.D.; van Dam, R.M.; Slavik, R. The search for an alternative to [^{68}Ga]Ga-DOTA-TATE in neuroendocrine tumor theranostics: Current state of ^{18}F-labeled somatostatin analog development. *Theranostics* **2019**, *9*, 1336–1347. [CrossRef]
146. Guhlke, S.; Wester, H.J.; Bruns, C.; Stöcklin, G. (2-[^{18}F]Fluoropropionyl-(D)phe^1)-octreotide, a potential radiopharmaceutical for quantitative somatostatin receptor imaging with PET: Synthesis, Radiolabeling, in vitro validation and biodistribution in mice. *Nucl. Med. Biol.* **1994**, *21*, 819–825. [CrossRef]
147. Hostetler, E.D.; Edwards, W.B.; Anderson, C.J.; Welch, M.J. Synthesis of 4-[^{18}F]fluorobenzoyl octreotide and biodistribution in tumour-bearing Lewis rats. *J. Label. Compd Radiopharm.* **1999**, *42*, S720–S722.
148. Wester, H.J.; Schottelius, M.; Poethko, T.; Bruus-Jensen, K.; Schwaiger, M. Radiolabeled Carbohydrated Somatostatin Analogs: A Review of the Current Status. *Cancer Biother. Radiopharm.* **2004**, *19*, 231–244. [CrossRef]
149. Maschauer, S.; Heilmann, M.; Wängler, C.; Schirrmacher, R.; Prante, O. Radiosynthesis and preclinical evaluation of ^{18}F-fluoroglycosylated octreotate for somatostatin receptor imaging. *Bioconjugate Chem.* **2016**, *27*, 2707–2714. [CrossRef]
150. Liu, Z.; Pourghiasian, M.; Bénard, F.; Pan, J.; Lin, K.S.; Perrin, D.M. Preclinical evaluation of a high-affinity ^{18}F-trifluoroborate octreotate derivative for somatostatin receptor imaging. *J. Nucl. Med.* **2014**, *55*, 1499–1505. [CrossRef]
151. Niedermoser, S.; Chin, J.; Wängler, C.; Kostikov, A.; Bernard-Gauthier, V.; Vogler, N.; Soucy, J.P.; McEwan, A.J.; Schirrmacher, R.; Wängler, B. In vivo evaluation of ^{18}F-SiFAlin-Modified TATE: A potential challenge for

^{68}Ga-DOTATATE, the clinical gold standard for somatostatin receptor imaging with PET. *J. Nucl. Med.* **2015**, *56*, 1100–1105. [CrossRef]

152. Allott, L.; Dubash, S.; Aboagye, E.O. [^{18}F]FET-βAG-TOCA: The Design, Evaluation and Clinical Translation of a Fluorinated Octreotide. *Cancers* **2020**, *12*, 865. [CrossRef] [PubMed]
153. Laverman, P.; McBride, W.J.; Sharkey, R.M.; Eek, A.; Joosten, L.; Oyen, W.J.G.; Goldenberg, D.M.; Boerman, O.C. A novel facile method of labeling octreotide with ^{18}F-fluorine. *J. Nucl. Med.* **2010**, *51*, 454–461. [CrossRef] [PubMed]
154. Meisetschlaeger, G.; Poethko, T.; Stahl, A.; Wolf, I.; Scheidhauer, K.; Schottelius, M.; Herz, M.; Wester, H.J.; Schwaiger, M. Gluc-Lys([^{18}F]FP)-TOCA PET in patients with SSTR-positive tumors: Biodistribution and diagnostic evaluation compared with [^{111}In]DTPA-octreotide. *J. Nucl. Med.* **2006**, *47*, 566–573.
155. Ilhan, H.; Lindner, S.; Todica, A.; Cyran, C.C.; Tiling, R.; Auernhammer, C.J.; Spitzweg, C.; Boeck, S.; Unterrainer, M.; Gildehaus, F.J.; et al. Biodistribution and first clinical results of ^{18}F-SiFAlin-TATE PET: A novel ^{18}F-labeled somatostatin analog for imaging of neuroendocrine tumors. *Eur. J. Nucl. Med. Mol. Imaging* **2020**, *47*, 870–880. [CrossRef] [PubMed]
156. Pauwels, E.; Cleeren, F.; Tshibangu, T.; Koole, M.; Serdons, K.; Dekervel, J.; Van Cutsem, E.; Verslype, C.; Van Laere, K.; Bormans, G.; et al. [^{18}F]AlF-NOTA-octreotide PET imaging: Biodistribution, dosimetry and first comparison with [^{68}Ga]Ga-DOTATATE in neuroendocrine tumour patients. *Eur. J. Nucl. Med. Mol. Imaging* **2020**. [CrossRef]
157. Kemerink, G.J.; Visser, M.G.; Franssen, R.; Beijer, E.; Zamburlini, M.; Halders, S.G.; Brans, B.; Mottaghy, F.M.; Teule, G.J. Effect of the positron range of ^{18}F, ^{68}Ga and ^{124}I on PET/CT in lung-equivalent materials. *Eur. J. Nucl. Med. Mol. Imaging* **2011**, *38*, 940–948. [CrossRef]
158. Uccelli, L.; Martini, P.; Cittanti, C.; Carnevale, A.; Missiroli, L.; Giganti, M.; Bartolomei, M.; Boschi, A. Therapeutic Radiometals: Worldwide Scientific Literature Trend Analysis (2008–2018). *Molecules* **2019**, *24*, 640. [CrossRef]
159. Cremonesi, M.; Ferrari, M.E.; Bodei, L.; Chiesa, C.; Sarnelli, A.; Garibaldi, C.; Pacilio, M.; Strigari, L.; Summers, P.E.; Orecchia, R.; et al. Correlation of dose with toxicity and tumour response to ^{90}Y- and ^{177}Lu-PRRT provides the basis for optimization through individualized treatment planning. *Eur. J. Nucl. Med. Mol. Imaging* **2018**, *45*, 2426–2441. [CrossRef]
160. Otte, A.; Mueller-Brand, J.; Dellas, S.; Nitzsche, E.U.; Herrmann, R.; Maecke, H.R. Yttrium-90 labeled somatostatin-analogue for cancer treatment. *Lancet* **1998**, *351*, 417–418. [CrossRef]
161. Otte, A.; Herrmann, R.; Heppeler, A.; Behe, M.; Jermann, E.; Powell, P.; Maecke, H.R.; Muller, J. Yttrium-90 DOTATOC: First clinical results. *Eur. J. Nucl. Med.* **1999**, *26*, 1439–1447. [CrossRef] [PubMed]
162. Vinjamuri, S.; Gilbert, T.M.; Banks, M.; McKane, G.; Maltby, P.; Poston, G.; Weissman, H.; Palmer, D.H.; Vora, J.; Pritchard, D.M.; et al. Peptide Receptor Radionuclide Therapy With ^{90}Y-DOTATATE/^{90}Y-DOTATOC in Patients with Progressive Metastatic Neuroendocrine Tumours: Assessment of Response, Survival and Toxicity. *Br. J. Cancer* **2013**, *108*, 1440–1448. [CrossRef] [PubMed]
163. Virgolini, I.; Britton, K.; Buscombe, J.; Moncayo, R.; Paganelli, G.; Riva, P. In- and Y-DOTA-lanreotide: Results and implications of the MAURITIUS trial. *Semin. Nucl. Med.* **2002**, *32*, 148–155. [CrossRef] [PubMed]
164. Bodei, L.; Cremonesi, M.; Grana, C.M.; Chinol, M.; Baio, S.M.; Severi, S.; Paganelli, G. Yttrium-labeled peptides for therapy of NET. *Eur. J. Nucl. Med. Mol. Imaging* **2012**, *39*, S93–S102. [CrossRef]
165. Gabriel, M.; Nilica, B.; Kaiser, B.; Virgolini, I.J. Twelve-Year Follow-up After Peptide Receptor Radionuclide Therapy. *J. Nucl. Med.* **2019**, *60*, 524–529. [CrossRef]
166. Baum, R.P.; Kluge, A.W.; Kulkarni, H.; Schorr-Neufing, U.; Niepsch, K.; Bitterlich, N.; van Echteld, C.J. [^{177}Lu-DOTA]^0-D-Phe^1-Tyr^3-Octreotide (^{177}Lu-DOTATOC) For Peptide Receptor Radiotherapy in Patients with Advanced Neuroendocrine Tumours: A Phase-II Study. *Theranostics* **2016**, *6*, 501–510. [CrossRef]
167. Esser, J.P.; Krenning, E.P.; Teunissen, J.J.; Kooij, P.P.; van Gameren, A.L.; Bakker, W.H.; Kwekkeboom, D.J. Comparison of [^{177}Lu-DOTA^0,Tyr^3]octreotate and [^{177}Lu-DOTA^0,Tyr^3]octreotide: Which peptide is preferable for PRRT? *Eur. J. Nucl. Med. Mol. Imaging* **2006**, *33*, 1346–1351. [CrossRef]
168. de Jong, M.; Breeman, W.A.; Valkema, R.; Bernard, B.F.; Krenning, E.P. Combination radionuclide therapy using ^{177}Lu- and ^{90}Y-labeled somatostatin analogs. *J. Nucl. Med.* **2005**, *46*, 13S–17S.
169. Kunikowska, J.; Królicki, L.; Hubalewska-Dydejczyk, A.; Mikołajczak, R.; Sowa-Staszczak, A.; Pawlak, D. Clinical results of radionuclide therapy of neuroendocrine tumours with ^{90}Y-DOTATATE and tandem

$^{90}Y/^{177}Lu$-DOTATATE: Which is a better therapy option? *Eur. J. Nucl. Med. Mol. Imaging* **2011**, *38*, 1788–1797. [CrossRef]

170. Kunikowska, J.; Zemczak, A.; Kołodziej, M.; Gut, P.; Łoń, I.; Pawlak, D.; Mikołajczak, R.; Kamiński, G.; Ruchała, M.; Kos-Kudła, B.; et al. Tandem peptide receptor radionuclide therapy using $^{90}Y/^{177}Lu$-DOTATATE for neuroendocrine tumors efficacy and side-effects—Polish multicenter experience. *Eur. J. Nucl. Med. Mol. Imaging* **2020**, *47*, 922–933. [CrossRef]
171. Brabander, T.; Nonnekens, J.; Hofland, J. The next generation of peptide receptor radionuclide therapy. *Endocr. Relat. Cancer* **2019**, *26*, C7–C11. [CrossRef] [PubMed]
172. Adant, S.; Shah, G.M.; Beauregard, J.M. Combination treatments to enhance peptide receptor radionuclide therapy of neuroendocrine tumours. *Eur. J. Nucl. Med. Mol. Imaging* **2020**, *47*, 907–921. [CrossRef] [PubMed]
173. Strosberg, J.; El-Haddad, G.; Wolin, E.; Hendifar, A.; Yao, J.; Chasen, B.; Mittra, E.; Kunz, P.L.; Kulke, M.H.; Jacene, H.; et al. Phase 3 Trial of 177Lu-Dotatate for Midgut Neuroendocrine Tumors. *N. Engl. J. Med.* **2017**, *376*, 125–135. [CrossRef] [PubMed]
174. Hennrich, U.; Kopka, K. Lutathera®: The First FDA- and EMA-Approved Radiopharmaceutical for Peptide Receptor Radionuclide Therapy. *Pharmaceuticals* **2019**, *12*, 114. [CrossRef]
175. Werner, R.A.; Bluemel, C.; Allen-Auerbach, M.S.; Higuchi, T.; Herrmann, K. ^{68}Gallium- and ^{90}Yttrium-/^{177}Lutetium: "theranostic twins" for diagnosis and treatment of NETs. *Ann. Nucl. Med.* **2015**, *29*, 1–7. [CrossRef]
176. Waseem, N.; Aparici, C.M.; Kunz, P.L. Evaluating the Role of Theranostics in Grade 3 Neuroendocrine Neoplasms. *J. Nucl. Med.* **2019**, *60*, 882–891. [CrossRef]
177. Sorbye, H.; Kong, G.; Grozinsky-Glasberg, S. PRRT in high-grade gastroenteropancreatic neuroendocrine neoplasms (WHO G3). *Endocr. Relat. Cancer* **2020**, *27*, R67–R77. [CrossRef]
178. Mak, I.Y.F.; Hayes, A.R.; Khoo, B.; Grossman, A. Peptide Receptor Radionuclide Therapy as a Novel Treatment for Metastatic and Invasive Phaeochromocytoma and Paraganglioma. *Neuroendocrinology* **2019**, *109*, 287–298. [CrossRef]
179. Vyakaranam, A.R.; Crona, J.; Norlén, O.; Granberg, D.; Garske-Román, U.; Sandström, M.; Fröss-Baron, K.; Thiis-Evensen, E.; Hellman, P.; Sundin, A. Favorable Outcome in Patients with Pheochromocytoma and Paraganglioma Treated with ^{177}Lu-DOTATATE. *Cancers* **2019**, *11*, 909. [CrossRef]
180. Lepareur, N.; Lacœuille, F.; Bouvry, C.; Hindré, F.; Garcion, E.; Chérel, M.; Noiret, N.; Garin, E.; Knapp, F.F.R., Jr. Rhenium-188 Labeled Radiopharmaceuticals: Current Clinical Applications in Oncology and Promising Perspectives. *Front. Med.* **2019**, *6*, 132. [CrossRef]
181. Zamora, P.O.; Gulhke, S.; Bender, H.; Diekmann, D.; Rhodes, B.A.; Biersack, H.J.; Knapp, F.F., Jr. Experimental radiotherapy of receptor-positive human prostate adenocarcinoma with ^{188}Re-RC-160, a directly-radiolabeled somatostatin analogue. *Int. J. Cancer* **1996**, *65*, 214–220. [CrossRef]
182. Zamora, P.O.; Bender, H.; Gulhke, S.; Marek, M.J.; Knapp, F.F., Jr.; Rhodes, B.A.; Biersack, H.J. Pre-clinical experience with Re-188-RC-160, a radiolabeled somatostatin analog for use in peptide-targeted radiotherapy. *Anticancer Res.* **1997**, *17*, 1803–1808. [PubMed]
183. Arteaga de Murphy, C.; Pedraza-López, M.; Ferro-Flores, G.; Murphy-Stack, E.; Chávez-Mercado, L.; Ascencio, J.A.; García-Salinas, L.; Hernández-Gutiérrez, S. Uptake of ^{188}Re-beta-naphthyl-peptide in cervical carcinoma tumours in athymic mice. *Nucl. Med. Biol.* **2001**, *28*, 319–326. [CrossRef]
184. Molina-Trinidad, E.M.; de Murphy, C.A.; Ferro-Flores, G.; Murphy-Stack, E.; Jung-Cook, H. Radiopharmacokinetic and dosimetric parameters of ^{188}Re-lanreotide in athymic mice with induced human cancer tumors. *Int. J. Pharm.* **2006**, *310*, 125–130. [CrossRef]
185. Molina-Trinidad, E.M.; de Murphy, C.A.; Jung-Cook, H.; Stack, E.M.; Pedraza-Lopez, M.; Morales-Marquez, J.L.; Serrano, G.V. Therapeutic ^{188}Re-lanreotide: Determination of radiopharmacokinetic parameters in rats. *J. Pharm. Pharmacol.* **2010**, *62*, 456–461. [CrossRef]
186. Cyr, J.E.; Pearson, D.A.; Wilson, D.M.; Nelson, C.A.; Guaraldi, M.; Azure, M.T.; Lister-James, J.; Dinkelborg, L.M.; Dean, R.T. Somatostatin receptor-binding peptides suitable for tumour radiotherapy with Re-188 or Re-186. Chemistry and initial biological studies. *J. Med. Chem.* **2007**, *50*, 1354–1364. [CrossRef]
187. Edelman, M.J.; Clamon, G.; Kahn, D.; Magram, M.; Lister-James, J.; Line, B.R. Targeted radiopharmaceutical therapy for advanced lung cancer: Phase I trial of rhenium Re188 P2045, a somatostatin analog. *J. Thorac. Oncol.* **2009**, *4*, 1550–1554. [CrossRef]

188. Nelson, C.A.; Azure, M.T.; Adams, C.T.; Zinn, K.R. The somatostatin analog ^{188}Re-P2045 inhibits the growth of AR42J pancreatic tumor xenografts. *J. Nucl. Med.* **2014**, *55*, 2020–2025. [CrossRef]
189. Champion, C.; Quinto, M.A.; Morgat, C.; Zanotti-Fregonara, P.; Hindié, E. Comparison between Three Promising ß-emitting Radionuclides, ^{67}Cu, ^{47}Sc and ^{161}Tb, with Emphasis on Doses Delivered to Minimal Residual Disease. *Theranostics* **2016**, *6*, 1611–1618. [CrossRef]
190. De Jong, M.; Breeman, W.A.; Bernard, B.F.; Rolleman, E.J.; Hofland, L.J.; Visser, T.J.; Setyono-Han, B.; Bakker, W.H.; van der Pluijm, M.E.; Krenning, E.P. Evaluation in vitro and in rats of ^{161}Tb-DTPA-octreotide, a somatostatin analogue with potential for intraoperative scanning and radiotherapy. *Eur. J. Nucl. Med.* **1995**, *22*, 608–616. [CrossRef]
191. Loveless, C.S.; Radford, L.L.; Ferran, S.J.; Queern, S.L.; Shepherd, M.R.; Lapi, S.E. Photonuclear production, chemistry, and in vitro evaluation of the theranostic radionuclide ^{47}Sc. *EJNMMI Res.* **2019**, *9*, 42. [CrossRef] [PubMed]
192. Tafreshi, N.K.; Doligalski, M.L.; Tichacek, C.J.; Pandya, D.N.; Budzevich, M.M.; El-Haddad, G.; Khushalani, N.I.; Moros, E.G.; McLaughlin, M.L.; Wadas, T.J.; et al. Development of Targeted Alpha Particle Therapy for Solid Tumors. *Molecules* **2019**, *24*, 4314. [CrossRef] [PubMed]
193. Nayak, T.; Norenberg, J.; Anderson, T.; Atcher, R. A comparison of high- versus low-linear energy transfer somatostatin receptor targeted radionuclide therapy in vitro. *Cancer Biother. Radiopharm.* **2005**, *20*, 52–57. [CrossRef] [PubMed]
194. Nayak, T.K.; Norenberg, J.P.; Anderson, T.L.; Prossnitz, E.R.; Stabin, M.G.; Atcher, R.W. Somatostatin-receptor-targeted α-emitting ^{213}Bi is therapeutically more effective than β^--emitting ^{177}Lu in human pancreatic adenocarcinoma cells. *Nucl. Med. Biol.* **2007**, *34*, 185–193. [CrossRef] [PubMed]
195. Chan, H.S.; de Blois, E.; Morgenstern, A.; Bruchertseifer, F.; de Jong, M.; Breeman, W.; Konijnenberg, M. In Vitro comparison of ^{213}Bi- and ^{177}Lu-radiation for peptide receptor radionuclide therapy. *PLoS ONE* **2017**, *12*, e0181473. [CrossRef]
196. Norenberg, J.P.; Krenning, B.J.; Konings, I.R.H.M.; Kusewitt, D.F.; Nayak, T.K.; Anderson, T.L.; de Jong, M.; Garmestani, K.; Brechbiel, M.W.; Kvols, L.K. ^{213}Bi-[DOTA^0, Tyr^3]Octreotide Peptide Receptor Radionuclide Therapy of Pancreatic Tumors in a Preclinical Animal Model. *Clin. Cancer Res.* **2006**, *12*, 897–903. [CrossRef]
197. Miederer, M.; Henriksen, G.; Alke, A.; Mossbrugger, I.; Quintanilla-Martinez, L.; Senekowitsch-Schmidtke, R.; Essler, M. Preclinical evaluation of the alpha-particle generator nuclide ^{225}Ac for somatostatin receptor radiotherapy of neuroendocrine tumors. *Clin. Cancer Res.* **2008**, *14*, 3555–3561. [CrossRef]
198. Chan, H.S.; Konijnenberg, M.W.; de Blois, E.; Koelewijn, S.; Baum, R.P.; Morgenstern, A.; Bruchertseifer, F.; Breeman, W.A.; de Jong, M. Influence of tumour size on the efficacy of targeted alpha therapy with ^{213}Bi-[DOTA^0,Tyr^3]-octreotate. *EJNMMI Res.* **2016**, *6*, 6. [CrossRef]
199. Kratochwil, C.; Giesel, F.L.; Bruchertseifer, F.; Mier, W.; Apostolidis, C.; Boll, R.; Murphy, K.; Haberkorn, U.; Morgenstern, A. ^{213}Bi-DOTATOC receptor-targeted alpha-radionuclide therapy induces remission in neuroendocrine tumours refractory to beta radiation: A first-in-human experience. *Eur. J. Nucl. Med. Mol. Imaging* **2014**, *41*, 2106–2119. [CrossRef]
200. Zhang, J.; Singh, A.; Kulkarni, H.R.; Schuchardt, C.; Müller, D.; Wester, H.J.; Maina, T.; Rösch, F.; van der Meulen, N.P.; Müller, C.; et al. From Bench to Bedside-The Bad Berka Experience with First-in-Human Studies. *Semin. Nucl. Med.* **2019**, *49*, 422–437. [CrossRef]
201. Ballal, S.; Yadav, M.P.; Bal, C.; Sahoo, R.K.; Tripathi, M. Broadening horizons with ^{225}Ac-DOTATATE targeted alpha therapy for gastroenteropancreatic neuroendocrine tumour patients stable or refractory to ^{177}Lu-DOTATATE PRRT: First clinical experience on the efficacy and safety. *Eur. J. Nucl. Med. Mol. Imaging* **2020**, *47*, 934–946. [CrossRef] [PubMed]
202. Stallons, T.A.R.; Saidi, A.; Tworowska, I.; Delpassand, E.S.; Torgue, J.J. Preclinical Investigation of ^{212}Pb-DOTAMTATE for Peptide Receptor Radionuclide Therapy in a Neuroendocrine Tumor Model. *Mol. Cancer Ther.* **2019**, *18*, 1012–1021. [CrossRef] [PubMed]
203. Tworowska, I.; Delpassand, E.S.; Bolek, L.; Shanoon, F.; Sgouros, G.; Frey, E.; He, B.; Muzammil, A.; Ghaly, M.; Stallons, T.; et al. Targeted Alpha-emitter Therapy of Neuroendocrine Tumors using ^{212}Pb-octreotate (AlphaMedix™). *J. Med. Imaging Radiat. Sci.* **2019**, *50*, S34. [CrossRef]
204. Guérard, F.; Gestin, J.F.; Brechbiel, M.W. Production of [^{211}At]-astatinated radiopharmaceuticals and applications in targeted α-particle therapy. *Cancer Biother. Radiopharm.* **2013**, *28*, 1–20. [CrossRef]
205. Vaidyanathan, G.; Boskovitz, A.; Shankar, S.; Zalutsky, M.R. Radioiodine and ^{211}At-labeled guanidinomethyl

halobenzoyl octreotate conjugates: Potential peptide radiotherapeutics for somatostatin receptor-positive cancers. *Peptides* **2004**, *25*, 2087–2097. [CrossRef] [PubMed]
206. Vaidyanathan, G.; Affleck, D.J.; Schottelius, M.; Wester, H.; Friedman, H.S.; Zalutsky, M.R. Synthesis and evaluation of glycosylated octreotate analogues labeled with radioiodine and ^{211}At via a tin precursor. *Bioconjugate Chem.* **2006**, *17*, 195–203. [CrossRef]
207. Zhao, B.; Qin, S.; Chai, L.; Lu, G.; Yang, Y.; Cai, H.; Yuan, X.; Fan, S.; Huang, Q.; Yu, F. Evaluation of astatine-211-labeled octreotide as a potential radiotherapeutic agent for NSCLC treatment. *Bioorg. Med. Chem.* **2018**, *26*, 1086–1091. [CrossRef]
208. Krenning, E.P.; Valkema, R.; Kooij, P.P.; Breeman, W.A.; Bakker, W.H.; de Herder, W.W.; van Eijck, C.H.; Kwekkeboom, D.J.; de Jong, M.; Pauwels, S. Scintigraphy and radionuclide therapy with [indium-111-labeled-diethyltriamine penta-acetic acid-D-Phe^1]-octreotide. *Ital. J. Gastroenterol. Hepatol.* **1999**, *31*, S219–S223.
209. Valkema, R.; De Jong, M.; Bakker, W.H.; Breeman, W.A.; Kooij, P.P.; Lugtenburg, P.J.; De Jong, F.H.; Christiansen, A.; Kam, B.L.; De Herder, W.W.; et al. Phase I study of peptide receptor radionuclide therapy with [In-DTPA]octreotide: The Rotterdam experience. *Semin. Nucl. Med.* **2002**, *32*, 110–122. [CrossRef]
210. Anthony, L.B.; Woltering, E.A.; Espenan, G.D.; Cronin, M.D.; Maloney, T.J.; McCarthy, K.E. Indium-111-pentetreotide prolongs survival in gastroenteropancreatic malignancies. *Semin. Nucl. Med.* **2002**, *32*, 123–132. [CrossRef]
211. Buscombe, J.R.; Caplin, M.E.; Hilson, A.J. Long-term efficacy of high-activity ^{111}In-pentetreotide therapy in patients with disseminated neuroendocrine tumors. *J. Nucl. Med.* **2003**, *44*, 1–6. [PubMed]
212. Lewington, V.J. Targeted radionuclide therapy for neuroendocrine tumours. *Endocr. Relat. Cancer* **2003**, *10*, 497–501. [CrossRef] [PubMed]
213. Capello, A.; Krenning, E.; Bernard, B.; Reubi, J.C.; Breeman, W.; de Jong, M. ^{111}In-labeled somatostatin analogues in a rat tumour model: Somatostatin receptor status and effects of peptide receptor radionuclide therapy. *Eur. J. Nucl. Med. Mol. Imaging* **2005**, *32*, 1288–1295. [CrossRef]
214. Ginj, M.; Zhang, H.; Waser, B.; Cescato, R.; Wild, D.; Wang, X.; Erchegyi, J.; Rivier, J.; Mäcke, H.R.; Reubi, J.C. Radiolabeled somatostatin receptor antagonists are preferable to agonists for in vivo peptide receptor targeting of tumors. *Proc. Natl. Acad. Sci. USA* **2006**, *103*, 16436–16441. [CrossRef] [PubMed]
215. Waser, B.; Tamma, M.L.; Cescato, R.; Maecke, H.R.; Reubi, J.C. Highly efficient in vivo agonist induced internalization of sst2 receptors in somatostatin target tissues. *J. Nucl. Med.* **2009**, *50*, 936941. [CrossRef] [PubMed]
216. Cescato, R.; Schulz, S.; Waser, B.; Eltschinger, V.; Rivier, J.E.; Wester, H.J.; Culler, M.; Ginj, M.; Liu, Q.; Schonbrunn, A.; et al. Internalization of sst2, sst3, and sst5 receptors: Effects of somatostatin agonists and antagonists. *J. Nucl. Med.* **2006**, *47*, 502–511. [PubMed]
217. Fani, M.; Peitl, P.K.; Velikyan, I. Current status of radiopharmaceuticals for the theranostics of neuroendocrine neoplasms. *Pharmaceuticals* **2017**, *10*, 30. [CrossRef] [PubMed]
218. Reubi, J.C.; Waser, B.; Mäcke, H.; Rivier, J. Highly Increased ^{125}I-JR11 Antagonist Binding In Vitro Reveals Novel Indications for sst2 Targeting in Human Cancers. *J. Nucl. Med.* **2017**, *58*, 300–306. [CrossRef]
219. Dude, I.; Zhang, Z.; Rousseau, J.; Hundal-Jabal, N.; Colpo, N.; Merkens, H.; Lin, K.S.; Bénard, F. Evaluation of agonist and antagonist radioligands for somatostatin receptor imaging of breast cancer using positron emission tomography. *EJNMMI Radiopharm. Chem.* **2017**, *2*, 4. [CrossRef]
220. Rylova, S.N.; Stoykow, C.; Del Pozzo, L.; Abiraj, K.; Tamma, M.L.; Kiefer, Y.; Fani, M.; Maecke, H.R. The somatostatin receptor 2 antagonist ^{64}Cu-NODAGA-JR11 outperforms ^{64}Cu-DOTA-TATE in a mouse xenograft model. *PLoS ONE* **2018**, *13*, e0195802. [CrossRef]
221. Krebs, S.; Pandit-Taskar, N.; Reidy, D.; Beattie, B.J.; Lyashchenko, S.K.; Lewis, J.S.; Bodei, L.; Weber, W.A.; O'Donoghue, J.A. Biodistribution and radiation dose estimates for ^{68}Ga-DOTA-JR11 in patients with metastatic neuroendocrine tumors. *Eur. J. Nucl. Med. Mol. Imaging* **2019**, *46*, 677–685. [CrossRef] [PubMed]
222. Wild, D.; Fani, M.; Behe, M.; Brink, I.; Rivier, J.E.; Reubi, J.C.; Maecke, H.R.; Weber, W.A. First clinical evidence that imaging with somatostatin receptor antagonists is feasible. *J. Nucl. Med.* **2011**, *52*, 1412–1417. [CrossRef] [PubMed]
223. Fani, M.; Del Pozzo, L.; Abiraj, K.; Mansi, R.; Tamma, M.L.; Cescato, R.; Waser, B.; Weber, W.A.; Reubi, J.C.; Maecke, H.R. PET of somatostatin receptor-positive tumors using ^{64}Cu- and ^{68}Ga-somatostatin antagonists: The chelate makes the difference. *J. Nucl. Med.* **2011**, *52*, 1110–1118. [CrossRef] [PubMed]

224. Fani, M.; Braun, F.; Waser, B.; Beetschen, K.; Cescato, R.; Erchegyi, J.; Rivier, J.E.; Weber, W.A.; Maecke, H.R.; Reubi, J.C. Unexpected sensitivity of sst2 antagonists to N-terminal radiometal modifications. *J. Nucl. Med.* **2012**, *53*, 1481–1489. [CrossRef]
225. Reubi, J.C.; Erchegyi, J.; Cescato, R.; Waser, B.; Rivier, J.E. Switch from antagonist to agonist after addition of a DOTA chelator to a somatostatin analog. *Eur. J. Nucl. Med. Mol. Imaging* **2010**, *37*, 15511558. [CrossRef]
226. Radford, L.; Gallazzi, F.; Watkinson, L.; Carmack, T.; Berendzen, A.; Lewis, M.R.; Jurisson, S.S.; Papagiannopoulou, D.; Hennkens, H.M. Synthesis and evaluation of a ^{99m}Tc tricarbonyl-labeled somatostatin receptor-targeting antagonist peptide for imaging of neuroendocrine tumors. *Nucl. Med. Biol.* **2017**, *47*, 4–9. [CrossRef]
227. Wild, D.; Fani, M.; Fischer, R.; Del Pozzo, L.; Kaul, F.; Krebs, S.; Fischer, R.; Rivier, J.E.; Reubi, J.C.; Maecke, H.R.; et al. Comparison of somatostatin receptor agonist and antagonist for peptide receptor radionuclide therapy: A pilot study. *J. Nucl. Med.* **2014**, *55*, 1248–1252. [CrossRef]
228. Fani, M.; Nicolas, G.P.; Wild, D. Somatostatin Receptor Antagonists for Imaging and Therapy. *J. Nucl. Med.* **2017**, *58*, 61S–66S. [CrossRef]
229. Mansi, R.; Fani, M. Design and development of the theranostic pair ^{177}Lu-OPS201/^{68}Ga-OPS202 for targeting somatostatin receptor expressing tumors. *J. Label. Compd. Radiopharm.* **2019**, *62*, 635–645. [CrossRef]
230. Nicolas, G.P.; Beykan, S.; Bouterfa, H.; Kaufmann, J.; Bauman, A.; Lassmann, M.; Reubi, J.C.; Rivier, J.E.F.; Maecke, H.R.; Fani, M.; et al. Safety, Biodistribution, and Radiation Dosimetry of ^{68}Ga-OPS202 in Patients with Gastroenteropancreatic Neuroendocrine Tumors: A Prospective Phase I Imaging Study. *J. Nucl. Med.* **2018**, *59*, 909–914. [CrossRef]
231. Nicolas, G.P.; Schreiter, N.; Kaul, F.; Uiters, J.; Bouterfa, H.; Kaufmann, J.; Erlanger, T.E.; Cathomas, R.; Christ, E.; Fani, M.; et al. Sensitivity Comparison of ^{68}Ga-OPS202 and ^{68}Ga-DOTATOC PET/CT in Patients with Gastroenteropancreatic Neuroendocrine Tumors: A Prospective Phase II Imaging Study. *J. Nucl. Med.* **2018**, *59*, 915–921. [CrossRef] [PubMed]
232. Reidy-Lagunes, D.; Pandit-Taskar, N.; O'Donoghue, J.A.; Krebs, S.; Staton, K.D.; Lyashchenko, S.K.; Lewis, J.S.; Raj, N.; Gönen, M.; Lohrmann, C.; et al. Phase I Trial of Well-Differentiated Neuroendocrine Tumors (NETs) with Radiolabeled Somatostatin Antagonist ^{177}Lu-Satoreotide Tetraxetan. *Clin. Cancer Res.* **2019**, *25*, 6939–6947. [CrossRef] [PubMed]
233. Rangger, C.; Haubner, R. Radiolabeled Peptides for Positron Emission Tomography and Endoradiotherapy in Oncology. *Pharmaceuticals* **2020**, *13*, 22. [CrossRef] [PubMed]
234. Villard, L.; Romer, A.; Marincek, N.; Brunner, P.; Koller, M.T.; Schindler, C.; Ng, Q.K.T.; Mäcke, H.R.; Müller-Brand, J.; Rochlitz, C.; et al. Cohort study of somatostatin-based radiopeptide therapy with [^{90}Y-DOTA]-TOC versus [^{90}Y-DOTA]-TOC plus [^{177}Lu-DOTA]-TOC in neuroendocrine cancers. *J. Clin. Oncol.* **2012**, *30*, 1100–1106. [CrossRef]
235. Gill, M.R.; Falzone, N.; Du, Y.; Vallis, K.A. Targeted radionuclide therapy in combined-modality regimens. *Lancet Oncol.* **2017**, *18*, e414–e423. [CrossRef]
236. Hartrampf, P.E.; Hänscheid, H.; Kertels, O.; Schirbel, A.; Kreissl, M.C.; Flentje, M.; Sweeney, R.A.; Buck, A.K.; Polat, B.; Lapa, C. Long-term results of multimodal peptide receptor radionuclide therapy and fractionated external beam radiotherapy for treatment of advanced symptomatic meningioma. *Clin. Transl. Radiat. Oncol.* **2020**, *22*, 29–32. [CrossRef]
237. Reubi, J.C.; Maecke, H.R. Approaches to multireceptor targeting: Hybrid radioligands, radioligand cocktails, and sequential radioligand applications. *J. Nucl. Med.* **2017**, *58*, 10S–16S. [CrossRef]
238. Ghosh, S.C.; Rodriguez, M.; Carmon, K.S.; Voss, J.; Wilganowski, N.L.; Schonbrunn, A.; Azhdarinia, A. A Modular Dual-Labeling Scaffold That Retains Agonistic Properties for Somatostatin Receptor Targeting. *J. Nucl. Med.* **2017**, *58*, 1858–1864. [CrossRef]
239. Langbein, T.; Weber, W.A.; Eiber, M. Future of Theranostics: An Outlook on Precision Oncology in Nuclear Medicine. *J. Nucl. Med.* **2019**, *60*, 13S–19S. [CrossRef]
240. Jones, W.; Griffiths, K.; Barata, P.C.; Paller, C.J. PSMA Theranostics: Review of the Current Status of PSMA-Targeted Imaging and Radioligand Therapy. *Cancers* **2020**, *12*, 1367. [CrossRef]

7

Involvement of Differentially Expressed microRNAs in the PEGylated Liposome Encapsulated ^{188}Rhenium-Mediated Suppression of Orthotopic Hypopharyngeal Tumor

Bing-Ze Lin [1,†], Shen-Ying Wan [1,2,†], Min-Ying Lin [1], Chih-Hsien Chang [1,3], Ting-Wen Chen [4,5,6], Muh-Hwa Yang [7,8,9] and Yi-Jang Lee [1,7,*]

1 Department of Biomedical Imaging and Radiological Sciences, National Yang-Ming University, No. 155, Sec. 2, Linong St. Beitou District, Taipei 11221, Taiwan; innovationmark1012@gmail.com (B.-Z.L.); sywang@mail.femh.org.tw (S.-Y.W.); milo841120@gmail.com (M.-Y.L.); chchang@iner.gov.tw (C.-H.C.)
2 Department of Nuclear Medicine, Far Eastern Memorial Hospital, New Taipei City 22000, Taiwan
3 Isotope Application Division, Institute of Nuclear Energy Research, Taoyuan 32546, Taiwan
4 Institute of Bioinformatics and Systems Biology, National Chiao Tung University, Hsinchu 30068, Taiwan; dodochen@nctu.edu.tw
5 Department of Biological Science and Technology, National Chiao Tung University, Hsinchu 30068, Taiwan
6 Center For Intelligent Drug Systems and Smart Bio-devices (IDS2B), National Chiao Tung University, Hsinchu 30068, Taiwan
7 Cancer Progression Research Center, National Yang-Ming University, Taipei 11221, Taiwan; mhyangymu@gmail.com
8 Institute of Clinical Medicine, National Yang-Ming University, Taipei 11221, Taiwan
9 Division of Medical Oncology, Department of Oncology, Taipei Veteran General Hospital, Taipei 11217, Taiwan
* Correspondence: yjlee2@ym.edu.tw
† These authors contributed equally to this work.

Academic Editor: Krishan Kumar

Abstract: Hypopharyngeal cancer (HPC) accounts for the lowest survival rate among all types of head and neck cancers (HNSCC). However, the therapeutic approach for HPC still needs to be investigated. In this study, a theranostic ^{188}Re-liposome was prepared to treat orthotopic HPC tumors and analyze the deregulated microRNA expressive profiles. The therapeutic efficacy of ^{188}Re-liposome on HPC tumors was evaluated using bioluminescent imaging followed by next generation sequencing (NGS) analysis, in order to address the deregulated microRNAs and associated signaling pathways. The differentially expressed microRNAs were also confirmed using clinical HNSCC samples and clinical information from The Cancer Genome Atlas (TCGA) database. Repeated doses of ^{188}Re-liposome were administrated to tumor-bearing mice, and the tumor growth was apparently suppressed after treatment. For NGS analysis, 13 and 9 microRNAs were respectively up-regulated and down-regulated when the cutoffs of fold change were set to 5. Additionally, miR-206-3p and miR-142-5p represented the highest fold of up-regulation and down-regulation by ^{188}Re-liposome, respectively. According to Differentially Expressed MiRNAs in human Cancers (dbDEMC) analysis, most of ^{188}Re-liposome up-regulated microRNAs were categorized as tumor suppressors, while down-regulated microRNAs were oncogenic. The KEGG pathway analysis showed that cancer-related pathways and olfactory and taste transduction accounted for the top pathways affected by ^{188}Re-liposome. ^{188}Re-liposome down-regulated microRNAs, including miR-143, miR-6723, miR-944, and miR-136 were associated with lower survival rates at a high expressive level. ^{188}Re-liposome could suppress the HPC tumors in vivo, and the therapeutic efficacy was associated with the deregulation of microRNAs that could be considered as a prognostic factor.

Keywords: hypopharyngeal cancer; ^{188}Re-liposome; repeated therapy; NGS; microRNA

1. Introduction

Hypopharyngeal cancer (HPC) represents malignant growth in the hypopharynx region and accounts for about 5% of all head and neck cancers (HNSCC) [1]. As HPC is a rare cancer type with a late occurrence of symptoms and tumor spreading, it is not uncommon for it to be detected at advanced stages with a high mortality rate and poor prognosis [2]. HPC can be treated by conventional surgery, radiotherapy and chemotherapy, while radiotherapy alone is usually used at an early stage [3]. On the other hand, a combination of different therapeutic modalities can improve the five-year survival of this disease [4]. Several lines of evidence have claimed that a combination of radiotherapy and chemotherapy would provide better control of locoregional recurrence compared to surgical procedures [4,5]. A radiopharmaceutical named ^{99m}Tc-MIBI (methoxy-isobutyl-isonitrile) has been reported to detect HPC with up to a 95% sensitivity using single photon emission computed tomography (SPECT) [6]. However, nuclear medicine has not been reported to have assessed or monitored the efficacy of HPC therapy as mentioned above.

Radiopharmaceuticals are not only used for diagnostic purposes but also therapeutic purposes, so-called radiotheranostics [7]. Rhenium-188 (^{188}Re) belongs to this type of radionuclide as it emits 85% high-energy β-particles (2.12MeV) and 15% γ-rays (155keV) [8]. The average soft tissue penetration distance of β-particles is only around 3.8mm, suggesting that ^{188}Re is suitable for tumor ablation and will not have significant side effects on distant normal tissues [9,10]. ^{188}Re has been conjugated to hydroxyethylidene diphosphonate (HEDP) for bone pain palliation [11,12]. The antibody conjugated ^{188}Re has also been reported to treat different cancers [13]. Additionally, low immunogenic peptides such as somatostatin derivative conjugated ^{188}Re, have been investigated in clinics for patients with advanced pulmonary cancer [14]. ^{188}Re-labeled lipiodol and microspheres were used for the treatment of hepatocellular carcinoma [15–17]. ^{188}Re-labelled radiocolloids have also been developed to treat skin cancers within a brachytherapy device [18]. ^{188}Re-loaded lipid nanocapsules, also called ^{188}Re-liposome, have been demonstrated to be biocompatible and subjected to a phase 0 clinical study for patients with metastatic tumors [19]. ^{188}Re-liposome has shown a theranostic efficacy in various human cancers, including colorectal cancer, glioblastomas, lung cancer, ovarian cancer, esophageal cancer and head and neck cancer using xenograft tumor models [20–26]. The molecular mechanisms of rhenium-188 labelled radiopharmaceuticals are of interest for investigation aimed at interpreting the potent therapeutic efficacy.

Radiogenomics is defined as connecting radiomics and genetic profiles to apply the feature of medical imaging in radiation-mediated molecular responses [27]. The purpose of this discipline is to predict the association between gene expression and the radiotherapy-induced toxic effects of tumors [28]. Next-generation sequencing (NGS) analysis is the most cutting-edge technology that can decipher dramatic amounts of gene expressive alterations in tumors, with or without therapies [29,30]. NGS applications include RNA sequencing (RNA-Seq) that can analyze the expression of various RNA populations (mRNA, microRNA, long non-coding RNA, etc.) and their modification forms generated from alternative splicing, mutations or gene fusion [31]. Compared to the conventional cDNA expression microarray, RNA-Seq has a broader spectrum for finding novel and unidentified transcripts [32]. This method is important for providing more detailed and quantitative data for bioinformatics analysis of genetic profiling in novel drug development and predicting the signaling pathways of toxicity and therapeutic effects [33]. As a radioactive compound, ^{188}Re-liposome is believed to influence the genetic profile of tumors. However, related studies have rarely been reported.

In this study, we investigated the effects of ^{188}Re-liposome on the miRNA expressive profiles of HPC derived xenograft tumors using RNA-Seq technology. The changed miRNA profiles were analyzed using the Kyoto Encyclopedia of Genes and Genomes (KEGG) pathway database and Ingenuity Pathway

Analysis (IPA). The total expressive amount of miRNA from ^{188}Re-liposome-treated tumors was about 10% lower than that of untreated tumor. The changed miRNA profile led to 4498 differentially expressed genes (DEGs) that influenced 30 molecular pathways, including olfactory transduction, the cancer pathway, and taste transduction, which accounted for the top three pathways. We also found that ^{188}Re-liposome up-regulated several tumor suppressor microRNAs, such as miR-34-5p, miR-193a-5p, miR-125b-5p, miR-133a-5p, and miR-133b-5p. Concomitantly, several oncomirs, including miR-21-5p, miR-32-5p and miR-205-5p were down-regulated by ^{188}Re-liposome. An online Kaplan-Meier (K-M) plotter with The Cancer Genome Atlas (TCGA) database was also used to compare the expression of these miRNA and the survival of head and neck cancer patients. The results of ^{188}Re-liposome-induced miRNA dysregulation detected by RNA-Seq were discussed.

2. Results

2.1. *Effects of ^{188}Re-Liposome on HPC Derived Orthotopic Tumors Using the Repeated Dose Regime*

A flowchart of ^{188}Re-liposomal manufacturing and the chemical structures of the ^{188}Re-perrhenate precursor and BMEDA chelator are illustrated in Figure 1. The timeline was schemed for the establishment of HPC tumor-bearing mice using FaDu-3R cells (Supplementary Figure S2), the administration of ^{188}Re-liposome, the optical imaging of tumor responses, tumor resection for RNA extraction, and NGS analysis (Figure 2A). The growth of orthotopic tumors was significantly suppressed by ^{188}Re-liposome but not saline as detected using bioluminescent imaging (Figure 2B,C). The size of resected tumors also exhibited obvious differences between the saline control and ^{188}Re-liposome-treated mice after 30 days of initial implantation (Figure 2D). The body weights of tumor-bearing mice were not significantly affected by ^{188}Re-liposome (Figure 2E). Furthermore, we showed that DNA damage marker γ-H2AX was significantly up-regulated by ^{188}Re-liposome treatment (Figure 2F,G). These data suggest that the regime of ^{188}Re-liposome treatment with repeated doses exhibited therapeutic efficacy, with little systemic toxicity.

2.2. *Use of NGS Analysis to Investigate the microRNA Expressive Profile of HPC Tumor Treated with ^{188}Re-Liposome*

The resected FaDu HPC tumors treated with saline or repeated doses of ^{188}Re-liposome were subjected to RNA extraction to obtain a high quality of total RNA for RNA-seq analysis (Supplementary Figure S3). The quality of raw data obtained by this analysis was determined by the GC content, by which the raw data quality of the saline control and ^{188}Re-liposome-treated tumor was shown to be similar (Supplementary Figure S4). To confirm the expressive change in microRNA in tumors treated with or without ^{188}Re-liposome, the reads number of small RNA (15–55 mers) was extracted and counted using a Small RNA Analysis tool (see Materials and Methods). The average lengths of small RNA after extraction were 32.9 and 32 mers for the control and ^{188}Re-liposome treated tumor, respectively. Under this condition, the total reads number of the control and ^{188}Re-liposome treated tumor was 10,612,998 and 9,844,775, respectively. The reads were then subjected to the miRBase database (release 21) for the annotation of small RNA using the Annotate and Merge Count of Small RNA Analysis software. The annotated small RNAs of saline-treated tumors and ^{188}Re-liposome treated tumors were 639 and 572, respectively. The differentially expressed microRNAs were clustered in a heatmap for a comparison of saline-treated and ^{188}Re-liposome treated HPC tumor models (Supplementary Figure S5). Furthermore, we set the cutoff at five-fold change ($\log_2$) of microRNA and showed that 13 microRNA and 9 microRNA with mature forms were up-regulated and down-regulated by ^{188}Re-liposome normalized to the saline control, respectively (Table 1). The 13 up-regulated microRNAs ranked from highest to lowest fold change were miR-206-3p, mir668-3p, mit-485-3p, miR-382-5p, miR-1268b-5p, miR-193a-5p, miR-7-1-5p, miR-378a-5p, miR-1266-5p, miR-4510-5p, miR-370-3p, miR-34a-5p, and miR-342-5p. The nine down-regulated microRNAs ranked from highest to lowest fold change were miR-142-5p, miR-6723-5p, miR-944-3p, miR-142-3p, miR-136-3p, miR-151b-3p, miR-194-2-5p, miR-143-5p, and miR-3960-3p. According to the online analysis of dbDEMC, ^{188}Re-liposome-up-regulated microRNAs were mostly naturally down-regulated in HNSCC and were predicted as tumor suppressors (Table 2). MiR-193a, miR-7-1-5p and miR-342-5p were up-regulated in HNSCC, but could still be tumor suppressors in different types of cancer (see references in Table 2). For the nine ^{188}Re-liposome down-regulated microRNAs, only four of them (miR-136-3p, miR-142-3p, miR-944-3p, and miR-142-5p) were reported in the HNSCC of dbDEMC database. Interestingly, three out of these four microRNAs were found to be up-regulated in HNSCC and predicted as oncogenes (Table 3). However, most of the ^{188}Re-liposome-down-regulated microRNAs contain oncogenic properties (see references in Table 3). These results suggested that the therapeutic efficacy of ^{188}Re-liposome was associated with the deregulation of tumor-suppressive and/or oncogenic microRNAs.

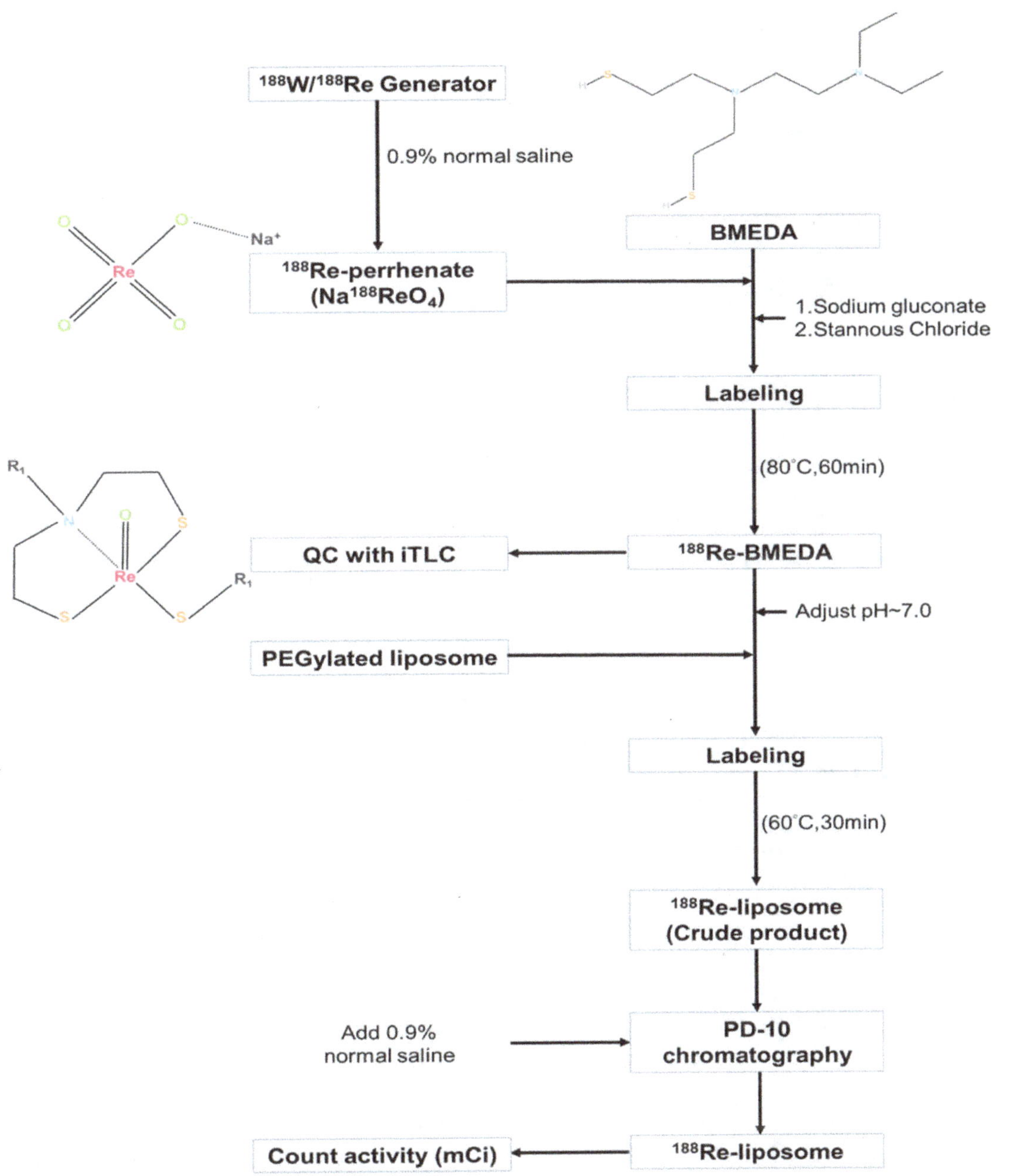

Figure 1. The flowchart of ^{188}Re-liposomal preparation. The chemical structures of $Na^{188}ReO_4$, BMEDA and formed ^{188}Re-BMEDA were also illustrated.

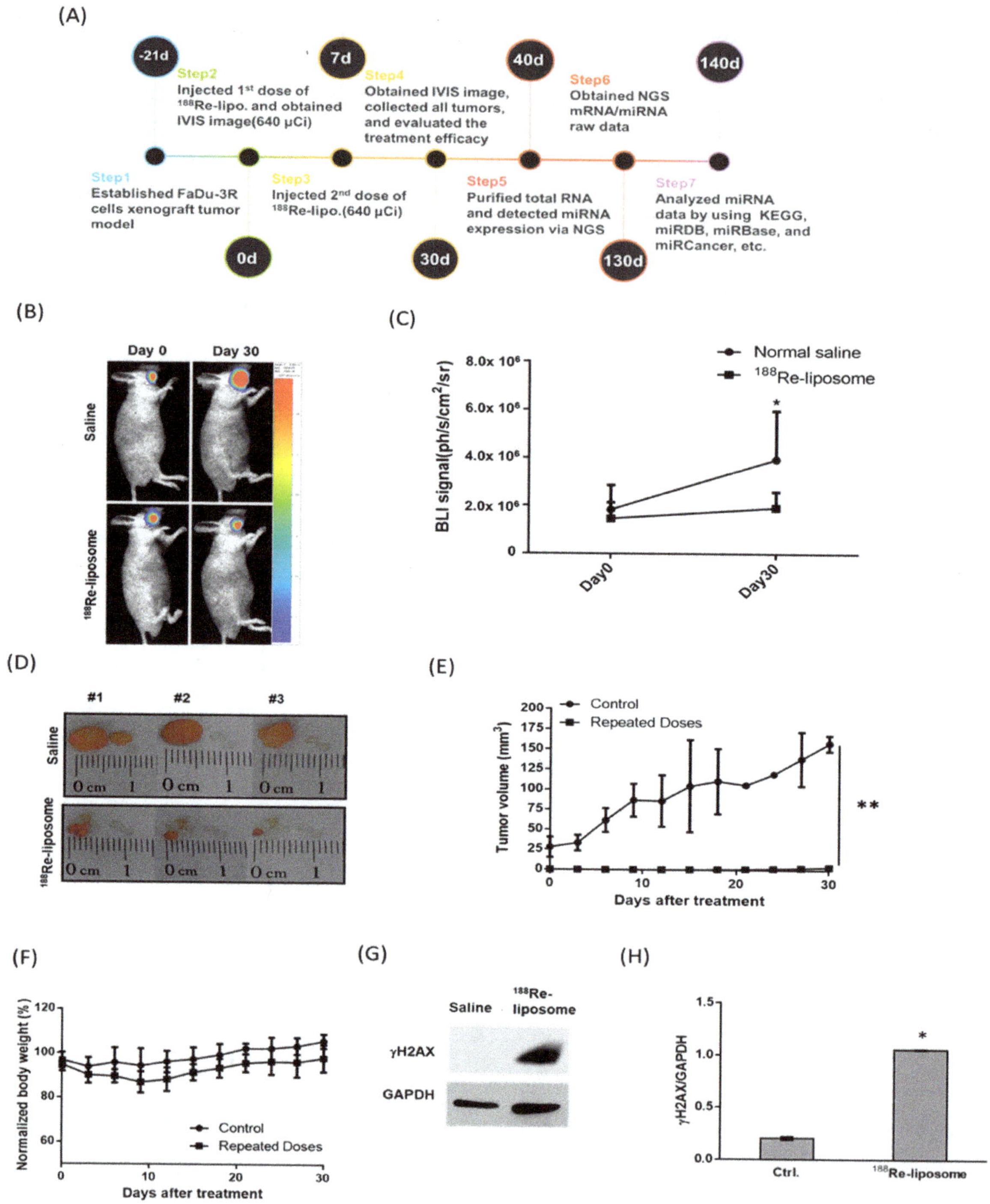

Figure 2. Comparison of PEGylated ^{188}Re-liposomal accumulation in orthotopic hypopharyngeal cancer (HPC) tumors after repeated injections. **(A)** The experimental scheme for ^{188}Re-liposome treatment and analysis. **(B)** Reporter gene imaging of tumor growth responding to repeated doses of ^{188}Re-liposome, and the saline-treated control. **(C)** Quantification of bioluminescent imaging (BLI) signals. *: $p < 0.05$. **(D)** Representative photos of excised orthotropic tumors with or without the treatment of ^{188}Re-liposomes. **(E)** Caliper measurement of tumor volumes. Data are represented as means ± S.D. **: $p < 0.01$. **(F)** Measurement of body weights of mice. **(G)** Comparison of the γ-H2AX protein expression in tumors with or without the treatment of ^{188}Re-liposomes. **(H)** Densitometric quantification of Western blots. *: $p < 0.05$.

Table 1. Expression of microRNAs in human hypopharyngeal tumor model treated with 188Re-liposome.

MicroRNA	Fold Change (188Re-lipo./Ctrl.) [a]	Ctrl. Norm. by TMM [b]	^{188}Re-lipo. Norm.by TMM	Ctrl. RPM [c]	^{188}Re-lipo. RPM
Hsa-miR-206-3p	40.19	76.05	3056.53	2.92	90.71
Hsa-miR-668-3p	11.16	2.45	27.38	0.09	0.81
Hsa-miR-485-3p	9.77	2.45	23.96	0.09	0.71
Hsa-miR-382-5p	9.15	22.08	201.94	0.85	5.99
Hsa-miR-1268b-5p	8.37	2.45	20.54	0.09	0.61
Hsa-miR-193a-5p	6.28	4.91	30.8	0.19	0.91
Hsa-miR-7-1-5p	6.28	9.81	61.61	0.38	1.83
Hsa-miR-378a-5p	5.78	51.52	297.78	1.98	8.84
Hsa-miR-1266-5p	5.58	2.45	13.69	0.09	0.41
Hsa-miR-4510-5p	5.58	2.45	13.69	0.09	0.41
Hsa-miR-370-3p	5.58	4.91	27.38	0.19	0.81
Hsa-miR-34a-5p	5.15	127.57	657.17	4.9	19.5
Hsa-miR-342-5p	5.12	7.36	37.65	0.28	1.12
Hsa-miR-3960-3p	−5.73	117.76	20.54	4.52	0.61
Hsa-miR-143-5p	−5.73	19.63	3.42	0.75	0.1
Hsa-miR-194-2-5p	−5.73	19.63	3.42	0.75	0.1
Hsa-miR-151b-3p	−6.45	22.08	3.42	0.85	0.1
Hsa-miR-136-3p	−7.17	24.53	3.42	0.94	0.1
Hsa-miR-142-3p	−7.88	26.99	3.42	1.04	0.1
Hsa-miR-944-3p	−9.32	31.89	3.42	1.22	0.1
Hsa-miR-6723-5p	−10.03	34.35	3.42	1.32	0.1
Hsa-miR-142-5p	−10.14	242.88	23.96	9.33	0.7

[a]—Fold change in microRNA over 5 or below −5 were selected. [b]—TMM: Trimmed mean of M values. [c]—RPM: Reads of exon model per million mapped reads. (ExonMappedReads × 10^6/TotalMapped Reads).

2.3. Validation of microRNA Identified in NGS Data Using qPCR

We next used qPCR to validate up-regulated and down-regulated microRNA in the FaDu HPC tumor model treated with ^{188}Re-liposome. We selected microRNAs that displayed over five-fold deregulation with the highest RPM, including miR-206-3p, miR-382-5p, miR-378a-5p, miR-3960-3p, and miR-142-5p to be validated. The results showed that the expressive patterns of these microRNAs obtained by qPCR were consistent with the observations of NGS analysis (Figure 3).

2.4. Investigation of Differentially Expressed microRNAs in Clinical Samples

As ^{188}Re-liposome could influence the expression of certain microRNAs that may correlate with the tumor-suppressive effect of the HPC model, we were interested in examining the status of these microRNAs in clinical HNSCC tumors. First, we obtained clinical HNSCC tissues from patients (n = 6) to investigate the differential expression of microRNAs in tumor tissues and adjacent normal tissues using qPCR analysis. We selected miR-206-3p, miR-378a-5p and miR-142-5p as they exhibited the highest differential deregulation by ^{188}Re-liposome (Figure 3). The results showed that the expression of miR-206-3p and miR-378a-5p was down-regulated (Figure 4A,B), while miR-142-5p was up-regulated in tumors compared to normal tissues (Figure 4C). Additionally, we employed the clinical information of HNSCC in the TCGA database to compare the differentially expressed microRNAs in HNSCC and normal tissues. Because the number of cases of hypopharynx cancer was too low to be analyzed, here we used clinical information on larynx cancer types instead. A heatmap was generated for the microRNAs displaying over five-fold change caused by ^{188}Re-liposome (Supplementary Figure S6). Accordingly, we found that miR-206 (equivalent to miR-206-3p) and miR-378a-5p were significantly down-regulated, while miR-143-5p, miR-142-3p, and miR-944 were significantly up-regulated in tumors (Figure 4D). MiR-142-5p also exhibited a trend of up-regulation, although the significance was marginal. This suggests that ^{188}Re-liposome can reverse the expression of the microRNAs that were originally deregulated in HNSCC.

Table 2. Functional prediction algorithm for microRNAs of human hypopharyngeal tumor model up-regulated by ^{188}Re-liposome.

MiRNAs up-Regulated in HPC	Original Change in HNSCC [a]	Role Prediction	Functional Importance	GEO ID	References [b]
Hsa-miR-206-3p	down-regulation	Tumor suppressor	Weaks cell proliferation, migration, invasion, promotes S phase cell arrest. Inhibits cell aggressiveness	TCGA_HNSC	[34,35]
Hsa-miR-668-3p	down-regulation	Tumor suppressor	Induces growth arrest and premature senescence	- [c]	[36,37]
Hsa-miR-485-3p	down-regulation	Tumor suppressor	Inhibits mitochondrial biogenesis or promotes cancer growth and migration	GSE75630	[38–40]
Hsa-miR-382-5p	down-regulation	Tumor Suppressor	Promotes lymph node metastasis and TNM stage; inhibition of proliferation and EMT in glioma cells	TCGA_HNSC	[41,42]
Hsa-miR-1268b-5p	-	Tumor suppressor	Increases chemosensitivity	-	[43]
Hsa-miR-193a-5p	up-regulation	Tumor Suppressor	Suppresses the growth and the metastasis of cancer cells	TCGA_HNSC	[44,45]
Hsa-miR-7-1-5p	up-regulation	Tumor suppressor	Inhibits proliferation, invasion and induces apoptosis in cancer cells	TCGA_HNSC	[46,47]
Hsa-miR-378a-5p	down-regulation	Tumor suppressor	Inhibits cellular proliferation and colony formation.	TCGA_HNSC	[48,49]
Hsa-miR-1266-5p	down-regulation	Tumor suppressor	Induces apoptosis and reduces proliferation	TCGA_HNSC	[50,51]
Hsa-miR-4510-5p	-	Tumor suppressor	Down-regulation in recurrent cancer and a potential cancer biomarker	-	[52,53]
Hsa-miR-370-3p	down-regulation	Tumor suppressor	Potential cancer biomarker	TCGA_HNSC	[54]
Hsa-miR-34a-5p	down-regulation	Tumor suppressor	Inhibits tumorigenesis and progression	TCGA_HNSC	[55,56]
Hsa-miR-342-5p	up-regulation	Tumor suppressor	Reduces cell cycle progression	TCGA_HNSC	[57,58]

[a]—The change of microRNA was determined by the dbDEMC online databases. [b]—The selected references may be not HPC or HNSCC related. [c]—The tumor suppressive function was concluded from clinical patients.

Table 3. Target prediction algorithm for microRNAs of human hypopharyngeal tumor model down-regulated by ^{188}Re-liposome.

MiRNAs Down-Regulated in HPC	Original Change in HNSCC	Role Prediction	Functional Importance	GEO ID	Reference
Hsa-miR-3960-3p	-	-	-	-	-
Hsa-miR-143-5p	-	Both	cell viability, colony formation	-	[59,60]
Hsa-miR-194-2-5p	-	Oncogene	cell proliferation, migration and invasion	-	[61,62]
Hsa-miR-151b-3p	-	Oncogene? [a]	Biomarker of sarcoma	-	[63]
Hsa-miR-136-3p	down-regulation	Oncogene	Biomarker of bladder cancer, promote cancer growth and migration	TCGA-HNSC	[64,65]
Hsa-miR-142-3p	up-regulation	Oncogene	Over-expression in OSCC, association with cancer growth and migration	TCGA-HNSC	[66,67]
Hsa-miR-944-3p	up-regulation	Oncogene	A biomarker of poor prognosis/Regulation of chemoresistance	TCGA-HNSC	[68,69]
Hsa-miR-6723-5p	-	-	-	-	-
Hsa-miR-142-5p	up-regulation	Oncogene	Deregulation of cell proliferation; SMAD3/TGF-β	GSE31277	[70,71]

[a] No direct evidence, but just an implication.

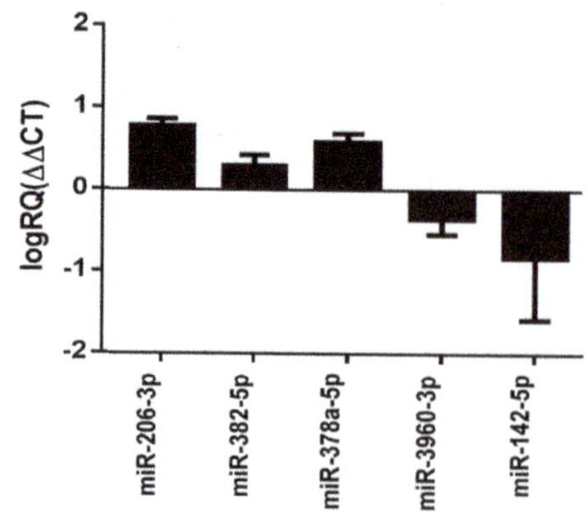

Figure 3. Validation of the next-generation sequencing (NGS) results of the HPC tumor model by qPCR analysis. The results were each microRNA of ^{188}Re-liposome-treated HPC normalized to that of untreated controls.

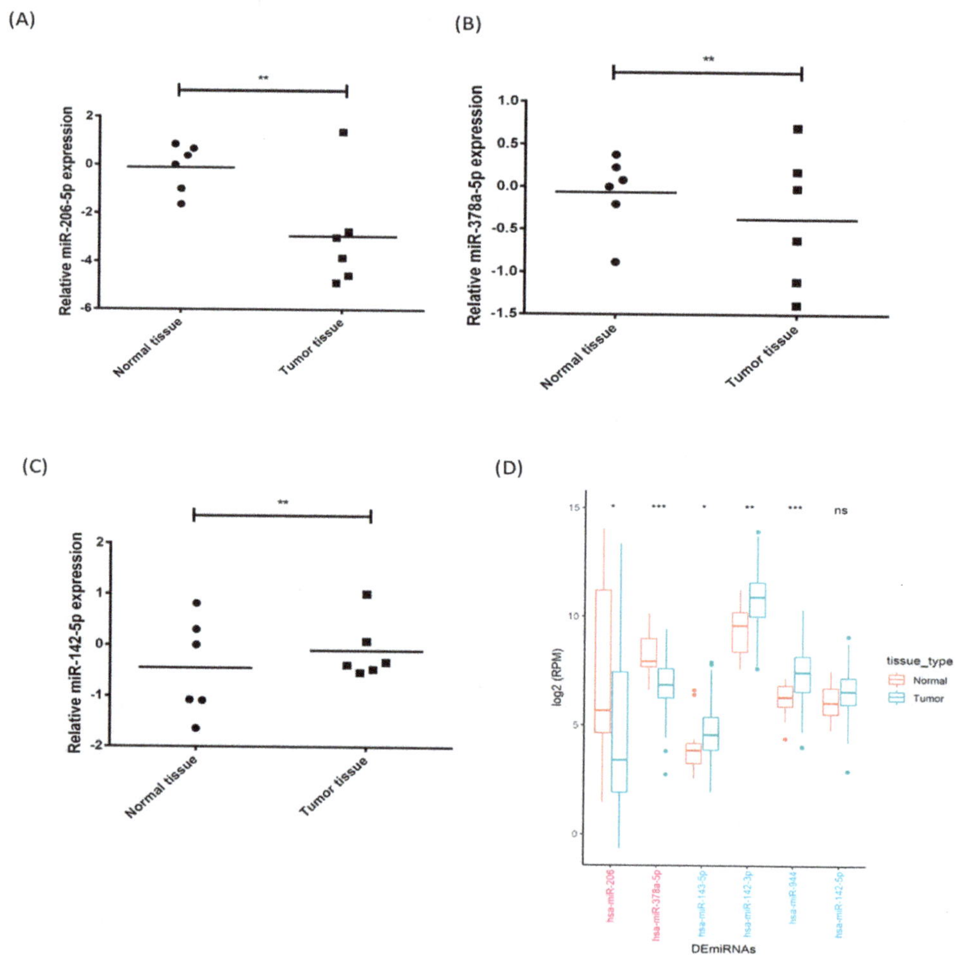

Figure 4. Comparison of the microRNA expression in clinical head and neck cancer (HNSCC) tissues and adjacent normal tissues by qPCR analysis. (**A**) MiR-206-3p. (**B**) MiR-378a-5p (**C**) MiR-142-5p. (**D**) Differentially expressed microRNA (DEmiRNA) in larynx tumor and normal tissues using the clinical information of The Cancer Genome Atlas (TCGA). *: $p < 0.05$, **: $p < 0.01$. ***: $p < 0.001$.

2.5. Prediction of Genes Targeted by ^{188}Re-Liposome-Deregulated microRNAs

We next examined the potent target genes that might be affected by ^{188}Re-liposome deregulated microRNAs. The miRDB online database was employed to rank the numbers of predicted genes targeted by microRNAs that were deregulated by ^{188}Re-liposome (see Materials and Methods). The ranking of target numbers affected by ^{188}Re-liposome up-regulated and down-regulated microRNAs was obtained, respectively (Figure 5A,B). Furthermore, miR-34a, miR-206-3p and miR-4510-5p were used to draw the Venn diagrams as their predicted target genes were ranked as the top three in ^{188}Re-liposome up-regulated microRNAs. Only one target, named *SLC44A2* encoded choline transporter-like protein 2 was co-regulated by these three microRNAs (Figure 5C). The same logic was used for ^{188}Re-liposome down-regulated microRNAs, and an only one target, named *U2SURP* encoded U2 snRNP-associated SURP motif-containing protein, was co-regulated by miR-142-5p, miR-194-5p and miR-944-3p (Figure 5D). Therefore, these bioinformatics analyses suggest that microRNAs and associated target genes of HPC tumors oppositely regulated by ^{188}Re-liposome are distinct.

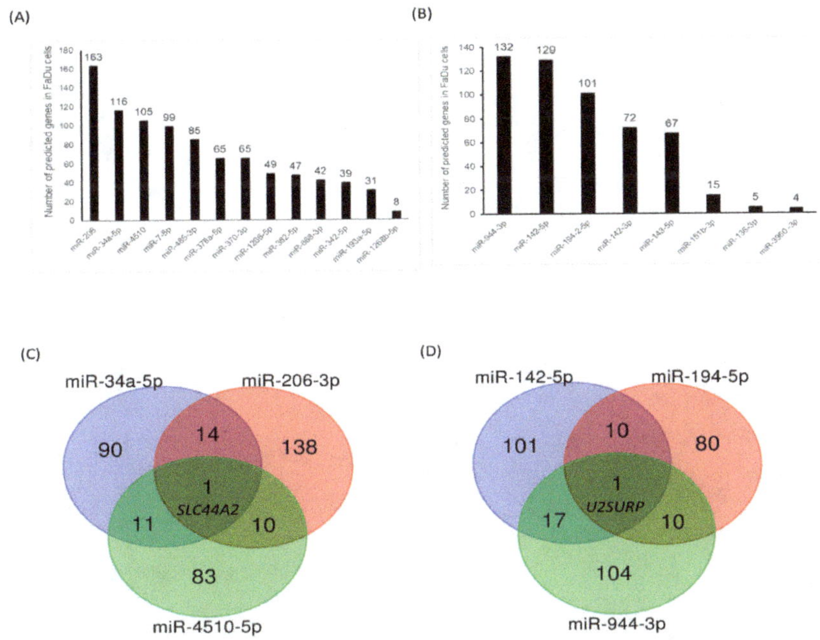

Figure 5. Analysis of miRNA-target interactions. (**A**) The individual target number of microRNAs up-regulated by ^{188}Re-liposome. (**B**) The individual target number of microRNAs down-regulated by ^{188}Re-liposome. (**C**,**D**) The Venn diagram calculated and drawn by the three microRNAs with the most targets.

2.6. Analysis of the Molecular Pathways Regulated by ^{188}Re-Liposome-Affected microRNA

We next used the pathview R package to investigate the genes influenced by microRNAs regulated by ^{188}Re-liposome. MicroRNA samples exhibiting over two-fold change were selected, and the affected target genes were subjected to the KEGG pathway database for determining the potent molecular pathways disturbed by ^{188}Re-liposome. We found that thirty pathways in resected HPC tumors were significantly affected by ^{188}Re-liposome ($p < 0.05$). The top three pathways with the lowest p values were genes involved in olfactory transduction, pathways in cancer, and taste transduction (Table 4). Additionally, ^{188}Re-liposome-influenced pathways could be categorized as cancer and carcinogenesis, cell adhesion and cytoskeletal organization, drug metabolism via cytochrome P450, tumor suppression and oncogenes. An integrated cancer pathway involved in the KEGG database was shown to demonstrate the related genes that could be regulated by ^{188}Re-liposome-induced or -suppressed microRNA expression (Figure 5). This revealed that genes associated with cell cycle progression, proliferation, and apoptosis were affected by ^{188}Re-liposome, including the down-regulation of *cyclin D*, *cyclin E*, cyclin-dependent kinase (*CDK*) *4/6*, *E2F* transcription factor, and *bcl-2* anti-apoptotic factor, and the up-regulation of *p15*, *p16*, and *p27* cell cycle inhibitors and the *Rb* tumor suppressor gene (Figure 6). This pathway analysis provides a potent profile of the molecular mechanism for ^{188}Re-liposome regulated microRNA expression and tumor suppression of the HPC tumor model.

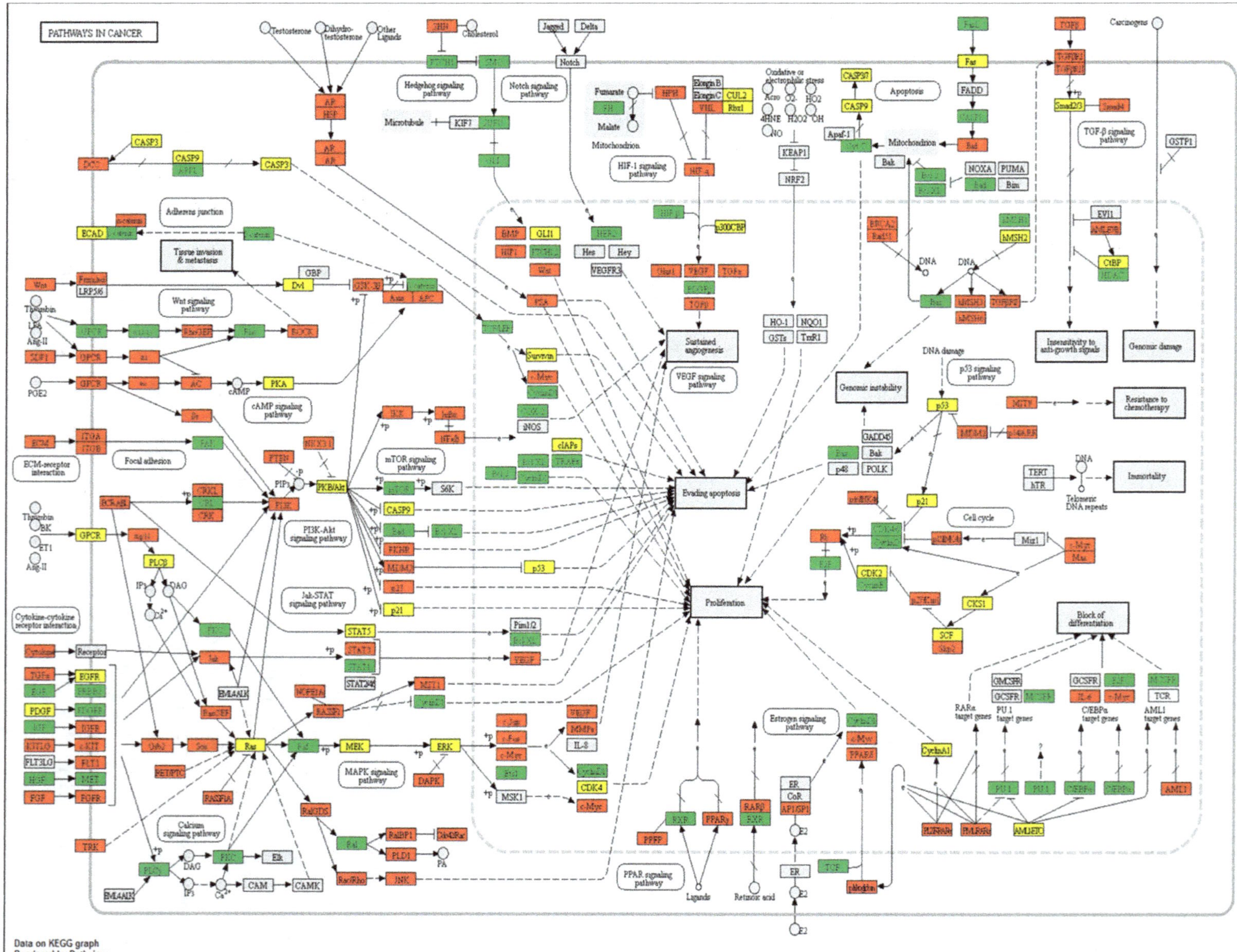

Figure 6. Use of the Kyoto Encyclopedia of Genes and Genomes (KEGG) database to display cancer pathway-associated genes affected by ^{188}Re-liposome mediated miRNA expression in HPC. Red: Up-regulated genes; green: down-regulated genes; yellow: unknown regulated genes; gray: unchanged genes.

Table 4. Thirty significant changed pathways after repeated doses of ^{188}Re-liposome treatment.

Pathways Description	No. of DEGs with Annotated Pathways (4498) [a]	Percentage of DEGs with Annotated Pathways (4498)	Down Regulated Gene	Up Regulated Gene	Unknown Regulated Gene	No. of All Genes with Annotated Pathways (6883)	Percentage of All Genes with Annotated Pathways (6883)	p-Value [b]
Olfactory transduction	51	1.13%	14	33	4	415	6.03%	6.37×10^{-45}
Pathways in cancer	329	7.31%	95	184	50	397	5.77%	0.00127
Taste transduction	16	0.36%	2	11	3	52	0.76%	0.00373
HTLV-I infection	217	4.82%	61	117	39	258	3.75%	0.00623
Proteoglycans in cancer	176	3.91%	60	93	23	203	2.95%	0.00739
Neuroactive ligand-receptor interaction	139	3.09%	40	84	15	277	4.02%	0.00779
MicroRNAs in cancer	151	3.36%	41	89	21	297	4.31%	0.00885
Viral carcinogenesis	175	3.89%	47	90	38	205	2.98%	0.0103
Chemical carcinogenesis	32	0.71%	4	21	7	81	1.18%	0.01124
Hippo signaling pathway	135	3.00%	34	82	19	154	2.24%	0.01459
Focal adhesion	174	3.87%	55	90	29	207	3.01%	0.01626
MAPK signaling pathway	209	4.65%	53	128	28	255	3.70%	0.01732
Drug metabolism - cytochrome P450	27	0.60%	5	17	5	68	0.99%	0.01947
Metabolism of xenobiotics by cytochrome P450	30	0.67%	4	20	6	74	1.08%	0.01954
ErbB signaling pathway	82	1.82%	30	40	12	87	1.26%	0.02121
Signaling pathways regulating pluripotency of stem cells	124	2.76%	29	80	15	142	2.06%	0.02202
Endocytosis	208	4.62%	65	116	27	258	3.75%	0.02587
FoxO signaling pathway	117	2.60%	32	75	10	134	1.95%	0.02612
Ras signaling pathway	185	4.11%	50	109	26	227	3.30%	0.0272
Neurotrophin signaling pathway	106	2.36%	28	64	14	120	1.74%	0.02764
Regulation of actin cytoskeleton	175	3.89%	49	98	28	214	3.11%	0.03031
Chronic myeloid leukemia	70	1.56%	22	40	8	73	1.06%	0.03053
Transcriptional misregulation in cancer	149	3.31%	43	80	26	179	2.60%	0.03365
Glioma	63	1.40%	23	30	10	65	0.94%	0.03554
Pancreatic cancer	64	1.42%	19	35	10	66	0.96%	0.03682
Colorectal cancer	60	1.33%	17	30	13	62	0.90%	0.03971
Acute myeloid leukemia	56	1.24%	17	28	11	57	0.83%	0.04123
Protein processing in endoplasmic reticulum	140	3.11%	40	78	22	169	2.46%	0.04447
Prostate cancer	80	1.78%	26	38	16	89	1.29%	0.04703
TGF-beta signaling pathway	76	1.69%	23	46	7	84	1.22%	0.04999

[a] DEG: Differentially expressed genes. [b] Only $p < 0.05$ was counted.

2.7. Association of ^{188}Re-Liposome-Regulated microRNA and Patients' Survival Rate

As ^{188}Re-liposome could up-regulate tumor suppressive microRNA or down-regulate oncogenic microRNA of the HPC tumor model, we considered whether these microRNAs could be considered as prognostic factors for patients' survival rates. The microRNAs deregulated by ^{188}Re-liposome that displayed over five-fold change were examined. Notably, the online dataset only includes precursor forms of microRNAs for an analysis of patients' survival. For ^{188}Re-liposome up-regulated microRNAs in the HPC model, only miR-342 and miR-378a potentially exhibited an increase in the survival rate in HNSCC patients, with a marginal significance (Figure 7A,B). Interestingly, a high expression of miR-342 was significantly associated with a better survival rate in female patients (HR = 0.61, 95% CI = 0.38–0.98, p = 0.038). On the other hand, ^{188}Re-liposome down-regulated microRNAs, including miR-143, miR-6723, miR-944, and miR-136 were associated with a reduced survival rate in HNSCC patients when they were highly expressed (Figure 7C–F). Additionally, miR-3960 was also associated with reduced survival, yet the expression was too low for meaningful analysis (data not shown). These data suggest that specific miRNAs affected by ^{188}Re-liposome may be important for perspective clinical evaluation.

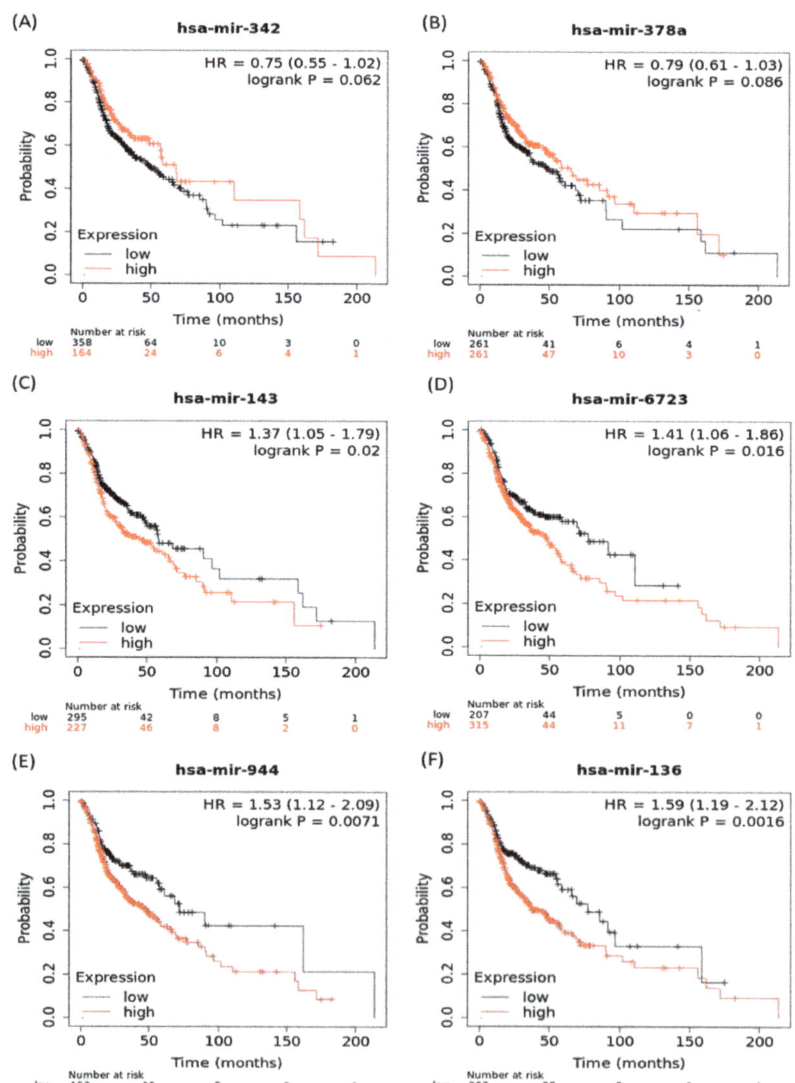

Figure 7. The association of ^{188}Re-liposome deregulated microRNAs with the survival rates of HNSCC patients. Kaplan–Meier (K-M) plot (**A**) hsa-miR-342; (**B**) hsa-miR-378a; (**C**) hsa-miR-143; (**D**) hsa-miR-6723; (**E**) hsa-miR-944; (**F**) hsa-miR-136.

3. Discussion

HPC mostly originates from mucosal squamous cells with a low incident rate. Because of unapparent early symptoms and a high metastatic ability, HPC accounts for the lowest survival rate of all head and neck cancers [72]. The FaDu cell line is a squamous cell carcinoma of the human hypopharynx commonly used for the study of molecular mechanisms of head and neck cancer in vitro and in vivo [73]. We have previously established an orthotopic tumor model using this cell line and found that *let-7* microRNA was associated with the therapeutic efficacy of ^{188}Re-liposome nanoparticles [24,74]. In this study, we used NGS analysis and found additional microRNAs that might be involved in the therapeutic efficacy of ^{188}Re-liposome after repeated administration. The expressions of the total RNA number and annotated small RNA were reduced in ^{188}Re-liposome treated tumors, suggesting that ^{188}Re-liposome would suppress gene transcription and expression.

As ^{188}Re is a high-energy β particles-emitter, it is expected to induce DNA damage. Indeed, the DNA damage marker γ H2AX was significantly induced by ^{188}Re-liposome compared to an untreated control. Interestingly, γ H2AX has been reported to be a tumor suppressor because of its role in the maintenance of genomic stability [75]. In our study, we found that ^{188}Re-liposome induced γ H2AX in HPC tumors. In the RNA-seq dataset, we also found that miR-138-2-5p, a potent inhibitor of H2AX [76], was down-regulated by over two-fold by ^{188}Re-liposome treatment. Together, these results are partially consistent with previous reports that might account for the therapeutic mechanisms of ^{188}Re-liposome from the viewpoint of γ-H2AX-mediated DNA damage responses.

According to the results of RNA-seq, ^{188}Re-liposome induced more than 200 microRNA to change their levels. To raise the selective criteria, we focused on the microRNA species exhibiting over five-fold up-regulation or down-regulation induced by ^{188}Re-liposome by comparing them to the untreated controls. The top three up-regulated microRNAs (miR-206-3p, miR-668-3p, and miR-485-3p) and down-regulated microRNAs (miR-142-5p, miR-944-3p, and miR-142-3p) displaying fold-change were categorized as tumor suppressors and oncogenes, respectively (Tables 2 and 3). Although miR-6723-5p was also highly suppressed by ^{188}Re-liposome, its role in cancer has not been interpreted in the dbDEMC database or microRNA Cancer association database (miRCancer) [77]. Most of the microRNAs deregulated by ^{188}Re-liposome were expressed oppositely in HNSCC, and they were reported to be potent tumor suppressors or oncogenes in different types of cancers. However, there were no available data for miR-4510-5p, miR-1268b-5p miR-6723-5p, miR-151b-3p, miR-143-5p, miR-194-2-5p and miR3960-3p in the database. As NGS is prominently used to find unknown genes that can be induced by treatment agents, the uncharacterized microRNAs shown to be significantly influenced by ^{188}Re-liposome treatment would be of interest for investigating their roles in the future.

The NGS analysis identified highly differentially expressed microRNAs that were also validated using FaDu tumors with or without ^{188}Re-liposome treatment, and clinical HNSCC samples using qPCR. The expression of analyzed microRNAs was consistent in these two different resources, although the case number of clinical samples was limited. The clinical information of the TCGA database could only be employed to analyze larynx cancer because the number of cases of HPC was too low to have normal tissues for analysis. Even so, we still found several microRNAs (e.g., miR-206-3p, miR-378-5p, and miR-142-5p) that were consistent with the results of NGS analysis and our clinical samples (Figure 4). In addition to ^{188}Re, ^{177}Lu is also a radionuclide that can emit 86% of β-particles and 14% of photons with a lower energy but longer half-life period. ^{177}Lu-octreotate has been reported to differentially regulate 57 specific microRNAs in mouse renal cortical tissue identified by the Mouse miRNA Oligo chip 4plex [78]. However, little microRNA was overlapped between their results and ours. Besides different types of radionuclides, the different animal models and microRNA mining methods may also account for the distinct observations in these two studies. Therefore, the differentially expressed microRNAs in the HPC model could be considered as specific prognostic factors for ^{188}Re-liposome treatment.

The predicted genes targeted by microRNAs were also analyzed by the miRDB public database. For the ^{188}Re-liposome up-regulated and down-regulated top three microRNAs, the *SLC44A2* gene and *U2SURP* gene were the targets recognized by these oppositely regulated microRNAs, respectively. Hence, it is expected that *SLC44A2* would exhibit an oncogenic property and *U2SURP* should be a tumor suppressor gene. *SLC44A2*, first discovered in the inner ear, is a member of the choline transporter-like protein family of membrane transporter proteins [79,80]. *U2SURP* is involved in RNA splicing as it is part of spliceosomes [81]. However, little is known about the association of these two genes with human cancers. It would be an interesting target gene to investigate for its role in mediating the efficacy of ^{188}Re-liposome.

Using the KEGG pathway database, we found that 30 pathways in orthotopic HPC tumors were significantly influenced by ^{188}Re-liposome treatment. Although the cancer-suppression-related pathways were expected to be regulated by ^{188}Re-liposome, most of the affected genes in the annotated pathway displayed olfactory transduction. Radiation therapy has been reported to cause olfactory loss in head and neck cancer patients [82]. However, the conclusion is that radiation can damage olfactory cells. The position of hypopharyngeal cancer was not in the olfactory tract, yet FaDu cells were orthotopically injected into the buccal position of the mouse. This operation was based on the fact that FaDu cells are also buccal carcinoma cells [83]. Whether the microenvironmental difference influences the gene regulatory pathway of tumors is unclear. We believed that the excised tumor should not be contaminated by olfactory cells because the human tumor was very small after ^{188}Re-liposome treatment, that is, the tumor size was not big enough to reach the olfactory tract.

An assessment of the correlation between the gene expression and survival rate of patients is important for evaluating the clinical relevance of preclinical study for novel genes and drugs. Here we used the Kaplan–Meier plotter online tool that includes the datasets of TCGA program, the Gene Expression Omnibus (GEO) and the European Genome-Phenome Archive (EGA) to find the ^{188}Re-liposome regulated primary microRNAs and their association with patients' survival rates [84]. Although several potent tumor suppressive or oncogenic microRNAs were influenced by ^{188}Re-liposome, only part of these microRNAs exhibited the expected association with patients' survival probability in HNSCC. For instance, ^{188}Re-liposome suppressed miR-142 exhibited higher survival probabilities in HNSCC when they were expressed at higher levels, although they were expected to be oncogenic microRNAs [85]. A potent limitation is the sample size (523 cases) of HNSCC patients, which may be too small to draw conclusions on the role of microRNAs in patients' survival rates. Besides, the online K-M plotter only analyzes the effects of precursor microRNA on patients' survival rate. The association of mature miRNAs with the survival rate remains unknown. Whether different forms of the same microRNAs will differentially influence the results of the survival rate remains to be addressed.

In summary, current data suggest that the de-regulation of microRNAs correlates with the therapeutic efficacy of ^{188}Re-liposome on human HPC tumors. Using NGS, we also found several microRNAs that have not been fully characterized for their roles in cancer development and therapy. Whether these microRNAs are important for mediating the efficacy of ^{188}Re-liposome would be interesting to further investigate. Additionally, the KEGG pathway analysis showed that not only cancer pathways but also olfactory and taste transduction were significantly changed in HPC tumors after they were treated by ^{188}Re-liposome. Although no clinical evidence showing that patients treated with ^{188}Re-liposome will lose olfactory and gustatory sensation, olfactory sensory dysfunction and gustatory impairment often occur after patients are treated with radiotherapy in the head and neck area [82,86–89]. To the best of our knowledge, this is the first study uncovering the therapeutic mechanisms of ^{188}Re-liposome by an investigation of the pan-expression of microRNA. As ^{188}Re-liposome has entered the clinical trial stage, these data may further extend the concept of precise medicine using this radiotheranostic agent and allow the affected microRNAs to be prognostic factors after cancer treatment.

4. Materials and Methods

4.1. Cell Lines and Plasmid

Human FaDu HPC cells (American Type Culture Collection, Manassas, VA, USA) were cultured in RPMI-1640 (Life Technologies Inc., Carlsbad, CA, USA) containing 10% fetal bovine serum (FBS) (Thermo Fisher Scientific Inc., Waltham, MA, USA), 1% penicillin (Sigma-Aldrich Co., St. Louis, MO, USA), and 1% L-glutamine (Sigma-Aldrich Co., St. Louis, MO, USA). FaDu-3R cells harboring multiple reporter genes were used and cultured as reported previously [24]. Cells were incubated at 37°C in a humidified incubator with 5% CO_2 and passaged every two days.

4.2. Preparation of ^{188}Re-Liposome

The procedure of ^{188}Re-liposomal preparation has been reported before [23]. In brief, ^{188}Re was milked from the ^{188}W/^{188}Re generator system (Institute National des Radioelements, Fleurus, Belgium) and conjugated with sodium perrhenate. Moreover, ^{188}Re was conjugated with *N*,*N*-bis(2-mercapatoethly)-*N′*,*N′*-diethylenediamine (BMEDA, ABX GmbH, Radeberg, Germany), and the quality of ^{188}Re-BMEDA was validated by using the instant thin-layer chromatography (iTLC) followed by a radioactive scanner (Bioscan AR2000; Bioscan, TriFoil Imaging Inc., Chatsworth, CA, USA). Furthermore, PEGylated liposome (NanoX; Taiwan Liposome Co. Ltd., Taipei, Taiwan) was used to encapsulate ^{188}Re-BMEDA and eluted using the PD-10 column (GE Health BioSciences, Pittsburgh, PA, USA) (Supplementary Figure S1). The average molecular weight of polyethylene glycol (PEG) was 2000. The particle size (84.6 ± 4.12 nm) and surface charge (1.1 ± 1.9 mV) were measured by the dynamic light scattering apparatus (Zetasizer Nano ZS90, Malvern Panalytical Ltd., Malvern, UK). The in vitro stabilities of ^{188}Re-liposome in normal saline and rat plasma were, respectively, over 92% and 82% in 72 h as reported before [20].

4.3. Establishment of HPC Orthotopic Tumor Model for Evaluating the Therapeutic Efficacy of ^{188}Re-Liposome

Six-week-old male BALB/c nude mice (*N* = 5 for each experimental group) were purchased from National Laboratory Animal Center, Taipei, Taiwan and used for the establishment of orthotopic HPC tumor model. FaDu-3R cells (1×10^6) were resuspended in 50 μL of OPTI-MEM (Sigma-Aldrich, St. Louis, MO, USA) and then injected into the buccal position of each mouse at right side using a 27 G insulin needle. For intravenous injection of ^{188}Re-liposome, 23.68 MBq (640 μCi) corresponding to 80% maximum tolerated dose (MTD), as we mentioned before [23]. To evaluate the therapeutic efficacy, the tumor viability and growth rate were measured using the luciferase reporter gene imaging and caliper measurement. The luminescent signals were acquired by the In Vivo Imaging System (*Optima*, Biospace Lab Inc., Paris, France). The tumor volume was calculated by the formula: $(\text{width}^2 \times \text{length})/2$ after caliper measurement every three days [90]. The animal experiments were approved by the Institutional Animal Care and Utilization Committee (IACUC) of National Yang-Ming University (No. 1061010).

4.4. Tumor Collection and Next-Generation Sequencing (NGS)

Tumors were harvested from tumor-bearing mice after four weeks of ^{188}Re-liposome treatment. Total RNA of both saline control and ^{188}Re-liposome treated group were extracted using the QIAGEN RNA mini kit (Thermo Fisher Scientific Inc., Waltham, MA, USA) according to manufacturer's instructions. Furthermore, the quality of RNA was detected using the Nanodrop spectrophotometer (Nanodrop Technologies LLC, Wilmington, DE, USA). The integrity and concentration of RNA samples were determined using the Agilent 2100 Bioanalyzer (Agilent Technologies, Santa Clara, CA, USA) with RNA 6000 nano kit (Agilent Technologies, Santa Clara, CA, USA). The TruSeq Small RNA Library kit (Illumina, Inc., San Diego, CA, USA) was then used to ligate RNA with adapters followed by the reverse transcription-PCR to generate cDNA library. The library was then sequenced by the HiSeq

4000 Sequencing System (2 × 150 bp paired-end Sequencing) and the results were processed with the Illumina software (Illumina, Inc., San Diego, CA, USA). To qualify the results of small RNA sequencing, the sequences were applied to the CLC Genomics Workbench v10 to obtain the qualified reads [91]. CLC Genomics Workbench counts different types of small RNAs in the data and compares them to databases of microRNAs or other small RNAs [92].

4.5. MicroRNA Expression Analysis

The 'miRBase' online source was used for the annotation of small RNA [93]. In the next step, all of the miRNAs were normalized by TMM (trimmed mean of M values) method using edgeR (R package: v.3.10.5) (Bioconductor, New York City, NY, USA) [94]. For a two-group experiment, we used the 'Fold Change' to tell how many times bigger the mean expression value in ^{188}Re-liposome group is relative to that of saline-only group. If the mean expression value in ^{188}Re-liposome group is small than that in saline-only group, the value will present negative sign, and vice versa. The criteria for microRNAs selection were fold change >5.

4.6. Western Blot Analysis

Tumors were collected from the tumor-bearing mice after 4 weeks of ^{188}Re-liposome treatment, and lysed in T-PER^{TM} Tissue Protein Extraction Reagent (Thermo Fisher Scientific, Waltham, MA, USA) containing 1% protease inhibitor cocktail (Sigma-Aldrich Co., St. Louis, MO, USA). Protein lysates (50 µg) were run on 8–12% SDS-PAGE, electro-transferred to nitrocellulose membrane, blocking and incubated with antibody as reported previously [95]. The primary antibodies were anti-γH2AX (GTX628789, GeneTex Inc., Irvine, CA, USA), and anti-glyceraldehyde3-phosphate dehydrogenase (GAPDH) (MA5-15738, Invitrogen Inc., Carlsbad, CA, USA).

4.7. Validation of microRNA Expression Using qPCR

To validate miRNA levels before and after HPC tumor treated with ^{188}Re-liposome and to compare normal tissue to HNSCC tissues using clinical samples, quantitative PCR (qPCR) of targeted miRNA was performed. Briefly, complementary DNA (cDNA) was generated from 2 µg total RNA using SuperScript II reverse transcriptase (Life-Technologies Co., Carlsbad, CA, USA). Then, the cDNA products were mixed with the Fast SYBR Green Master Mix (Life-Technologies Co., Carlsbad, CA, USA) and subjected to the StepOnePlus Real-time PCR System (Life-Technologies Co., Carlsbad, CA, USA) following the manufacturer's instructions. The sequences of stem loop primers, forward primers and universal primer used for miR-206-3p, miR-382-5p, miR-378a-5p, miR-3960-3p, and miR-142-5p amplification were summarized in Table 5. Use of human tissue samples was approved by the Institutional Review Board (No. 2019-01-010BC).

4.8. Heatmap Analysis of NGS Data

To gain the heatmap of total microRNAs' expression, 'TreeView' (v1.1.6r4) was used [96]. The heatmap analysis was based on the small RNA that has twice difference between individuals with or without the treatment of ^{188}Re-liposome, and then took Log2 value to draw out.

4.9. Analysis of microRNA Using the Cancer Genome Atlas (TCGA)

The expression levels of miRNAs and clinical information for TCGA Head-Neck Squamous Cell Carcinoma (HNSC) were downloaded from Broad GDAC Firehose [97]. The miRNA expression values for samples having anatomic subdivision labeled as normal larynx tissue (12 cases), larynx cancers (117 cases) or hypopharynx cancers (10 cases) were used. In house R scripts were used to parse and generate heatmap and boxplots [98]. The difference between normal and tumor samples were tested with Wilcoxon signed-rank test.

Table 5. The list of stem loop primers, forward primers, and reverse primer used for qPCR of microRNAs.

MicroRNA	Stem Loop Primer Sequence
miR-206-3p	5′-GTCGTATCCAGTGCAGGGTCCGAG GTATTCGCACTGGATACGACCCACAC-3′
miR-382-5p	5′-GTCGTATCCAGTGCAGGGTCCGA GGTATTCGCACTGGATACGACCGAATC-3′
miR-378a-5p	5′-GTCGTATCCAGTGCAGGGTCCGAG GTATTCGCACTGGATACGACACACAG-3′
miR-3960-3p	5′-GTCGTATCCAGTGCAGGGTCCGAG GTATTCGCACTGGATACGACCCCCCG-3′
miR-142-5p	5′-GTCGTATCCAGTGCAGGGTCCGAG GTATTCGCACTGGATACGACAGTAGT-3′
MicroRNA	**Forward Primer Sequence**
miR-206-3p	5′-CACGCATGGAATGTAAGGAAGT-3′
miR-382-5p	5′-CACGCAGAAGTTGTTCGTGGTG-3′
miR-378a-5p	5′-TGATTACTCCTGACTCCAGGTC-3′
miR-3960-3p	5′-TAATTATGGCGGCGGCGGAG-3′
miR-142-5p	5′-CACGCGCATAAAGTAGAAAGCA-3′
MicroRNA	**Reverse Primer Sequence**
Universal reverse primer	5′-CCAGTGCAGGGTCCGAGGT-3′

4.10. Characterization of miRNAs

The miRNA of interests were subjected to a Database of Differentially Expressed MiRNAs in human Cancer 2.0 (dbDEMC v2.0) that collects the data sets of Gene Expression Omnibus (GEO) and The Cancer Genome Atlas (TCGA) to exhibit differentially expressed miRNAs in human cancers detected by high throughput method [99]. The roles of miRNAs belonging to tumor suppressor genes or oncogenes were predicted accordingly. The miRDB online database for prediction of miRNA targets by a MirTarget bioinformatics tool was used to analyze putative downstream genes influenced by the miRNAs of interests [100,101]. Each microRNA was selected for target expression analysis for FaDu cells, and the targets expression level over 20 was counted as they were most relevant to FaDu cells. Target expression level was determined by RNA-Seq using the RPKM method (Reads Per Kilobase of transcript, per Million mapped reads). An online Venn diagrams drawing tool was exploited to calculate the intersections of list of miRNA targets [102].

4.11. The Pathway Analysis

The 'pathview' (R package: v1.4.2) software (Bioconductor, New York City, NY, USA) was used to draw pathways and find significant gene change (Fold change > 2) with the Kyoto Encyclopedia of Genes and Genomes (KEGG) [103,104]. Moreover, the pathways would be regarded significant if the p-value < 0.05.

4.12. Statistical Analysis

Statistical analysis was performed using GraphPad Prism 6.0 (GraphPad Software, San Diego, CA, USA). All data were represented as the means ± standard deviation (SD) with independent experiments. The Student's t-test was used for statistical analysis. Two-way Analysis of

Variance (ANOVA) was used to compare the tumor growth curves. The Kaplan–Meier method with the log-rank test was used to analyze the association of miRNAs and patients' survival rates using the online K-M plotter with public datasets [84].

Author Contributions: Conceptualization, Y.-J.L. and S.-Y.W.; methodology, B.-Z.L.; software, T.-W.C.; validation, B.-Z.L., M.-Y.L. and Y.-J.L.; formal analysis, B.-Z.L.; investigation, B.-Z.L.; resources, C.-H.C. and M.-H.Y.; data curation, M.-Y.L.; writing—original draft preparation, Y.-J.L.; writing—review and editing, Y.-J.L.; supervision, Y.-J.L. and S.-Y.W.; funding acquisition, Y.-J.L. and S.-Y.W. All authors have read and agreed to the published version of the manuscript.

Acknowledgments: We thanked Shen-Nan Lo, Ming-Hsuan Lin for helping the ^{188}Re preparation, production, and quality assurance. We thank Liang-Ting Lin for discussion of references. We also thank the Taiwan Animal Consortium (MOST 106-2319-B-001-004)—Taiwan Mouse Clinic which is funded by the Ministry of Science and Technology (MOST) of Taiwan for technical support in in vivo imaging experiments. We also thank the support from the Cancer Progression Research Center, National Yang-Ming University, from the Featured Areas Research Center Program within the framework of the Higher Education Sprout Project by the Ministry of Education (MOE) in Taiwan.

References

1. Patel, R.S.; Goldstein, D.P.; Brown, D.; Irish, J.; Gullane, P.J.; Gilbert, R.W. Circumferential pharyngeal reconstruction: History, critical analysis of techniques, and current therapeutic recommendations. *Head Neck* **2010**, *32*, 109–120. [CrossRef] [PubMed]
2. Chu, P.Y.; Chang, S.Y. Reconstruction of the hypopharynx after surgical treatment of squamous cell carcinoma. *J. Chin. Med. Assoc.* **2009**, *72*, 351–355. [CrossRef]
3. Iwamoto, H. Operative treatment of cancer of the hypopharynx. *Gan No Rinsho* **1968**, *14*, 660–662. [PubMed]
4. Kim, S.; Wu, H.G.; Heo, D.S.; Kim, K.H.; Sung, M.W.; Park, C.I. Advanced hypopharyngeal carcinoma treatment results according to treatment modalities. *Head Neck* **2001**, *23*, 713–717. [CrossRef] [PubMed]
5. Mura, F.; Bertino, G.; Occhini, A.; Benazzo, M. Surgical treatment of hypopharyngeal cancer: A review of the literature and proposal for a decisional flow-chart. *Acta Otorhinolaryngol. Ital.* **2013**, *33*, 299–306. [PubMed]
6. Medvedeva, A.; Chernov, V.; Zeltchan, R.; Sinilkin, I.; Bragina, O.; Chijevskaya, S.; Choynzonov, E.; Goldberg, A. Nuclear medicine imaging of locally advanced laryngeal and hypopharyngeal cancer. In *AIP Conference Proceedings*; AIP Publishing LLC: Melville, NY, USA, 2017; Volume 1882.
7. Jadvar, H.; Chen, X.; Cai, W.; Mahmood, U. Radiotheranostics in Cancer Diagnosis and Management. *Radiology* **2018**, *286*, 388–400. [CrossRef]
8. Argyrou, M.; Valassi, A.; Andreou, M.; Lyra, M. Rhenium-188 production in hospitals, by w-188/re-188 generator, for easy use in radionuclide therapy. *Int. J. Mol. Imaging* **2013**, *2013*, 290750. [CrossRef]
9. Liepe, K.; Hliscs, R.; Kropp, J.; Gruning, T.; Runge, R.; Koch, R.; Knapp, F.F., Jr.; Franke, W.G. Rhenium-188-HEDP in the palliative treatment of bone metastases. *Cancer Biother. Radiopharm.* **2000**, *15*, 261–265. [CrossRef]
10. Zhang, H.; Tian, M.; Li, S.; Liu, J.; Tanada, S.; Endo, K. Rhenium-188-HEDP therapy for the palliation of pain due to osseous metastases in lung cancer patients. *Cancer Biother. Radiopharm.* **2003**, *18*, 719–726. [CrossRef]
11. Guerra Liberal, F.D.C.; Tavares, A.A.S.; Tavares, J. Palliative treatment of metastatic bone pain with radiopharmaceuticals: A perspective beyond Strontium-89 and Samarium-153. *Appl. Radiat. Isot.* **2016**, *110*, 87–99. [CrossRef]
12. Maxon, H.R., III; Schroder, L.E.; Washburn, L.C.; Thomas, S.R.; Samaratunga, R.C.; Biniakiewicz, D.; Moulton, J.S.; Cummings, D.; Ehrhardt, G.J.; Morris, V. Rhenium-188(Sn)HEDP for treatment of osseous metastases. *J. Nucl. Med.* **1998**, *39*, 659–663. [PubMed]
13. Uccelli, L.; Martini, P.; Pasquali, M.; Boschi, A. Monoclonal Antibodies Radiolabeling with Rhenium-188 for Radioimmunotherapy. *BioMed Res. Int.* **2017**, *2017*, 5923609. [CrossRef] [PubMed]
14. Edelman, M.J.; Clamon, G.; Kahn, D.; Magram, M.; Lister-James, J.; Line, B.R. Targeted radiopharmaceutical therapy for advanced lung cancer: Phase I trial of rhenium Re188 P2045, a somatostatin analog. *J. Thorac. Oncol.* **2009**, *4*, 1550–1554. [CrossRef] [PubMed]
15. Kumar, A.; Bal, C.; Srivastava, D.N.; Thulkar, S.P.; Sharma, S.; Acharya, S.K.; Duttagupta, S. Management

of multiple intrahepatic recurrences after radiofrequency ablation of hepatocellular carcinoma with rhenium-188-HDD-lipiodol. *Eur. J. Gastroenterol. Hepatol.* **2006**, *18*, 219–223. [CrossRef] [PubMed]

16. Lambert, B.; Bacher, K.; De Keukeleire, K.; Smeets, P.; Colle, I.; Jeong, J.M.; Thierens, H.; Troisi, R.; De Vos, F.; Van de Wiele, C. 188Re-HDD/lipiodol for treatment of hepatocellular carcinoma: A feasibility study in patients with advanced cirrhosis. *J. Nucl. Med.* **2005**, *46*, 1326–1332. [PubMed]
17. Nowicki, M.L.; Cwikla, J.B.; Sankowski, A.J.; Shcherbinin, S.; Grimmes, J.; Celler, A.; Buscombe, J.R.; Bator, A.; Pech, M.; Mikolajczak, R.; et al. Initial study of radiological and clinical efficacy radioembolization using 188Re-human serum albumin (HSA) microspheres in patients with progressive, unresectable primary or secondary liver cancers. *Med. Sci. Monit.* **2014**, *20*, 1353–1362. [CrossRef]
18. Jeong, J.M.; Lee, Y.J.; Kim, E.H.; Chang, Y.S.; Kim, Y.J.; Son, M.; Lee, D.S.; Chung, J.K.; Lee, M.C. Preparation of (188) Re-labeled paper for treating skin cancer. *Appl. Radiat. Isot.* **2003**, *58*, 551–555. [CrossRef]
19. Wang, S.J.; Huang, W.S.; Chuang, C.M.; Chang, C.H.; Lee, T.W.; Ting, G.; Chen, M.H.; Chang, P.M.; Chao, T.C.; Teng, H.W.; et al. A phase 0 study of the pharmacokinetics, biodistribution, and dosimetry of (188)Re-liposome in patients with metastatic tumors. *Ejnmmi. Res.* **2019**, *9*, 46. [CrossRef]
20. Chang, Y.J.; Chang, C.H.; Chang, T.J.; Yu, C.Y.; Chen, L.C.; Jan, M.L.; Luo, T.Y.; Lee, T.W.; Ting, G. Biodistribution, pharmacokinetics and microSPECT/CT imaging of 188Re-bMEDA-liposome in a C26 murine colon carcinoma solid tumor animal model. *Anticancer Res.* **2007**, *27*, 2217–2225.
21. Chang, C.H.; Liu, S.Y.; Chi, C.W.; Yu, H.L.; Chang, T.J.; Tsai, T.H.; Lee, T.W.; Chen, Y.J. External beam radiotherapy synergizes (1)(8)(8)Re-liposome against human esophageal cancer xenograft and modulates (1)(8)(8)Re-liposome pharmacokinetics. *Int. J. Nanomed.* **2015**, *10*, 3641–3649. [CrossRef]
22. Huang, F.Y.; Lee, T.W.; Chang, C.H.; Chen, L.C.; Hsu, W.H.; Chang, C.W.; Lo, J.M. Evaluation of 188Re-labeled PEGylated nanoliposome as a radionuclide therapeutic agent in an orthotopic glioma-bearing rat model. *Int. J. Nanomed.* **2015**, *10*, 463–473. [CrossRef]
23. Lin, L.T.; Chang, C.H.; Yu, H.L.; Liu, R.S.; Wang, H.E.; Chiu, S.J.; Chen, F.D.; Lee, T.W.; Lee, Y.J. Evaluation of the therapeutic and diagnostic effects of PEGylated liposome-embedded 188Re on human non-small cell lung cancer using an orthotopic small-animal model. *J. Nucl. Med.* **2014**, *55*, 1864–1870. [CrossRef]
24. Lin, L.T.; Chang, C.Y.; Chang, C.H.; Wang, H.E.; Chiou, S.H.; Liu, R.S.; Lee, T.W.; Lee, Y.J. Involvement of let-7 microRNA for the therapeutic effects of Rhenium-188-embedded liposomal nanoparticles on orthotopic human head and neck cancer model. *Oncotarget* **2016**, *7*, 65782–65796. [CrossRef]
25. Shen, Y.A.; Lan, K.L.; Chang, C.H.; Lin, L.T.; He, C.L.; Chen, P.H.; Lee, T.W.; Lee, Y.J.; Chuang, C.M. Intraperitoneal (188)Re-Liposome delivery switches ovarian cancer metabolism from glycolysis to oxidative phosphorylation and effectively controls ovarian tumour growth in mice. *Radiother. Oncol.* **2016**, *119*, 282–290. [CrossRef]
26. Chang, C.M.; Lan, K.L.; Huang, W.S.; Lee, Y.J.; Lee, T.W.; Chang, C.H.; Chuang, C.M. 188Re-Liposome Can Induce Mitochondrial Autophagy and Reverse Drug Resistance for Ovarian Cancer: From Bench Evidence to Preliminary Clinical Proof-of-Concept. *Int. J. Mol. Sci.* **2017**, *18*, 903. [CrossRef]
27. Rutman, A.M.; Kuo, M.D. Radiogenomics: Creating a link between molecular diagnostics and diagnostic imaging. *Eur. J. Radiol.* **2009**, *70*, 232–241. [CrossRef]
28. Kang, J.; Rancati, T.; Lee, S.; Oh, J.H.; Kerns, S.L.; Scott, J.G.; Schwartz, R.; Kim, S.; Rosenstein, B.S. Machine Learning and Radiogenomics: Lessons Learned and Future Directions. *Front. Oncol.* **2018**, *8*, 228. [CrossRef]
29. Lawrence, M.S.; Stojanov, P.; Mermel, C.H.; Robinson, J.T.; Garraway, L.A.; Golub, T.R.; Meyerson, M.; Gabriel, S.B.; Lander, E.S.; Getz, G. Discovery and saturation analysis of cancer genes across 21 tumour types. *Nature* **2014**' *505*, 495–501. [CrossRef]
30. Schulze, K.; Nault, J.C.; Villanueva, A. Genetic profiling of hepatocellular carcinoma using next-generation sequencing. *J. Hepatol.* **2016**, *65*, 1031–1042. [CrossRef]
31. Wang, Z.; Gerstein, M.; Snyder, M. RNA-Seq: A revolutionary tool for transcriptomics. *Nat. Rev. Genet.* **2009**, *10*, 57–63. [CrossRef]
32. Roh, S.W.; Abell, G.C.; Kim, K.H.; Nam, Y.D.; Bae, J.W. Comparing microarrays and next-generation sequencing technologies for microbial ecology research. *Trends Biotechnol.* **2010**, *28*, 291–299. [CrossRef]
33. Doostparast Torshizi, A.; Wang, K. Next-generation sequencing in drug development: Target identification and genetically stratified clinical trials. *Drug Discov. Today* **2018**, *23*, 1776–1783. [CrossRef]
34. Liu, F.; Zhao, X.; Qian, Y.; Zhang, J.; Zhang, Y.; Yin, R. MiR-206 inhibits Head and neck squamous cell

carcinoma cell progression by targeting HDAC6 via PTEN/AKT/mTOR pathway. *Biomed. Pharm.* **2017**, *96*, 229–237. [CrossRef]

35. Koshizuka, K.; Hanazawa, T.; Fukumoto, I.; Kikkawa, N.; Matsushita, R.; Mataki, H.; Mizuno, K.; Okamoto, Y.; Seki, N. Dual-receptor (EGFR and c-MET) inhibition by tumor-suppressive miR-1 and miR-206 in head and neck squamous cell carcinoma. *J. Hum. Genet.* **2017**, *62*, 113–121. [CrossRef]
36. Momen-Heravi, F.; Trachtenberg, A.J.; Kuo, W.P.; Cheng, Y.S. Genomewide Study of Salivary MicroRNAs for Detection of Oral Cancer. *J. Dent. Res.* **2014**, *93*, 86S–93S. [CrossRef]
37. Shin, K.H.; Pucar, A.; Kim, R.H.; Bae, S.D.; Chen, W.; Kang, M.K.; Park, N.H. Identification of senescence-inducing microRNAs in normal human keratinocytes. *Int. J. Oncol.* **2011**, *39*, 1205–1211. [CrossRef]
38. Lou, C.; Xiao, M.; Cheng, S.; Lu, X.; Jia, S.; Ren, Y.; Li, Z. MiR-485-3p and miR-485-5p suppress breast cancer cell metastasis by inhibiting PGC-1alpha expression. *Cell Death Dis.* **2016**, *7*, e2159. [CrossRef]
39. Wang, Z.Q.; Zhang, M.Y.; Deng, M.L.; Weng, N.Q.; Wang, H.Y.; Wu, S.X. Low serum level of miR-485-3p predicts poor survival in patients with glioblastoma. *PLoS ONE* **2017**, *12*, e0184969. [CrossRef]
40. Zhang, Y.; Sui, R.; Chen, Y.; Liang, H.; Shi, J.; Piao, H. Downregulation of miR-485-3p promotes glioblastoma cell proliferation and migration via targeting RNF135. *Exp. Med.* **2019**, *18*, 475–482. [CrossRef]
41. Wang, J.; Chen, C.; Yan, X.; Wang, P. The role of miR-382-5p in glioma cell proliferation, migration and invasion. *Onco. Targets* **2019**, *12*, 4993–5002. [CrossRef]
42. Feng, J.; Qi, B.; Guo, L.; Chen, L.Y.; Wei, X.F.; Liu, Y.Z.; Zhao, B.S. miR-382 functions as a tumor suppressor against esophageal squamous cell carcinoma. *World J. Gastroenterol.* **2017**, *23*, 4243–4251. [CrossRef]
43. Zhu, W.J.; Chen, X.; Wang, Y.W.; Liu, H.T.; Ma, R.R.; Gao, P. MiR-1268b confers chemosensitivity in breast cancer by targeting ERBB2-mediated PI3K-AKT pathway. *Oncotarget* **2017**, *8*, 89631–89642. [CrossRef]
44. Pu, Y.; Zhao, F.; Cai, W.; Meng, X.; Li, Y.; Cai, S. MiR-193a-3p and miR-193a-5p suppress the metastasis of human osteosarcoma cells by down-regulating Rab27B and SRR, respectively. *Clin. Exp. Metastasis* **2016**, *33*, 359–372. [CrossRef]
45. Chou, N.H.; Lo, Y.H.; Wang, K.C.; Kang, C.H.; Tsai, C.Y.; Tsai, K.W. MiR-193a-5p and -3p Play a Distinct Role in Gastric Cancer: miR-193a-3p Suppresses Gastric Cancer Cell Growth by Targeting ETS1 and CCND1. *Anticancer Res.* **2018**, *38*, 3309–3318. [CrossRef]
46. Yin, C.Y.; Kong, W.; Jiang, J.; Xu, H.; Zhao, W. miR-7-5p inhibits cell migration and invasion in glioblastoma through targeting SATB1. *Oncol. Lett.* **2019**, *17*, 1819–1825. [CrossRef]
47. Shi, Y.; Luo, X.; Li, P.; Tan, J.; Wang, X.; Xiang, T.; Ren, G. miR-7-5p suppresses cell proliferation and induces apoptosis of breast cancer cells mainly by targeting REGgamma. *Cancer Lett.* **2015**, *358*, 27–36. [CrossRef]
48. Wang, Z.; Ma, B.; Ji, X.; Deng, Y.; Zhang, T.; Zhang, X.; Gao, H.; Sun, H.; Wu, H.; Chen, X.; et al. MicroRNA-378-5p suppresses cell proliferation and induces apoptosis in colorectal cancer cells by targeting BRAF. *Cancer Cell Int.* **2015**, *15*, 40. [CrossRef]
49. Li, H.; Dai, S.; Zhen, T.; Shi, H.; Zhang, F.; Yang, Y.; Kang, L.; Liang, Y.; Han, A. Clinical and biological significance of miR-378a-3p and miR-378a-5p in colorectal cancer. *Eur. J. Cancer.* **2014**, *50*, 1207–1221. [CrossRef]
50. Ostadrahimi, S.; Abedi Valugerdi, M.; Hassan, M.; Haddad, G.; Fayaz, S.; Parvizhamidi, M.; Mahdian, R.; Fard Esfahani, P. miR-1266-5p and miR-185-5p Promote Cell Apoptosis in Human Prostate Cancer Cell Lines. *Asian Pac. J. Cancer Prev.* **2018**, *19*, 2305–2311. [CrossRef]
51. Shen, X.P.; Ling, X.; Lu, H.; Zhou, C.X.; Zhang, J.K.; Yu, Q. Low expression of microRNA-1266 promotes colorectal cancer progression via targeting FTO. *Eur. Rev. Med. Pharm. Sci.* **2018**, *22*, 8220–8226. [CrossRef]
52. Hironaka-Mitsuhashi, A.; Matsuzaki, J.; Takahashi, R.U.; Yoshida, M.; Nezu, Y.; Yamamoto, Y.; Shiino, S.; Kinoshita, T.; Ushijima, T.; Hiraoka, N.; et al. A tissue microRNA signature that predicts the prognosis of breast cancer in young women. *PLoS ONE* **2017**, *12*, e0187638. [CrossRef] [PubMed]
53. Chen, L.; Yuan, L.; Wang, G.; Cao, R.; Peng, J.; Shu, B.; Qian, G.; Wang, X.; Xiao, Y. Identification and bioinformatics analysis of miRNAs associated with human muscle invasive bladder cancer. *Mol. Med. Rep.* **2017**, *16*, 8709–8720. [CrossRef] [PubMed]
54. Pedersen, N.J.; Jensen, D.H.; Lelkaitis, G.; Kiss, K.; Charabi, B.W.; Ullum, H.; Specht, L.; Schmidt, A.Y.; Nielsen, F.C.; von Buchwald, C. MicroRNA-based classifiers for diagnosis of oral cavity squamous cell carcinoma in tissue and plasma. *Oral. Oncol.* **2018**, *83*, 46–52. [CrossRef] [PubMed]
55. Wang, X.; Zhao, Y.; Lu, Q.; Fei, X.; Lu, C.; Li, C.; Chen, H. MiR-34a-5p Inhibits Proliferation, Migration,

Invasion and Epithelial-mesenchymal Transition in Esophageal Squamous Cell Carcinoma by Targeting LEF1 and Inactivation of the Hippo-YAP1/TAZ Signaling Pathway. *J. Cancer* **2020**, *11*, 3072–3081. [CrossRef] [PubMed]
56. Gao, J.; Li, N.; Dong, Y.; Li, S.; Xu, L.; Li, X.; Li, Y.; Li, Z.; Ng, S.S.; Sung, J.J.; et al. miR-34a-5p suppresses colorectal cancer metastasis and predicts recurrence in patients with stage II/III colorectal cancer. *Oncogene* **2015**, *34*, 4142–4152. [CrossRef] [PubMed]
57. Yang, H.; Li, Q.; Niu, J.; Li, B.; Jiang, D.; Wan, Z.; Yang, Q.; Jiang, F.; Wei, P.; Bai, S. microRNA-342-5p and miR-608 inhibit colon cancer tumorigenesis by targeting NAA10. *Oncotarget* **2016**, *7*, 2709–2720. [CrossRef]
58. Soriano, A.; Masanas, M.; Boloix, A.; Masia, N.; Paris-Coderch, L.; Piskareva, O.; Jimenez, C.; Henrich, K.O.; Roma, J.; Westermann, F.; et al. Functional high-throughput screening reveals miR-323a-5p and miR-342-5p as new tumor-suppressive microRNA for neuroblastoma. *Cell Mol. Life Sci.* **2019**, *76*, 2231–2243. [CrossRef]
59. He, Z.; Yi, J.; Liu, X.; Chen, J.; Han, S.; Jin, L.; Chen, L.; Song, H. MiR-143-3p functions as a tumor suppressor by regulating cell proliferation, invasion and epithelial-mesenchymal transition by targeting QKI-5 in esophageal squamous cell carcinoma. *Mol. Cancer* **2016**, *15*, 51. [CrossRef]
60. Jin, X.; Chen, X.; Hu, Y.; Ying, F.; Zou, R.; Lin, F.; Shi, Z.; Zhu, X.; Yan, X.; Li, S.; et al. LncRNA-TCONS_00026907 is involved in the progression and prognosis of cervical cancer through inhibiting miR-143-5p. *Cancer Med.* **2017**, *6*, 1409–1423. [CrossRef]
61. Yang, F.; Xiao, Z.; Zhang, S. Knockdown of miR-194-5p inhibits cell proliferation, migration and invasion in breast cancer by regulating the Wnt/beta-catenin signaling pathway. *Int. J. Mol. Med.* **2018**, *42*, 3355–3363. [CrossRef]
62. Jiang, M.J.; Chen, Y.Y.; Dai, J.J.; Gu, D.N.; Mei, Z.; Liu, F.R.; Huang, Q.; Tian, L. Dying tumor cell-derived exosomal miR-194-5p potentiates survival and repopulation of tumor repopulating cells upon radiotherapy in pancreatic cancer. *Mol. Cancer* **2020**, *19*, 68. [CrossRef] [PubMed]
63. Kosela-Paterczyk, H.; Paziewska, A.; Kulecka, M.; Balabas, A.; Kluska, A.; Dabrowska, M.; Piatkowska, M.; Zeber-Lubecka, N.; Ambrozkiewicz, F.; Karczmarski, J.; et al. Signatures of circulating microRNA in four sarcoma subtypes. *J. Cancer* **2020**, *11*, 874–882. [CrossRef] [PubMed]
64. Gullu Amuran, G.; Tinay, I.; Filinte, D.; Ilgin, C.; Peker Eyuboglu, I.; Akkiprik, M. Urinary micro-RNA expressions and protein concentrations may differentiate bladder cancer patients from healthy controls. *Int. Urol. Nephrol.* **2020**, *52*, 461–468. [CrossRef] [PubMed]
65. Chen, X.; Huang, Z.; Chen, R. Microrna-136 promotes proliferation and invasion ingastric cancer cells through Pten/Akt/P-Akt signaling pathway. *Oncol. Lett.* **2018**, *15*, 4683–4689. [CrossRef] [PubMed]
66. Li, Y.; Chen, D.; Jin, L.U.; Liu, J.; Li, Y.; Su, Z.; Qi, Z.; Shi, M.; Jiang, Z.; Yang, S.; et al. Oncogenic microRNA-142-3p is associated with cellular migration, proliferation and apoptosis in renal cell carcinoma. *Oncol. Lett.* **2016**, *11*, 1235–1241. [CrossRef] [PubMed]
67. Zhang, H.; Li, T.; Zheng, L.; Huang, X. Biomarker MicroRNAs for Diagnosis of Oral Squamous Cell Carcinoma Identified Based on Gene Expression Data and MicroRNA-mRNA Network Analysis. *Comput. Math Methods Med.* **2017**, *2017*, 9803018. [CrossRef]
68. Park, S.; Kim, J.; Eom, K.; Oh, S.; Kim, S.; Kim, G.; Ahn, S.; Park, K.H.; Chung, D.; Lee, H. microRNA-944 overexpression is a biomarker for poor prognosis of advanced cervical cancer. *Bmc Cancer* **2019**, *19*, 419. [CrossRef]
69. He, H.; Tian, W.; Chen, H.; Jiang, K. MiR-944 functions as a novel oncogene and regulates the chemoresistance in breast cancer. *Tumour Biol.* **2016**, *37*, 1599–1607. [CrossRef]
70. Ma, Z.; Liu, T.; Huang, W.; Liu, H.; Zhang, H.M.; Li, Q.; Chen, Z.; Guo, A.Y. MicroRNA regulatory pathway analysis identifies miR-142-5p as a negative regulator of TGF-beta pathway via targeting SMAD3. *Oncotarget* **2016**, *7*, 71504–71513. [CrossRef]
71. Islam, F.; Gopalan, V.; Vider, J.; Lu, C.T.; Lam, A.K. MiR-142-5p act as an oncogenic microRNA in colorectal cancer: Clinicopathological and functional insights. *Exp. Mol. Pathol.* **2018**, *104*, 98–107. [CrossRef]
72. Lamperska, K.M.; Kolenda, T.; Teresiak, A.; Kowalik, A.; Kruszyna-Mochalska, M.; Jackowiak, W.; Blizniak, R.; Przybyla, W.; Kapalczynska, M.; Kozlowski, P. Different levels of let-7d expression modulate response of FaDu cells to irradiation and chemotherapeutics. *PLoS ONE* **2017**, *12*, e0180265. [CrossRef] [PubMed]
73. Rangan, S.R. A new human cell line (FaDu) from a hypopharyngeal carcinoma. *Cancer* **1972**, *29*, 117–121. [CrossRef]
74. Chang, C.Y.; Chen, C.C.; Lin, L.T.; Chang, C.H.; Chen, L.C.; Wang, H.E.; Lee, T.W.; Lee, Y.J. PEGylated

liposome-encapsulated rhenium-188 radiopharmaceutical inhibits proliferation and epithelial-mesenchymal transition of human head and neck cancer cells in vivo with repeated therapy. *Cell Death Discov.* **2018**, *4*, 100. [CrossRef] [PubMed]

75. Bonner, W.M.; Redon, C.E.; Dickey, J.S.; Nakamura, A.J.; Sedelnikova, O.A.; Solier, S.; Pommier, Y. GammaH2AX and cancer. *Nat. Rev. Cancer* **2008**, *8*, 957–967. [CrossRef]
76. Wang, Y.; Huang, J.W.; Li, M.; Cavenee, W.K.; Mitchell, P.S.; Zhou, X.; Tewari, M.; Furnari, F.B.; Taniguchi, T. MicroRNA-138 modulates DNA damage response by repressing histone H2AX expression. *Mol. Cancer Res.* **2011**, *9*, 1100–1111. [CrossRef]
77. Xie, B.; Ding, Q.; Han, H.; Wu, D. miRCancer: A microRNA-cancer association database constructed by text mining on literature. *Bioinformatics* **2013**, *29*, 638–644. [CrossRef]
78. Schuler, E.; Parris, T.Z.; Helou, K.; Forssell-Aronsson, E. Distinct microRNA expression profiles in mouse renal cortical tissue after 177Lu-octreotate administration. *PLoS ONE* **2014**, *9*, e112645. [CrossRef]
79. Zajic, G.; Nair, T.S.; Ptok, M.; Van Waes, C.; Altschuler, R.A.; Schacht, J.; Carey, T.E. Monoclonal antibodies to inner ear antigens: I. Antigens expressed by supporting cells of the guinea pig cochlea. *Hear. Res.* **1991**, *52*, 59–71. [CrossRef]
80. He, L.; Vasiliou, K.; Nebert, D.W. Analysis and update of the human solute carrier (SLC) gene superfamily. *Hum. Genom.* **2009**, *3*, 195–206. [CrossRef]
81. De Maio, A.; Yalamanchili, H.K.; Adamski, C.J.; Gennarino, V.A.; Liu, Z.; Qin, J.; Jung, S.Y.; Richman, R.; Orr, H.; Zoghbi, H.Y. RBM17 Interacts with U2SURP and CHERP to Regulate Expression and Splicing of RNA-Processing Proteins. *Cell Rep.* **2018**, *25*, 726–736.e7. [CrossRef]
82. Bramerson, A.; Nyman, J.; Nordin, S.; Bende, M. Olfactory loss after head and neck cancer radiation therapy. *Rhinology* **2013**, *51*, 206–209. [CrossRef] [PubMed]
83. Reiss, M.; Stash, E.B.; Vellucci, V.F.; Zhou, Z.L. Activation of the autocrine transforming growth factor alpha pathway in human squamous carcinoma cells. *Cancer Res.* **1991**, *51*, 6254–6262. [PubMed]
84. Nagy, A.; Lanczky, A.; Menyhart, O.; Gyorffy, B. Author Correction: Validation of miRNA prognostic power in hepatocellular carcinoma using expression data of independent datasets. *Sci. Rep.* **2018**, *8*, 11515. [CrossRef] [PubMed]
85. Chang, S.S.; Jiang, W.W.; Smith, I.; Poeta, L.M.; Begum, S.; Glazer, C.; Shan, S.; Westra, W.; Sidransky, D.; Califano, J.A. MicroRNA alterations in head and neck squamous cell carcinoma. *Int. J. Cancer* **2008**, *123*, 2791–2797. [CrossRef] [PubMed]
86. Sagar, S.M.; Thomas, R.J.; Loverock, L.T.; Spittle, M.F. Olfactory sensations produced by high-energy photon irradiation of the olfactory receptor mucosa in humans. *Int. J. Radiat. Oncol. Biol. Phys.* **1991**, *20*, 771–776. [CrossRef]
87. Hua, M.S.; Chen, S.T.; Tang, L.M.; Leung, W.M. Olfactory function in patients with nasopharyngeal carcinoma following radiotherapy. *Brain Inj.* **1999**, *13*, 905–915. [CrossRef] [PubMed]
88. Ruo Redda, M.G.; Allis, S. Radiotherapy-induced taste impairment. *Cancer Treat. Rev.* **2006**, *32*, 541–547. [CrossRef]
89. Epstein, J.B.; Smutzer, G.; Doty, R.L. Understanding the impact of taste changes in oncology care. *Support. Care Cancer* **2016**, *24*, 1917–1931. [CrossRef]
90. Carlsson, G.; Gullberg, B.; Hafström, L. Estimation of liver tumor volume using different formulas—An experimental study in rats. *J. Cancer Res. Clin. Oncol.* **1983**, *105*, 20–23. [CrossRef]
91. Andrews, S.; Krueger, F.; Segonds-Pichon, A.; Biggins, L.; Krueger, C.; Wingett, S.; Montgomery, J. Babraham Bioinformatics-Fastqc a Quality Control Tool For High Throughput Sequence Data. Available online: http://www.bioinformatics.babraham.ac.uk/projects/fastqc/ (accessed on 22 January 2019).
92. Creighton, C.J.; Reid, J.G.; Gunaratne, P.H. Expression profiling of microRNAs by deep sequencing. *Brief. Bioinform.* **2009**, *10*, 490–497. [CrossRef]
93. Ambros, V.; Bartel, B.; Bartel, D.P.; Burge, C.B.; Carrington, J.C.; Chen, X.; Dreyfuss, G.; Eddy, S.R.; Griffiths-Jones, S.; Marshall, M.; et al. A uniform system for microRNA annotation. *RNA* **2003**, *9*, 277–279. [CrossRef] [PubMed]
94. Robinson, M.D.; McCarthy, D.J.; Smyth, G.K. edgeR: A Bioconductor package for differential expression analysis of digital gene expression data. *Bioinformatics* **2010**, *26*, 139–140. [CrossRef] [PubMed]
95. Tsai, C.H.; Lin, L.T.; Wang, C.Y.; Chiu, Y.W.; Chou, Y.T.; Chiu, S.J.; Wang, H.E.; Liu, R.S.; Wu, C.Y.; Chan, P.C.; et al. Over-expression of cofilin-1 suppressed growth and invasion of cancer cells is associated with

up-regulation of let-7 microRNA. *Biochim. Biophys. Acta* **2015** *1852*, 851–861. [CrossRef] [PubMed]
96. Saldanha, A.J. Java Treeview-extensible visualization of microarray data. *Bioinformatics* **2004**, *20*, 3246–3248. [CrossRef]
97. Deng, M.; Bragelmann, J.; Kryukov, I.; Saraiva-Agostinho, N.; Perner, S. FirebrowseR: An R client to the Broad Institute's Firehose Pipeline. *Database* **2017**, *2017*, baw160. [CrossRef]
98. Wickham, H. *ggplot2: Elegant Graphics for Data Analysis*; Springer: New York, NY, USA, 2016.
99. Yang, Z.; Wu, L.; Wang, A.; Tang, W.; Zhao, Y.; Zhao, H.; Teschendorff, A.E. dbDEMC 2.0: Updated database of differentially expressed miRNAs in human cancers. *Nucleic. Acids Res.* **2017**, *45*, D812–D818. [CrossRef]
100. Chen, Y.; Wang, X. miRDB: An online database for prediction of functional microRNA targets. *Nucleic Acids Res.* **2020**, *48*, D127–D131. [CrossRef]
101. Liu, W.; Wang, X. Prediction of functional microRNA targets by integrative modeling of microRNA binding and target expression data. *Genome Biol.* **2019**, *20*, 18. [CrossRef]
102. Lieven Sterck, V.d.P.Y. Draw Venn Diagram-Bioinformatics.psb.ugent.be. Available online: http://bioinformatics.psb.ugent.be/webtools/Venn/ (accessed on 25 June 2020).
103. Kanehisa, M.; Sato, Y.; Kawashima, M.; Furumichi, M.; Tanabe, M. KEGG as a reference resource for gene and protein annotation. *Nucleic Acids Res.* **2016**, *44*, D457–D462. [CrossRef]
104. Kanehisa, M.; Sato, Y.; Morishima, K. BlastKOALA and GhostKOALA: KEGG Tools for Functional Characterization of Genome and Metagenome Sequences. *J. Mol. Biol.* **2016**, *428*, 726–731. [CrossRef]

8

The Influence of Cell Type and Culture Medium on Determining Cancer Selectivity of Cold Atmospheric Plasma Treatment

Eline Biscop [1], Abraham Lin [1,2], Wilma Van Boxem [1], Jinthe Van Loenhout [2], Joey De Backer [3], Christophe Deben [2], Sylvia Dewilde [3], Evelien Smits [2] and Annemie Bogaerts [1,*]

1 PLASMANT Research Group, Department of Chemistry, University of Antwerp, 2610 Antwerp, Belgium
2 Center for Oncological Research, University of Antwerp, 2610 Antwerp, Belgium
3 Department of Biomedical Sciences, University of Antwerp, 2610 Antwerp, Belgium
* Correspondence: annemie.bogaerts@uantwerpen.be

Abstract: Increasing the selectivity of cancer treatments is attractive, as it has the potential to reduce side-effects of therapy. Cold atmospheric plasma (CAP) is a novel cancer treatment that disrupts the intracellular oxidative balance. Several reports claim CAP treatment to be selective, but retrospective analysis of these studies revealed discrepancies in several biological factors and culturing methods. Before CAP can be conclusively stated as a selective cancer treatment, the importance of these factors must be investigated. In this study, we evaluated the influence of the cell type, cancer type, and cell culture medium on direct and indirect CAP treatment. Comparison of cancerous cells with their non-cancerous counterparts was performed under standardized conditions to determine selectivity of treatment. Analysis of seven human cell lines (cancerous: A549, U87, A375, and Malme-3M; non-cancerous: BEAS-2B, HA, and HEMa) and five different cell culture media (DMEM, RPMI1640, AM, BEGM, and DCBM) revealed that the tested parameters strongly influence indirect CAP treatment, while direct treatment was less affected. Taken together, the results of our study demonstrate that cell type, cancer type, and culturing medium must be taken into account before selectivity of CAP treatment can be claimed and overlooking these parameters can easily result in inaccurate conclusions of selectivity.

Keywords: cold atmospheric plasma; selectivity; plasma-treated liquid; dielectric barrier discharge

1. Introduction

Chemotherapy and radiotherapy are two major pillars in the management of cancer. Significant efforts to make these treatments more selective are ongoing, with the intention of reducing side-effects of therapy [1]. Despite the remarkable evolution of conventional cancer therapies, they are still met with limitations as evidenced by the fact that cancer remains the second leading cause of death worldwide [2]. As a result, new alternative or additional cancer treatment methods are also under investigation to support current treatment strategies.

Cold atmospheric plasma (CAP) has been investigated as novel cancer treatment strategy, and interest in the use of CAP for cancer treatment has been growing [3]. CAP is an ionized gas near room temperature, composed of various molecules, radicals, ions, electrons, and excited species [4]. Over the past decade, the anti-cancer capacity of CAP has been reported for multiple cancer types in vitro [5–11], while in animal models, CAP treatment has reduced tumor burden in mice and increased survival [12,13]. Nowadays, several CAP devices are being used in the clinic for treatment of cancerous lesions [14–16].

The current understanding of CAP mechanisms for effecting biological response is that the reactive oxygen and nitrogen species (RONS) generated by CAP elicit oxidative damage to the cell, resulting in cell death [17,18]. According to this understanding, CAP treatment has been hypothesized to be selective for cancer, as the disturbance of the oxidative balance occurs more easily in cancer cells compared to healthy cells [19,20]. Additionally, cancer cells have more aquaporins and less cholesterol in their cellular membrane, which contributes to the diffusion of certain CAP-generated RONS through the membrane and facilitates pore formation, respectively [21–24]. Furthermore, Bauer and Graves proposed a theory where the initial concentration of singlet oxygen, produced by the plasma, triggers cells to generate higher concentrations of secondary singlet oxygen, which leads to the inactivation of catalase in the cell membrane [25]. The inactivation of catalase can also play an important role in the selectivity, as this allows reactivation of intercellular ROS/RNS-dependent, apoptosis-inducing signaling within the population of tumor cells [25]. To date, however, the underlying mechanisms of CAP selectivity are not yet fully understood, and furthermore, the selectivity has not been fully validated.

While several papers claim that CAP selectively kills cancer cells in vitro, retrospective analysis of these papers reveals that definitive proof is rather scarce. This is largely due to the discrepancies between treatment conditions for cancerous and non-cancerous cells. In several cases, the cell culture media used for cancerous and non-cancerous cells were not the same, while in other studies, the cell culture media was not specified at all [8,26–30]. It is understandable that non-cancerous cells normally require more advanced cell culture media with additional organic compounds compared to cancer cells, but the different media have disparate buffering and antioxidant capacities [31]. In fact, the stability of RONS in different liquids has been thoroughly investigated [32,33] and Yan et. al showed that the presence of cysteine and methionine can significantly degrade CAP-generated RONS [31]. Since the working mechanism of CAP involves disrupting the oxidative balance of cells via RONS generation, changes in media composition could impede their production and delivery, subsequently affecting biological outcome. Therefore, the observed selectivity of CAP treatment could actually result from variation in media and not from intrinsic sensitivity of cancerous and normal cells. In other studies, the selectivity of CAP treatment was claimed, but comparisons were made with different cell types (e.g., epithelial cancer cells with non-cancerous fibroblast cells) and even tissue types (e.g., comparison of ovarian cancer cells with non-cancerous lung cells) [27,30,34–36]. Due to the different physiological characteristics of distinct tissues [37], comparisons between equivalent cell types must also be made before selectivity of treatment can be claimed [37].

Taken together, in order to avoid false claims of selectivity for CAP treatment, the potentially confounding factors found in previous work, must be investigated. Therefore, our goals in this study were to address the following: What are the influences of the cell and cancer types on selectivity experiments? What are the influences of cell culture medium on selectivity experiments? Finally, when the proper comparisons are made, is CAP treatment more selective against cancerous cells compared to their normal, non-cancerous counterparts? In this study, two well-established methods of CAP treatment were studied—'direct' and 'indirect' treatment [38]. In the direct case, CAP was generated directly onto cells, while in the indirect case, a liquid (e.g., saline) was enriched with RONS following CAP treatment, and this plasma-treated liquid (PTL) was then delivered to cells or tissue. The selectivity of both treatment methods for three different cancer types (lung cancer, skin cancer, and brain cancer) was analyzed by comparing their survival 24 hours after treatment with that of their non-cancerous counterparts. Next, the cytotoxic effects of CAP treatment on cells using five different cell culture media—i.e., two 'standard' cell culture media and three 'more advanced' cell culture media for cancerous and non-cancerous cells, respectively, were analyzed. Our results showed that both the cell type and cancer type, as well as the cell culture medium, can have a substantial influence on the outcome of experiments. When analyzing selectivity of CAP treatment in the correct way (with cancerous and non-cancerous cells from the same tissue, the same cell type, and cultured in the same medium), appreciable selectivity was not observed in this study.

2. Results

2.1. Influence of Cell Type and Cancer Type on Cell Viability

Since different cell types have different responses to oxidative stress [39], we first investigated the cytotoxic effect of CAP on two human malignant melanoma cell types: an epithelial cell line (A375, derived from skin) and a fibroblast cell line (Malme-3M, derived from a metastatic site on the lung), according to the American Type Culture Collection (ATCC). As these cells were cultured in the same medium and under the same conditions, the cell type was the only variable in this experiment. Our results showed that while there was no significant difference in sensitivity for the cell lines with direct CAP treatment, the epithelial cells were more sensitive to indirect treatment compared to malignant fibroblasts (Figure 1a). To further evaluate the cytotoxic effects of CAP on different cancer types, we treated two additional human epithelial cells, U87 glioblastoma and A549 lung carcinoma. All cancer types were equally sensitive to direct CAP treatment, but the U87 was less sensitive to indirect treatment (Figure 1b). Therefore, it is clear that cell sensitivity to indirect CAP treatment is influenced by both cell type and cancer type, while this impact seems not present with direct treatment.

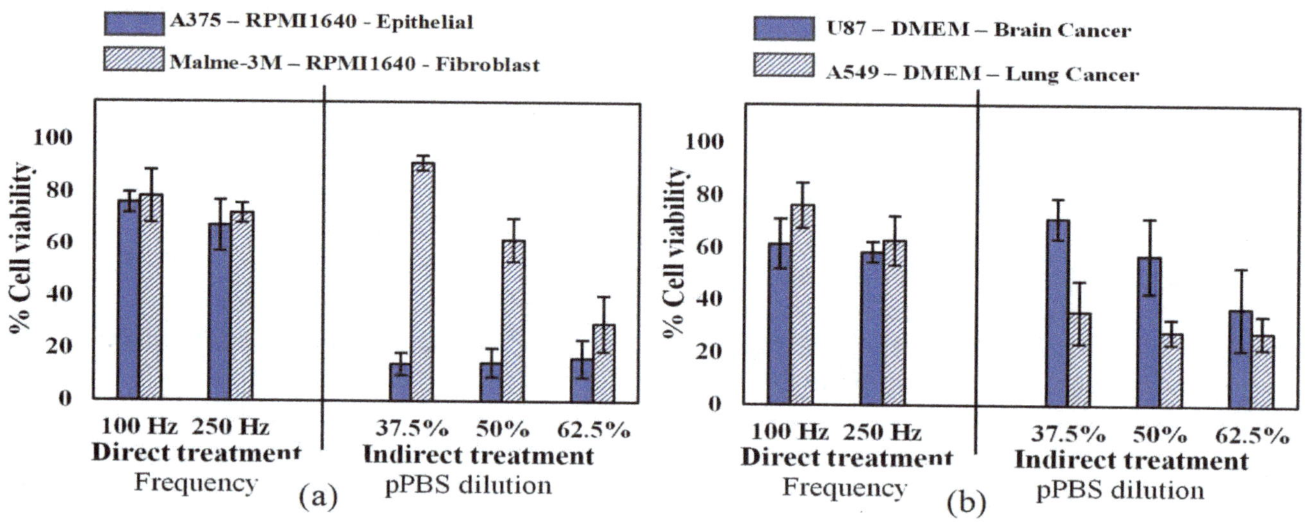

Figure 1. Analysis of the influence of the cell type and cancer type on both direct treatment (FE-DBD at two different frequencies) and indirect treatment (pPBS in three different dilutions). (**a**) Comparison of an epithelial cell line (A375) with a fibroblast cell line (Malme-3M), which are both skin cancer cell lines. (**b**) Comparison of a brain cancer cell line (U87) with a lung cancer cell line (A549). For both figures, the cells were cultured in the same cell culture medium and treated with exactly the same conditions. Therefore, the only variables tested were (**a**) cell type and (**b**) cancer type. Data are represented as mean ± standard deviation (SD) of three independent experiments with at least two replicates. Statistical significance of all treatment conditions was compared to untreated. *$p < 0.05$, **$p < 0.01$, and ***$p < 0.005$ (one-way ANOVA).

2.2. Influence of Cell Culture Media on Cell Viability

To determine the importance and influence of cell culture medium when assessing selectivity of treatment, we evaluated the cytotoxicity of both direct and indirect treatment for the A549 and A375 cell lines, in five different media. In order to ensure that the different media alone did not significantly affect cell growth and death, the cytotoxicity assay was performed on cells 24 hours after incubation and cell density in the different media was compared to that of their recommended medium: DMEM for A549 and RPMI for A375 (Figure S1, Supplementary Information). The A375 cells were able to grow in all media with a similar growth rate to that in RPMI1640. However, there was a statistically significant decrease in cell growth of the A549 cells in BEGM compared to DMEM. This suggests that even without CAP treatment, certain cell processes are strongly influenced by the components of the cell culture medium. Due to this discrepancy on cell growth, selectivity of treatment cannot be determined for cases where normal, non-cancerous cells are grown in the BEGM medium. This was further validated when A549 and their normal counterparts (BEAS-2B) were cultured in the BEGM medium and treated with direct and indirect CAP (Figure S2, Supplementary Information). Therefore, this medium was removed from all subsequent experiments. For the other three media, the difference in growth rate was not significant ($p > 0.05$, details in Supplementary Information).

The effect of direct CAP treatment was unaffected by the cell culture medium (Figure 2a), as the cell culture medium was removed during treatment. These results further indicated that the effect of direct CAP treatment was initiated during treatment and unaffected by the scavenging effects of the cell culture media added immediately afterwards. For the indirect treatment, cytotoxicity was significantly influenced by the cell culture media (Figure 2b). Cancer cells treated in the standard media (DMEM and RPMI1640) resulted in ≥50% cytotoxicity, but were unaffected when treated in advanced media used to culture normal, non-cancerous cells (AM and DCBM).

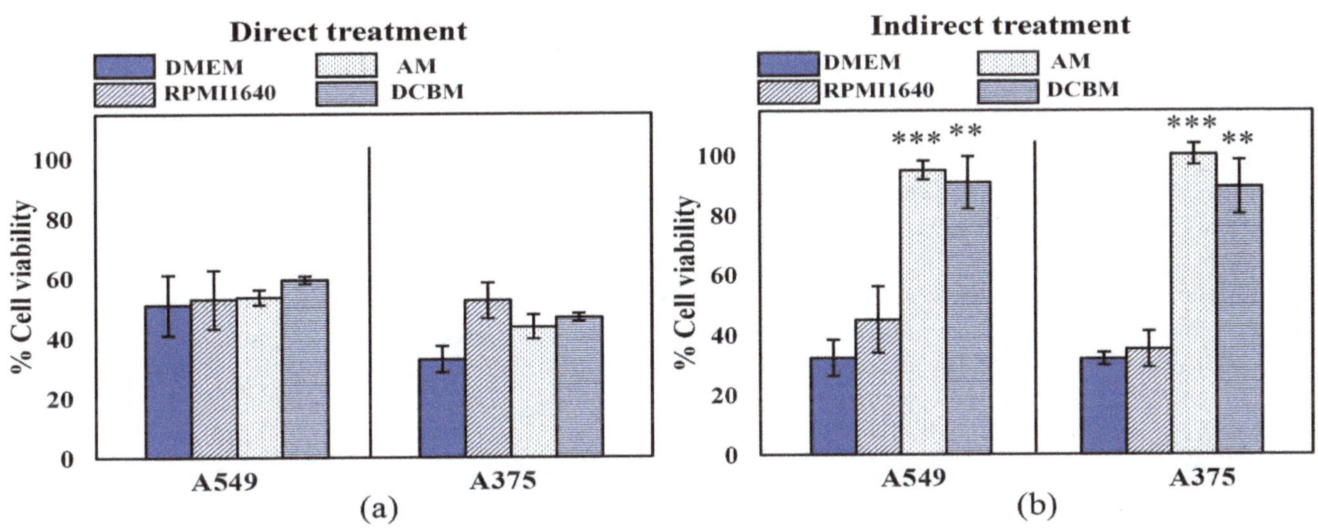

Figure 2. Influence of the cell culture medium on the direct and indirect plasma treatment of two cancer cell lines. (**a**) The direct plasma treatment was performed for 10 s, with a frequency of 500 Hz and a gap of 1 mm. (**b**) The indirect treatment was performed for 7 min treatment, with a gas flow rate of 3 slm and a gap of 10 mm. Data are represented as mean ± standard deviation (SD) of three independent experiments with at least two replicates. Statistical significance of all treatment conditions was compared to untreated. *$p < 0.05$, **$p < 0.01$, and ***$p < 0.005$ (one-way ANOVA).

2.3. *Influence of Cell Culture Media on Selectivity Evaluation of Indirect CAP Treatment*

To further validate selectivity of indirect CAP treatment and the influence of cell culture media, we compared cytotoxicity for the cancerous cell lines with their non-cancerous, complimentary cell lines (astrocytes and melanocytes for glioblastoma and melanoma, respectively) in both standard and advanced media. Experiments were performed with cells seeded in their recommended medium and with cells seeded in the same medium. As non-cancerous cells were incapable of being cultured in standard media, cancerous cells were grown in the more advanced media of their non-cancerous counterparts. When cultured and treated in their recommended media (different media), as commonly done in literature, it would appear that pPBS treatment resulted in significant selectivity (Figure 3). However, when both cell lines were cultured in the same media, selectivity was diminished. Only the A375 cell line showed cytotoxic effect in the more advanced media, but this was also reduced compared to treatment in standard media.

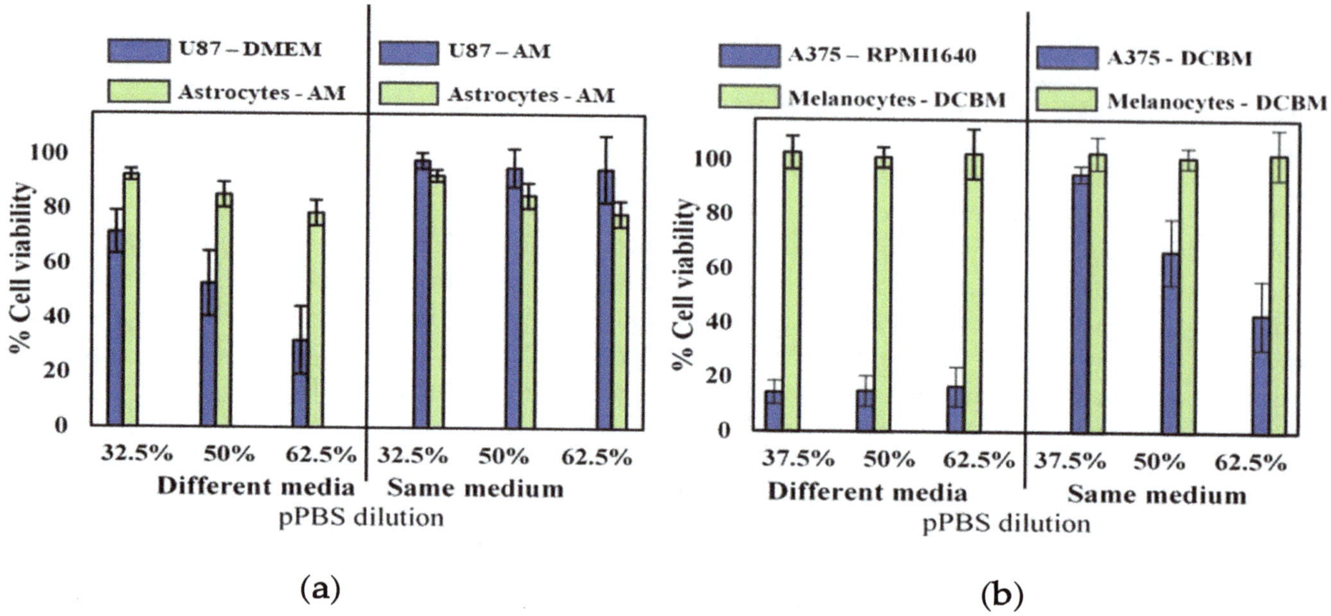

Figure 3. Analysis of the selectivity with the indirect treatment for brain cancer and skin cancer. A 5-min treatment with a gas flow rate of 1 slm and a gap of 6 mm was used to create the pPBS, which we further diluted. Comparison of (**a**) brain and (**b**) skin cancer cells in their common medium (blue solid bars on the left side) with non-cancerous cells in their common medium (green solid bar on the left side) appeared to show selectivity in all cases. However, when compared to the cancer cells in the advanced media (on the right side of the graph), the selectivity was not found. Hence, this clearly shows that the selectivity was affected by the cell culture medium. This is important to realize, to avoid drawing false conclusions. Data are represented as mean ± standard deviation (SD) of three independent experiments with at least two replicates. Statistical significance of all treatment conditions was compared to untreated. $^{*}p < 0.05$, $^{**}p < 0.01$, and $^{***}p < 0.005$ (one-way ANOVA).

2.4. Influence of Cell Culture Media on Selectivity Evaluation of Direct CAP Treatment

Following previous Sections 2.1–2.3, it is clear that cell type, cancer type, and culture media are critical parameters for indirect CAP treatment. These parameters were also standardized for direct CAP treatment to evaluate their effect on selectivity.

Though we observed that the influence of different cell culture medium was not pronounced for direct CAP treatment, as described in Section 2.2, to be correct, we still performed our selectivity analysis of cancerous versus non-cancerous cell lines in both the same and different culture media. No selectivity was observed when cancerous and normal cells were cultured in their own recommended medium (Figure 4, different media), but when cancer cells were cultured and treated in the medium used for their non-cancerous counterparts, slight selectivity was observed in the U87 glioblastoma cell line, and the A375 melanoma cell line at lower intensity CAP treatment (Figure 4, same medium). However, at higher intensity treatment (250 Hz), no such selectivity was observed, as the difference was within error. Interestingly, our results suggest that there is an optimal regime for direct CAP treatment where selectivity can be achieved, above which the oxidative burden becomes too overwhelming for even normal cells to manage.

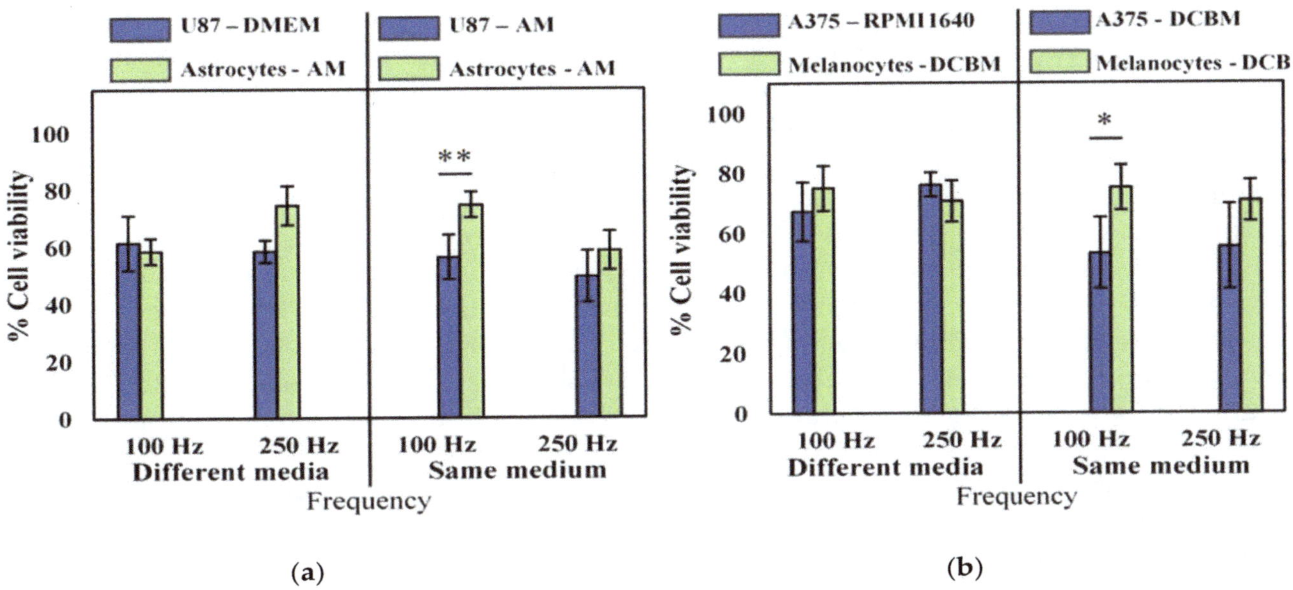

Figure 4. Analysis of selectivity with the direct treatment for brain cancer and skin cancer. A 10 second treatment with a gap of 1 mm and a frequency of either 100 Hz or 250 Hz was used to treat (**a**) brain and (**b**) skin cancer and non-cancerous cells. Data are represented as mean ± standard deviation (SD) of three independent experiments with at least two replicates. Statistical significance of all treatment conditions was compared to untreated. *$p < 0.05$, **$p < 0.01$, and ***$p < 0.005$ (one-way ANOVA).

3. Discussion

Selectivity of CAP treatment for cancer is an important topic of research, but it has often been misconcluded. Multiple research groups claim to have found treatment conditions which selectively kill cancerous cells and leave non-cancerous cells unharmed. When examining those articles in more detail, we found critical discrepancies between the treatment conditions and origins of the cancerous and non-cancerous cells [8,26–30,34,35]. To ensure that these comparisons are not confounded by the discrepancies we identified, we analyzed their influence on cell viability after CAP treatment.

An important parameter often neglected in past studies, is the difference in cell type or cancer type [27,30,34,35]. For example, in one article, the authors compared ovarian cancer cells with non-cancerous lung cells [35]. In comparing the responses of two cell lines for both ovarian adenocarcinoma and non-cancerous lung tissue, they concluded that the cancer cell lines were more sensitive to the treatment than the non-cancerous cell line. However, Giordano et al. has reported a difference in gene expression profiles between lung cancer and ovarian cancer [40], which can result in differential responses to CAP treatment. Furthermore, the cell type of the cancerous cell lines and non-cancerous cell lines was different. The two ovarian cancerous cell lines used in that study, SKOV-3 and HRA, were epithelial cell lines, while the two non-cancerous lung cell lines, WI-38 and MRC-5, were fibroblasts. Epithelial cells and fibroblasts show different gene expression levels and can therefore give a different response to CAP treatment [41]. To analyze the influence of these parameters, we examined the difference in cell type and cancer type by comparing an epithelial and fibroblast cell line from the same cancer type and by comparing two epithelial cell lines from different cancer types. According to our results, both cell type and cancer type had an effect on sensitivity to CAP treatment. In light of these findings, it is clear that for analyzing selectivity, cells of the same cancer type and cell type should be chosen, and discrepancies between these two biological parameters could lead to misdirected conclusions of selectivity.

The influence of the cell culture medium is another important parameter often overlooked when determining the selectivity of CAP treatment. Therefore, the influence hereof on cell viability after CAP treatment was also investigated. The effect of two commonly used cell culture media (DMEM and RPMI1640) was compared with two more advanced cell culture media required for culturing non-cancerous cells (AM and DCBM). Our results showed that, when cells were cultured in the more advanced media, indirect CAP treatment was ineffective. This was likely in part due to the presence of more organic components in the advanced media, as non-cancerous cells require more nutrients and are much harder to grow in vitro [39]. RONS produced by CAP can react with these organic components before reaching the cells [31]. One component commonly added to most advanced media is sodium pyruvate, a known H_2O_2-scavenger [42,43]. For DMEM and RPMI1640, we ensured that no sodium pyruvate was present, but for the other two cell culture media, the composition was not specified by the manufacturer [44–46]. This would also explain why the cell culture media did not significantly influence cell viability following direct CAP treatment, as it was removed prior to treatment. These results highlight the influence of cell culture media on downstream biological effects following indirect CAP treatment. Taken together, it is clear that selectivity of CAP treatment cannot be evaluated for indirect plasma treatment when the cancer cells are cultured in medium different to that of non-cancerous cells.

Several papers claiming that CAP selectively kills cancerous cells cultured their cells in different media [8,26–30]. For example, one study cultured the A549 cells in DMEM, while their normal BEAS-2B cells were cultured in BEGM [30]. Since the authors saw more response to the treatment in their A549 cell line compared to the BEAS-2B cell line, they stated that their indirect CAP treatment was more selective. However, as evident from our results above, the sensitivity of A549 cells to indirect CAP treatment was reduced when cultured in BEGM compared to DMEM (Figure S2, Supplementary Information). Therefore, the reported selectivity was not cell line specific, but due to the different medium used to culture the cells. This strongly highlights the fact that cell culture medium plays an important role in indirect CAP treatment and must be standardized before claims of selectivity can be made.

Since the influence of the cell culture medium was less important for direct CAP treatment, we used this treatment method to analyze the selectivity of treatment for two cancer types: melanoma and glioblastoma. Interestingly, we observed that direct treatment preferentially affected cancer cells at lower intensity treatments (Figure 4), suggesting that selectivity depends on optimizing CAP treatment conditions that exploit the differences between normal and cancerous tissue. It is widely known that cancer cells have a higher proliferation rate, compared to non-cancerous cells. Healthy cells primarily produce energy through mitochondrial oxidative phosphorylation, while cancer cells predominantly produce their energy through a high rate of glycolysis followed by lactic acid fermentation, which benefits this high proliferation rate [47,48]. To sustain this fast growth rate, cancer cells require a 'hyper metabolism', which results in a higher level of basal intracellular ROS [49,50]. Simultaneously, cancer cells also maintain a high level of antioxidant activity, mainly reduced nicotinamide adenine dinucleotide phosphate (NADPH) and glutathione (GSH), to prevent build-up of ROS [47,49]. However, once the levels of ROS become excessively high through the addition of extra ROS, detrimental oxidative stress can occur, leading to cell death [51,52]. While randomized control clinical trials using pro-oxidant therapy are still ongoing, increasing evidence suggests that raising ROS levels through small molecules can selectively induce cancer cell death by disabling antioxidants [50,53,54]. Taken together with our observations, this would mean that the aim to reach selectivity of CAP treatment lies in the optimization of parameters and conditions to produce sufficient ROS to overwhelm the oxidative threshold in cancer cells, without reaching this threshold in the healthy cells.

It must be noted here that selectivity of CAP treatment may also depend on the RONS generated and delivered to the biological target. This is particularly important as direct and indirect CAP treatments generate a different cocktail of reactive species. With the indirect CAP treatment, a liquid is treated with CAP and then transferred to cells or tissue. Due to the time delay between treatment and application, only the long-lived species (mostly H_2O_2, NO_2^-, NO_3^-) remain in the liquid and reach the cells [36]. In the case of direct CAP treatment, the liquid is removed before treatment in order for CAP to be generated directly onto the cells, thereby enabling both the long-lived and short-lived (•OH, $^1O_2$,

O, O_3, •NO, $ONOO^-$) species to interact with the biological target [55]. Several reports have already demonstrated the importance of these short-lived species in direct CAP treatment for effecting cell death [55–57], though further fundamental investigations are still required, including the type of cell death modalities elicited.

The experiments performed in this study used cancer cell lines in 2D cultures. Cancer cell lines are derived from primary patient material and have provided important knowledge for cancer research. However, care must be taken when interpreting the results, as cell lines are genetically manipulated and therefore do not always accurately reflect the responses of primary cells [58]. Furthermore, comparison between two cell lines often involves comparison between two patient sources. To further investigate the selectivity in a more realistic manner, the cancer and healthy cells should be derived from the same patient [58]. Hasse et al. analyzed CAP treatment on cancer and healthy human tissue samples from head and neck cancer patients [58]. They found that CAP treatment of tumor tissue induced more apoptotic cells than in healthy tissue. This was accompanied by elevated extracellular cytochrome c levels in the tumor tissue [59]. Though this is probably the most representative in vitro model, human tissue samples cannot be preserved long-term and are therefore much more difficult to work with [60]. Another recently developed in vitro model is organoids [61,62]. These are 3D self-organizing organotypic structures, grown from tissue-derived adult stem cells. Organoids can be expanded long-term without losing their genetic and phenotypical stability [61,62]. Such 3D cell culture systems feature increased complexity for increased faithfulness to the in vivo environment and are above all fairly easy to work with [60]. When comparing these 3D organoids from healthy and cancerous tissue from the same patient, more representative results concerning the selectivity can be obtained compared to those obtained with 2D models.

The results from Hasse et al. are encouraging as it suggests that CAP treatment may indeed be selective when operated at certain regimes. As more studies using primary patient tissue and the proper 3D models start to emerge, the selectivity capacity of CAP treatment will become more clear. However, as it stands, it is evident from this study, several biological factors must be standardized and the proper comparisons must be made before these conclusions can be made.

4. Materials and Methods

4.1. Cell Culture and Plating

To evaluate the selectivity of the CAP treatment, we used three non-cancerous human cell lines as a model for healthy tissue (BEAS-2B—lung epithelial cell line, ATCC, Virginia; HA—human astrocytes, Sciencell, California; and HEMa—human epidermal melanocytes, ATCC, Virginia) and four cancer human cell lines (A549—Non-Small-Cell Lung Cancer cell line, ATCC, Virginia; U87—glioblastoma cell line, ATCC, Virginia; and A375, Malme-3M—melanoma cell lines, ATCC, Virginia). A549 and U87 were cultured in Dulbecco's modified Eagle medium (DMEM) (Life Technologies, California, 10938025), A375 and Malme-3M were cultured in Roswell Park Memoriam Institute 1640 (RPMI1640) (Life Technologies, 52400025), BEAS-2B was cultured in Bronchial Epithelial Growth Medium (BEGM) (Lonza, Basel, CC-3170), the astrocytes were cultured in Astrocyte Medium (AM) (Sciencell, California, 1801) and the melanocytes were cultured in Dermal Cell Basal Medium DCBM (ATCC®, Virginia, PCS-200030TM). DMEM and RPMI1640 were supplemented with 10% Fetal Bovine Serum (FBS) (Gibco™ FBS, Life Technologies, 10270098), 2 mM L-glutamine (Gibco™, Life Technologies, 25030081), 100 units/mL penicillin, and 100 µg/mL streptomycin (Life Technologies, 15140163). According to the manufacturer's protocol, BEGM was supplemented with 2 mL Bovine Pituitary Extract (BPE), 0.50 mL insulin, 0.50 mL hydrocortisone, 0.50 mL GA-1000, 0.50 mL retinoic acid, 0.50 mL transferrin, 0.50 mL triiodothyronine, 0.50 mL epinephrine, and 0.50 mL human epidermal growth factor (hEGF) (Lonza, CC-4175), AM was supplemented with 2% fetal bovine serum (Sciencell, 0010), 5 mL astrocyte growth supplement (Sciencell, 1852), and 5 mL of a penicillin/streptomycin solution (Sciencell, 0503). Finally, DCBM was supplemented with 5 µg/mL recombinant human insulin, 50 µg/mL ascorbic acid, 1 µM epinephrine, 1.5 mM calcium chloride, 1 mL peptide growth factor, and 5 mL M8 supplement (ATCC®, PCS-200042TM). The cells were incubated at 37 °C in a 5% CO2 humidified atmosphere. All media were prepared according to the recommendation for each cell line [44–46].

For the indirect treatment, the cells were seeded in 96-well plates with a density of 2500 cells per well for A549, BEAS-2B, and A375; 3000 cells per well for U87; and 6000 cells per well for the astrocytes and melanocytes, in 150 μL of cell culture medium. The densities were chosen for each cell lines based on their growth rate, in order to achieve comparable densities for all cell lines at the time of treatment. For the direct treatment, the cells were seeded in a 24-well plate with a density of 8333 cells per well for A549, BEAS-2B, and A375; 10,000 cells per well for U87; and 20,000 cells per well for the astrocytes and melanocytes, in 500 μL of cell culture medium.

4.2. Plasma Sources

We studied both direct and indirect plasma treatment. For the indirect treatment, we used the kINPen®IND plasma jet (INP Greifswald/Neoplas tools GmbH, Greifswald, Germany). This is an atmospheric pressure argon plasma jet, made of a central pin electrode (1 mm diameter), shielded by a dielectric quartz capillary (internal diameter 1.6 mm and outer diameter 2 mm), which is connected to a grounded ring electrode. The distance from the tip of the central electrode to the exit nozzle is about 3.5 mm (Figure 5). Plasma is generated by applying a sinusoidal voltage to the central electrode with a frequency between 1.0 and 1.1 MHz, and a maximum power of 3.5 W. This voltage creates a gas discharge between both electrodes, which generates the reactive species inside the capillary. These species are carried out with the argon gas flow, creating a plasma effluent with a length of 9–12 mm and a diameter of about 1 mm.

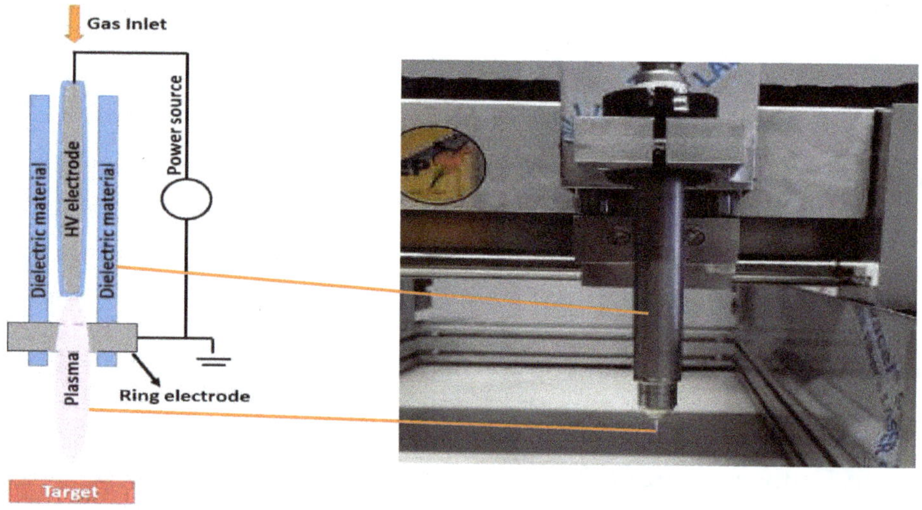

Figure 5. Schematic representation and picture of the kINPen®IND used in the experiments.

For the direct plasma treatment, we used a floating-electrode dielectric barrier discharge (FE-DBD) operated at atmospheric pressure in air. A DBD normally consists of a pair of electrodes, of which at least one is shielded with a dielectric material, separated by a small gap filled with a gas [63]. High voltage (HV) is applied to one electrode, while the target, in our case cells in a well on a grounded metal plate, functions as the second electrode. As the discharge takes place in the gap between the HV electrode and the target, no additional carrier gas was used with this plasma source (Figure 6). The plasma was generated by applying microsecond-pulses to the HV electrode from a pulse generator (Advanced Plasma Solutions, Malvern, PA, USA) with an amplitude in the range of 17 kV and a varying frequency between 100 Hz and 500 Hz in our experiments.

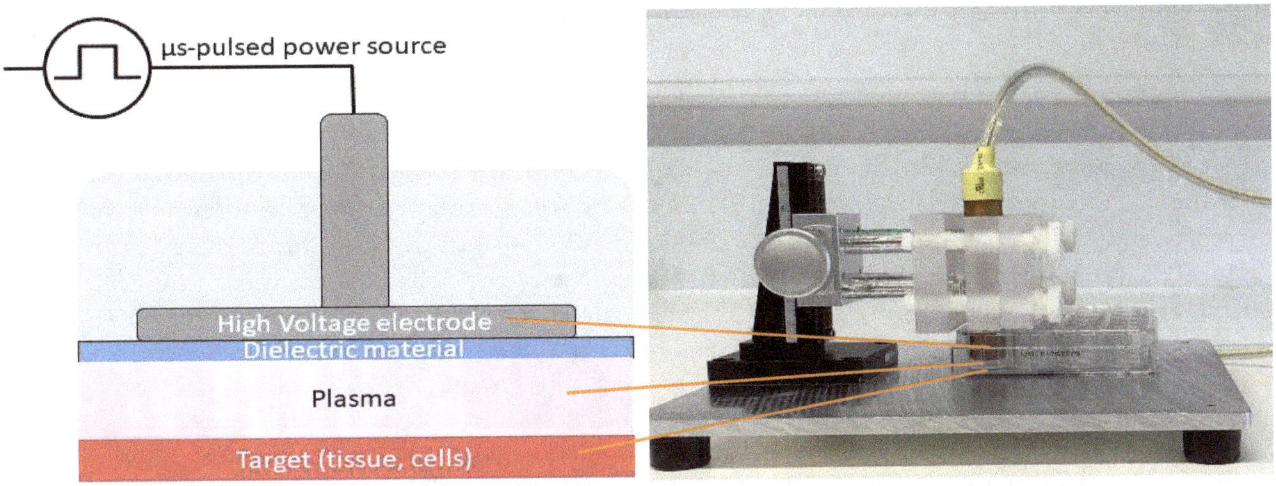

Figure 6. Schematic representation and picture of the FE-DBD used in the experiments.

4.3. Indirect Plasma Treatment

We used the kINPen®IND to treat 2 mL phosphate-buffered saline (PBS) (pH 7.3) in a 12-well plate. A gap of 6 mm between the tip of the plasma source and the liquid, a gas flow rate of 1 slm, and a treatment time of 5 min was used. In this case, the gap was small enough to have discharges at the liquid surface, as discharge streamers were visible between the head of the plasma jet and the liquid interface. Here, the liquid surface acts as a third electrode, and the electrons interact with the liquid, resulting in electron impact reactions, which affect the generation of RONS. In our experiments comparing all cell culture media on cancer cells, a gap of 30 mm, a gas flow rate of 3 slm, and a treatment time of 7 min was used. Here, the gap was sufficiently large to avoid the generation of these discharges at the liquid surface. Before treatment of cells with plasma-treated PBS (pPBS), the cells were seeded in a 96 well-plate and incubated for 24 h at 37 °C and 5% CO_2. For treatment, we applied 30 µL of (diluted) pPBS to each well of the 96-well plate. We also used a control sample, where 30 µL of untreated PBS was added.

4.4. Direct Plasma Treatment

After cell seeding into 24-well plates and incubating for 24 h at 37 °C and 5% CO2, the cells were treated with the FE-DBD as stated in our previous work [55]. The cell culture medium was first removed, after which cells were washed with PBS and treated for 10 s at a distance of 1 mm and a frequency varying between 100 Hz and 500 Hz. Immediately after treatment, 500 µL of fresh cell culture medium was added to each well. The control sample was handled in exactly the same way, but without turning on the power source and applying high voltage.

4.5. Cell Viability Assay

After treatment, the cells were incubated for 24 h at 37 °C and 5% CO_2 before the further viability analysis with the sulforhodamine B-method (SRB). The cell culture medium was removed from each well and the cells were first fixed to the plate using 10% trichloro acetic acid (TCA) (Fischer Scientific, A322), 100 µL for a 96-well plate and 400 µL for a 24-well plate. The plates were placed at 4 °C for 1 h, after which the TCA was thoroughly washed away with deionized water. The wells were dried, and a SRB-solution (0.1 w/v % in 1% (v/v) acetic acid, Sigma-Aldrich®, Missouri, s1402) was added (100 µL for a 96-well plate and 400 µL for a 24-well plate). After 30 min, the SRB was washed away with 1% acetic acid. The cells were dried again, and tris(hydrocymethyl)aminomethane (TRIS)-buffer (Sigma-Aldrich®, 252859) was added to each well (100 µL for a 96 well-plate and 400 µL for a 24-well plate). After 30 min, the absorbance was measured at 540 nm, using a BIO-RAD iMark™ Microplate reader for the 96-well plates and a Tecan Infinite F Plex Microplate reader for the 24-well plates. The cell viability was determined by comparing the absorbance of the treated groups with the untreated control sample.

4.6. Analysis of the Influence of the Cell Culture Medium

Since the cancerous cell lines and non-cancerous cell lines have different optimal culture media, it was important to analyze the influence of the media on the plasma treatment results. For this purpose, we tested two of the cancer cell lines—i.e., A549 and A375—with the five different cell culture media (DMEM, RPMI1640, BEGM, AM, and DCBM). We cultured the cells in their recommended medium, but at the moment of seeding, we seeded them in the different media. Both the direct (FE-DBD at 500 Hz) and indirect (pPBS, condition 2) treatment were tested.

4.7. Statistical Analysis

All experiments were performed in triplicate, and the results are expressed as the mean with associated standard deviation. Statistical significance was determined using Students *t*-test with Welch's correction (assuming unequal standard deviation) and displayed on the figure plots as $^{*}p < 0.05$, $^{**}p < 0.01$, and $^{***}p < 0.005$.

5. Conclusions

In this study, we evaluated the influence of the cell type, cancer type, and cell culture medium on the cytotoxic effects of both direct and indirect CAP treatment for cancer. In all cases, we found that the influence of these biological parameters was more pronounced for indirect CAP treatment compared to direct CAP treatment.

When analyzing the influence of the cell type, we found that fibroblasts are more resistant to indirect CAP treatment. Also, the different cancer types gave different responses to CAP treatment, where the lung cancer cell line, A549, was more sensitive, compared to the brain cancer cell line, U87.

For the indirect CAP treatment, we observed a large influence of the cell culture medium on cell cytotoxicity, as the more advanced media virtually negated the effects of treatment. Thus, when comparing the viability of cancerous cells in their standard media with the non-cancerous cells in their advanced media, it is tempting to conclude significant selectivity of treatment for all the cancer types. However, when cytotoxicity was compared for cancerous and non-cancerous cells cultured in the same media, it was obvious that this apparent selectivity was due to the cell culture media and genuine differential sensitivity to indirect CAP. This is an important conclusion, which must be kept in mind to avoid drawing false conclusions in cancer cell selectivity studies.

Taken together, the results of our study demonstrate that biological factors—including cell type, cancer type, and culturing medium—must be taken into account before selectivity of CAP treatment can be claimed. Overlooking these parameters can easily result in misdirected conclusions and false claims of selectivity.

Supplementary Materials:
Figure S1: Comparison of the cell densities of A375 and A549 in the different cell culture media. The results are normalized to the recommended media for the cell line (DMEM for A549 and RPMI1640 for A375) indicated by the blue bars. Data are represented as mean ± standard deviation (SD) of three independent experiments with at least two replicates. Statistical significance of all treatment conditions was compared to untreated. $^{*}p < 0.05$ (One-way ANOVA). Figure S2: Selectivity analysis for lung cancer using (a) indirect and (b) direct CAP treatment. For the indirect treatment we used different dilutions of plasma-treated PBS (pPBS), using the first condition (5 min treatment with a gas glow rate of 1 slm and a gap of 6 mm) and for the direct treatment we used a 10 second treatment with a gap of 1 mm and two different frequencies of the FE-DBD.

Author Contributions: Conceptualization, E.B. and W.V.B.; Methodology, E.B. and W.V.B.; Software, E.B.; Validation, E.B.; Formal analysis, E.B. and W.V.B.; Investigation, E.B. and W.V.B.; Resources, J.V.L. and J.D.B.; Data curation, E.B.; Writing—original draft preparation, E.B.; Writing—review and editing, A.L., J.V.L., J.D.B., C.D., S.D., E.S., and A.B.; Visualization, E.B.; Supervision, W.V.B., A.L., A.B., and E.S.; Project administration, E.B. and W.V.B.; Funding acquisition, W.V.B., A.B., and E.S.

References

1. Mokhtari, R.B.; Homayouni, T.S.; Baluch, N.; Morgatskaya, E.; Kumar, S.; Das, B.; Yeger, H. Combination Therapy in Combating Cancer. *Oncotarget* **2017**, *8*, 38022–38043. [CrossRef] [PubMed]
2. Nagai, H.; Kim, Y.H. Cancer Prevention from the Perspective of Global Cancer Burden Patterns. *J. Thorac. Dis.* **2017**, *9*, 448–451. [CrossRef] [PubMed]
3. Yan, D.; Sherman, J.H.; Keidar, M. Cold Atmospheric Plasma, a Novel Promising Anti-Cancer Treatment Modality. *Oncotarget* **2017**, *8*, 15977–15995. [CrossRef] [PubMed]
4. Hoffmann, C.; Berganza, C.; Zhang, J. Cold Atmospheric Plasma: Methods of Production and Application in Dentistry and Oncology. *Med. Gas Res.* **2013**, *3*, 1–15. [CrossRef] [PubMed]
5. Huang, J.; Chen, W.; Li, H.; Wang, X.; Lv, G.; Khohsa, M.L.; Guo, M.; Feng, K.; Wang, P.; Yang, S. Needle Deactivation of A549 Cancer Cells in Vitro by a Dielectric Barrier Discharge Plasma Needle. *J. Appl. Phys.* **2011**, *109*, 053305. [CrossRef]
6. Kim, S.J.; Chung, T.H.; Bae, S.H.; Leem, S.H. Induction of Apoptosis in Human Breast Cancer Cells by a Pulsed Atmospheric Pressure Plasma Jet. *Appl. Phys. Lett.* **2010**, *97*, 203702. [CrossRef]
7. Hattori, N.; Yamada, S.; Torii, K.; Takeda, S.; Nakamura, K.; Tanaka, H.; Kajiyama, H.; Kanda, M.; Fujii, T.; Nakayama, G.; et al. Effectiveness of Plasma Treatment on Pancreatic Cancer Cells. *Int. J. Oncol.* **2015**, *47*, 1655–1662. [CrossRef] [PubMed]
8. Tanaka, H.; Mizuno, M.; Ishikawa, K.; Nakamura, K.; Kajiyama, H.; Kano, H.; Kikkawa, F.; Hori, M. Plasma-Activated Medium Selectively Kills Glioblastoma Brain Tumor Cells by Down-Regulating a Survival Signaling Molecule, AKT Kinase. *Plasma Med.* **2011**, *1*, 265–277. [CrossRef]
9. Yonson, S.; Coulombe, S.; Leveille, V.; Leask, R.L. Cell Treatment and Surface Functionalization Using a Miniature Atmospheric Pressure Glow Discharge. *J. Phys. D. Appl. Phys.* **2006**, *39*, 3508–3513. [CrossRef]
10. Leduc, M.; Guay, D.; Leask, R.L.; Coulombe, S. Cell Permeabilization Using a Non-Thermal Plasma. *New J. Phys.* **2009**, *11*, 115021. [CrossRef]
11. Vermeylen, S.; De Waele, J.; Vanuytsel, S.; De Backer, J.; Ramakers, M.; Leyssens, K.; Marcq, E.; Van Der Paal, J.; Smits, E.L.J.; Dewilde, S.; et al. Cold Atmospheric Plasma Treatment of Melanoma and Glioblastoma Cancer Cells. *Plasma Process. Polym.* **2016**, *13*, 1195–1205. [CrossRef]
12. Vandamme, M.; Robert, E.; Dozias, S.; Sobilo, J.; Lerondel, S.; Le Pape, A.; Pouvesle, J.M. Response of Human Glioma U87 Xenografted on Mice to Non Thermal Plasma Treatment. *Plasma Med.* **2011**, *1*, 27–43. [CrossRef]
13. Vandamme, M.; Rie, D.; Martel, E.; Robert, E.; Brulle, L.; Richard, S.; Pouvesle, J.; Pape, A.L. Effects of a Non Thermal Plasma Treatment Alone or in Combination with Gemcitabine in a MIA PaCa2-Luc Orthotopic Pancreatic Carcinoma Model. *PLoS ONE* **2012**, *7*, e52653.
14. Metelmann, H.; Seebauer, C.; Miller, V.; Fridman, A.; Bauer, G.; Graves, D.B.; Pouvesle, J.; Rutkowski, R.; Schuster, M.; Bekeschus, S.; et al. Clinical Experience with Cold Plasma in the Treatment of Locally Advanced Head and Neck Cancer. *Clin. Plasma Med.* **2018**, *9*, 6–13. [CrossRef]
15. Friedman, P.C.; Miller, V.; Fridman, G.; Lin, A.; Fridman, A. Successful Treatment of Actinic Keratoses Using Nonthermal Atmospheric Pressure Plasma: A Case Series. *J. Am. Acad. Dermatol.* **2017**, *76*, 349–350. [CrossRef]
16. Miller, V.; Lin, A.; Fridman, G.; Fridman, A.; Friedman, P. Nanosecond-Pulsed DBD Plasma For A Clinical Trial Of Actinic Keratosis. *Clin. Plasma Med.* **2018**, *9*, 44. [CrossRef]
17. Fridman, A.; Friedman, G. *Plasma Medicine*; John Wiley & Sons: Chichester, UK, 2013.
18. Dubuc, A.; Monsarrat, P.; Virard, F.; Merbahi, N.; Sarrette, J.; Laurencin-dalicieux, S.; Cousty, S. Use of Cold-Atmospheric Plasma in Oncology: A Concise Systematic Review. *Ther. Adv. Med. Oncol.* **2018**, *10*, 1–12. [CrossRef]
19. Ratovitski, E.A.; Cheng, X.; Yan, D.; Sherman, J.H.; Canady, J.; Trink, B.; Keidar, M. Anti-Cancer Therapies of 21st Century: Novel Approach to Treat Human Cancers Using Cold Atmospheric Plasma. *Plasma Process. Polym.* **2014**, *11*, 1128–1137. [CrossRef]
20. Keidar, M. Plasma for Cancer Treatment. *Plasma Sources Sci. Technol.* **2015**, *24*, 1–20. [CrossRef]
21. Maksudbek, Y.; Dayun, Y.; Cordeiro, R.M.; Bogaerts, A. Atomic Scale Simulation of H_2O_2 Permeation through Aquaporin: Toward the Understanding of Plasma-Cancer Treatment. *J. Phys. D. Appl. Phys.* **2018**, *12*, 125401.
22. Yan, D.; Xiao, H.; Zhu, W.; Nourmohammadi, N.; Zhang, L.G.; Bian, K.; Keidar, M. The Role of Aquaporins in the Anti- Glioblastoma Capacity of the Cold Plasma-Stimulated Medium. *J. Phys. D. Appl. Phys.* **2017**, *50* 055401. [CrossRef]

23. Van Der Paal, J.; Verheyen, C.; Neyts, E.C.; Bogaerts, A. Hampering Effect of Cholesterol on the Permeation of Reactive Oxygen Species through Phospholipids Bilayer: Possible Explanation for Plasma Cancer Selectivity. *Sci. Rep.* **2017**, *7*, 1–11.
24. Van Der Paal, J.; Neyts, E.C.; Verlackt, C.C.W.; Bogaerts, A. Chemical Science Permeability of Cancer and Normal Cells Subjected to Oxidative Stress. *Chem. Sci.* **2016**, *7*, 489–498. [CrossRef] [PubMed]
25. Bauer, G. Cold Atmospheric Plasma and Plasma-Activated Medium: Antitumor Cell Effects with Inherent Synergistic Potential. *Plasma Med.* **2019**, *9*, 57–88. [CrossRef]
26. Zucker, S.N.; Zirnheld, J.; Bagati, A.; Disanto, T.M.; Des Soye, B.; Wawrzyniak, J.A.; Etemadi, K.; Nikiforov, M.; Berezney, R. Preferential Induction of Apoptotic Cell Death in Melanoma Cells as Compared with Normal Keratinocytes Using a Non-Thermal Plasma Torch. *Cancer Biol. Ther.* **2012**, *13*, 1299–1306. [CrossRef] [PubMed]
27. Kim, S.J.; Chung, T.H. Cold Atmospheric Plasma Jet-Generated RONS and Their Selective Effects on Normal and Carcinoma Cells. *Sci. Rep.* **2016**, *6*, 1–14. [CrossRef] [PubMed]
28. Wang, M.; Holmes, B.; Cheng, X.; Zhu, W.; Keidar, M.; Zhang, L.G. Cold Atmospheric Plasma for Selectively Ablating Metastatic Breast Cancer Cells. *PLoS ONE* **2013**, *8*, 1–11. [CrossRef] [PubMed]
29. Guerrero-preston, R.; Ogawa, T.; Uemura, M.; Shumulinsky, G.; Valle, B.L.; Pirini, F.; Ravi, R.; Sidransky, D.; Keidar, M.; Trink, B. Cold Atmospheric Plasma Treatment Selectively Targets Head and Neck Squamous Cell Carcinoma Cells. *Int. J. Mol. Med.* **2014**, *34*, 941–946. [CrossRef] [PubMed]
30. Georgescu, N.; Lupu, A.R. Tumoral and Normal Cells Treatment With High-Voltage Pulsed Cold Atmospheric Plasma Jets. *IEEE Trans. Plasma Sci.* **2010**, *38*, 1949–1955. [CrossRef]
31. Yan, D.; Nourmohammadi, N.; Bian, K.; Murad, F.; Sherman, J.H.; Keidar, M. Stabilizing the Cold Plasma-Stimulated Medium by Regulating Medium' s Composition. *Sci. Rep.* **2016**, *6*, 26016. [CrossRef]
32. Heirman, P.; Van Boxem, W.; Bogaerts, A. Reactivity and Stability of Plasma-Generated Oxygen and Nitrogen Species in Buffered Water Solution: A Computational Study. *Phys. Chem. Chem. Phys.* **2019**. [CrossRef] [PubMed]
33. Van Boxem, W.; Van Der Paal, J.; Gorbanev, Y.; Vanuytsel, S.; Smits, E.; Dewilde, S.; Bogaerts, A. Anti-Cancer Capacity of Plasma-Treated PBS: Effect of Chemical Composition on Cancer Cell Cytotoxicity. *Sci. Rep.* **2017**, *7*, 1–15. [CrossRef] [PubMed]
34. Kim, J.Y.; Kim, S.; Wei, Y.; Li, J. A Flexible Cold Microplasma Jet Using Biocompatible Dielectric Tubes for Cancer Therapy A Flexible Cold Microplasma Jet Using Biocompatible Dielectric Tubes. *Appl. Phys. Lett.* **2010**, *96*, 203701. [CrossRef]
35. Iseki, S.; Nakamura, K.; Hayashi, M.; Tanaka, H.; Kondo, H.; Kajiyama, H.; Kano, H.; Kikkawa, F.; Hori, M. Selective Killing of Ovarian Cancer Cells through Induction of Apoptosis by Nonequilibrium Atmospheric Pressure Plasma Selective Killing of Ovarian Cancer Cells through Induction of Apoptosis by Nonequilibrium Atmospheric Pressure Plasma. *Appl. Phys. Lett.* **2012**, *100*, 113702. [CrossRef]
36. Laroussi, M. Effects of PAM on Select Normal and Cancerous Epithelial Cells. *Plasma Res. Express* **2019**, *1*, 1–7. [CrossRef]
37. Zhang, L.; Zhou, W.; Velculescu, V.E.; Kern, S.E.; Hruban, R.H.; Hamilton, S.R.; Vogelstein, B.; Kinzler, K.W. Gene Expression Profiles in Normal and Cancer Cells. *Science* **1997**, *276*, 1268–1272. [CrossRef] [PubMed]
38. Saadati, F.; Mahdikia, H.; Abbaszadeh, H.; Abdollahifar, M.; Khoramgah, M.S.; Shokri, B. Comparison of Direct and Indirect Cold Atmospheric-Pressure Plasma Methods in the B 16 F 10 Melanoma Cancer Cells Treatment. *Sci. Rep.* **2018**, *8*, 1–15. [CrossRef] [PubMed]
39. Cooper, G.M. The Development and Causes of Cancer. In *The Cell: A Molecular Approach*, 2nd ed.; Sinauer Associates: Sunderland, MA, USA, 2000.
40. Giordano, T.J.; Shedden, K.A.; Schwartz, D.R.; Kuick, R.; Taylor, J.M.G.; Lee, N.; Misek, D.E.; Greenson, J.K.; Kardia, S.L.R.; Beer, D.G.; et al. Organ-Specific Molecular Classification of Primary Lung, Colon, and Ovarian Adenocarcinomas Using Gene Expression Profiles. *Am. J. Pathol.* **2001**, *159*, 1231–1238. [CrossRef]
41. Mallinjoud, P.; Villemin, J.; Mortada, H.; Espinoza, M.P.; Desmet, F.-O.; Samaan, S.; Chautard, E.; Tranchevent, L.-C.; Auboeuf, D. Endothelial, Epithelial, and Fibroblast Cells Exhibit Specific Splicing Programs Independently of Their Tissue of Origin. *Genome Res.* **2014**, *24*, 511–521. [CrossRef]
42. Jagtap, J.C.; Chandele, A.; Chopde, B.A.; Shastry, P. Sodium Pyruvate Protects against H_2O_2 Mediated Apoptosis in Human Neuroblastoma Cell Line-SK-N-MC. *J. Chem. Neuroanat.* **2003**, *26*, 109–118. [CrossRef]
43. Wang, X.; Perez, E.; Liu, R.; Yan, L.; Mallet, R.T.; Yang, S. Pyruvate Protects Mitochondria from Oxidative Stress in Human Neuroblastoma SK-N-SH Cells. *Brain Res.* **2007**, *1132*, 1–9. [CrossRef] [PubMed]

44. Astrocyte Medium—Sciencell. Available online: https://www.sciencellonline.com/astrocyte-medium.html, (accessed on 20 August 2019).
45. BEGMTM Bronchial Epithelial Cell Growth Medium BulletKitTM. Available online: https://bioscience.lonza.com/lonza_bs/CH/en/Primary-and-Stem-Cells/p/000000000000185308/BEGM-Bronchial-Epithelial-Cell-Growth-Medium-BulletKit, (accessed on 20 August 2019).
46. Dermal Cell Basal Medium(ATCC®PCS-200-030™). Available online: https://www.lgcstandards-atcc.org/products/all/PCS-200-030.aspx?geo_country=be, (accessed on 20 August 2019).
47. Vander Heiden, M.G.; Cantley, L.C.; Thompson, C.B.; Mammalian, P.; Exhibit, C.; Metabolism, A. Understanding the Warburg Effect: The Metabolic Requirements of Cell Proliferation. *Science*. **2009**, *324*, 1029–1033. [CrossRef] [PubMed]
48. Fadaka, A.; Ajiboye, B.; Ojo, O.; Adewale, O.; Olayide, I.; Emuowhochere, R. Biology of Glucose Metabolization in Cancer Cells. *J. Oncol. Sci.* **2017**, *3*, 45–51. [CrossRef]
49. Cairns, R.A.; Harris, I.S.; Mak, T.W. Regulation of Cancer Cell Metabolism. *Nat. Rev.* **2011**, *11*, 85. [CrossRef] [PubMed]
50. Hanahan, D.; Weinberg, R.A. Hallmarks of Cancer: The Next Generation. *Cell* **2011**, *144*, 646–674. [CrossRef] [PubMed]
51. Schieber, M.; Chandel, N.S. ROS Function in Redox Signaling and Oxidative Stress. *Curr. Biol.* **2014**, *24*, R453–R462. [CrossRef]
52. Redza-dutordoir, M.; Averill-bates, D.A. Activation of Apoptosis Signalling Pathways by Reactive Oxygen Species. *Biochem. Biophys. Acta* **2016**, *1863*, 2977–2992. [CrossRef]
53. Shaw, A.T.; Winslow, M.M.; Magendantz, M.; Ouyang, C.; Dowdle, J. Selective Killing of K-Ras Mutant Cancer Cells by Small Molecule Inducers of Oxidative Stress. *PNAS*. **2011**, *108*, 8773–8778. [CrossRef]
54. Glasauer, A.; Sena, L.A.; Diebold, L.P.; Mazar, A.P.; Chandel, N.S. Targeting SOD1 Reduces Experimental Non–Small-Cell Lung Cancer. *J. Clin. Investig.* **2014**, *124*, 117–128. [CrossRef]
55. Lin, A.; Gorbanev, Y.; De Backer, J.; Van Loenhout, J.; Van Boxem, W.; Lemière, F.; Cos, P.; Dewilde, S.; Smits, E.; Bogaerts, A. Non-Thermal Plasma as a Unique Delivery System of Short-Lived Reactive Oxygen and Nitrogen Species for Immunogenic Cell Death in Melanoma Cells. *Adv. Sci.* **2019**, *6*, 1802062. [CrossRef]
56. Lin, A.; Truong, B.; Patel, S.; Kaushik, N.; Choi, E.H.; Fridman, G.; Fridman, A.; Miller, V. Nanosecond-Pulsed DBD Plasma-Generated Reactive Oxygen Species Trigger Immunogenic Cell Death in A549 Lung Carcinoma Cells through Intracellular Oxidative Stress. *Int. J. Mol. Sci.* **2017**, *18*, 966. [CrossRef] [PubMed]
57. Lin, A.; Chernets, N.; Han, J.; Alicea, Y.; Dobrynin, D.; Fridman, G.; Freeman, T.A.; Fridman, A.; Miller, V. Non-Equilibrium Dielectric Barrier Discharge Treatment of Mesenchymal Stem Cells: Charges and Reactive Oxygen Species Play the Major Role in Cell Death A. *Plasma Process. Polym.* **2015**, *12*, 1117–1127. [CrossRef]
58. Kaur, G.; Dufour, J.M. Cell Lines, Valuable Tools or Useless Artifacts. *Spermatogenesis* **2012**, *2*, 1–5. [CrossRef] [PubMed]
59. Hasse, S.; Seebauer, C.; Wende, K.; Schmidt, A.; Metelmann, H.; Von Woedtke, T.; Bekeschus, S. Cold Argon Plasma as Adjuvant Tumour Therapy on Progressive Head and Neck Cancer: A Preclinical Study. *Appl. Sci.* **2019**, *9*, 2061. [CrossRef]
60. Grizzle, W.E.; Bell, W.C.; Sexton, K.C. Issues in Collecting, Processing and Storing Human Tissues and Associated Information to Support Biomedical Research. *Cancer Biomarkers* **2010**, *9*, 531–549. [CrossRef]
61. Xu, H.; Lyu, X.; Yi, M.; Zhao, W.; Song, Y.; Wu, K. Organoid Technology and Applications in Cancer Research. *J. Hematol. Oncol.* **2018**, *1*, 116. [CrossRef]
62. Drost, J.; Clevers, H. Organoids in Cancer Research. *Nat. Rev. Cancer* **2018**, *18*, 407–418. [CrossRef]
63. Barrier, D.; Dbd, D.; Bibinov, N.; Rajasekaran, P.; Mertmann, P. Basics and Biomedical Applications of DBD. Available online: http://cdn.intechweb.org/pdfs/12799.pdf (accessed on 1 August 2019).

9

Cold Plasma-Treated Ringer's Saline: A Weapon to Target Osteosarcoma

Miguel Mateu-Sanz [1,2,3], Juan Tornín [1,2,3], Bénédicte Brulin [4], Anna Khlyustova [1,2,3], Maria-Pau Ginebra [1,2,3,5], Pierre Layrolle [4] and Cristina Canal [1,2,3,*]

1 Biomaterials, Biomechanics and Tissue Engineering Group, Department Materials Science and Metallurgy, Technical University of Catalonia (UPC), Escola d'Enginyeria Barcelona Est (EEBE), c/Eduard Maristany 14, 08019 Barcelona, Spain; miguel.mateu@upc.edu (M.M.-S.); juan.tornin@upc.edu (J.T.); avlada5577@gmail.com (A.K.); maria.pau.ginebra@upc.edu (M.-P.G.)
2 Barcelona Research Center in Multiscale Science and Engineering, UPC, 08019 Barcelona, Spain
3 Research Centre for Biomedical Engineering (CREB), UPC, 08019 Barcelona, Spain
4 Inserm, UMR 1238, PHY-OS, Laboratory of Bone Sarcomas and Remodeling of Calcified Tissues, Faculty of Medicine, University of Nantes, 44035 Nantes, France; benedicte.brulin@univ-nantes.fr (B.B.); pierre.layrolle@univ-nantes.fr (P.L.)
5 Institute for Bioengineering of Catalonia (IBEC), Barcelona Institute of Science and Technology (BIST), c/Baldiri i Reixach 10-12, 08028 Barcelona, Spain
* Correspondence: cristina.canal@upc.edu

Abstract: Osteosarcoma (OS) is the main primary bone cancer, presenting poor prognosis and difficult treatment. An innovative therapy may be found in cold plasmas, which show anti-cancer effects related to the generation of reactive oxygen and nitrogen species in liquids. In vitro models are based on the effects of plasma-treated culture media on cell cultures. However, effects of plasma-activated saline solutions with clinical application have not yet been explored in OS. The aim of this study is to obtain mechanistic insights on the action of plasma-activated Ringer's saline (PAR) for OS therapy in cell and organotypic cultures. To that aim, cold atmospheric plasma jets were used to obtain PAR, which produced cytotoxic effects in human OS cells (SaOS-2, MG-63, and U2-OS), related to the increasing concentration of reactive oxygen and nitrogen species generated. Proof of selectivity was found in the sustained viability of hBM-MSCs with the same treatments. Organotypic cultures of murine OS confirmed the time-dependent cytotoxicity observed in 2D. Histological analysis showed a decrease in proliferating cells (lower Ki-67 expression). It is shown that the selectivity of PAR is highly dependent on the concentrations of reactive species, being the differential intracellular reactive oxygen species increase and DNA damage between OS cells and hBM-MSCs key mediators for cell apoptosis.

Keywords: bone cancer; osteosarcoma; cold atmospheric plasma; reactive species; plasma-activated liquid; Ringer's saline; organotypic model

---

1. Introduction

Osteosarcoma (OS) is the most common primary malignant bone tumor and it mainly affects children, adolescents, and young adults. It usually appears as an osteoid-producing solid tumor in the metaphysis of long bones, which experience rapid growth during childhood and adolescence [1]. Despite the low incidence of OS, it is ranked among the most frequent cause of cancer-related child death [2,3]. Current OS therapy consists in surgical resection of the tumor, combined with radiotherapy and/or systemic chemotherapy. Although chemotherapeutic drugs have increased patient survival, this survival rate is still relatively low (50–60%) [4] and many patients develop drug-resistance [5]. On the other hand, chemotherapeutics displays unspecific toxicity with undesired side-effects. For these reasons, innovative therapies are of interest, and thus, cold plasmas could be an interesting approach.

Cold atmospheric plasmas (CAP) are created by generating an electrical discharge and applying it to a gas, and are a source of reactive molecules, ions, electrons, free radicals, UV and electromagnetic fields that have shown a variety of biological effects such as antimicrobial sterilization [6,7], blood coagulation [8] and wound healing [9,10]. CAPs have also been suggested to selectively target cancer cells, showing their efficiency in more than 20 types of cancer without damaging healthy cells and surrounding tissues [11,12].

Plasma-generated electrical fields may induce cell membrane permeabilization and even its disruption [13]. This can act synergistically with the reactive oxygen and nitrogen species (RONS) generated by CAP. There is a wide variety of RONS that can be generated by CAP, which can include short-lived species ($ONOO^-$, OH^-, NO, O_2^-, etc.) and long-lived species (O_3, H_2O_2, NO_2^-, etc.), and which are thought to be key players in its anticancer effect [14–16]. The induction of the increase of intracellular RONS in cancer cells have been reported as a potential target for cancer therapies [17]. Many species are involved in the cellular effects of CAP; for instance, increased levels of hydrogen peroxide are well-known to induce double strand breaks, chromosomal fragmentation and apoptosis in cancer cells [18,19]. In addition, NO_2^- is a precursor for intracellular formation of NO, which induces protein and lipid oxidation, leading to cell death [20].

The selectivity of CAP is suggested to be produced due to the higher sensibility of cancer cells to oxidative stress as a result of their high metabolic rate. This selectivity has been reported to be highly dependent on the composition of RONS generated, which depends on different parameters such as treatment time [21,22], plasma device configuration [23] or gas employed to generate the plasma discharge. The properties of the cancer cells, such as their "activation" state by CAP can also affect their sensitivity to the RONS generated by plasma [24]. For this reason, in this work, two different plasma devices with different design and working gas have been employed to obtain different characteristics of the discharge and of the treated liquid.

In an in vitro situation, RONS produced in the plasma are transported to the liquid covering the cells and react with this liquid forming secondary reactive species [25]. In this sense, the effects of plasma can be triggered by direct application over cells or by previous treatment of the liquid media as an indirect treatment [26,27]. This second approach is more interesting for OS, as it would avoid the open surgery needed to expose the tumor to CAP. Taking into account that in clinics drugs are supplied dissolved in saline solutions, the possibility of using this kind of solutions as plasma-activated liquids is an attractive therapeutic option that has been explored with interest for glioblastoma, cervical and ovarian [11] and pancreatic [28] cancers (among others) but is still unexplored for OS, and is undertaken in this work.

In recent years, CAP have shown lethal in vitro efficiency by direct treatment as well as by plasma-treated cell culture medium in different OS cell lines and by different plasma devices [22,23, 29–31]. OS is a heterogeneous disease characterized by presenting different subtypes and high levels of genomic instability [32,33], making it difficult to assess the clinical relevance of new therapeutic options for the different cases. For example, two main tumor suppressor proteins (P53 and pRB,) are suggested to be altered in over 50% of patients [34], and are involved in cell cycle arrest, DNA repair and induction of apoptosis [35]. Given the heterogeneity of OS, it is of paramount interest to evaluate OS cell lines with different genomic profiles in views of assessing the real applicability of plasma-activated liquids in OS. Our previous work employing SaOS-2 cells (which are p53 and pRB null), highlighted the importance of an equilibrated cocktail of RONS for anticancer selectivity of the plasma-activated medium and revealed the critical role of H_2O_2 in these cytotoxic effects [36].

From another point of view, up to now, cytotoxicity of CAPs or plasma-activated media in OS cell lines have been investigated only in adherent cell cultures [22,23,29–31,36,37]. This kind of in vitro models provides limited clinically relevant information. In 2D models, some key aspects like the impact of stroma and cell-to-cell interaction are lacking [38–40]. The effects of CAP have been reported to be highly dependent of the number of cells and 3D spatial distribution [41,42]. In order to evaluate the applicability of CAP-based therapies, it is necessary to move from 2D cell cultures to 3D models to have a more relevant situation.

In light of the facts discussed above, the objective of this work is to investigate for the first time the cytotoxic effects of plasma-activated Ringer's saline (PAR) in OS cell cultures and its possible translation to a 3D OS model while providing insights on the mechanism potentially involved. To that aim, firstly, the cytotoxic potential of PAR obtained from two different atmospheric pressure plasma jets is evaluated in human OS cell lines with different genetic profile; SaOS-2 (p53−/pRB−), U2-OS (p53+/pRB−) and MG-63 (p53−/pRB+) [43], and in human Bone Marrow Mesenchymal Stem Cells (hBM-MSCs). This is investigated with regard to the RONS generated in PAR by plasma jets and their intracellular effects. Secondly, a tumor was generated in mice by paratibial injection of MOS-J cells and the effects of PAR are investigated in sections of the tumor through organotypic cultures.

2. Results

2.1. *Characterization of the Plasma Gas Phase and Effects Producing PAR*

Two different plasma devices were employed in this work to treat Ringer's saline and obtain PAR; a single-electrode needle device operating in helium that will herein be designated as atmospheric pressure plasma jet (APPJ) and the kINPen, which is a pin-type electrode with a grounded outer electrode operating with Argon.

Optical Emission Spectra were obtained for both plasma jets employing the same parameters of gas flow (1 L/min) and distance between the nozzle of the jet and the surface of the liquid (10 mm) during treatment of the Ringer's saline (Figure 1A). Apart from the main differences regarding the Helium or Argon emission bands in APPJ or kINPen respectively, both jets show emission bands from oxygen and nitrogen species. The most intense bands in APPJ come from Nitrogen, namely N_2 2nd positive system, N_2^+ 1st negative, are recorded, as well as monoatomic oxygen (at 777 nm) (Figure 1(Ai)). kINPen shares only N_2 2nd positive in its emission bands, while other relevant species appear: OH and γ-NO radicals (Figure 1(Aii)).

Secondly, the evolution of pH with plasma treatment time was measured in Ringer's saline, which progressively decreased from pH 7.4 to 3 with both plasma jets (Figure 1(Bi)). Addition of 10% FBS right after plasma treatment (necessary for cell culture studies) buffered the plasma-induced decrease, so pH after 5 min of plasma treatment was recorded to be 7.15 (Figure 1(Bii)).

The concentration of NO_2^- and H_2O_2 and total reactive oxygen species (ROS) in situ production were measured in Ringer's saline treated by APPJ and kINPen from 1 to 5 min just after the addition of 10% FBS (Figure 1C). The generation of H_2O_2 and NO_2^- and their concentration increase were treatment time-dependent in PAR with both devices. Few differences were recorded among APPJ or kINPen in the concentration of NO_2^-, which was much lower than that of H_2O_2 (Figure 1(Ci)). The amount of H_2O_2 generated was significantly higher ($p < 0.05$) with kINPen than APPJ, ranging from 40 μM to 150 μM for APPJ and from 60 μM to 220 μM for kINPen (Figure 1(Cii)). Total reactive oxygen species (ROS) were measured in plasma-treated Ringer's saline in situ, following the same trend observed for peroxides, with significantly higher amounts formed with kINPen than with APPJ up to 5 min ($p < 0.01$ for 1 min and $p < 0.05$ for 2.5 and 5 min) (Figure 1(Ciii)).

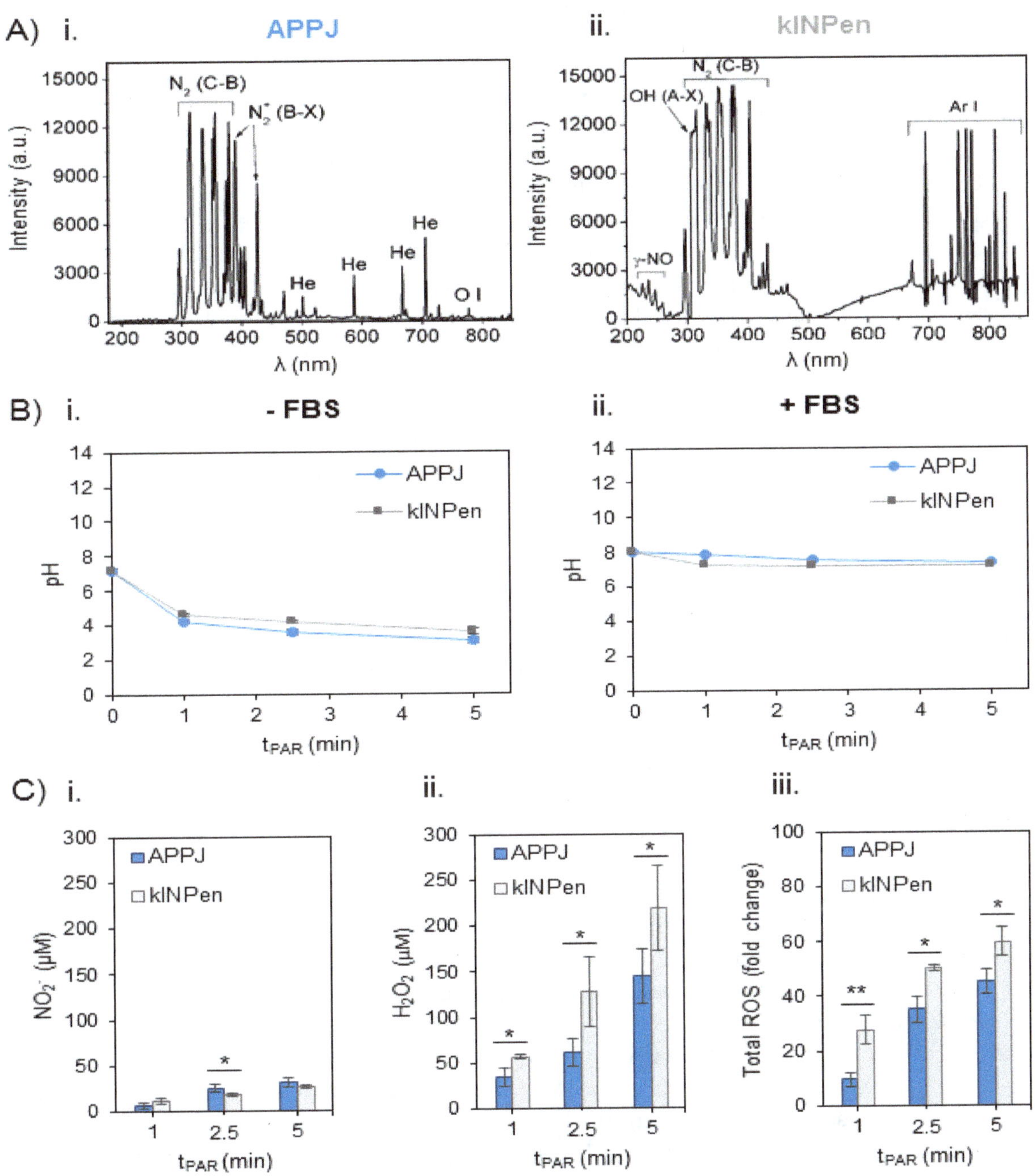

Figure 1. Reactive oxygen and nitrogen species in the plasma gas phase and time-dependent concentration generated in Ringer's saline at 1 L/min of gas flow, 10 mm of distance between the nozzle of the plasma jet and the surface of the liquid (2 mL in 24 well-plates). (**A**) Optical Emission Spectra (OES) of the plasma gas phase in (**Ai**) atmospheric pressure plasma jet (APPJ) and (**Aii**) kINPen during treatment of Ringer's saline. (**B**) pH evolution in Ringer's saline treated by APPJ and kINPen at increasing treatment time (**Bi**) without and (**Bii**) with addition of 10% FBS after treatment. (**C**) Concentration of (**Ci**) NO_2^-, (**Cii**) H_2O_2 and (**Ciii**) total reactive oxygen species (ROS) measured in situ and relativized to untreated plasma-activated Ringer's saline (PAR). Reactive oxygen and nitrogen species (RONS) created by both plasmas in 2 mL of Ringer's saline were measured right after plasma treatment and addition of 10% of FBS. Asterisks represent statistically significance differences between APPJ and kINPen for each time-point ($n = 3$; * p-value < 0.05; ** p-value < 0.01; two-sided Student's t-test).

2.2. Effects of PAR on 2D Cultures of Human OS Cell Lines and hBM-MSCs

PAR was obtained from Ringer's saline treated with APPJ and kINPen at increasing treatment times and, after addition of 10% FBS, it was placed in contact with adherent OS cells for 2 h. Metabolic activity of SaOS-2, U2-OS, MG6-3 and healthy hBM-MSCs (Figure 2) revealed interesting effects: On the one hand, both plasma jets efficiently reduced metabolic activity in all human OS cell lines 24 h after exposition in a plasma treatment time-dependent manner (Figure 2A). The effects of this single treatment with PAR were fostered at 72 h, being more evident in MG-63 cells which attained complete cell death already with a 2.5 min treatment (Figure 2B). The cytotoxicity induced by PAR obtained from either two of the plasma jets employed followed essentially the same trends. Nevertheless, kINPen seemed to produce more cytotoxic PAR than APPJ, as it yielded slightly lower metabolic activity, especially at 24 h, with MG-63 cells already dead in 2.5 and 5 min treatments (Figure 2(Aii)).

On the other hand, healthy hBM-MSCs display completely distinct behavior following contact with APPJ-treated PAR (Figure 2(Ai,Bi)); they show significantly higher cell viability than OS cell lines, between 100 and 80% up to 5 min of treatment at 24 h ($p < 0.005$ for all treatment times) and recovering their complete viability and even proliferating between 120 and 130% after 72 h ($p < 0.005$). Conversely, kINPen–treated PAR induced deleterious effects in hBM-MSCs treated with PAR from 2.5 min of plasma treatment at all incubation times, while hBM-MSCs treated with 1 min PAR kept their complete viability. Given the interest in developing selective treatments, subsequent experiments focused on APPJ-treated PAR as it ensured healthy cell survival while being lethal for OS.

The levels of intracellular ROS were measured in the cells exposed to 5 min-treated PAR with APPJ, revealing differential effects between OS and hBM-MSCs 2 h after exposure to PAR (Figure 3A): while PAR induced an increase in intracellular ROS in both OS cells and healthy cells, in OS the rise was 7–8 times higher than the control. In contrast, a much more moderate increase was recorded in hBM-MSCs 4 times higher than control, finding significant differences between OS and hBM-MSCs ($p < 0.05$). Given the increased cytotoxic effects in MG-63 and similar intracellular ROS generated by exposition to PAR, this cell line was selected for subsequent analysis of the possible mechanisms involved.

In the first place, DNA damage was evaluated by immunostaining of γH2AX foci in MG-63 and hBM-MSCs 6 h after the treatment with PAR (Figure 3B). As reflected in the image, only PAR-treated cells display green immunostaining indicating DNA damage in the nuclei; this was quantified by the increase of γH2AX/DAPI ratio being significantly higher in MG-63 cells (51 ± 18%) than in hBM-MSCs (20 ± 7%) ($p < 0.001$) (Figure 3C).

Secondly, the mechanism of cell death was evaluated by flow cytometry in MG-63 and hBM-MSCs cells exposed to increasing treatment times of PAR. PAR treatment decreased the percentage of alive (Anx−/PI−) cells in a dose-dependent manner (Figure 3D), leaving less than 10% of alive cells in 5 min treated PAR. Treatment time of PAR up to 2.5 min progressively led to pre-apoptotic cells (Anx+; $p < 0.005$). The percentage of late-apoptotic cells (Anx+/PI+) was above 70% with 5 min-treated PAR ($p < 0.005$), and no necrotic cells (Anx−/PI+) were recorded in any case (Supplementary Figure S1A). In contrast, hBM-MSCs just showed a minor decrease in cell viability (70% of Anx−/PI− up to 5 min; $p < 0.005$), still displaying essentially apoptotic cell death mechanisms (Figure S2B).

2.3. Effects of PAR in a 3D Model: Murine OS Tumor Sections

In this section the effects of PAR were evaluated on organotypic cultures to count with a 3D model of bone cancer. An OS tumor generated in intramuscular paratibial site of mice was excised and after obtaining regular tumor sections they were exposed to PAR (Figure 4). A significant reduction of metabolic activity was observed by exposition of the tumor sections to PAR as a function of plasma treatment time, beyond the values obtained with cisplatin 24 h after treatment ($p < 0.005$) (Figure 5A), especially for PAR treated during 15 and 20 min. Metabolic activity was completely abrogated 72 h after the treatment, both with PAR or with Cisplatin. No significant effects were observed by 500 μM H_2O_2, which was an equivalent concentration to PAR treated for 15 min (Figure S2B).

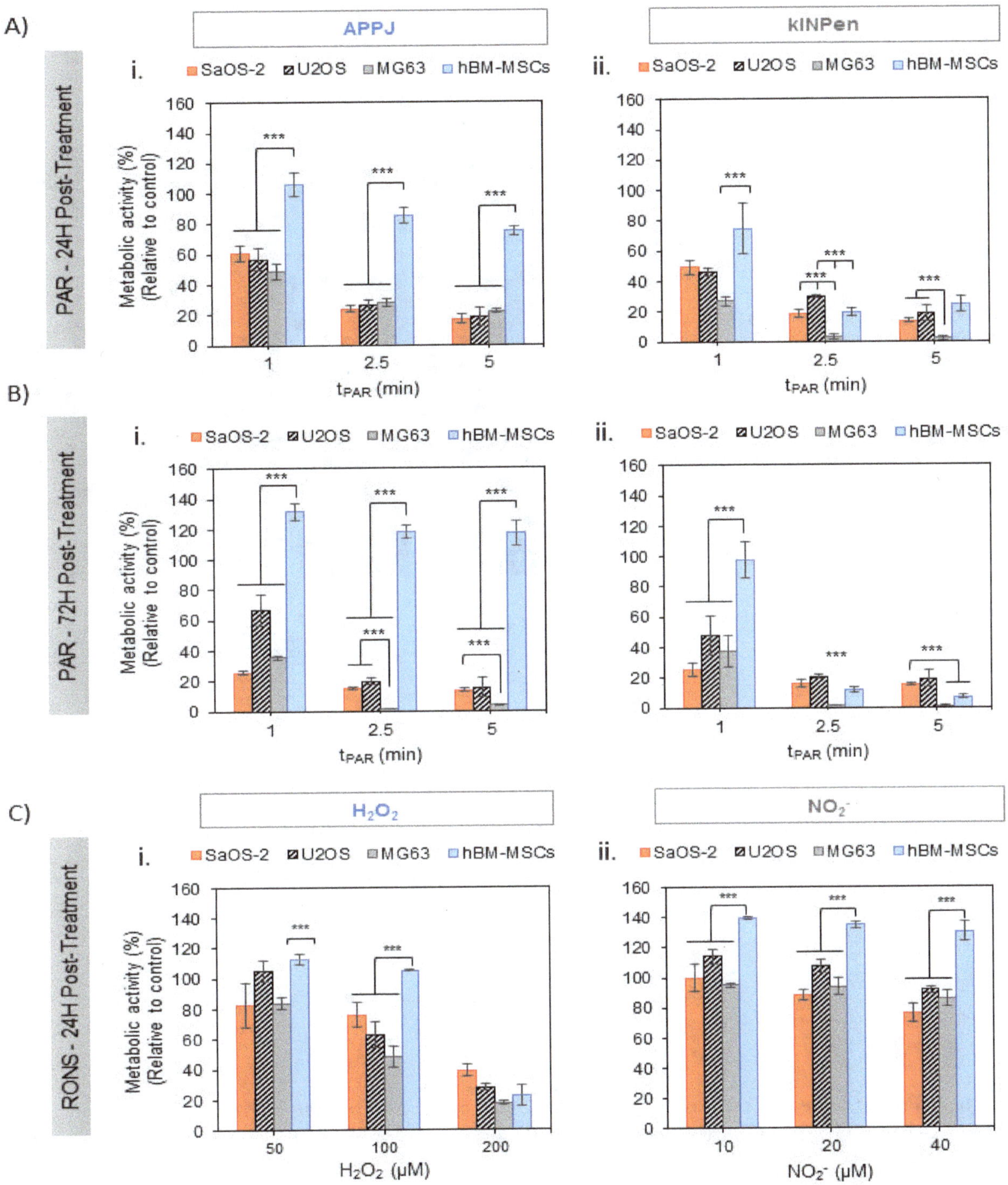

Figure 2. Effects of PAR on the metabolic activity of human OS cell lines (SaOS-2, MG-63, U2-OS) and healthy hBM-MSC with treatment time. Cells in adherent culture were exposed during 2 h to PAR treated by APPJ or kINPen for 1, 2.5 and 5 min. After that, PAR was replaced by fresh medium. Metabolic activity was determined 24 h (**A**) and 72 h (**B**) after PAR exposure by WST-1 test. (**C**) Cells were also exposed during 2 h to increasing concentrations of H_2O_2 and NO_2^- standards in Ringer's saline with 10% FBS (which match with concentrations determined in Figure 1), corresponding to 50, 100 and 200 μM for H_2O_2 (**Ci**) and 10, 20 and 40 μM for NO_2^- (**Cii**) and metabolic activity was determined 24 h after exposure. Values were relativized to cells exposed to untreated PAR. Asterisks represent statistically significant differences among cell lines for the same PAR treatment time-point. ($n = 3$; *** p-value < 0.005, ANOVA and two-sided Student's t-test).

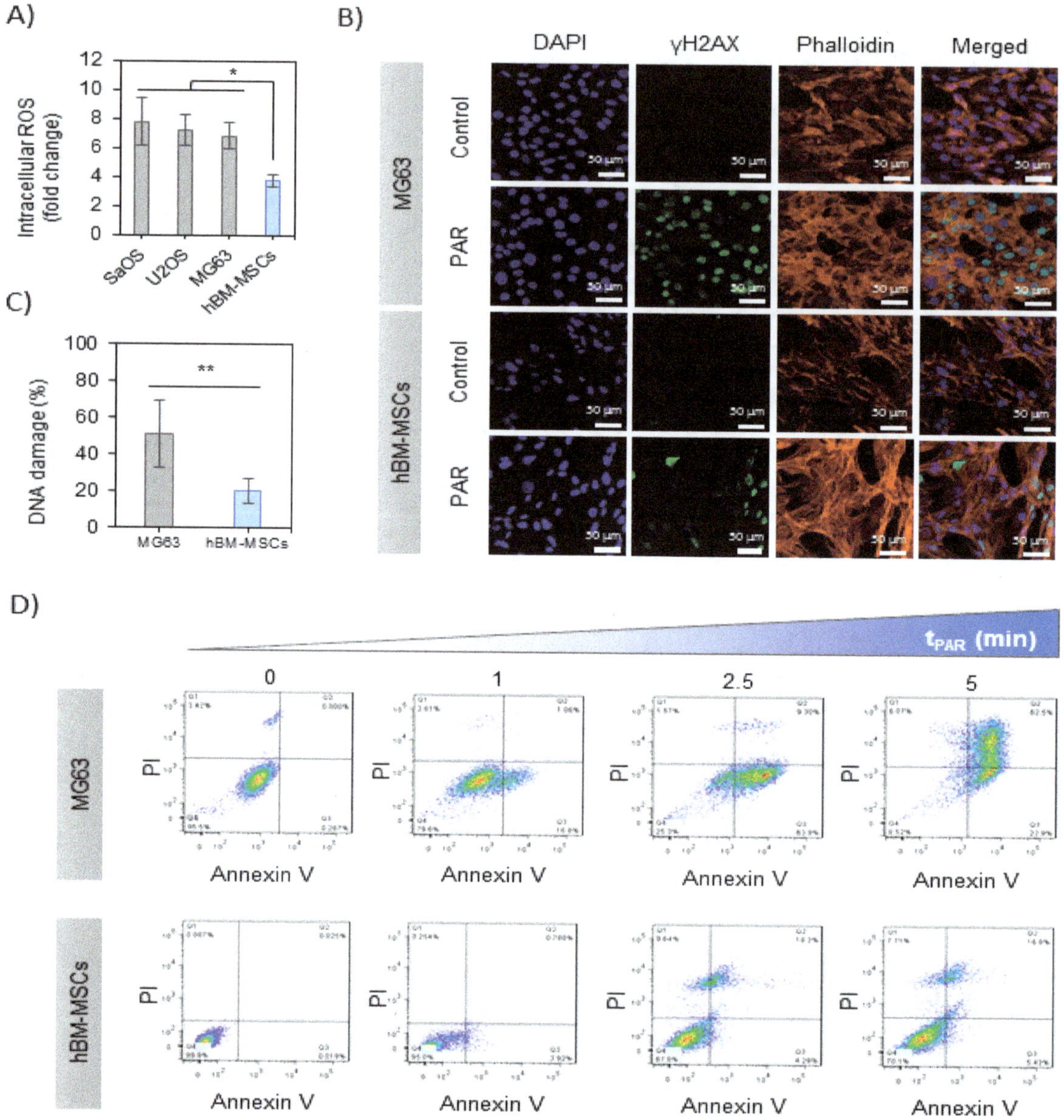

Figure 3. PAR-induced selective cell death in MG-63 cells rather than in hBM-MSCs. (**A**) Intracellular ROS measurement; OS cell lines and hBM-MSCs were incubated with dichlorofluorescin diacetate (DCFH-DA) and exposed during 2 h to PAR treated during 5 min by APPJ and after that fluorescence was measured. Values were relativized to negative control. (**B**) % of DNA damage quantification (positive γH2AX area relativized to DAPI area; images: $n = 5$, mean of 70 nuclei per image). Asterisks represent statistically significance ($n = 3$; * p-value < 0.05; ** p-value < 0.01; ANOVA and two-sided Student's t-test). (**C**) Representative images of MG-63 and hBM-MSCs cells after 2 h of exposition to 5 min-treated PAR by APPJ. Cells were labelled with DAPI (nuclei, blue), phalloidin (F-actin, orange) and anti-γH2AX (DNA damage reporter, green). Scale bar = 50 μM. (**D**) MG-63 and hBM-MSCs cultures were exposed during 2 h to untreated PAR and treated during 1, 2.5 and 5 min with APPJ. After that, PAR was replaced by fresh medium. Cells were collected 24 h after PAR exposure and then they were stained with Annexin-V/PI and analyzed by flow cytometry. This assay was done in triplicate.

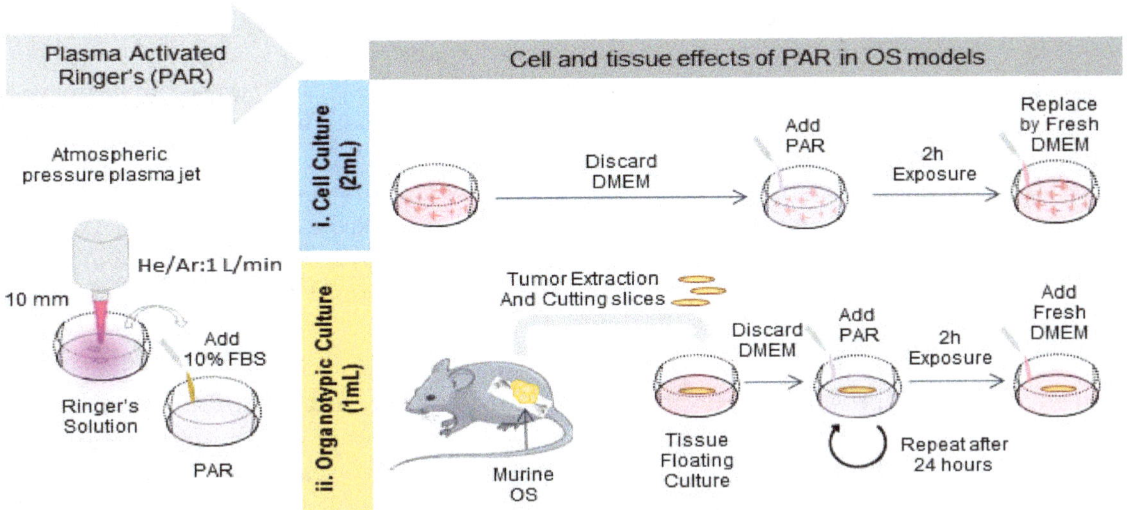

Figure 4. Protocol followed for the generation of PAR and the treatment of cell and organotypic cultures. Briefly, PAR was obtained by treatment of Ringer's saline at different times followed by adding 10% FBS. For cell cultures (**i**), cells were placed with 2 mL-treated PAR and incubated during 2 h; after that PAR was replaced by fresh medium. For organotypic cultures (**ii**), murine OS tumors were cut in slices and placed in floating culture; then samples were placed with 1 mL-treated PAR during 2 h and after that, PAR was diluted at 25% in fresh medium. In this case, treatment was repeated after 24 h.

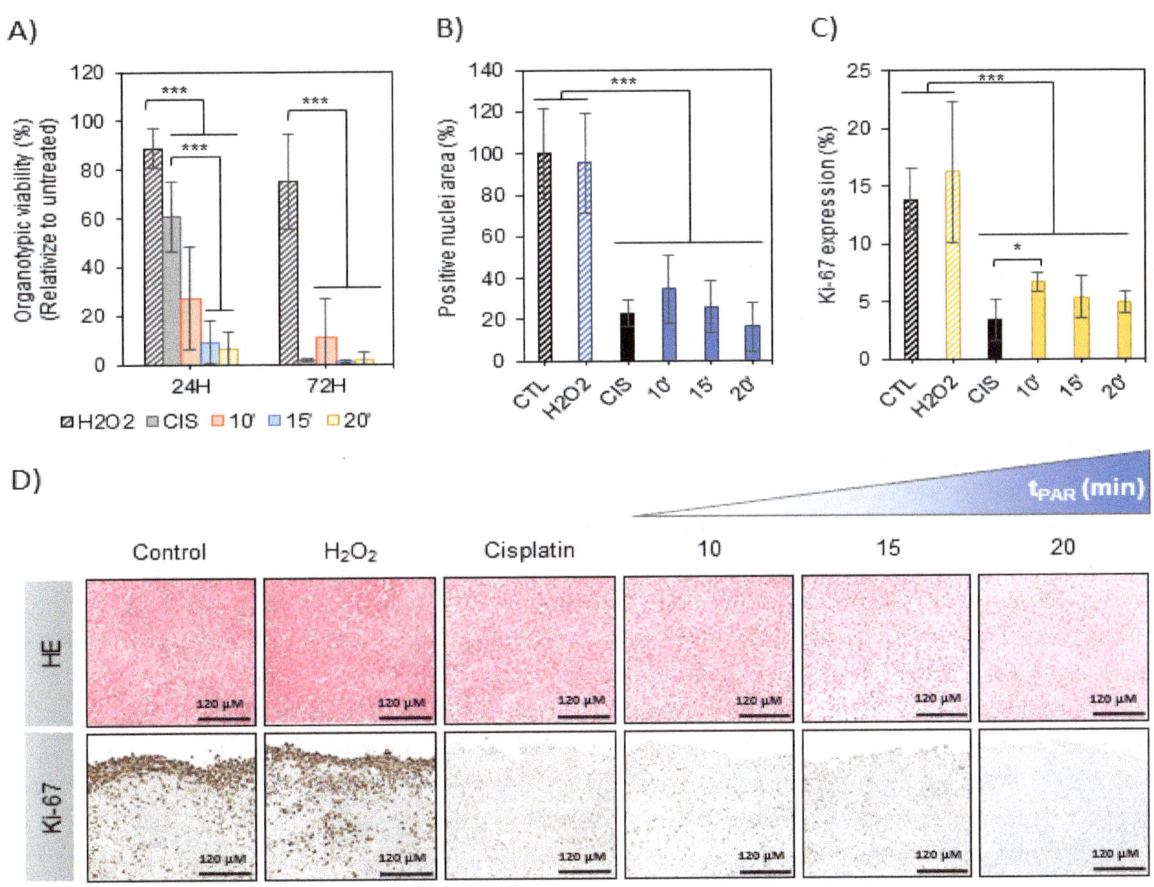

Figure 5. PAR effects in mouse organotypic OS model. Mouse OS tumor sections in floating culture were treated with PAR at increasing treatment times (10, 15 and 20 min) or by 100 µM of Cisplatin (CIS)

or 500 μM of H_2O_2. (**A**) Metabolic activity was determined by resazurin 24 and 72 h after PAR exposure. In this assay, four sections were analyzed per condition, and the assay was performed in three independent experiments. Values were relativized to tumor sections exposed to untreated PAR. Tumor sections were fixed 72 h after treatment and processed for histological analysis. Samples were stained with haematoxylin/eosin (HE) and immunostained for Ki-67. (**B**) HE quantification of positive nuclei stained areas (values relativized to control). (**C**) Percentage of positive Ki-67 stained nuclei. For statistical analysis, 5 well-distributed images were taken at X40 and were analyzed. Asterisks represent statistically significance between different conditions ($n = 3$; * p-value < 0.05; *** p-value < 0.005; ANOVA and two-sided Student's t-test). (**D**) Representative images for HE and Ki-67 immunostaining for each condition (Scale bar = 120 μm).

Haematoxylin/Eosin (HE) and Ki-67 immunostaining allowed to evaluate histological effects of PAR in tumor tissues after 72 h of treatment (Figure 5D). A significant reduction of relative nuclei area (HE staining) was observed to be induced by PAR with increasing plasma treatment times ($p < 0.005$) (Figure 5B). This reduction was also observed in Cisplatin-treated samples, being of more than 70% (Figure 5B). A high number of proliferating cells (Ki-67 stained) were observed in the first 40 μm of tumor section margins in the control (Figure 5D), with less percentage of Ki-67 cells in the rest of the section (14 ± 3%) (Figure 5C). Proliferation in tumor margins was abrogated by both PAR and Cisplatin at 72 h (Figure 5D); the percentage of Ki-67 expressing cells was significantly reduced by PAR treatment, being of 5–7% for PAR-exposed sections (Figure 5C; $p < 0.005$). The reduction of proliferating cells by Cisplatin was equivalent to 15–20 min of PAR. In contrast with the results in 2D, no effects were observed to be induced by H_2O_2 added at the 500 μM of concentration neither in proliferation nor in nuclei area.

3. Discussion

We report here on the effects of saline solutions activated by plasma in 2D adherent and on 3D organotypic OS cultures, employing a clinically compatible Ringer's saline. Cold atmospheric plasmas have been highlighted as a potential therapy against many types of cancers. However, most studies up to now were conducted in vitro (95%), mostly in 2D cultures, and only 26% evaluated the effects of plasma-activated liquids on the cells (as opposed to directly treating the cells with plasma) [44]. The direct application of plasma and the homogeneity of the treatment may depend on tumor size and body location, restricting the possibility of treating tumors hard to reach. Employing plasma-activated liquids can allow injection to the tumor site, and thus provide a minimally invasive approach for this therapy [11].

The reactivity transfer from the plasma gas phase to the liquid phase has been highlighted as being of prime importance for its biological effects [21]. Despite employing here two jets that use noble gases (Helium in APPJ or Ar in kINPen), an important part of the reactivity of these jets derives from mixing of the plasma gas phase with air. The gas phase of the APPJ during treatment of Ringer's included different nitrogen species, monoatomic oxygen, and hydroxyl radicals, as recorded by optical emission spectroscopy (Figure 1(Ai)), as similarly observed during treatment of cell culture medium [22,36]. Both plasma jets have been extensively characterized in [45,46]. In contrast, kINPen produced two other oxygen-containing species: γ-NO and OH (Figure 1(Aii)). These species in the gas phase were related to a progressive increase of RONS in Ringer's with plasma treatment time. In fact, while similar amounts of NO_2^- were generated with both jets, much higher concentrations of H_2O_2 and of total ROS were recorded in PAR produced from kINPen (Figure 1C).

In the presence of air, short-lived reactive nitrogen species such as (NO or $ONOO^-$) are formed in liquid medium. These nitrogen oxides subsequently react in water forming acids, which affect the conductivity and pH of plasma-treated liquids and based on pH dissociate to nitrite (NO_2^-) (Figure 1C) and nitrate (NO_3^-) ions. In fact, decrease of pH (from 7.3) to non-physiological values (3–4) was recorded after treatment, in a dose-dependent manner (Figure 1(Bi)), as observed in other works employing water or non-buffered saline solutions [47,48]. An important body of literature led by Hori et al. have proposed clinical-compatible saline solutions to be activated by cold plasmas, such as Ringer lactate solutions [11]. These solutions present some experimental limitations for in vitro conditions, mainly the lack of nutrients to sustain cell viability [15,48]. For this reason, here 10% of FBS was added to Ringer's to mimic nutrient tumor environment and allow further treatment of cells with this liquid. To avoid altering the reactivity of FBS with plasma [41], it was added just after plasma treatment. The addition of 10% of FBS after treatment stabilized the pH between 7.8 and 7.1 (Figure 1(Bii)), which allowed isolating the cell effects due only to the concentration and kind of RONS generated in the liquid, as in non-buffered solutions high pH decrease induced by plasma treatment is also reported to severely compromise cell viability [12,48].

It was shown in previous works [36,49] that long treatment time of cell culture medium may produce a lethal concentration of H_2O_2 which overwhelms cell defense mechanisms and kills both OS and healthy cells [36]. In line with these data, to obtain an equilibrated cocktail of RONS, plasma treatments only up to 5 min were selected (Figure 1C). Due to the low stability of NO_2^- produced by plasma (Figure S1), cell cultures were exposed to PAR just after production. In our experiments, incubation of cell cultures or tumor sections in contact with PAR for only 2 h was enough to induce cytotoxic effects in SaOS-2, MG-63 and U2-OS cells (Figure 2). The different p53 and pRB status of these human OS cell lines (p53−/pRB− for SaOS-2, p53+/pRB− for U2-OS and p53−/pRB+ for MG-63) [44] indicates that plasma-activated Ringer's cytotoxic action possibly follows a p53 and pRB− independent mechanism of cell death.

Cold atmospheric plasmas are reported to act selectively targeting cancer cell lines without affecting their healthy homologues [50,51]. This can be explained by the gap between cancer cells and normal cells, due to an increased cell metabolism and intracellular production of RONS [52] which oversaturates antioxidant system, making cancer cells more sensitive to oxidative stress [53]. The ability of PAR targeting different OS cell lines but without deleterious effects in hBM-MSCs is clearly observed in this study, in Ringer's obtained from treatment with APPJ but not with kINPen (Figure 2). At discussed earlier, under these working conditions kINPen produced higher amount of total ROS and H_2O_2 (i.e., 219 ± 46 μM at 5 min) than APPJ (143 ± 30 μM at 5 min), but without significant differences in the production of NO_2^-. This higher concentration of H_2O_2 produced in PAR by kINPen in contrast with APPJ may compromise PAR selectivity. However, the fact that the concentration of H_2O_2 produced by kINPen at 2.5 min treatment is equivalent to that of 5 min of APPJ treatment but the selectivity of the treatment is lost only for kINPen indicates that other species apart from those measured here are formed in Ringer's that are important for cell survival. As mentioned earlier, it has been described that a wide variety of the species generated by CAP can be of influence in its anticancer effects (i.e., $ONOO^-$, OH^-, NO, O_2^-, O_3, H_2O_2, NO_2^-, NO_3^-, etc.) [14–16].

Controls were prepared with artificially added H_2O_2 or NO_2^- at concentrations equivalent to those of kINPen and showed that NO_2^- does not affect cell toxicity in OS cell lines and increase cell viability in healthy cells (Figure 2C). Equivalent concentrations of H_2O_2 induced less cytotoxic effects than PAR in OS, suggesting again that other RONS are contributing to the cytotoxic effects produced by PAR. Recent studies have shown that artificially added H_2O_2 and NO_2^-, which lead to the formation of peroxinitrite, act synergistically and produce higher cytotoxic effects than each species separately [54].

The highest H_2O_2 concentration leads, as in kINPen-treated PAR, to a loss of selectivity (hBM-MSC cell death). To obtain an equilibrated cocktail of RONS and avoiding a loss of anti-cancer selectivity [36], for further work we selected APPJ-treated PAR. In order to adjust the production of RONS, plasma parameters like gas flow [36,55], distance of the nozzle [7,36,55], working gas composition [56–59] and here, device configuration [60,61] are of paramount importance to adjust the composition of RONS generated in the liquid, and the conditions selected here followed previous works of our group [36,62].

The genotoxic potential of PAR was evaluated by analyzing the levels of intracellular ROS and γH2AX and apoptosis activation. The three OS lines analyzed display similar 7-fold increase in intracellular ROS, while the rise recorded in healthy cells is only about half of that from OS cells (Figure 3A), which can be explained by the decreased antioxidant ability of cancer cells [17]. APPJ-treated PAR induced an increase in the level of γH2AX in both healthy and OS cells after treatment (Figure 3B,C), in line with previous works [36,56,63]. The lower levels of γH2AX recorded after PAR treatment in hBM-MSCs indicate that PAR induces DNA damage mainly in human OS cells. Following the mentioned results, there seems to be a clear correlation between the increase in the intracellular ROS and the induction of DNA damage. A relevant fact is APPJ-treated PAR induces apoptosis in MG-63 cells (Figure 3D), as observed in previous works for other OS cells treated with plasma-activated cell culture media or even directly with plasma [22,36]. On the other hand, hBM-MSCs are clearly less affected, with little induction of late apoptosis and necrosis at longer APPJ treatment times on PAR (this is quantified in Figure S2).

In recent years, 3D cultures are gaining increasing interest due to the need to recapitulate the complexity of the in vivo situation. As reported in previous studies, tumor complexity regarding the presence of stroma, cell-to-cell contact [64], and tumor heterogeneity [65,66] have a high impact in chemotherapy efficiency [67,68] and also on the penetration of RONS [69]. To take all this into account, the treatments on tumors were performed by two doses of PAR separated by 24 h, and to obtain higher concentration of RONS in plasma-activated media, plasma treatment was performed in lower volume of saline solution and longer treatment times (Figure S3). The treatment profile designed showed effectiveness to completely reduce metabolic activity of tumor sections up to 72 h (Figure 5A).

We confirmed the anti-tumoral potential of PAR by Hematoxylin-Eosin (HE) and Ki-67 immunodetection, showing that PAR can induce cell death and decrease of proliferation in a similar way than 100 μm Cisplatin (Figure 5A–C). In 2D we observed that concentrations of H_2O_2 equivalent to those generated with plasma treatment had clear cytotoxic effects (Figure 2C), so 500 μM H_2O_2 was employed as a positive control (Figure 5B–D). In the 3D organotypic cultures it was clear that H_2O_2 did not induce any cell death, nor decrease on Ki-67 (Figure 5A–C). It was also observed that caspase-3 (caspase protein involved in mitochondrial apoptotic pathway) was induced by Cisplatin but not by PAR (Figure S4), suggesting a caspase-3 independent mechanism (which does not exclude apoptosis, but rather indicates that other markers are involved in the process). Our results reflect on the important effect of PAR as potential anti-tumoral therapy, which reduces the viability of the ex vivo tumor sections by reducing cell proliferation in a similar way to high doses of Cisplatin on OS models with the advantage of not affecting healthy hMSCs.

4. Materials and Methods.

4.1. Cell Lines

Sarcoma osteogenic SaOS-2, MG-63 and U2-OS cells (ATCC, Manassas, VA, USA) were cultured in DMEM (Gibco™, Carlsbad, CA, USA) supplemented with 10% of fetal bovine serum (FBS), 2 mM L-glutamine and penicillin/streptomycin (50 U/mL and 50 μg/mL, respectively), all from Gibco™. Cells from passages 1–29 were used in all experiments. hBM-MSCs (ATCC, USA) were expanded in Advanced DMEM (Gibco™) supplemented with 10% of FBS, 2 mM L-glutamine and penicillin/streptomycin. Cells from passages 1–9 were used in all experiments. MOS-J cell line, established from spontaneous C57BL/6J mouse OS by Joliat, M.J. et al. [70], were expanded in DMEM with glucose at 4.5 g/L (Lonza, Walkersville, MA, USA), supplemented with 1% of FBS, and 1% penicillin/streptomycin. For organotypic culture, DMEM with 15% FBS and 1% penicillin/streptomycin was prepared and glucose was added to the medium to each a final concentration of 6 g/L. The same medium was used for 2D and 3D plasma treatments. All cell lines were maintained and expanded at 37 °C in a 95% humidified atmosphere containing 5% of CO_2.

4.2. Atmospheric Pressure Plasma Jets

Two atmospheric pressure plasma jets were employed: An atmospheric pressure plasma jet (APPJ) was created using He (5.0 Linde, Spain) as plasma carrier gas in a jet design with a single electrode as described elsewhere [46]. The discharge electrode was a copper wire with a diameter of 0.1 mm inserted inside of a 1.2 mm inner diameter quartz capillary tube, covered by a polytetrafluoroethylene (PTFE) holder. The electrode was connected to a commercial high voltage power supply from Conrad Electronics (nominally 6 W power consumption). The discharge was operating with sinusoidal waveform at 25 kHz with (U) ~2 kV and (I) ~3 mA. Helium flow in the capillary was regulated by a Bronkhorst MassView flow controller [22].

kINPen®® IND (Neoplas tools GmbH, Greifswald, Germany) is a commercial plasma jet tool that consists of a hand-held unit that discharges plasma under atmospheric conditions, employing a DC power unit and Argon gas to generate the plasma. In the centre of a ceramic capillary (inner diameter 1.6 mm) a pin-type electrode (1 mm diameter) is mounted, and a ring around the dielectric as grounded counter-electrode. The needle is powered by a small RF generator producing a sinusoidal voltage waveform ranging from 2 kV to 3 kV amplitude peak at a frequency of 1 MHz and modulated with 2.5 kHz and a plasma duty cycle of 1:1 [71,72].

Both plasma jets operated with a gas flow of 1 L/min, based on a previous work [36] at a distance of 10 mm between the surface of the liquid and the jet nozzle.

4.3. Optical Emission Spectroscopy (OES)

OES was used to determine the main plasma emitting species. The equipment used was a spectrometer F600-UVVIS-SR (StellarNet, Tampa, FL, USA), which was connected to an optical fiber (QP600-2SR-Ocean Optics) with lens that collected information from the measure point near the plasma jet (integration time 10,000 ms, average of 5 scans). Measurements were conducted close to the surface. For data processing, the SpectraWiz software (StellarNet, Tampa, FL, USA) was used.

4.4. Plasma Treatment

To produce the plasma-activated Ringer's saline (PAR), 2 mL of sterile Ringer's saline (8.6 g/L NaCl, 0.33 g/L $CaCl_2$ and 0.3 g/L KCl) were placed under the jet at room temperature at a distance of 10 mm from the jet nozzle in sterile conditions. The liquid was placed in multiple well plates of 1.9 cm^2 of surface (24 well-plates). Plasma treatment times between 1–5 min were investigated. A 10% of FBS was added immediately after treatment. The protocol followed is schematized in Figure 4. For treatment of organotypic cultures, 1 mL of Ringer's saline were treated with APPJ between 10–20 min at same conditions.

4.5. Characterization of PAR

For characterization of PAR, each parameter was measured immediately after plasma treatment and addition of FBS. pH was measured using an MM 41 Crison multimeter. The H_2O_2 produced by plasma was measured using an Amplex Red/horseradish peroxidase method (all from Sigma) and by monitoring the peak of fluorescence at λex/em of 560/590 nm. H_2O_2 concentrations were determined using a calibration curve constructed from known stock H_2O_2 solutions (0–10 μM). NO_2^- were quantified by using the Griess reagent method and using a calibration curve from known $NaNO_2$ stock solutions (0–100 μM). Griess reagent is prepared from sulphanilamide (1%), *N*-(1-naphtyl) ethylene diamine (NEED) (0.1%) (both from Sigma), phosphoric acid (1.2%) (Panreac) and distilled water (97.7%). The absorbance was measured at 540 nm. For total ROS detection, 2′,7′-dichlorofluorescin diacetate (DCFH-DA; Sigma) was used. Briefly, 150 μL of sample were placed in black 96 well-plates and 1 μL of DCFH-DA at 2 mM in DMSO was added to each sample. Samples were incubated for 30 min at 37 °C and then fluorescence intensity was read at a λex/em of 485/528 nm. Total ROS increase was expressed as a fold change. In total ROS detection all the reactive oxygen species present in the media are considered, therefore including short and long-lived species (i.e., H_2O_2, NO_2^-, HOO *, * OH, NO *, ONOO *, etc.). Absorbance and fluorescence were measured using a Synergy HTX multi-mode microplate reader (BioTek Instruments, Winooski, VT, USA). From all techniques, samples were measured in triplicate.

4.6. Metabolic Activity

Subconfluent SaOS-2, MG-63, U2-OS and hBM-MSCs were trypsinized, centrifuged and seeded in a 48-well plate at a density of 15x 10^3 cells/well, and incubated in 300 μL of their corresponding medium for 24 h. After incubation, the culture medium was replaced in each cell line by 300 μL of PAR treated during 1, 2.5 or 5 min where 10% FBS had been added immediately after treatment. Cells were incubated during two hours with PAR for each condition in triplicate. As a positive control, each cell line was incubated during two hours with untreated PAR. Afterwards, PAR was replaced by fresh complete DMEM. The experimental protocol is shown in Figure 5. Cells were then incubated at 37 °C for 24 h and 72 h. Cell metabolism was evaluated by WST-1 assay (Roche, Mannheim, Germany) 18 μL of WST-1 were employed per mL of culture medium. As a negative control, WST-1 was incubated without cells. The absorbance was measured at 440 nm and absorbance from negative control was subtracted. Absorbance of each treated condition was referenced to positive control.

4.7. Immunofluorescence

For immunofluorescence staining, MG63 and hBM-MSCs cells were incubated during 2 h with PAR treated during 5 min. After incubation, PAR was removed and changed by fresh medium, cells were incubated during 6 h and then fixed with 4% of paraformaldehyde (Sigma) for 20 min at room temperature. Then, cells were washed, twice with PBS, permeabilized with 0.1% Triton X-100 in PBS and blocked with 5% BSA in PBS-0.1% Tween-20 10X (blocking solution) with agitation during 3 h. Then, cells were washed and incubated with mouse Anti-phospho-Histone γH2AX (Ser139) Antibody, clone JBW301 (Merk Millipore, Burlington, MS, USA) (1:500 in blocking solution) in agitation at 4 °C overnight and after washing with PBS, cells were incubated with secondary antibody Alexa Fluor 488 goat anti-mouse (Invitrogen) for 30 min in the dark. After that cells were washed with PBS and incubated with Alexa Fluor 546 Phalloidin (1:300 in PBS-0.1% Tween-20) (Invitrogen Carlsbad, CA, USA) during 1 h in dark. Cells were washed with 20 mM glycine in PBS and samples were mounted with ProLong™ Gold Antifade Mountant with DAPI (LifeTechnologies, Carlsbad, CA, USA). Images were captured using Zeiss laser scanning microscope. For % of DNA damage, total positive area for γH2AX foci and DAPI stain were quantified using ImageJ software and total γH2AX-positive area were relativized to total DAPI area ($n = 5$, with a mean of 70 nuclei per image).

4.8. Intracellular ROS Measurement

Intracellular levels of ROS were measured using DCFH-DA. SaOS-2, MG63, U2OS and hBM-MSCs cells were cultured in black 96-well plates at a density of 5000 cells/well in their corresponding medium for 24 h. After that, cells were incubated before treatment during 1 h with 40 μM of DCFH-DA in DPBS, prepared from 2 mM of DCFH-DA solved in DMSO. Afterwards, cells were washed in DPBS and treated with PAR for 2 h following the protocol in Figure 4i. To quantify of intracellular ROS levels, fluorescence was measured after 2 h of incubation with PAR replacing it by 50 μL of DPBS. The $\lambda_{ex/em}$ was of 490/530 nm. As a negative control, fluorescence of cells without DCFH-DA was measured in DPBS and then subtracted. Values were relativized to the positive control (untreated cells) and intracellular ROS increased was expressed as a fold change.

4.9. Flow Cytometry

MG63 and hBM-MSCs were seeded on 6-well plate at a density of 2×10^5 per 2 mL of culture medium and incubated during 24 h. After that, cells were exposed during 2 h to 1 mL of PAR treated during 1, 2.5 and 5 min following the protocol in Figure 5. 24 h after treatment, cells were stained with Cell Death Apoptosis Kit with Annexin V Alexa Fluor™ 488 & Propidium Iodide (PI) (Invitrogen, cat.no 10257392, Carlsbad, CA, USA) following the manufacturer's protocol. Cell counts were determined by flow cytometer BD LSR II and data analysis was performed with FlowJo Software. Each condition was done in triplicate.

4.10. Murine OS Organotypic Model

35 days old C57BL/6J mice were injected with 2 million MOS-J cells in 50 μL of DPBS by intramuscular paratibial injection. 17 days after injections, mice with 900–1200 mm^3 tumor size were selected and sacrificed. Tumor sections of (2 × 2 × 0.2 mm) were obtained using LeicaVT 1200S vibratome under sterile conditions and sections were maintained in 2 mL of DMEM high glucose in 24 ultra-low attachment well-plates during 24 h. After that, tumor sections were exposed during 2 h to 1 mL Ringer's saline that had been previously treated for 10, 15 or 20 min and then, PAR was diluted at $\frac{1}{4}$ in DMEM high glucose. Tumor sections were also exposed during 2 h to 500 μM H_2O_2 in Ringer's saline with 10% of FBS and also were maintained with 100 μM Cisplatin (Santa Cruz, CA, USA) in DMEM high glucose. After 24 h of incubation, each treatment was repeated and tumor sections were kept in these for 48 more hours, being 72 h at the end. Sections from three different tumours were exposed to different conditions and 4 Sections were used per condition to estimate the mean. Tumor sections were incubated with resazurin solution (0.5 g/L Resazurin from Sigma in PBS) at 20% in DMEM high glucose during 3 h to measure metabolic activity. This was done before treatments and 24 and 72 h after first treatment. Fluorescence were measured with λex/em of 530/600 nm. As a negative control, fluorescence of resazurin without cells or tumor sections were measured and subtracted. Each value was relativized to control.

4.11. Histological Analysis

For histological analysis, tumor sections at 72 h after treatment were fixed in 4% formol overnight at 4 °C. After fixation, sections were dehydrated, included in paraffin, sectioned with microtome and deparaffinized before being rehydrated for histological analysis. Haematoxylin/eosin staining were performed to observe tissue structure and number of nuclei. For immunohistochemistry, sections were incubated in citrate buffer at 96 °C for 20 min and then blocked in PBS-Triton 0.05% with 1% BSA during 1 h at room temperature. After that, samples were washed with TBS-Tween 20 0.05% and then incubated with hydrogen peroxide 3% for 15 min to inhibit endogenous peroxidase. Sections were incubated with monoclonal rabbit anti-Ki-67 (Abcam, Cambrigde, UK) overnight at 4 °C. After that, samples were washed and incubated with secondary goat anti-rabbit biotinylated (Dako, E0432, Santa Clara, CA, USA) for one hour at room temperature. Then samples were incubated with streptavidin/peroxidase (Dako, P0397, Santa Clara, CA, USA) TBS-Tween 20 0.05% for one hour at room temperature. Diaminobenzidine (DAB) was used to visualize positive staining. Samples were countercolored with hematoxyline, washed and then mounted with Pertex. Images were taken by NanoZoomer (Hamamatsu Photonics). For positive nuclei area quantification and percentage of positive Ki-67 nuclei, 5 well-distributed high magnification pictures (X40) were taken for each condition in triplicate and analysed with ImageJ. For positive nuclei area, values were relativized to positive control. For percentage of positive Ki-67 nuclei, positive nuclei were quantified and relativized to total number of nuclei excluding the first 40 μm of tumor section (proliferating margins).

4.12. Statistical Analysis

All data are presented as means ± SD. Statistical analysis of the data was performed using ANOVA to compare conditions within the same experimental group and Student's t-test to compare couple of conditions between them. p-values < 0.05 were considered statistically significant. For the case of viability and flow cytometry studies, p-values < 0.005 were considered statistically significant

5. Conclusions

Many studies reported that saline solutions activated by cold atmospheric plasma can offer a potential therapy against cancer, but there are very few works than demonstrate its effects in 3D and no studies in osteosarcoma models. The main aim of the present study was to demonstrate the cytotoxic effects of PAR in human and mouse osteosarcoma, employing 2D and organotypic cultures. Our data show that plasma-activated saline solutions could be used for the treatment of OS, by investigating the implication of RONS for the anti-cancer effect and cellular mechanisms involved in selective cell death. First, PAR induces cell death in adherent cell cultures, related to the increase in the intracellular ROS that triggers DNA damage and subsequent apoptosis, and not being related directly to H_2O_2 concentration. This kind of mechanism produced clearly higher lethal effects in osteosarcoma cells than in hBM-MSCs, that were significantly less affected. Second, PAR reduces OS tumor viability and proliferation, displaying a reduction of metabolic activity, number of nuclei and Ki-67 expressing cells. Although further investigations are needed, the results of the present work provide evidence of PAR as a promising tool for clinical use for OS treatment.

Author Contributions: Conceptualization, J.T. and C.C.; Formal analysis, M.M.-S. and J.T.; Funding acquisition, C.C.; Investigation, M.M.-S., J.T., B.B., A.K., P.L. and C.C.; Methodology, M.M.-S., B.B. and P.L.; Project administration, C.C.; Supervision, J.T., M.-P.G. and C.C.; Validation, J.T.; Writing—original draft, M.M.-S.; Writing—review & editing, J.T., A.K., M.-P.G., P.L. and C.C. All authors have read and agreed to the published version of the manuscript.

References

1. Gill, J.; Ahluwalia, M.K.; Geller, D.; Gorlick, R. New targets and approaches in osteosarcoma. *Pharmacol. Ther.* **2013**, *137*, 89–99. [CrossRef] [PubMed]
2. Ottaviani, G.; Jaffe, N.; Ottaviani, M.D.G. *The Epidemiology of Osteosarcoma*; Springer: Boston, MA, USA, 2009; Volume 152, pp. 3–13.
3. Botter, S.M.; Neri, D.; Fuchs, B. Recent advances in osteosarcoma. *Curr. Opin. Pharmacol.* **2014**, *16*, 15–23. [CrossRef] [PubMed]
4. Longhi, A.; Errani, C.; De Paolis, M.; Mercuri, M.; Bacci, G. Primary bone osteosarcoma in the pediatric age: State of the art. *Cancer Treat. Rev.* **2006**, *32*, 423–436. [CrossRef]
5. Van Driel, M.; Van Leeuwen, J.P. Cancer and bone: A complex complex. *Arch. Biochem. Biophys.* **2014**, *561*, 159–166. [CrossRef]
6. Lackmann, J.W.; Bandow, J.E. Inactivation of microbes and macromolecules by atmospheric-pressure plasma jets. *Appl. Microbiol. Biotechnol.* **2014**, *98*, 6205–6213. [CrossRef]
7. Wiegand, C.; Beier, O.; Horn, K.; Pfuch, A.; Tölke, T.; Hipler, U.C.; Schimanski, A. Antimicrobial Impact of Cold Atmospheric Pressure Plasma on Medical Critical Yeasts and Bacteria Cultures. *Skin Pharmacol. Physiol.* **2014**, *27*, 25–35. [CrossRef]
8. Mashayekh, S.; Rajaee, H.; Akhlaghi, M.; Shokri, B.; Hassan, Z.M. Atmospheric-pressure plasma jet characterization and applications on melanoma cancer treatment (B/16-F10). *Phys. Plasmas* **2015**, *22*, 93508. [CrossRef]
9. Xu, G.M.; Shi, X.M.; Cai, J.F.; Chen, S.L.; Li, P.; Yao, C.W.; Chang, Z.S.; Zhang, G.J. Dual effects of atmospheric pressure plasma jet on skin wound healing of mice. *Wound Repair Regen.* **2015**, *23*, 878–884. [CrossRef]
10. Arndt, S.; Unger, P.; Wacker, E.; Shimizu, T.; Heinlin, J.; Li, Y.F.; Thomas, H.M.; Morfill, G.E.; Zimmermann, J.L.; Bosserhoff, A.K.; et al. Cold Atmospheric Plasma (CAP) Changes Gene Expression of Key Molecules of the Wound Healing Machinery and Improves Wound Healing In Vitro and In Vivo. *PLoS ONE* **2013**, *8*, e79325. [CrossRef]
11. Tanaka, H.; Nakamura, K.; Mizuno, M.; Ishikawa, K.; Takeda, K.; Kajiyama, H.; Utsumi, F.; Kikkawa, F.; Hori, M. Non-thermal atmospheric pressure plasma activates lactate in Ringer's solution for anti-tumor effects. *Sci. Rep.* **2016**, *6*, 36282. [CrossRef]
12. Kaushik, N.K.; Ghimire, B.; Li, Y.; Adhikari, M.; Veerana, M.; Kaushik, N.; Jha, N.; Adhikari, B.; Lee, S.J.; Masur, K.; et al. Biological and medical applications of plasma-activated media, water and solutions. *Biol. Chem.* **2018**, *400*, 39–62. [CrossRef] [PubMed]
13. Steuer, A.; Wolff, C.M.; Von Woedtke, T.; Weltmann, K.D.; Kolb, J.F. Cell stimulation versus cell death induced by sequential treatments with pulsed electric fields and cold atmospheric pressure plasma. *PLoS ONE* **2018**, *13*, e0204916. [CrossRef] [PubMed]
14. Yan, X.; Xiong, Z.; Zou, F.; Zhao, S.; Lu, X.; Yang, G.; He, G.; Ostrikov, K. (Ken) Plasma-Induced Death of HepG2 Cancer Cells: Intracellular Effects of Reactive Species. *Plasma Process. Polym.* **2011**, *9*, 59–66. [CrossRef]
15. Yan, D.; Cui, H.; Zhu, W.; Nourmohammadi, N.; Milberg, J.; Zhang, L.G.; Sherman, J.H.; Keidar, M. The

Specific Vulnerabilities of Cancer Cells to the Cold Atmospheric Plasma-Stimulated Solutions. *Sci. Rep.* **2017**, *7*, 4479. [CrossRef]

16. Graves, D.B. Reactive Species from Cold Atmospheric Plasma: Implications for Cancer Therapy. *Plasma Process. Polym.* **2014**, *11*, 1120–1127. [CrossRef]
17. Moloney, J.N.; Cotter, T.G. ROS signalling in the biology of cancer. *Semin. Cell Dev. Biol.* **2018**, *80*, 50–64. [CrossRef]
18. Nerush, A.; Shchukina, K.; Balalaeva, I.; Orlova, A. Hydrogen peroxide in the reactions of cancer cells to cisplatin. *Biochim. Biophys. Acta BBA Gen. Subj.* **2019**, *1863*, 692–702. [CrossRef]
19. Ma, E.; Chen, P.; Wilkins, H.M.; Wang, T.; Swerdlow, R.H.; Chen, Q. Pharmacologic ascorbate induces neuroblastoma cell death by hydrogen peroxide mediated DNA damage and reduction in cancer cell glycolysis. *Free. Radic. Biol. Med.* **2017**, *113*, 36–47. [CrossRef]
20. Kamm, A.; Przychodzen, P.; Kuban-Jankowska, A.; Jacewicz, D.; Dabrowska, A.M.; Nussberger, S.; Wozniak, M.; Gorska-Ponikowska, M. Nitric oxide and its derivatives in the cancer battlefield. *Nitric Oxide* **2019**, *93*, 102–114. [CrossRef]
21. Khlyustova, A.; Labay, C.; Machala, Z.; Ginebra, M.P.; Canal, C. Important parameters in plasma jets for the production of RONS in liquids for plasma medicine: A brief review. *Front. Chem. Sci. Eng.* **2019**, *13*, 238–252. [CrossRef]
22. Canal, C.; Fontelo, R.; Hamouda, I.; Guillem-Marti, J.; Cvelbar, U.; Ginebra, M.P. Plasma-induced selectivity in bone cancer cells death. *Free Radic. Biol. Med.* **2017**, *110*, 72–80. [CrossRef]
23. Gümbel, D.; Suchy, B.; Wien, L.; Gelbrich, N.; Napp, M.; Kramer, A.; Ekkernkamp, A.; Daeschlein, G.; Stope, M.B. Comparison of Cold Atmospheric Plasma Devices' Efficacy on Osteosarcoma and Fibroblastic In Vitro Cell Models. *Anticancer Res.* **2017**, *37*, 5407–5414.
24. Yan, D.; Xu, W.; Yao, X.; Lin, L.; Sherman, J.H.; Keidar, M. The Cell Activation Phenomena in the Cold Atmospheric Plasma Cancer Treatment. *Sci. Rep.* **2018**, *8*, 15418. [CrossRef]
25. Hamaguchi, S. Chemically reactive species in liquids generated by atmospheric-pressure plasmas and their roles in plasma medicine. *AIP Conf. Proc.* **2013**, *1545*, 214–222.
26. Wada, N.; Ikeda, J.I.; Tanaka, H.; Sakakita, H.; Hori, M.; Ikehara, Y.; Morii, E. Effect of plasma-activated medium on the decrease of tumorigenic population in lymphoma. *Pathol. Res. Pract.* **2017**, *213*, 773–777. [CrossRef]
27. Chen, C.Y.; Cheng, Y.C.; Cheng, Y.J. Synergistic effects of plasma-activated medium and chemotherapeutic drugs in cancer treatment. *J. Phys. D Appl. Phys.* **2018**, *51*. [CrossRef]
28. Bekeschus, S.; Käding, A.; Schröder, T.; Wende, K.; Hackbarth, C.; Liedtke, K.R.; Van Der Linde, J.; Von Woedtke, T.; Heidecke, C.D.; Partecke, L.I. Cold Physical Plasma-Treated Buffered Saline Solution as Effective Agent Against Pancreatic Cancer Cells. *Anticancer Agents Med. Chem.* **2018**, *18*, 824–831. [CrossRef]
29. Gümbel, D.; Gelbrich, N.; Napp, M.; Daeschlein, G.; Sckell, A.; Ender, S.A.; Kramer, A.; Burchardt, M.; Weiss, M.; Ekkernkamp, A.; et al. New Treatment Options for Osteosarcoma – Inactivation of Osteosarcoma Cells by Cold Atmospheric Plasma. *Anticancer Res.* **2016**, *36*, 5915–5922. [CrossRef]
30. Gümbel, D.; Gelbrich, N.; Napp, M.; Daeschlein, G.; Kramer, A.; Sckell, A.; Burchardt, M.; Ekkernkamp, A.; Stope, M.B. Peroxiredoxin Expression of Human Osteosarcoma Cells Is Influenced by Cold Atmospheric Plasma Treatment. *Anticancer Res.* **2017**, *37*, 1031–1038.
31. Haralambiev, L.; Wien, L.; Gelbrich, N.; Kramer, A.; Mustea, A.; Burchardt, M.; Ekkernkamp, A.; Stope, M.B.; Gümbel, D. Effects of Cold Atmospheric Plasma on the Expression of Chemokines, Growth Factors, TNF Superfamily Members, Interleukins, and Cytokines in Human Osteosarcoma Cells. *Anticancer Res.* **2018**, *39*, 151–157. [CrossRef]
32. Kansara, M.; Teng, M.W.; Smyth, M.J.; Thomas, D.M. Translational biology of osteosarcoma. *Nat. Rev. Cancer* **2014**, *14*, 722–735. [CrossRef] [PubMed]
33. Morrow, J.J.; Khanna, C. Osteosarcoma Genetics and Epigenetics: Emerging Biology and Candidate Therapies. *Crit. Rev. Oncog.* **2015**, *20*, 173–197. [CrossRef] [PubMed]
34. Chen, X.; Bahrami, A.; Pappo, A.; Easton, J.; Dalton, J.; Hedlund, E.; Ellison, D.; Shurtleff, S.; Wu, G.; Wei, L.; et al. Recurrent somatic structural variations contribute to tumorigenesis in pediatric osteosarcoma. *Cell Rep.* **2014**, *7*, 104–112. [CrossRef] [PubMed]
35. Ozaki, T.; Nakagawara, A. p53: The attractive tumor suppressor in the cancer research field. *J. Biomed. Biotechnol.* **2011**, *2011*, 603925. [CrossRef]

36. Tornin, J.; Mateu-Sanz, M.; Rodríguez, A.; Labay, C.; Rodríguez, R.; Canal, C. Pyruvate Plays a Main Role in the Antitumoral Selectivity of Cold Atmospheric Plasma in Osteosarcoma. *Sci. Rep.* **2019**, *9*, 10681. [CrossRef]
37. Gümbel, D.; Bekeschus, S.; Gelbrich, N.; Napp, M.; Ekkernkamp, A.; Kramer, A.; Stope, M.B. Cold Atmospheric Plasma in the Treatment of Osteosarcoma. *Int. J. Mol. Sci.* **2017**, *18*, 2004. [CrossRef]
38. Cortini, M.; Avnet, S.; Baldini, N. Mesenchymal stroma: Role in osteosarcoma progression. *Cancer Lett.* **2017**, *405*, 90–99. [CrossRef]
39. Zhang, Y.; Yao, Y.; Zhang, Y. Three-Dimensional Bone Extracellular Matrix Model for Osteosarcoma. *J. Vis. Exp.* **2019**, e59271. [CrossRef]
40. Salo, T.; Dourado, M.R.; Sundquist, E.; Apu, E.H.; Alahuhta, I.; Tuomainen, K.; Vasara, J.; Al-Samadi, A. Organotypic three-dimensional assays based on human leiomyoma-derived matrices. *Philos. Trans. R. Soc. B Boil. Sci.* **2018**, *373*. [CrossRef]
41. Boehm, D.; Heslin, C.; Cullen, P.J.; Bourke, P. Cytotoxic and mutagenic potential of solutions exposed to cold atmospheric plasma. *Sci. Rep.* **2016**, *6*, 21464. [CrossRef]
42. Griseti, E.; Kolosnjaj-Tabi, J.; Gibot, L.; Fourquaux, I.; Rols, M.P.; Yousfi, M.; Merbahi, N.; Golzio, M. Pulsed Electric Field Treatment Enhances the Cytotoxicity of Plasma-Activated Liquids in a Three-Dimensional Human Colorectal Cancer Cell Model. *Sci. Rep.* **2019**, *9*, 7583. [CrossRef]
43. Pereira, B.P.; Zhou, Y.; Gupta, A.; Leong, D.T.; Aung, K.Z.; Ling, L.; Pho, R.W.H.; Galindo, M.; Salto-Tellez, M.; Stein, G.S.; et al. Runx2, p53, and pRB status as diagnostic parameters for deregulation of osteoblast growth and differentiation in a new pre-chemotherapeutic osteosarcoma cell line (OS1). *J. Cell. Physiol.* **2009**, *221*, 778–788. [CrossRef]
44. Dubuc, A.; Monsarrat, P.; Virard, F.; Merbahi, N.; Sarrette, J.P.; Laurencin-Dalicieux, S.; Cousty, S. Use of cold-atmospheric plasma in oncology: A concise systematic review. *Ther. Adv. Med Oncol.* **2018**, *10*. [CrossRef]
45. Reuter, S.; Von Woedtke, T.; Weltmann, K.D. The kINPen—A review on physics and chemistry of the atmospheric pressure plasma jet and its applications. *J. Phys. D Appl. Phys.* **2018**, *51*. [CrossRef]
46. Zaplotnik, R.; Biščan, M.; Kregar, Z.; Cvelbar, U.; Mozetic, M.; Milošević, S. Influence of a sample surface on single electrode atmospheric plasma jet parameters. *Spectrochim. Acta Part B At. Spectrosc.* **2015**, *103*, 124–130. [CrossRef]
47. Ikawa, S.; Kitano, K.; Hamaguchi, S. Effects of pH on Bacterial Inactivation in Aqueous Solutions due to Low-Temperature Atmospheric Pressure Plasma Application. *Plasma Process. Polym.* **2010**, *7*, 33–42. [CrossRef]
48. Van Boxem, W.; Van Der Paal, J.; Gorbanev, Y.; Vanuytsel, S.; Smits, E.; Dewilde, S.; Bogaerts, A. Anti-cancer capacity of plasma-treated PBS: Effect of chemical composition on cancer cell cytotoxicity. *Sci. Rep.* **2017**, *7*, 16478. [CrossRef]
49. Balzer, J.; Heuer, K.; Demir, E.; Hoffmanns, M.A.; Baldus, S.; Fuchs, P.C.; Awakowicz, P.; Suschek, C.V.; Opländer, C. Non-Thermal Dielectric Barrier Discharge (DBD) Effects on Proliferation and Differentiation of Human Fibroblasts Are Primary Mediated by Hydrogen Peroxide. *PLoS ONE* **2015**, *10*, e0144968. [CrossRef]
50. Dai, X.; Bazaka, K.; Richard, D.J.; Thompson, E.R.W.; Ostrikov, K.K. The Emerging Role of Gas Plasma in Oncotherapy. *Trends Biotechnol.* **2018**, *36*, 1183–1198. [CrossRef]
51. Reiazi, R.; Akbari, M.E.; Norozi, A.; Etedadialiabadi, M.; Akbari, M.E. Application of Cold Atmospheric Plasma (CAP) in Cancer Therapy: A Review. *Int. J. Cancer Manag.* **2017**, *10*, e8728. [CrossRef]
52. Tong, L.; Chuang, C.C.; Wu, S.; Zuo, L. Reactive oxygen species in redox cancer therapy. *Cancer Lett.* **2015**, *367*, 18–25. [CrossRef]
53. Assi, M. The differential role of reactive oxygen species in early and late stages of cancer. *Am. J. Physiol. Integr. Comp. Physiol.* **2017**, *313*, R646–R653. [CrossRef]
54. Bauer, G. The synergistic effect between hydrogen peroxide and nitrite, two long-lived molecular species from cold atmospheric plasma, triggers tumor cells to induce their own cell death. *Redox Biol.* **2019**, *26*, 101291. [CrossRef]
55. Akhlaghi, M.; Rajayi, H.; Mashayekh, A.S.; Khani, M.; Hassan, Z.M.; Shokri, B. On the design and characterization of a new cold atmospheric pressure plasma jet and its applications on cancer cells treatment. *Biointerphases* **2015**, *10*, 29510. [CrossRef]
56. Choi, J.Y.; Joh, H.M.; Park, J.M.; Kim, M.J.; Chung, T.H.; Kang, T.H. Non-thermal plasma-induced apoptosis

is modulated by ATR- and PARP1-mediated DNA damage responses and circadian clock. *Oncotarget* **2016**, *7*, 32980–32989. [CrossRef]

57. Virard, F.; Cousty, S.; Cambus, J.P.; Valentin, A.; Kémoun, P.; Clément, F. Cold Atmospheric Plasma Induces a Predominantly Necrotic Cell Death via the Microenvironment. *PLoS ONE* **2015**, *10*, e0133120. [CrossRef]
58. Iuchi, K.; Morisada, Y.; Yoshino, Y.; Himuro, T.; Saito, Y.; Murakami, T.; Hisatomi, H. Cold atmospheric-pressure nitrogen plasma induces the production of reactive nitrogen species and cell death by increasing intracellular calcium in HEK293T cells. *Arch. Biochem. Biophys.* **2018**, *654*, 136–145. [CrossRef]
59. Shi, X.M.; Chang, Z.S.; Wu, X.L.; Zhang, G.J.; Peng, Z.Y.; Dong, Z.Y.; Shao, X.J. Inactivation Effect of Argon Atmospheric Pressure Low-Temperature Plasma Jet on Murine Melanoma Cells. *Plasma Process. Polym.* **2013**, *10*, 808–816. [CrossRef]
60. Chen, Z.; Simonyan, H.; Cheng, X.; Gjika, E.; Lin, L.; Canady, J.; Sherman, J.H.; Young, C.; Keidar, M. A Novel Micro Cold Atmospheric Plasma Device for Glioblastoma Both In Vitro and In Vivo. *Cancers* **2017**, *9*, 61. [CrossRef]
61. Isbary, G.; Shimizu, T.; Li, Y.F.; Stolz, W.; Thomas, H.M.; Morfill, G.E.; Zimmermann, J.L. Cold atmospheric plasma devices for medical issues. *Expert Rev. Med Devices* **2013**, *10*, 367–377. [CrossRef]
62. Labay, C.; Hamouda, I.; Tampieri, F.; Ginebra, M.P.; Canal, C. Production of reactive species in alginate hydrogels for cold atmospheric plasma-based therapies. *Sci. Rep.* **2019**, *9*, 16160. [CrossRef]
63. Hirst, A.M.; Simms, M.S.; Mann, V.M.; Maitland, N.J.; O'Connell, D.; Frame, F.M. Low-temperature plasma treatment induces DNA damage leading to necrotic cell death in primary prostate epithelial cells. *Br. J. Cancer* **2015**, *112*, 1536–1545. [CrossRef]
64. Wei, Q.; Hariharan, V.; Huang, H. Cell-Cell Contact Preserves Cell Viability via Plakoglobin. *PLoS ONE* **2011**, *6*, e27064. [CrossRef]
65. Burrell, R.A.; Swanton, C. Tumour heterogeneity and the evolution of polyclonal drug resistance. *Mol. Oncol.* **2014**, *8*, 1095–1111. [CrossRef]
66. Junior, P.L.D.S.; Câmara, D.A.D.; Porcacchia, A.S.; Fonseca, P.M.M.; Jorge, S.D.; Araldi, R.P.; Ferreira, A.K. The Roles of ROS in Cancer Heterogeneity and Therapy. *Oxidative Med. Cell. Longev.* **2017**, *2017*, 2467940.
67. Aljitawi, O.S.; Li, D.; Xiao, Y.; Zhang, D.; Ramachandran, K.; Stehno-Bittel, L.; Van Veldhuizen, P.; Lin, T.L.; Kambhampati, S.; Garimella, R. A novel three-dimensional stromal-based model for in vitro chemotherapy sensitivity testing of leukemia cells. *Leuk. Lymphoma* **2013**, *55*, 378–391. [CrossRef]
68. Houshmand, M.; Soleimani, M.; Atashi, A.; Saglio, G.; Abdollahi, M.; Zarif, M.N. Mimicking the Acute Myeloid Leukemia Niche for Molecular Study and Drug Screening. *Tissue Eng. Part C Methods* **2017**, *23*, 72–85. [CrossRef]
69. Gorska, M.; Krzywiec, P.B.; Kuban-Jankowska, A.; Zmijewski, M.; Wozniak, M.; Wierzbicka, J.; Piotrowska, A.; Siwicka, K. Growth Inhibition of Osteosarcoma Cell Lines in 3D Cultures: Role of Nitrosative and Oxidative Stress. *Anticancer Res.* **2016**, *36*, 221–229.
70. Joliat, M.J.; Umeda, S.; Lyons, B.L.; Lynes, M.A.; Shultz, D. Establisment and characterization of a new osteogenic cell line (MOS-J) from a spontaneous C57BL/6J mouse osteosarcoma. *In Vivo* **2002**, *16*, 223–228.
71. Schuster, M.; Seebauer, C.; Rutkowski, R.; Hauschild, A.; Podmelle, F.; Metelmann, C.; Metelmann, B.; Von Woedtke, T.; Hasse, S.; Weltmann, K.D.; et al. Visible tumor surface response to physical plasma and apoptotic cell kill in head and neck cancer. *J. Cranio Maxillofacial Surg.* **2016**, *44*, 1445–1452. [CrossRef]
72. Weltmann, K.D.; Kindel, E.; Brandenburg, R.; Meyer, C.; Bussiahn, R.; Wilke, C.; Von Woedtke, T. Atmospheric Pressure Plasma Jet for Medical Therapy: Plasma Parameters and Risk Estimation. *Contrib. Plasma Phys.* **2009**, *49*, 631–640. [CrossRef]

10

Cold-Atmospheric Plasma Induces Tumor Cell Death in Preclinical In Vivo and In Vitro Models of Human Cholangiocarcinoma

Javier Vaquero [1,2,3,4,*], Florian Judée [2], Marie Vallette [1], Henri Decauchy [2], Ander Arbelaiz [1], Lynda Aoudjehane [1,5], Olivier Scatton [1,5,6], Ester Gonzalez-Sanchez [1,3,4], Fatiha Merabtene [1], Jérémy Augustin [1], Chantal Housset [1,5,7], Thierry Dufour [2,*,†] and Laura Fouassier [1,*,†]

1 Institut National de la Santé et de la Recherche Médicale (Inserm), Centre de Recherche Saint-Antoine, CRSA, Sorbonne Université, 75012 Paris, France; marie-v@neuf.fr (M.V.); aarbelaizcossio@gmail.com (A.A.); lynda.aoudjehane@gmail.com (L.A.); olivier.scatton@gmail.com (O.S.); m.gonzalezsanchez@idibell.cat (E.G.-S.); fatiha.merabtene@inserm.fr (F.M.); jrm.augustin@gmail.com (J.A.); chantal.housset@inserm.fr (C.H.)

2 LPP (Laboratoire de Physique des Plasmas, UMR 7648), Sorbonne Université, Centre National de la Recherche Scientifique (CNRS), Ecole Polytechnique, 75005 Paris, France; florian.judee@uca.fr (F.J.); henri.decauchy@sorbonne-universite.fr (H.D.)

3 TGF-β and Cancer Group, Oncobell Program, Bellvitge Biomedical Research Institute (IDIBELL), 08908 Barcelona, Spain

4 Oncology Program, CIBEREHD, National Biomedical Research Institute on Liver and Gastrointestinal Diseases, Instituto de Salud Carlos III, 28029 Madrid, Spain

5 Inserm, Institute of Cardiometabolism and Nutrition (ICAN), Sorbonne Université, 75013 Paris, France

6 Department of Hepatobiliary Surgery and Liver Transplantation, Pitié-Salpêtrière Hospital, Assistance Publique-Hôpitaux de Paris (AP-HP), 75013 Paris, France

7 Department of Hepatology, Reference Center for Inflammatory Biliary Diseases and Autoimmune Hepatitis (Centre de Référence Maladies Rares (CRMR), Maladies Inflammatoires des Voies Biliaires et Hépatites Auto-Immunes (MIVB-H), AP-HP, 75012 Paris, France

* Correspondence: jvaquero@idibell.cat (J.V.); thierry.dufour@sorbonne-universite.fr (T.D.); laura.fouassier@inserm.fr (L.F.)

† Co-senior authors.

Abstract: Through the last decade, cold atmospheric plasma (CAP) has emerged as an innovative therapeutic option for cancer treatment. Recently, we have set up a potentially safe atmospheric pressure plasma jet device that displays antitumoral properties in a preclinical model of cholangiocarcinoma (CCA), a rare and very aggressive cancer emerging from the biliary tree with few efficient treatments. In the present study, we aimed at deciphering the molecular mechanisms underlying the antitumor effects of CAP towards CCA in both an in vivo and in vitro context. In vivo, using subcutaneous xenografts into immunocompromised mice, CAP treatment of CCA induced DNA lesions and tumor cell apoptosis, as evaluated by 8-oxoguanine and cleaved caspase-3 immunohistochemistry, respectively. The analysis of the tumor microenvironment showed changes in markers related to macrophage polarization. In vitro, the incubation of CCA cells with CAP-treated culture media (i.e., plasma-activated media, PAM) led to a dose response decrease in cell survival. At molecular level, CAP treatment induced double-strand DNA breaks, followed by an increased phosphorylation and activation of the cell cycle master regulators CHK1 and p53, leading to cell cycle arrest and cell death by apoptosis. In conclusion, CAP is a novel therapeutic option to consider for CCA in the future.

Keywords: cholangiocarcinoma; cold plasma; innovative therapy; tumor cells; macrophages; plasma selectivity; plasma jet

1. Introduction

Cholangiocarcinoma (CCA) is a tumor of the biliary tree with poor prognosis that is characterized by a dense desmoplastic stroma [1]. CCA is a rare tumor. Currently, CCA accounts for 3% of all gastrointestinal cancers, but overall its incidence tends to increase worldwide. So far, surgical resection of the tumor is the only curative and effective therapeutic option. However, this cancer is usually diagnosed at advanced stage, so that this treatment is feasible in a small proportion of patients and recurrence is high. When tumor resection is not possible or when recurrence occurs, the therapeutic alternatives consist in palliative treatments based on chemotherapy regimens with poor results [2]. Hence, there is a need for new therapeutic approaches.

Cold atmospheric plasma (CAP) (named also non-thermal plasma or low temperature plasma) is a weakly ionized gas that is created by electrical discharges, composed of transient, energetic, and chemical active species (electrons, ions, metastables, radicals) that displays radiation, gas dynamics and electric field properties. Today, CAP interaction with biological systems (cells, tissues, tumors) is studied to address medical issues, such as blood clotting, wound healing, dentistry, repair surgery, cosmetics, infectious and inflammatory diseases, and oncology [3]. CAP science and technology appear as a new research avenue to provide breakthrough solutions where conventional therapies in cancer appear limited [3]. Indeed, plasmas can reduce the cell proliferation or tumor volume in preclinical mice models, in several types of cancers, including skin, pancreatic, bladder, and colon [4,5]. Therefore, plasmas have major potential in driving antitumor effects, notably in resistant tumors, such as CCA. The primary action of CAP is to generate long-lived molecules, such as reactive oxygen and nitrogen species (RONS), mainly from nitrogen and oxygen in atmospheric air or solution. This action can be either beneficial or deleterious on living tissues, depending on their concentrations. RONS are primarily responsible for the anti-tumor activity of CAP. They drive cell cycle arrest and cell death by damaging DNA and regulating cancer-relevant molecules, such as the tumor suppressor p53 [6,7].

To date, only two studies addressed the potential of CAP to treat liver tumors [5,8]. In these studies, CAP was tested on hepatocellular carcinoma cell lines and induced cell death. We previously engineered a new cold plasma jet device that showed significant antitumor effects in a mouse CCA model, without inducing toxic effects on heathy tissue, in order to investigate CAP as a potential new therapeutic option [9]. Here, we aim to gain insight into the molecular mechanisms by which CAP halts CCA development and progression in vivo and in vitro. In addition, we investigated whether CAP has an effect on non-tumoral cells notably hepatocytes, the parenchymal liver cells. Evidence was previously provided to indicate that CAP induced cell death selectively in tumor cells and not in non-malignant cells [3]. The tumor itself is a complex tissue structure, including cells of the tumor microenvironment, such as cancer-associated fibroblasts (CAF), endothelial cells (EC), and tumor-associated macrophages (TAM). Therefore, we also evaluated in vivo the impact of CAP on these cell populations.

2. Results

2.1. Cold Atmospheric Plasma Treatment Reduces Cholangiocarcinoma Progression in a Murine Xenograft Model

We previously compared two CAP generating devices, i.e., Plasma Gun (PG) and Plasma Tesla Jet (PTJ), showing that both devices were safe, but differed with respect to anticancer properties [9]. Only PTJ (Figure 1a) displayed a significant therapeutic efficacy in a subcutaneous xenograft model of CCA [9]. In the present study, we used the same model to further analyze the molecular mechanisms accounting for PTJ effects in the same preclinical model. In order to better assess the effect of CAP on CCA growth, we compared its effect with that of gemcitabine, one of the chemotherapeutic drugs currently used in CCA patient treatment.

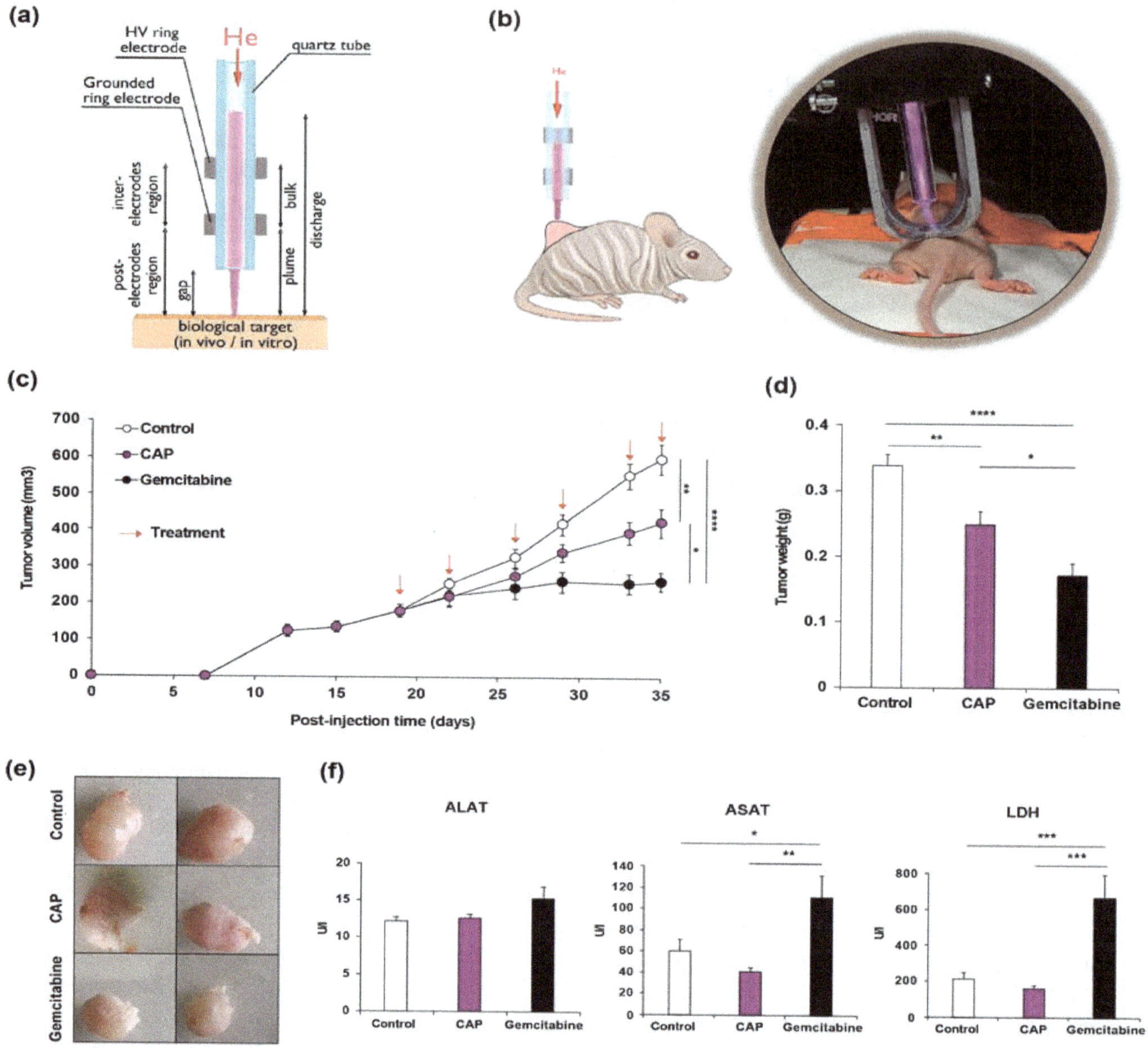

Figure 1. (**a**) Experimental setup of the Plasma Tesla Jet device (PTJ). (**b**) Schematic representation and representative image of the cold atmospheric plasma (CAP) application to subcutaneous xenograft cholangiocarcinoma (CCA) tumors. (**c**) Tumor volume of mice bearing CCA developed from EGI-1 cells treated with gemcitabine (120 mg/kg, black circles), CAP (1 min. at 9 kV of amplitude, frequency = 30 kHz, duty cycle = 14%, gap = 10 mm, purple circles) or untreated (control, white circles). Arrows indicate treatments points with CAP and gemcitabine. (**d**) Tumor weight at sacrifice (day 35). (**e**) Representative images of tumors from each group at sacrifice. (**f**) Plasmatic concentrations of alanine aminotransferase (ALAT), aspartate aminotransferase (ASAT) and lactate dehydrogenase (LDH). Values are expressed as means ± SEM. *, $p < 0.05$; **, $p < 0.01$; ***, $p < 0.001$; ****, $p < 0.0001$.

EGI-1 CCA cells were injected to induce tumors in the flank of immunodeficient mice and, once the tumors reached an arbitrary volume of 200 mm^3, we applied CAP directly on the tumors (Figure 1b) or we administrated gemcitabine by intraperitoneal injection twice a week for three weeks (see red arrows in Figure 1c). Animals were sacrificed 2 h after the last treatment. Tumor size and growth rate were significantly reduced after the application of CAP (Figure 1c–e) consistently with our previous results [9]. The well-established antitumoral effect of gemcitabine was evident and it exceeded that of CAP [10]. We measured the plasma concentrations of alanine aminotransferase (ALAT) and aspartate aminotransferase (ASAT) as well as lactate dehydrogenase (LDH) in treated mice to verify that local CAP treatment did not induce side effects in the whole organism. No significant difference of concentration was observed between CAP treated animals and controls (Figure 1f). By contrast, ASAT and LDH were significantly increased in the animals that received gemcitabine, indicating liver damage (Figure 1f). These results show the advantage of direct CAP treatment, which remains local over the systemic effects of gemcitabine, but also less toxic. If, at first sight, CAP might appear less efficient than gemcitabine, one has to underline that CAP exposure times were as low as 1 min., while the lifetime of gemcitabine injected in the organism is several hours.

2.2. *Cold Atmospheric Plasma Induces Apoptosis in Cholangiocarcinoma Cells In Vivo*

We performed a histological analysis of the tumors to further evaluate the effect of CAP on CCA xenografts. A deep analysis revealed the presence of purple round structures that represent calcifications (Figure 2a,b). These calcifications are often associated with apoptotic bodies and they may represent a late state of condensed apoptotic structures. The quantification showed an increased number of calcifications in tumors treated with CAP or gemcitabine when compared to the controls (Figure 2c).

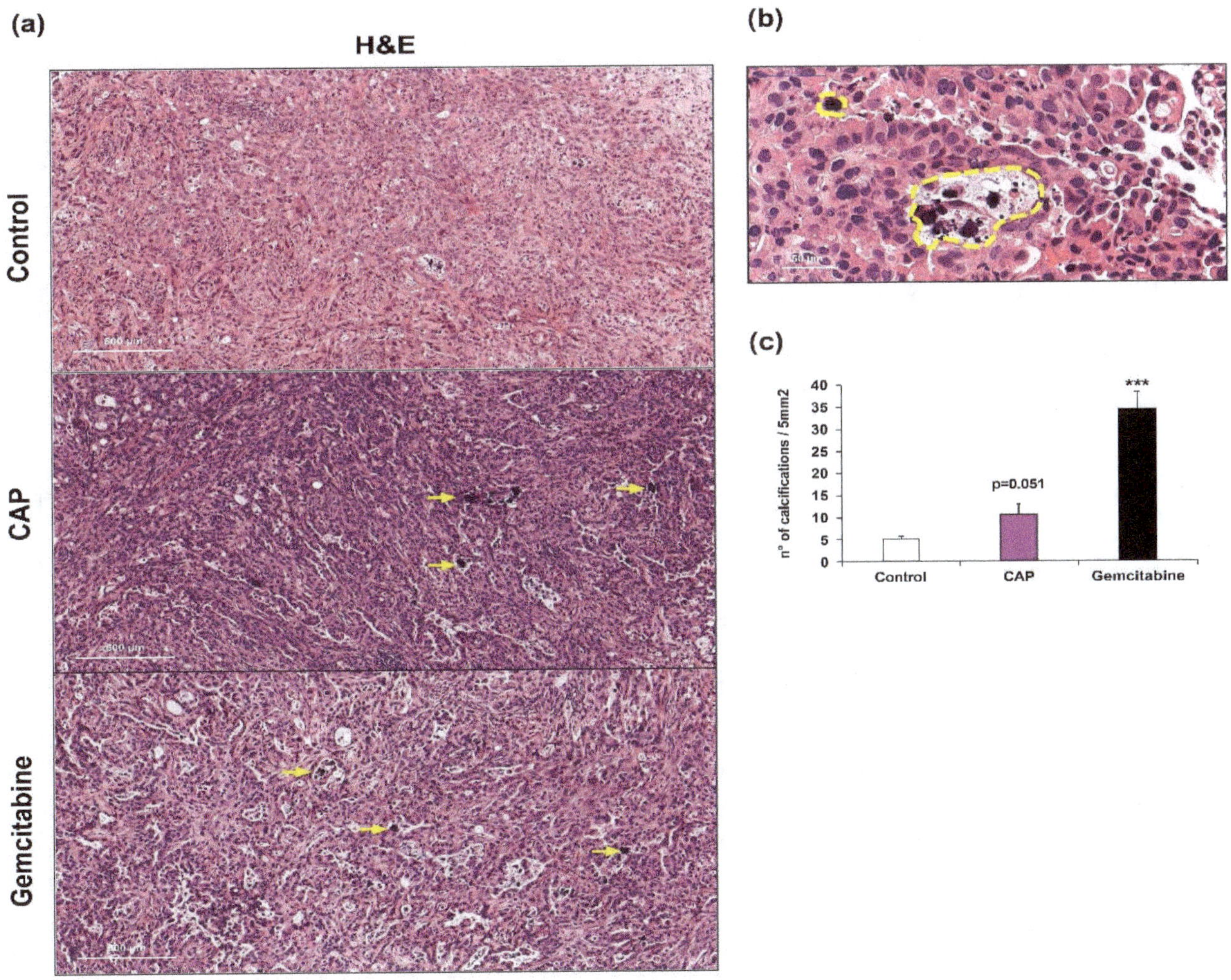

Figure 2. (**a**) Representative HE staining of control (upper panel), CAP (middle panel) and gemcitabine (bottom panel) treated xenograft tumors. Magnification ×125. Scale: 500 μm. (**b**) Magnification (×1000) of calcifications corresponding to apoptotic bodies (outlined in yellow). Scale: 50 μm. (**c**) Quantification of apoptotic structures. ***, $p < 0.001$; compared with control tumors.

The presence of these calcifications prompted us to study apoptosis, the main type of cell death related to CAP, by performing immunostaining against cleaved caspase-3 (cCaspase-3), a critical executioner of apoptosis that is responsible for the cleavage of many key proteins. Animals treated with CAP showed an intense staining of cCaspase-3 in some areas of the tumors when compared to the controls, as shown in Figure 3 (left panels). This staining was also present, but weaker in animals that received gemcitabine. These differences that can be explained by the time at which the animals were sacrificed, i.e., approximately 2 h after CAP or gemcitabine treatments. Since CAP is applied locally, its effects operate faster than drugs that are delivered intraperitoneally, such as gemcitabine. Indeed, this drug must be first absorbed and then transported to the tumors. In that latter case, the therapeutic effects of gemcitabine may be observed later than 2 h.

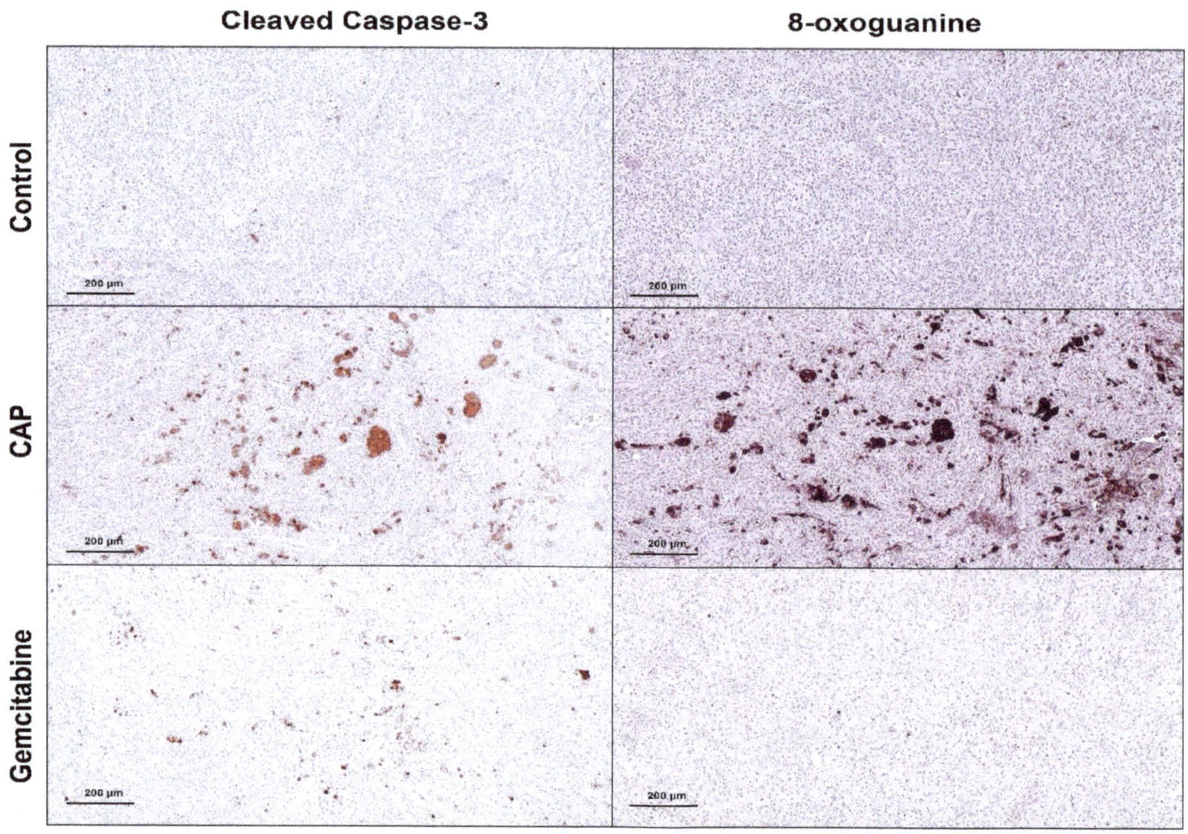

Figure 3. Representative IHC staining of cleaved caspase-3 and 8-oxoguanine in control (upper panel), CAP (middle panel) and gemcitabine (bottom panel) treated xenograft tumors. Magnification, ×250. Scale: 200 μm.

We evaluated the presence of cellular components altered as a result of reactive species overload, more specifically 8-oxoguanine, one of the major products of DNA oxidation, as an event that could unchain the signaling pathways leading to cell death by apoptosis, since one of the main effects of CAP is the production of RONS. CAP treatment was able to strongly induce DNA alterations, as shown in Figure 3 (right panels). In addition, it is worth noting that these alterations were colocalized with the areas positive for cleaved caspase-3 (left panels). This perfect overlapping enables us to bridge DNA damage with cell apoptosis. Interestingly, there was no staining of 8-oxoguanine in tumors from the group that received gemcitabine, showing that the main effects of this drug are not mediated by reactive species related molecular mechanisms.

2.3. *Cold Atmospheric Plasma Reduces Viability of Cholangiocarcinoma Cells but Not of Normal Hepatocytes In Vitro*

Next, we performed in vitro studies on CCA cell lines to further dissect the effects that are induced by CAP on tumor cells. First, we evaluated the effects of CAP treatment on the viability of two human CCA cell lines, EGI-1, the same cell line used for the induction of subcutaneous xenografts, and HuCCT1. Besides, to verify whether CAP treatment is biologically selective, non-malignant primary human hepatocytes, the main cell type in the liver, where isolated from patients. They were also exposed to the same CAP treatment to verify whether CAP might drive to side effects. We first treated by plasma a standard volume of fresh culture media (3 mL) in a standardized plastic support (6-well plates) for 3 min in order to standardize the application of CAP across the different in vitro experiments. Second, we incubated the resulting plasma-activated culture media (commonly called PAM) with either CCA cell lines or human hepatocytes in culture (Figure S1). Such indirect CAP treatment induced a decrease in the viability of CCA cells and this effect became stronger for CAP exposure times increasing from 1 to 10 min. (Figure 4a). In contrast, no effect was observed on the viability of human hepatocytes isolated from 3 different patients (Figure 4a), hence demonstrating a selective effect of CAP on tumor cells over non-malignant liver cells. Of note, similar experiments performed after exposure to gemcitabine showed a dose-dependent decrease in cell viability that was more pronounced in CCA cells, but reached an approximately 30% reduction in hepatocytes (Figure 4b), demonstrating a better selectivity of CAP over gemcitabine. We evaluated the production of RONS in media since CCA cell lines and primary hepatocytes need different culture media due to specific requirements of each cell type. More specifically, we determined the concentration of NO_2 and H_2O_2 in CAP-exposed culture media at different time points, the same used in cell viability studies. While the production of NO_2 remains overall the same over treatment time in both types of media (Figure 4c), production of H_2O_2, was approximately six times higher in hepatocyte media than in CCA media (Figure 4d). To get more insight on this issue we determined the generation of ROS in cell lysates from CCA cells and hepatocytes exposed to PAM. Interestingly, production of H_2O_2 was only increased in CCA cells exposed to PAM, while it remained unchanged in hepatocytes (Figure 4e). This observation led us to think about potential defense mechanisms protecting hepatocytes from ROS production, more specifically, ROS-scavenging enzymes. Indeed, further analysis revealed that the mRNA expression of several enzymes was strongly increased in hepatocytes when compared to both CCA cell lines (Figure 4f). Altogether, these results validate the selective effect of CAP-activated medium in CCA cells over hepatocytes.

2.4. *Cold Atmospheric Plasma Induces Cell Cycle Arrest and Apoptosis in Cholangiocarcinoma Cells*

CAP-derived RONS drive cell cycle arrest and cell death by damaging DNA, as previously underlined [6,7]. For the following experiments we used the IC50 from the viability assays (Figure 4a), corresponding to 3-min. treatment with CAP. Therefore, we evaluated the possibility of cell cycle arrest in our experimental conditions. Indeed, flow cytometry analysis of cell cycle distribution showed changes in the different phases (Figure 5). EGI-1 and HuCCT1 cells both experienced a decrease in the percentage of cells in G0/G1 phases and S, and an increase of the percentage of cells in G2/M phases.

The accumulation of cells in G2/M indicate that cells arrested the cell cycle at the G2/M DNA damage checkpoint, which serves to prevent cells with genomic DNA damage from entering the M phase. Therefore, our next step was to determine whether, as observed in vivo, CAP treatment could drive DNA damage in CCA cells in vitro. One of the most important proteins required for checkpoint-mediated cell cycle arrest and DNA repair following double-stranded DNA breaks is the histone H2AX. DNA damage that is caused by oxidative stress results in a rapid phosphorylation of H2AX (named γH2AX), which leads to the recruitment of several proteins in response to DNA damage. Immunofluorescence analysis showed a strong staining of phospho-histone H2AX in both EGI-1 and HuCCT1 cells at different times (i.e., 24 h, 48 h and 72 h) after exposure to CAP-activated culture medium compared to untreated cells (Figure 6a,d), being 72 h in EGI-1 and 48 h in HuCCT1 cells, the highest signal, as ascertained by western blot (Figure 6b,c,e,f and Figures S3–S10). Western blot analyses showed a clear correlation between the increase of histone H2AX phosphorylation and PARP cleavage (Figure 6b–e and Figures S3–S10), a marker of cell apoptosis.

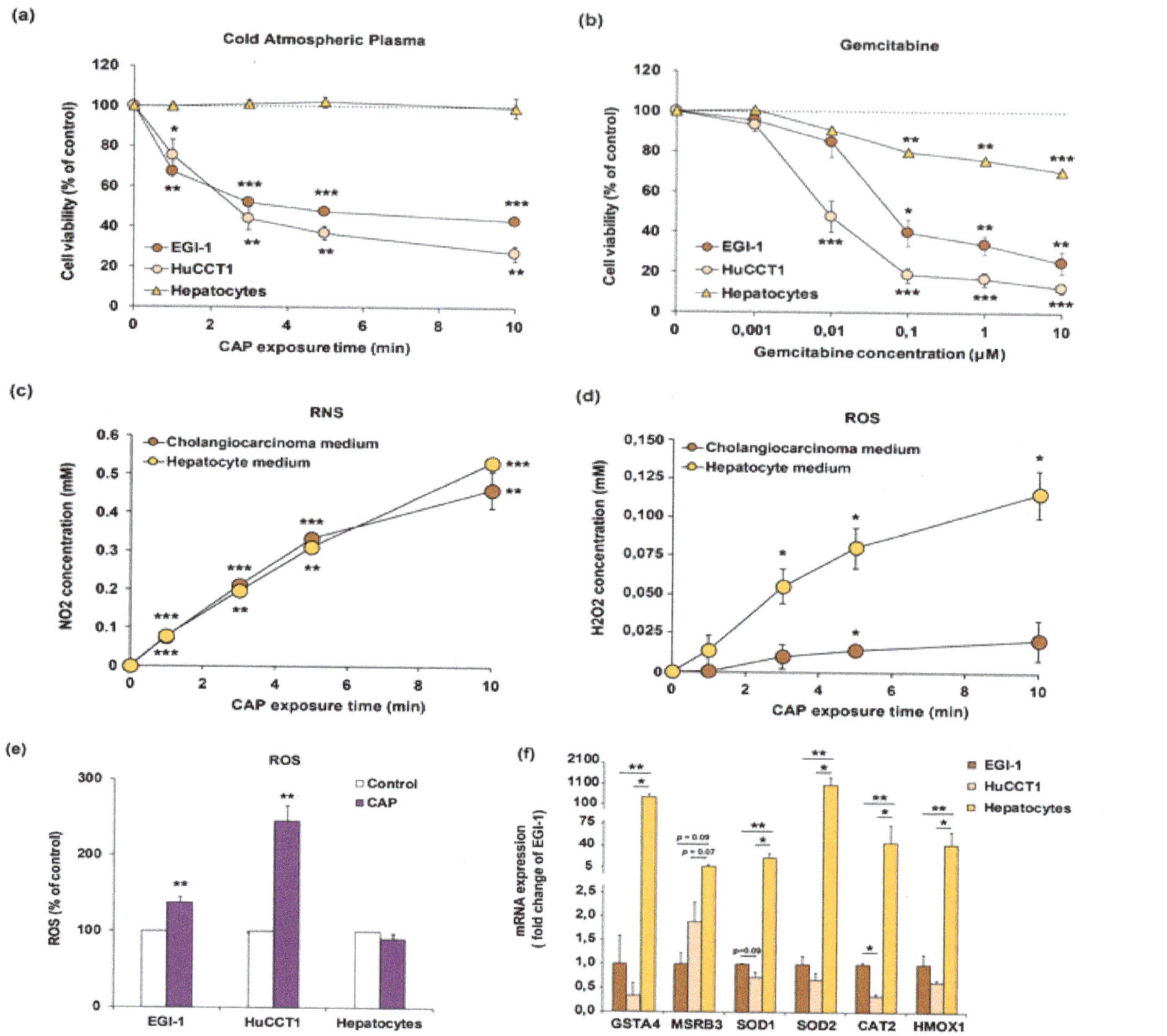

Figure 4. (**a**,**b**) Effect of CAP (**a**) and gemcitabine (**b**) on the viability of EGI-1 and HuCCT1 CCA cells and human primary hepatocytes. Cell viability was measured after incubation for 72 h with culture medium previously treated for 1, 3, 5, and 10 min. with CAP (9 kV, 30 kHz, 14%, gap of 7 mm). (**c**,**d**) NO_2 (**c**) and H_2O_2 (**d**) determination in culture media from CCA cells and primary hepatocytes. (**e**) H_2O_2 determination in cell lysates from CCA cells and primary hepatocytes exposed to PAM for 3 min. (**f**) Expression of GSTA4, MSRB3, SOD1, SOD2, CAT2, and HMOX1 at mRNA level in CCA cell and hepatocytes. Values are expressed as means ± SEM from at least three independent cultures. *, $p < 0.05$; **, $p < 0.01$; ***, $p < 0.001$; compared with untreated cells (0 min.).

We evaluated the activation of the two parallel signaling pathways that ultimately break the cell cycle once the DNA damage is sensed to better decipher the mechanism of cell cycle arrest in CCA cells treated with CAP. These signaling cascades that block the progression to mitosis are led by CHK kinases and p53, respectively. Western blot analysis from Figure 7b,c,e,f showed a strong phosphorylation of both CHK1 and p53 from 24 h to 72 h in both cell lines. These results suggest that the cell cycle is arrested soon after CAP-activated culture medium exposure, when DNA damage is first detected, but apoptosis is not induced until the accumulation of DNA damage is strong enough, which is 72 h after exposure to CAP in EGI-1 and 48 h in HuCCT1 cells. Interestingly, CAP exposure of hepatocytes showed a reduced expression of CHK1 and p53 when compared to CCA cells (Figures S2a and S11), probably due to the low proliferative capacity of these cells in primary culture. Additionally, no changes in H2AX phosphorylation or PARP cleavage were observed, indicating the absence of DNA damage and corroborating the selective capacity of CAP in hepatocytes (Figures S2a and S11).

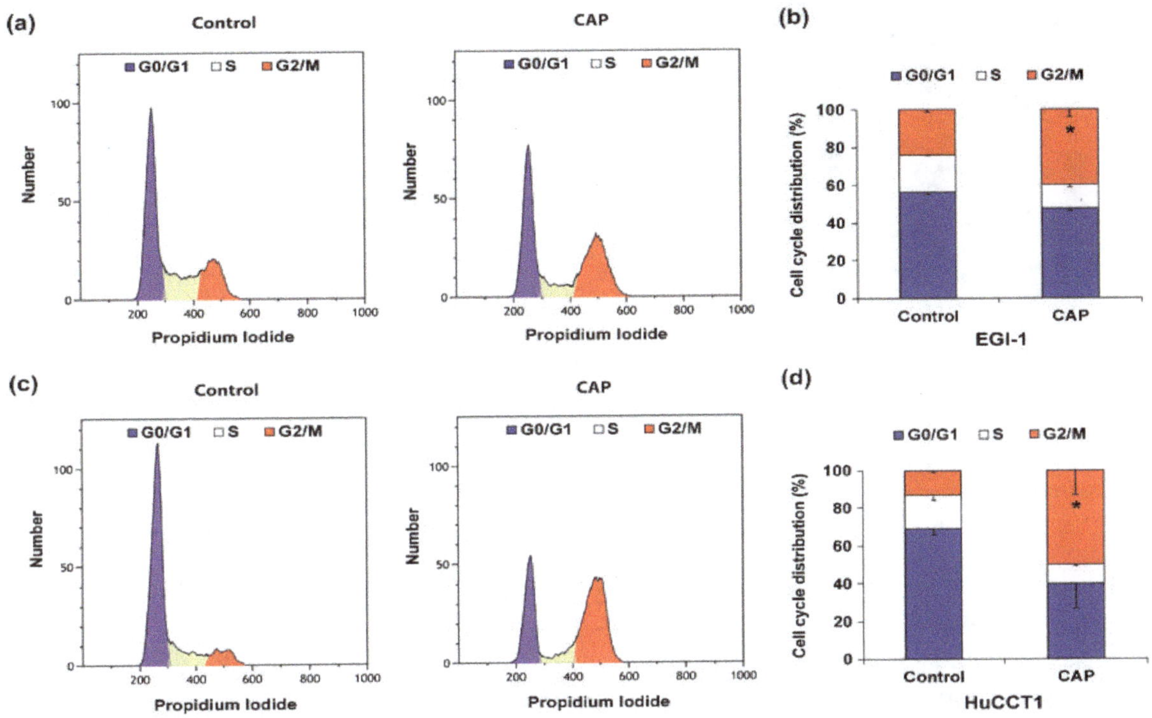

Figure 5. (**a**–**d**) Representative flow cytometry cell cycle measurement (**a**,**c**) and graphical representation of the cell cycle distribution (**b**,**d**) of EGI-1 (**a**,**b**) and HuCCT1 (**c**,**d**) CCA cells after 24 h of exposure to culture medium pretreated with CAP for 3 min. (9 kV, 30 kHz, 14%, gap of 7 mm). Cell populations in G0/G1, S, and G2/M phases are given as percentage of total cells. Values are expressed as means ± SEM from at least three independent cultures. *, $p < 0.05$; as compared with control cells.

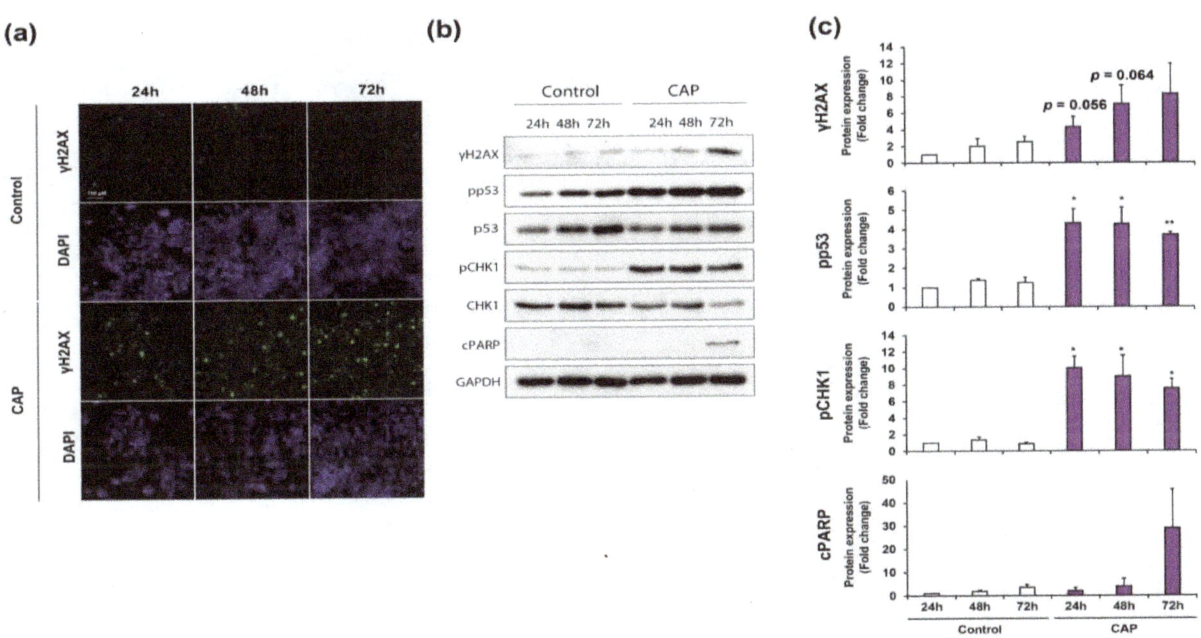

Figure 6. *Cont.*

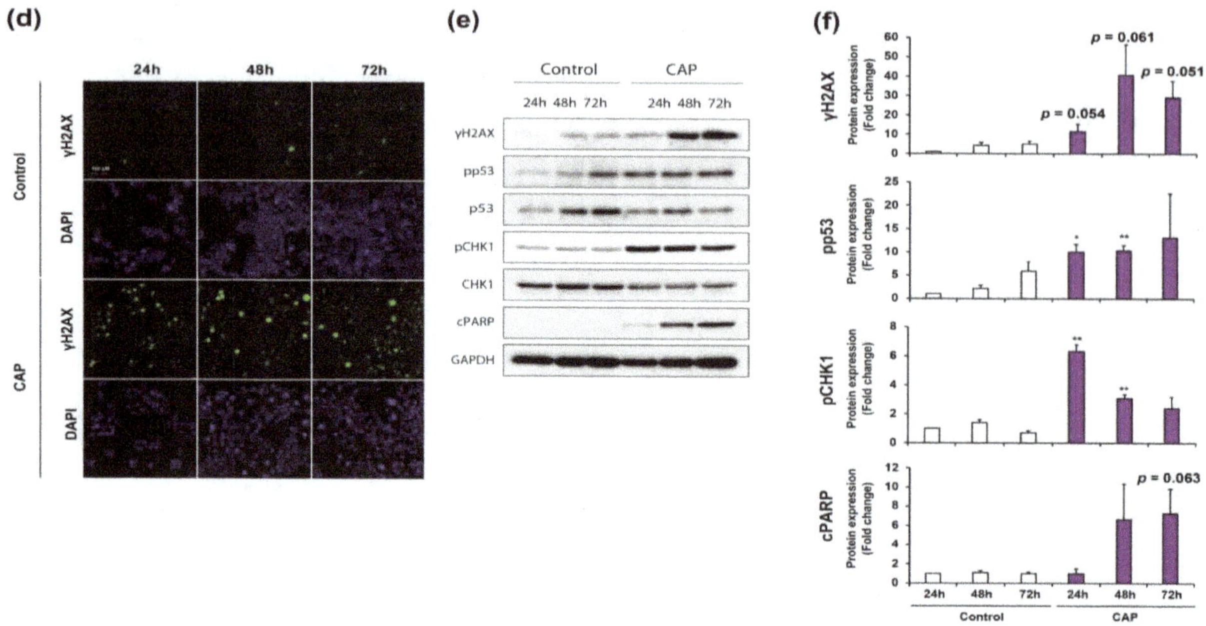

Figure 6. (**a**,**d**) Representative images of phosphorylated H2AX (γH2AX) analyzed by immunofluorescence in EGI-1 (**a**) and HuCCT1 (**d**) CCA cells after 24 h, 48 h and 72 h of exposure to culture medium pretreated with CAP for 3 min. (9 kV, 30 kHz, 14%, gap of 7 mm). Magnification, ×10. (**b**,**e**) Representative images of western blot analysis of cleaved PARP, phosphorylated and total p53, phosphorylated and total CHK1 and phosphorylated H2AX in EGI-1 (**b**) and HuCCT1 (**e**) cells treated in the same conditions. (**c**,**f**) Densitometry analysis of western blot from cleaved PARP, phosphorylated p53, phosphorylated CHK1, and phosphorylated H2AX. Values are expressed as means ± SEM from three independent cultures. *, $p < 0.05$; **, $p < 0.01$; compared with control cells.

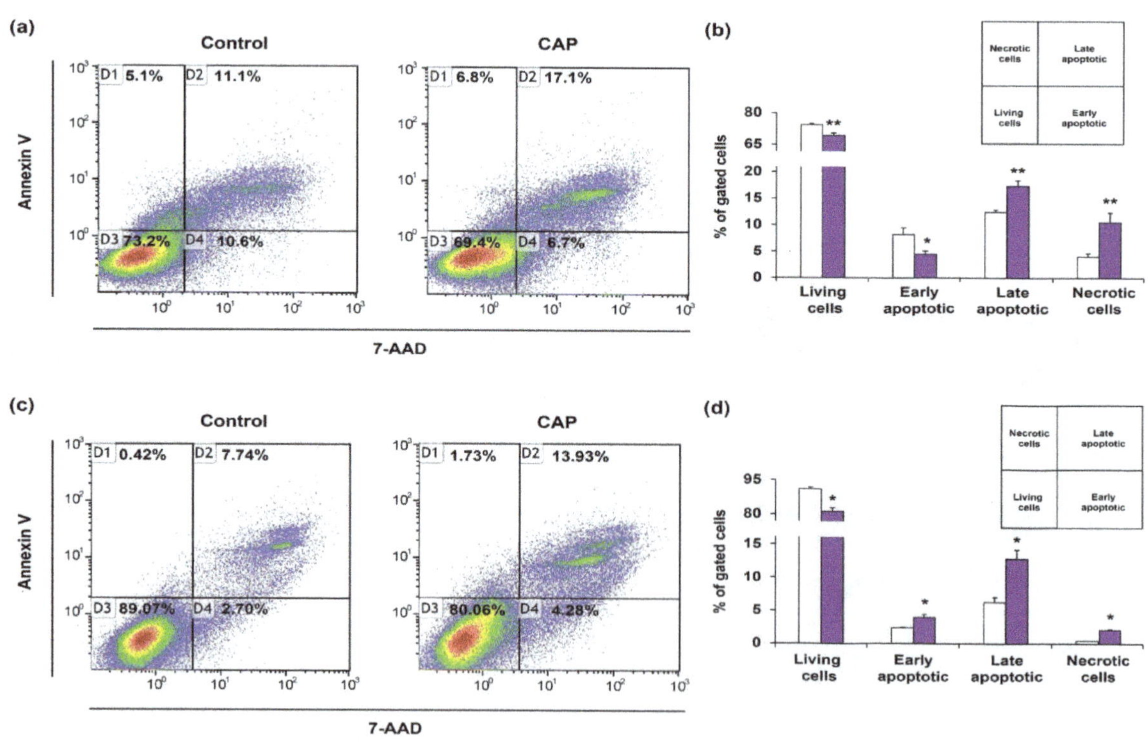

Figure 7. (**a–d**) Representative images (**a**,**c**) and quantification (**b**,**d**) of apoptosis by flow cytometry analysis of Annexin V/7AAD in EGI-1 (**a**,**b**) and HuCCT1 (**c**,**d**) CCA cells after 48 h of exposure to PAM for 3 min. (9 kV, 30 kHz, 14%, gap of 7 mm). Values are expressed as means ± SEM from at least three independent cultures. *, $p < 0.05$; **, $p < 0.01$; compared with control condition.

When these experiments were reproduced after exposure to gemcitabine, we observed similar results in terms of increase of H2AX, CHK1, and p53 phosphorylation, accompanied by PARP cleavage in both CCA cell lines (Figures S2b, S12 and S13). Interestingly, gemcitabine induces DNA damage in hepatocytes in a dose dependent manner (Figures S2c and S14), concordant with the decrease in viability that is observed in Figure 4b, and this DNA damage started as early as 24 h after exposure and was maintained until 72 h, as ascertained by H2AX phosphorylation (Figures S2d and S15). However, no change was observed in the phosphorylation of CHK1 and p53 or PARP cleavage, indicating that the reduction in hepatocyte viability induced by gemcitabine might not be related to cell cycle arrest and apoptosis, but other types of dead, such as necrosis or senescence.

Finally, we verified that the decrease in cell viability of EGI-1 and HuCCT1 after CAP treatment was due to apoptosis. Indeed, the exposure of cells to PAM reduces the number of viable cells and increases the populations in the quadrants corresponding to late-apoptotic and necrotic cells in both cell types (Figure 7a–d), as ascertained by Annexin V-7AAD quantification by flow cytometry. Of note, this increase in apoptotic cells was observed in HuCCT1 at 48 h, but it was not in EGI-1 at this time, only becoming evident at 72 h in the later. These results may corroborate that apoptosis is not induced until the accumulation of DNA damage is strong enough, that is 72 h after exposure to PAM in EGI-1 and 48 h in HuCCT1 cells.

2.5. Cold Atmospheric Plasma Affects the Phenotype of Tumor-Associated Macrophage

Besides the effects of CAP on tumor cells, we sought to determine whether CAP exposure might have any effect on the stroma of the EGI-1 subcutaneous xenograft model. This model has the advantage of providing the opportunity of evaluating the expression of human genes, corresponding to the injected tumor CCA cells, and murine genes, corresponding to the cells forming the stroma that are recruited by cancer cells during tumor formation. Therefore, we examined the mRNA expression of different specific markers corresponding to cancer-associated fibroblasts (CAF) (*Acta2*, coding alpha-SMA), endothelial cells (EC) (*Pecam1*, coding for CD31), and tumor-associated macrophages (TAM) (*Adgre1*, coding for F4/80). There were no significant changes in the mRNA of *Acta2* or *Pecam1* among the different groups (Figure 8a). However, the expression of *Adgre1* increased in the tumors from the animals that received CAP or gemcitabine treatment when compared to the controls, suggesting a potential enhanced recruitment and/or proliferation of TAM in the treated tumors (Figure 8a). The presence of TAM in tumor from the different groups was evidenced by immunohistochemical analyses of F4/80, as shown in representative images from each group (Figure 8b), although it was impossible to properly determine the differences in macrophage infiltration by F4/80 IHC quantification. However, we decided to perform a preliminary analysis to elucidate this point based on previous publications indicating a phenotypic change of macrophages in absence of changes in the total number of these cells after exposure to experimental therapies [11]. Analysis of *Ccl2* (coding for Monocyte chemotactic protein-1, MCP-1) and *Ccr2*, a chemokine and its receptor, respectively, which are major regulators of monocyte chemotaxis and macrophage trafficking, showed an increased expression in groups that were treated with CAP and gemcitabine when compared to the controls (Figure 8c), which might suggest changes in chemotactic response of resident TAM. In addition, CAP was able to increase the expression of several cytokines that are associated with the antitumor phenotype of macrophages and that are involved in the induction of apoptosis, i.e., *Tnfa* (coding for Tnfα), *Tnfsf1* (coding for TNF-related apoptosis-inducing ligand (Trail)) and *Il1b* (coding for Il1β) (Figure 8d). These results are in accordance with previous publications that link CAP treatment with the modulation of immune cells and together with the increasing interest of immunotherapies as cancer treatment validate the need for further investigation on this topic in CCA.

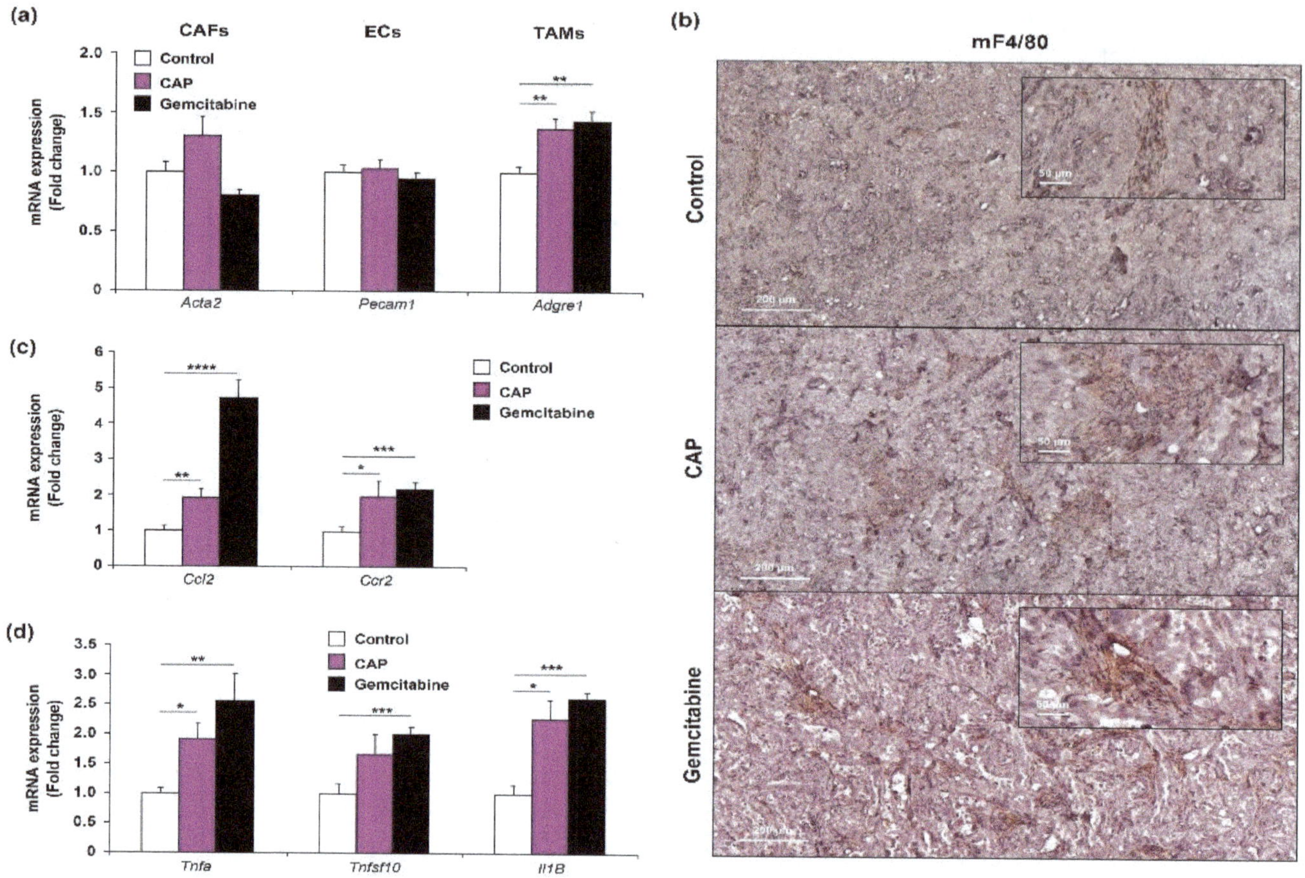

Figure 8. (**a**) Changes in mRNA expression of cell type markers (*Acta2*/α-SMA, a marker of cancer-associated fibroblasts CAFs, *Pecam1*/CD31, a marker of endothelial cells (EC) and *Adgre1*/F4/80, a marker of tumor-associated macrophages (TAM) in control (white bars), CAP (purple bars) and gemcitabine (black bars) treated xenograft tumors. (**c**) Representative IHC staining of F4/80 in the same tumors. Magnification ×250 (inserts ×1000). Scale: 200 μm. (**b**) Changes in mRNA expression of *Ccl2*/Mcp1 and *Ccr2* (c) in control (white bars), CAP (purple bars) and gemcitabine (black bars) treated xenograft tumors. (**d**) Changes in mRNA expression of pro-apoptotic cytokines (*Tnfa*/Tnfα, *Tnfsf1*/Trail and *Il1b*/Il1β) in control (white bars), CAP (purple bars), and gemcitabine (black bars) treated xenograft tumors. Values are expressed as means ± SEM. *, $p < 0.05$; **, $p < 0.01$; ***, $p < 0.001$; ****, $p < 0.0001$; compared with control tumors.

3. Discussion

In the present work, we analyzed the effects of CAP in vivo in a mouse xenograft model of CCA and in vitro on human CCA cell lines, as well as on non-malignant human hepatocytes. We found that local application of CAP on the tumor halts its growth without inducing systemic side effects. The analysis of tumors showed areas of calcification suggesting cell dead, which was confirmed by immunostaining of cleaved-caspase-3, a protein of the apoptotic pathway, along with DNA lesions due to plasma-originated reactive species. In vitro, CAP-activated medium contains reactive species (e.g., nitrites) that induced oxidative stress and reduced cell survival by arresting the cell cycle and inducing apoptosis in CCA cells but not in hepatocytes. Finally, preliminary analysis suggested changes in the surrounding stroma of CCA tumors after exposure to CAP.

Since the early 2000s, CAP have generated a lot of interest in cancer medicine as a promising treatment for cancer without inducing systemic toxic side effect. The anti-tumor properties of CAP are now well established and tumor volume reductions have been demonstrated in murine tumor models of several cancer types, including pancreatic [12,13], ovary [14], breast [15] and colon [16], melanoma [17], and glioblastoma [6,18]. We investigated if CAP might drive to anti-cancer effects in vivo since CCA is a very aggressive tumor with a limited therapeutic arsenal. We conducted further studies to decipher in a deeper way the cellular mechanisms behind CAP effect based on our previous work that aimed to set up a safe device with anti-tumor properties in CCA [9]. Up to date, the only two studies dealing with the effects of CAP on liver cancer were performed in hepatocellular carcinoma cell lines [5,8]. Thus, this study is the first conducted on CCA while using in vivo and in vitro preclinical models.

Only 5% of the studies published so far include in vivo experiments, owing to the emerging and highly multidisciplinary aspects of "cold plasma oncology" [19]. Most CAP studies in cancer have been achieved while using tumor cell lines originating from either solid or blood tumors and rarely on mouse tumor models. We conducted in vivo studies to analyze the effects of CAP on death and oxidative stress, and we compared this treatment to conventional treatment with gemcitabine. In our study, CAP demonstrated anti-tumor properties although a traditional chemotherapeutic agent such as gemcitabine showed higher efficiency. Interestingly, CAP was locally applied on a very small tumor surface for a very short period of time (1 min) demonstrating no side effects, while gemcitabine, which was applied intraperitoneally, was accompanied by an increased plasmatic concentration of markers indicating liver damage. Even if few studies have been performed in vivo, some of them confirmed that CAP has no systemic effects. Liedtle et al. have addressed this point through a complete study showing that CAP by using plasma-activated medium does not affect blood parameters, leucocyte distribution, or cytokine signature [20]. However, classical blood parameters to evaluate liver and cell toxicity, such as transaminases and LDH, were not measured, in contrast to our study. Studies using orthotopic CCA model are required to evaluate the direct effect of CAP on liver parenchyma in spite of our in vitro observation on primary hepatocytes and the absence of liver damage in vivo. Nevertheless, further investigation to improve the surface exposure and the time of treatment with CAP is crucial in order to obtain the maximum benefit from this new therapeutic tool.

At the cellular level, histology examination of the tumor showed signs of calcification, a reaction occurring in response to cell injury, indicating the presence of apoptotic tissue. The activation of signaling pathways involved in cell death was confirmed by the immunohistochemical analysis of cleaved caspase-3, suggesting an induction of caspase-3-dependent apoptosis in tumor cells. The induction of cell apoptosis is the primary mechanism of CAP action following the reactive species generated by CAP [19]. However, other cell death pathways have been recently evidenced, such as ferroptosis in tumor cells subjected to CAP treatment [21]. In CCA cell lines, we tested cell media that were first treated by CAP, i.e., PAM. Subsequently, PAM was immediately transferred to the cell culture. Indirect or direct treatment by CAP displays similar efficacy on tumor cell culture, and PAM is also able to reduce tumor burden without inducing side effects when injected intraperitoneally in a murine model of pancreatic cancer [20]. The intraperitoneal injection of PAM lead to reduced metastatic potential of ovarian and gastric cancer cells [22,23]. When we evaluated PAM on CCA cells, although PAM decreased cell survival in both CCA cell lines with similar efficacy, induction of apoptosis was lower in EGI-1 than in the HuCCT1 cells. Doses of CAP used to treat the medium matters and, as suggested in previous studies, low doses of CAP can inhibit cell proliferation without inducing apoptosis, but instead induce senescence [24,25] or autophagy [26,27]. In addition, CAP can affect other cell biology features, for example by inducing endoplasmic reticulum stress, depolarization of mitochondrial membrane potential, DNA damage, or by decreasing migratory and invasive properties [22,28,29], although these aspects deserve further characterization in CCA.

At the molecular level, we detected DNA double strand breaks in both CCA cell lines, along with DNA damage responses with an upregulation of the phosphorylation status of p53 and of CHK1, both regulating cell cycle checkpoints. We previously observed similar DNA damage in CCA cells that were subjected to oxidative stress with hydrogen peroxide [30], suggesting that, upon CAP treatment, CCA cells may undergo oxidative stress. The overload of RONS in CCA cells leads to DNA damage, attested by the phosphorylation of histone H2AX, triggering pathways that will ultimately kill the cancer cells [31]. Altogether, these results fit perfectly with previous finding in other tumors, such as oral cancer, were p53 signaling pathway was identified as one of the most deregulated pathways after exposure to PAM by using RNA-sequencing approaches [32].

Specifically targeting tumor cells without damaging healthy cells is a major challenge of anti-cancer treatment. CAP has the advantage to selectively induce cell cycle arrest and death of tumor cells, but not of healthy ones. Whatever the direct/indirect approach, the concept of plasma selectivity is a key issue in treatment. Pioneering studies from Babington et al. have shown that the plasma treatment of mice bearing subcutaneous glioblastoma led to a 56% decrease of tumor volume while maintaining the viability of healthy cells surrounding the tumor at 85% [33]. While CAP had a significant effect on CCA cancer cells by decreasing cell viability, it had no deleterious effect on non-malignant liver cells, i.e., primary human hepatocytes, suggesting a selectivity of CAP treatment. By killing primarily cancer cells, plasma treatment preserves healthy tissue and thereby tissue function. Keidar et al. were amongst the first to demonstrate a selectivity of CAP on the lung cancer cell lines vs. normal human bronchial epithelial cells [34]. This selectivity was also emphasized in melanoma cells compared to normal keratinocytes [35], and other cancer types (ovarian, glioblastoma), as a general property of CAP [36]. However, all of these studies deal with cell lines, but none with primary cells. In our studies, hepatocytes were isolated from human liver and cultured according to a well-defined protocol [37]. We found that CAP has no impact on hepatocyte survival or the induction of DNA damage or apoptotic regulatory signaling pathways, in contrast to CCA cell lines. We chose hepatocytes as non-tumor cells, because they are the most abundant cell type of the liver. Although the media composition, an essential parameter [36], was not the same between the two cell types, CAP generated the same profile of RNS in both media and higher ROS in hepatocyte media. Furthermore, hydrogen peroxide increased in CCA cell lines after exposure to PAM, as previously described for atmospheric pressure plasma jets [38], while it remained unchanged in hepatocytes. The cellular mechanisms by which CAP operates this selectivity are still poorly understood and indirect evidence exists to explain this crucial issue. Among the potential mechanisms given so far, aquaporins and anti-oxidant cellular defense systems seem to be the most plausible explanations [4]. Indeed, as happened in our study, elevated expression of ROS-scavenging enzymes, such as superoxide dismutase, catalase, and glutathione reductase, has been observed in healthy cells as compared to tumor cells, which might contribute to cellular defense against CAP-originated reactive species [4].

Finally, one major point that should be considered when CAP treats a tumor is its potential effect on the tumor microenvironment cells. Tumor is a mix of several cell types, including tumor cells, but also CAF, EC, and TAM. According to histological examination of CCA tumors treated with CAP, fibrotic stroma is not affected by CAP treatment, a result that is confirmed by unchanged mRNA expression level of a-SMA, a marker of CAF, between the treated and untreated conditions. As previously shown, fibroblasts are less affected by CAP when compared to cancer cells [20,39]. No obvious change in vascularization is observed, even if plasma has been shown to suppress neovascularization, but not pre-existing vessels, an effect that is partly independent of ROS [40]. Further studies must be conducted in the case of CCA to confirm or not a potential action of CAP on vascular system. Interestingly, one of the most promising views is that CAP treatment is able to activate the immune response in order to attack the tumor [16,41,42]. Indeed, our analysis on tumor xenografts showed changes in the expression of markers related to the TAM phenotype, suggesting a potential shift towards an anti-tumor phenotype of TAM, although this issue deserves further consideration and new research will be undertaken. In vitro studies performed by other groups are in agreement with our findings in vivo, suggesting that increasing the function of pro-inflammatory macrophages might help to control tumorigenesis that is caused by compromised immune response [41]. Taking into account that one of the most therapeutic strategies under study nowadays is the activation of the patient immune system to fight tumors, it is imperative to keep deepening the molecular mechanisms implicated in the effects of CAP on the immune system, especially in immunocompetent murine cancer models, in which not only macrophages, but also lymphocytes, could be potentially involved in this response.

4. Materials and Methods

4.1. Cell Culture and Treatment

HuCCT1 cells, which were derived from intrahepatic biliary tract, were kindly provided by Dr. G. Gores (Mayo Clinic, Rochester, MN, USA). EGI-1 cells, derived from extrahepatic biliary tract, were obtained from the German Collection of Microorganisms and Cell Cultures (DSMZ, Braunschweig, Germany). The cells were cultured in DMEM supplemented with 1 g/L glucose, 10 mmol/L HEPES, 10% fetal bovine serum (FBS), antibiotics (100 UI/mL penicillin and 100 mg/mL streptomycin), and antimycotic (0.25 mg/mL amphotericin B). Cell lines were routinely screened for the presence of mycoplasma and authenticated for polymorphic markers in order to prevent cross-contamination.

4.2. Isolation and Culture of Human Hepatocytes

Normal liver tissue was obtained from adult patients undergoing partial hepatectomy for the treatment of colorectal cancer metastases. Primary human hepatocyte isolation was performed on the ICAN Human HepCell platform, as previously described [43]. Ethical approval for the isolation of human hepatocytes was granted by the Persons Protection Committee (CPP Ile de France III) and by the French Ministry of Health (N°: COL 2929 and COL 2930). Hepatocytes were isolated while using an established two-step-perfusion protocol with collagenase. First, the tissue was rinsed with pre-warmed (37 °C) calcium-free buffer that was supplemented with 5 mmol/L ethylene glycol tetraacetic acid (Sigma, Saint-Quentin Fallavier, France). Subsequently, the liver sample was perfused with recirculating perfusion solution containing 5 mg/mL of collagenase (Sigma) at 37 °C. Afterwards, the tissue was transferred into a petri dish containing a Hepatocyte Wash Medium (Life technologies, Villebon sur Yvette, France). Tissue was mechanically disrupted by shaking and using tweezers to disrupt cells from the remaining scaffold structures. Cellular suspension was filtered through a gauze-lined funnel. The cells were centrifuged at low speed centrifugation (50 g). The supernatant was removed, and pelleted hepatocytes were re-suspended in Hepatocyte Wash Medium. Viability cell was determined by trypan blue exclusion test. Freshly isolated normal hepatocytes were suspended in Williams' medium E (Life Technologies) containing 10% fetal calf serum (FCS) (Eurobio, Courtaboeuf, France), penicillin-streptomycin (penicillin: 200 U/mL; streptomycin: 200 μg/mL), and insulin (0.1 U/mL). Afterwards, the cells were seeded in 6- and 96-well plates that were pre-coated with type I collagen at a density of 1.8×10^6 and 0.5×10^5 viable cells/well, respectively, and then incubated at 37 °C in a 5% CO_2 overnight. Then, the medium was replaced with fresh complete hepatocyte medium that was supplemented with 1 μmol/L hydrocortisone hemisuccinate (SERB, Paris, France) and the cells were left in this medium until treatment with plasma activated medium (PAM).

4.3. Xenograft Tumor Model

Animal experiments were performed in accordance with the French Animal Research Committee guidelines and a local ethic committee approved all of the procedures (No 10609). 2×10^6 of EGI-1 cells were suspended in 60 μL of PBS and 60 μL of Matrigel® growth factor reduced (Corning) and implanted subcutaneously into the flank of five-week-old female ATHYM-Foxn1 nu/nu mice (Janvier Labs, Le Genest-Saint-Isle, France). Mice were housed under standard conditions in individually ventilated cages enriched with a nesting material and kept at 22 °C on a 12 h light/12 h dark cycle with ad libitum access to food and tap water. Tumor growth was monitored by measuring every 2–3 days the tumor volume (V xenograft) with a caliper, as follows: V xenograft = $x \times y^2/2$ where x and y are the longest and shortest lateral diameters, respectively. Once the tumor volume reached approximately 200 mm^3, CAP and gemcitabine treatments were initiated. Gemcitabine was administered every Monday and Thursday during three weeks by intraperitoneal injection at a concentration of 120 mg/kg dissolved in saline solution (vehicle). Cold atmospheric plasma was administered, as explained in Section 4.4, the same days as gemcitabine.

4.4. Cold Atmospheric Plasma Treatment

The in vivo and the in vitro experiments were conducted while using the same atmospheric pressure plasma jet device, called PTJ, as sketched in Figure 1a. It is composed of a 10 cm long dielectric quartz tube presenting a 4 mm inner diameter and a 2 mm wall thickness. Its electrode configuration is made of two outer ring electrodes with inner and outer diameters of 8 mm and 12.8 mm, respectively, while the inter-ring distance is 50 mm. For all experiments, the lower ring electrode was connected to the ground, while the upper ring electrode was biased to the high voltage. The PTJ was supplied with helium gas (flow rate of 1 slm) and powered with a nanopulse high voltage generator device (model Nanogen 1) from RLC Electronic Company. For both in vivo and in vitro experiments, electrical parameters were fixed, as follows: 9 kV of amplitude, 14% of duty cycle, and 30 kHz of repetition frequency. The reasons explaining how these values were chosen as well as the physico-chemical characterizations of the PTJ device have already been published in [9]. For the in vivo studies, the cold atmospheric plasma was applied to the animals, as previously described [9], 9 kV, 30 kHz, 14%, maintaining a gap of 10 mm between the tube and the skin. For the in vitro studies, the cells were treated with PAM. In order to maintain reproducibility among different plastic supports, 3 mL of the corresponding culture media in a 6-well plate were treated with the same conditions (9 kV, 30 kHz, 14%) during 1, 3, 5, or 10 min. A gap of 7 mm between the tube and the surface of medium was constantly maintained. After treatments, PAM was transferred to 96-, 24-, or 6-well plates, according to the different analysis performed (Figure S1).

4.5. Biochemistry

The concentrations of alanine aminotransferase (ALAT), aspartate aminotransferase (ASAT), and lactate dehydrogenase (LDH) in the plasma of mice were measured on an Olympus AU400 Analyzer.

4.6. Histology and (Immuno)Histochemistry

Formalin-fixed paraffin-embedded tissue samples from mice xenografts were cut in 4 μm sections, deparaffined, and stained with hematoxylin and eosin to observe tissue histology.

For immunohistochemistry, the antigens were unmasked, as indicated in Table 1. For cleaved -caspase-3 and 8-oxoguanine, the sections were sequentially incubated with H_2O_2 for 5 min. (only for caspase3), with Protein Block (Novolink Polymer Detection System; Novocastra Laboratories Ltd., Nanterre, France) for 5 min., and with primary antibodies for 30 min. (overnight for 8-oxoguanine). Novolink Post Primary was applied for 15 min. The sections were finally washed and incubated with Novolink Polymer for 15 min. An automated staining system (Autostainer Plus, Dakocytomation, Les Ulis, France) was used to perform immunostaining. The color was developed while using amino-ethyl-carbazole (AEC peroxidase substrate kit; Vector Laboratories, Le Perray-en-Yvelines, France). The sections were counterstained with hematoxylin and then mounted with glycergel (Dako). For F4/80 immunostaining, sections were incubated with PBS 0.5% triton X-100 30 min. to increase the permeabilization of the tissue. Subsequently, they were blocked with horse serum 2.5% (Vector) during 1 h. After tissue blocking, the samples were immunostained with primary antibody overnight at 4 °C. Afterwards, endogenous peroxidase blocking was performed with hydrogen peroxide solution (Leica) during 1 h. The samples were developed with the ImPRESS Excel staining kit (Vector) following manufacturer instruction. Briefly, the tissue samples were incubated with anti-rabbit Ig secondary antibody for 90 min washed with PBS, and then incubated with an anti-goat amplifier antibody for 1 h. Finally, the samples were developed with peroxidase substrate for 3 min. and counterstained with Mayer's hematoxylin (Dako) for 5 min.

Table 1. Primary antibodies used for immunodetection.

Name	Species	Manufacturer	Reference	Dilution	Antigen Unmasking
8-oxoguanine	M	Abcam	ab206461	1/100 (IHC)	EDTA pH8
cCaspase3	R	CST	CST9664	1/100 (IHC)	Citrate pH6
cPARP	R	CST	CST5625	1/1000 (WB)	
CHK1	M	CST	CST2360	1/1000 (WB)	
pCHK1	R	CST	CST2348	1/1000 (WB)	
F4/80	R	Spring Bioscience	M4154	1/100 (IHC)	Citrate pH6
GAPDH	M	Santa Cruz	sc-32233	1/5000 (WB)	
p53	M	Santa Cruz	sc-126	1/500 (WB)	
pp53	R	CST	CST9284	1/1000 (WB)	
γH2A.X	R	CST	CST9718	1/1000 (WB), 1/200 (IF)	

M, mouse; R, rabbit; WB, western blot; IF, immunofluorescence; IHC, immunohistochemistry.

4.7. Cell Viability

5000 EGI-1 cells/well, 4000 HuCCT1 cells/well, and 50,000 hepatocytes/well were plated in 96-well plates. 24 h later, fresh culture medium, PAM, or gemcitabine replaced the medium. The cells were then incubated for 72 h before determining the viability by the crystal violet method. Absorbance was quantified with a spectrophotometer (Tecan) at 595 nm.

4.8. RONS Determination in Culture Media

Nitrites and H_2O_2 concentrations were measured using Griess reagent (Sigma Aldrich, Saint-Quentin Fallavier, France) and Titanium Sulfate $TiSO_4$ (Sigma-Aldrich, Saint-Quentin Fallavier, France), respectively, to verify whether reactive species are produced in PAM. In the presence of nitrite species, the Griess reagent shows an absorption peak at 518 nm (pink coloration), while, in the presence of peroxide, the $TiSO_4$ shows an absorption peak at 405 nm (yellow coloration) both measured with the Biotek Cytation 3 device. A two-steps protocol was followed: first, the media were placed in 6-well plates and exposed to plasma, as previously explained in Section 4.4. Second, plasma was switched off. For the nitrite determination, 25 mL of each culture media sample was mixed with 175 mL of distilled water and 50 mL of Griess reagent. For the peroxide determination, 250 mL of each culture media sample was mixed with 100 mL of $TiSO_4$.

4.9. ROS Determination in Cell Lysates

ROS production was assessed using the 2′,7′-dichlorofluorescein diacetate (H2DCFDA; Abcam cat number ab113851) according to the instructions. Briefly, the CCA cells and hepatocytes were plated at 2.5×10^5 cells/well and 0.5×10^5 cells/well, respectively, in black-walled, clear-bottom 96-well microplates, and then incubated for 24 h at 37 °C. The cells were incubated with CM-H2DCFDA (25 μM) in PBS for 30 min. and then with PAM for 30 min. The cells were washed with PBS, and fluorescence was measured at 485/535 nm (Tecan, Lyon, France). Normalization was done by the crystal violet method.

4.10. Apoptosis Assay

2×10^5 EGI-1 cells/well and 1.5×10^5 HuCCT1 cells/well were plated in 6-well plates. 24 h later, the medium was replaced by fresh culture medium or PAM. 48 h or 72 h later both cells from the supernatant and the plates were collected and stained while using the PE Annexin V Apoptosis Detection Kit with 7-AAD (BioLegend, London, UK), according to the manufacturer's instructions. Flow-cytometric analysis was performed using a Gallios flow cytometer (Beckman-Coulter, Villepinte, France) to calculate the apoptosis rate. The results were analyzed using Kaluza analysis software (Beckman-Coulter).

4.11. Immunofluorescence

Immunofluorescence assays were performed, as previously described [44]. Table 1 provides the primary antibodies. The cells were observed with an Olympus Bx 61 microscope (Olympus, Rungis, France).

4.12. Western Blot Analysis

For obtaining whole-cell lysates for WB, the cell cultures were lysed in RIPA buffer supplemented with 1 mmol/L orthovanadate and a cocktail of protease inhibitors. Proteins were quantified using a BCA kit (Pierce, Lllkirch, France). WB analyses were performed, as previously described [44]. Table 1 provides the primary antibodies.

4.13. Cell Cycle Analysis

0.6×10^5 EGI-1 cells/well and 0.5×10^5 HuCCT1 cells/well were seeded in 6-well plates and incubated for 24 h. The cells were then treated with PAM for 24 h. The cells are detached with trypsin, washed with cold PBS, pooled, and centrifuged before being fixed in 70% ice-cold ethanol during 30 min. at −20 °C, and stored at −20 °C if required. The cells are incubated with 100 μg/mL of RNase A and 40 μg/mL of propidium iodide in PBS buffer. The stained cells were analyzed with a CytoFLEX (Beckman-Coulter), and their distribution in different phases of the cell cycle was calculated using Kaluza analysis software 2.0 (Beckman Coulter, Brea, CA, USA).

4.14. RNA and Reverse Transcription-PCR

Total RNA extraction and RT-qPCR was performed as previously described [44]. Table 2 provides the primer sequences. Gene expression was normalized to Hprt1 mRNA content for mouse genes and was expressed relatively to the control condition of each experiment. The relative expression of each target gene was determined from replicate samples using the formula $2^{-\Delta\Delta Ct}$.

Table 2. Mouse primer used for quantitative real-time PCR.

Gene	Protein	Forward (5′→3′)	Reverse (5′→3′)
Acta2	α-Sma	CTGTCAGGAACCCTGAGACGCT	TACTCCCTGATGTCTGGGAC
Pecam1	CD31	AGCCTCCAGGCTGAGGAAAA	GATGTCCACAAGGCACTCCA
Ccr2	Ccr2	GGCCACCACACCGTATGACTA	AGAGATGGCCAAGTTGAGCAGATAG
Adgre1	F4-80	CTTTGGCTATGGGCTTCCAGTC	GCAAGGAGGACAGAGTTTATCGTG
Il1b	Il1β	GCAACTGTTCCTGAACTCAACT	ATCTTTTGGGGTCCGTCAACT
Ccl2	Mcp1	GCCTGCTGTTCACAGTTGC	CAGGTGAGTGGGGCGTTA
Tnfa	Tnfa	CCCTCACACTCAGATCATCTTCT	GCTACGACGTGGGCTACAG
Tnfsf10	Trail	GCTCCTGCAGGCTGTGTC	CCAATTTTGGAGTAATTGTCCTG
Hprt1	Hprt	TCAGTCAACGGGGGACATAA	TGCTTAACCAGGGAAAGCAAA

4.15. Statistics

The results were analyzed using the GraphPad Prism 5.0 statistical software (GraphPad Software, San Diego, CA, USA). Data are shown as means ± standard error of the mean (SEM). For comparisons between two groups, parametric Student t test or nonparametric Mann–Whitney test were used. For comparisons between more than two groups, parametric one-way ANOVA test followed by a posteriori Bonferroni test was used.

5. Conclusions

Our results indicate that CAP is able to reduce CCA progression through the induction of DNA damage, which leads to cell cycle arrest and apoptosis of tumor cells, together with potential effects in the immune microenvironment in terms of the phenotypic change of TAM. These evidences support the potential usefulness of CAP as a future tool to treat CCA. However, several questions remain to be solved before reaching application in CCA patients. First, the effect of CAP on healthy liver cells must be evaluated in preclinical orthotopic models of CCA to assess the level of side damaging effects after a direct CAP treatment to the liver. Moreover, to reach human applicability, the size of the CAP applicating device must be reduced and adapted to the human anatomy and localization of biliary tumors. Therefore, although CAP is a novel promising anticancer "agent", further investigation is needed to include it in the therapeutic arsenal of CCA in the future.

Supplementary Materials:

Figure S1: Schematic representation of in vitro treatment of CCA cell lines and hepatocytes with PAM, Figure S2: (a) Representative images of western blot analysis of cleaved PARP, phosphorylated and total p53, phosphorylated and total CHK1 and phosphorylated H2AX in hepatocytes after 24 h, 48 h and 72 h of exposure to culture medium pretreated with CAP for 3 min. (9 kV, 30 kHz, 14%, gap of 7 mm). (b) Representative images of western blot analysis of cleaved PARP, phosphorylated and total p53, phosphorylated and total CHK1 and phosphorylated H2AX in EGI-1 and HuCCT1 after 24 h, 48 h and 72 h of exposure to 0.1 and 0.01 μM of gemcitabine, respectively. (c) Representative images of western blot analysis of cleaved PARP, phosphorylated and total p53, phosphorylated and total CHK1 and phosphorylated H2AX in hepatocytes after 72 h of exposure to increasing doses of gemcitabine. (d) Representative images of western blot analysis of cleaved PARP, phosphorylated and total p53, phosphorylated and total CHK1 and phosphorylated H2AX in hepatocytes after 24 h, 48 h and 72 h of exposure to 10 μM of gemcitabine, Figures S3–S15: Detailed information of western blot.

Author Contributions: Conceptualization, J.V., F.J., T.D., and L.F.; methodology, J.V., F.J., M.V., H.D., A.A., L.A., E.G.-S., and F.M.; validation, J.V., F.J., H.D.; formal analysis, J.V., F.J., H.D., J.A., and T.D.; investigation, J.V., F.J., M.V., H.D., A.A., L.A., and F.M.; resources, J.V., F.J., M.V., H.D., L.A., O.S., T.D., and L.F.; data curation, J.V., M.V., H.D., A.A., L.A., T.D., and L.F.; writing—original draft preparation, J.V., T.D., and L.F; writing—review and editing, J.V., H.D., A.A., L.A., E.G.-S., C.H., T.D., and L.F.; visualization, J.V., T.D., and L.F.; supervision, J.V., T.D., and L.F.; project administration, J.V., T.D., and L.F.; funding acquisition, L.A., T.D., and L.F. All authors have read and agreed to the published version of the manuscript.

Acknowledgments: The authors acknowledge Tatiana Ledent and her team from Housing and experimental animal facility (HEAF), Centre de recherche Saint-Antoine (CRSA), Brigitte Solhonne from the histomorphology Platform, UMS 30 Lumic, Centre de recherche Saint-Antoine (CRSA). Annie Munier and Romain Morichon from the Flow cytometry-imaging platform UMS_30 LUMIC, CRSA, Haquima El-Mourabit, Nathalie Ferrand, Jean-Alain Martignoles and Maxime Tenon from CRSA for their help in flow cytometry, and Elisabeth Lasnier for plasma biochemistry dosages (Biochemistry Department Saint-Antoine Hospital).

References

1. Banales, J.M.; Cardinale, V.; Carpino, G.; Marzioni, M.; Andersen, J.B.; Invernizzi, P.; Lind, G.E.; Folseraas, T.; Forbes, S.J.; Fouassier, L.; et al. Expert consensus document: Cholangiocarcinoma: Current knowledge and future perspectives consensus statement from the European Network for the Study of Cholangiocarcinoma (ENS-CCA). *Nat. Rev. Gastroenterol. Hepatol.* **2016**, *13*, 261–280. [CrossRef] [PubMed]
2. Valle, J.; Wasan, H.; Palmer, D.H.; Cunningham, D.; Anthoney, A.; Maraveyas, A.; Madhusudan, S.; Iveson, T.; Hughes, S.; Pereira, S.P.; et al. Cisplatin plus gemcitabine versus gemcitabine for biliary tract cancer. *N. Engl. J. Med.* **2010**, *362*, 1273–1281. [CrossRef]
3. Dai, X.; Bazaka, K.; Richard, D.J.; Thompson, E.R.W.; Ostrikov, K.K. The Emerging Role of Gas Plasma in Oncotherapy. *Trends Biotechnol.* **2018**, *36*, 1183–1198. [CrossRef] [PubMed]
4. Yan, D.; Sherman, J.H.; Keidar, M. Cold atmospheric plasma, a novel promising anti-cancer treatment modality. *Oncotarget* **2017**, *8*, 15977–15995. [CrossRef] [PubMed]
5. Smolkova, B.; Lunova, M.; Lynnyk, A.; Uzhytchak, M.; Churpita, O.; Jirsa, M.; Kubinova, S.; Lunov, O.; Dejneka, A. Non-Thermal Plasma, as a New Physicochemical Source, to Induce Redox Imbalance and Subsequent Cell Death in Liver Cancer Cell Lines. *Cell. Physiol. Biochem.* **2019**, *52*, 119–140.
6. Vandamme, M.; Robert, E.; Lerondel, S.; Sarron, V.; Ries, D.; Dozias, S.; Sobilo, J.; Gosset, D.; Kieda, C.; Legrain, B.; et al. ROS implication in a new antitumor strategy based on non-thermal plasma. *Int. J. Cancer* **2012**, *130*, 2185–2194. [CrossRef]
7. Ahn, H.J.; Kim, K.I.; Hoan, N.N.; Kim, C.H.; Moon, E.; Choi, K.S.; Yang, S.S.; Lee, J.S. Targeting cancer cells with reactive oxygen and nitrogen species generated by atmospheric-pressure air plasma. *PLoS ONE* **2014**, *9*, e86173. [CrossRef]
8. Adachi, T.; Tanaka, H.; Nonomura, S.; Hara, H.; Kondo, S.; Hori, M. Plasma-activated medium induces A549

cell injury via a spiral apoptotic cascade involving the mitochondrial-nuclear network. *Free Radic. Biol. Med.* **2015**, *79*, 28–44. [CrossRef]

9. Judée, F.; Vaquero, J.; Guégan, S.; Fouassier, L.; Dufour, T. Atmospheric pressure plasma jets applied to cancerology: Correlating electrical configuration with in vivo toxicity and therapeutic efficiency. *J. Phys. D Appl. Phys.* **2019**, *52*, 245201. [CrossRef]
10. Lin, G.; Lin, K.J.; Wang, F.; Chen, T.C.; Yen, T.C.; Yeh, T.S. Synergistic antiproliferative effects of an mTOR inhibitor (rad001) plus gemcitabine on cholangiocarcinoma by decreasing choline kinase activity. *Dis. Model. Mech.* **2018**, *11*. [CrossRef]
11. Luo, X.Y.; Meng, X.J.; Cao, D.C.; Wang, W.; Zhou, K.; Li, L.; Guo, M.; Wang, P. Transplantation of bone marrow mesenchymal stromal cells attenuates liver fibrosis in mice by regulating macrophage subtypes. *Stem Cell Res. Ther.* **2019**, *10*, 16. [CrossRef] [PubMed]
12. Brulle, L.; Vandamme, M.; Ries, D.; Martel, E.; Robert, E.; Lerondel, S.; Trichet, V.; Richard, S.; Pouvesle, J.M.; Le Pape, A. Effects of a non thermal plasma treatment alone or in combination with gemcitabine in a MIA PaCa2-luc orthotopic pancreatic carcinoma model. *PLoS ONE* **2012**, *7*, e52653. [CrossRef] [PubMed]
13. Hattori, N.; Yamada, S.; Torii, K.; Takeda, S.; Nakamura, K.; Tanaka, H.; Kajiyama, H.; Kanda, M.; Fujii, T.; Nakayama, G.; et al. Effectiveness of plasma treatment on pancreatic cancer cells. *Int. J. Oncol.* **2015**, *47*, 1655–1662. [CrossRef] [PubMed]
14. Utsumi, F.; Kajiyama, H.; Nakamura, K.; Tanaka, H.; Mizuno, M.; Ishikawa, K.; Kondo, H.; Kano, H.; Hori, M.; Kikkawa, F. Effect of indirect nonequilibrium atmospheric pressure plasma on anti-proliferative activity against chronic chemo-resistant ovarian cancer cells in vitro and in vivo. *PLoS ONE* **2013**, *8*, e81576. [CrossRef] [PubMed]
15. Xiang, L.; Xu, X.; Zhang, S.; Cai, D.; Dai, X. Cold atmospheric plasma conveys selectivity on triple negative breast cancer cells both in vitro and in vivo. *Free Radic. Biol. Med.* **2018**, *124*, 205–213. [CrossRef] [PubMed]
16. Freund, E.; Liedtke, K.R.; van der Linde, J.; Metelmann, H.R.; Heidecke, C.D.; Partecke, L.I.; Bekeschus, S. Physical plasma-treated saline promotes an immunogenic phenotype in CT26 colon cancer cells in vitro and in vivo. *Sci. Rep.* **2019**, *9*, 634. [CrossRef]
17. Binenbaum, Y.; Ben-David, G.; Gil, Z.; Slutsker, Y.Z.; Ryzhkov, M.A.; Felsteiner, J.; Krasik, Y.E.; Cohen, J.T. Cold Atmospheric Plasma, Created at the Tip of an Elongated Flexible Capillary Using Low Electric Current, Can Slow the Progression of Melanoma. *PLoS ONE* **2017**, *12*, e0169457. [CrossRef]
18. Chen, Z.; Simonyan, H.; Cheng, X.; Gjika, E.; Lin, L.; Canady, J.; Sherman, J.H.; Young, C.; Keidar, M. A Novel Micro Cold Atmospheric Plasma Device for Glioblastoma Both In Vitro and In Vivo. *Cancers* **2017**, *9*, 61. [CrossRef]
19. Dubuc, A.; Monsarrat, P.; Virard, F.; Merbahi, N.; Sarrette, J.P.; Laurencin-Dalicieux, S.; Cousty, S. Use of cold-atmospheric plasma in oncology: A concise systematic review. *Ther. Adv. Med. Oncol.* **2018**, *10*. [CrossRef]
20. Liedtke, K.R.; Bekeschus, S.; Kaeding, A.; Hackbarth, C.; Kuehn, J.P.; Heidecke, C.D.; von Bernstorff, W.; von Woedtke, T.; Partecke, L.I. Non-thermal plasma-treated solution demonstrates antitumor activity against pancreatic cancer cells in vitro and in vivo. *Sci. Rep.* **2017**, *7*, 8319. [CrossRef]
21. Furuta, T.; Shi, L.; Toyokuni, S. Non-thermal plasma as a simple ferroptosis inducer in cancer cells: A possible role of ferritin. *Pathol. Int.* **2018**, *68*, 442–443. [CrossRef] [PubMed]
22. Nakamura, K.; Peng, Y.; Utsumi, F.; Tanaka, H.; Mizuno, M.; Toyokuni, S.; Hori, M.; Kikkawa, F.; Kajiyama, H. Novel Intraperitoneal Treatment With Non-Thermal Plasma-Activated Medium Inhibits Metastatic Potential of Ovarian Cancer Cells. *Sci. Rep.* **2017**, *7*, 6085. [CrossRef] [PubMed]
23. Takeda, S.; Yamada, S.; Hattori, N.; Nakamura, K.; Tanaka, H.; Kajiyama, H.; Kanda, M.; Kobayashi, D.; Tanaka, C.; Fujii, T.; et al. Intraperitoneal Administration of Plasma-Activated Medium: Proposal of a Novel Treatment Option for Peritoneal Metastasis From Gastric Cancer. *Ann. Surg. Oncol.* **2017**, *24*, 1188–1194. [CrossRef] [PubMed]
24. Arndt, S.; Wacker, E.; Li, Y.F.; Shimizu, T.; Thomas, H.M.; Morfill, G.E.; Karrer, S.; Zimmermann, J.L.; Bosserhoff, A.K. Cold atmospheric plasma, a new strategy to induce senescence in melanoma cells. *Exp. Dermatol.* **2013**, *22*, 284–289. [CrossRef]
25. Schneider, C.; Gebhardt, L.; Arndt, S.; Karrer, S.; Zimmermann, J.L.; Fischer, M.J.M.; Bosserhoff, A.K. Cold atmospheric plasma causes a calcium influx in melanoma cells triggering CAP-induced senescence. *Sci. Rep.* **2018**, *8*, 10048. [CrossRef]

26. Shi, L.; Ito, F.; Wang, Y.; Okazaki, Y.; Tanaka, H.; Mizuno, M.; Hori, M.; Hirayama, T.; Nagasawa, H.; Richardson, D.R.; et al. Non-thermal plasma induces a stress response in mesothelioma cells resulting in increased endocytosis, lysosome biogenesis and autophagy. *Free Radic. Biol. Med.* **2017**, *108*, 904–917. [CrossRef]
27. Ito, T.; Ando, T.; Suzuki-Karasaki, M.; Tokunaga, T.; Yoshida, Y.; Ochiai, T.; Tokuhashi, Y.; Suzuki-Karasaki, Y. Cold PSM, but not TRAIL, triggers autophagic cell death: A therapeutic advantage of PSM over TRAIL. *Int. J. Oncol.* **2018**, *53*, 503–514. [CrossRef]
28. Ruwan Kumara, M.H.; Piao, M.J.; Kang, K.A.; Ryu, Y.S.; Park, J.E.; Shilnikova, K.; Jo, J.O.; Mok, Y.S.; Shin, J.H.; Park, Y.; et al. Non-thermal gas plasma-induced endoplasmic reticulum stress mediates apoptosis in human colon cancer cells. *Oncol. Rep.* **2016**, *36*, 2268–2274. [CrossRef]
29. Chang, J.W.; Kang, S.U.; Shin, Y.S.; Kim, K.I.; Seo, S.J.; Yang, S.S.; Lee, J.S.; Moon, E.; Lee, K.; Kim, C.H. Non-thermal atmospheric pressure plasma inhibits thyroid papillary cancer cell invasion via cytoskeletal modulation, altered MMP-2/-9/uPA activity. *PLoS ONE* **2014**, *9*, e92198. [CrossRef]
30. Nguyen Ho-Bouldoires, T.H.; Claperon, A.; Mergey, M.; Wendum, D.; Desbois-Mouthon, C.; Tahraoui, S.; Fartoux, L.; Chettouh, H.; Merabtene, F.; Scatton, O.; et al. Mitogen-activated protein kinase-activated protein kinase 2 mediates resistance to hydrogen peroxide-induced oxidative stress in human hepatobiliary cancer cells. *Free Radic. Biol. Med.* **2015**, *89*, 34–46. [CrossRef]
31. Matt, S.; Hofmann, T.G. The DNA damage-induced cell death response: A roadmap to kill cancer cells. *Cell Mol. Life Sci.* **2016**, *73*, 2829–2850. [CrossRef] [PubMed]
32. Shi, L.; Yu, L.; Zou, F.; Hu, H.; Liu, K.; Lin, Z. Gene expression profiling and functional analysis reveals that p53 pathway-related gene expression is highly activated in cancer cells treated by cold atmospheric plasma-activated medium. *PeerJ* **2017**, *5*, e3751. [CrossRef] [PubMed]
33. Babington, P.; Rajjoub, K.; Canady, J.; Siu, A.; Keidar, M.; Sherman, J.H. Use of cold atmospheric plasma in the treatment of cancer. *Biointerphases* **2015**, *10*, 029403. [CrossRef] [PubMed]
34. Keidar, M.; Walk, R.; Shashurin, A.; Srinivasan, P.; Sandler, A.; Dasgupta, S.; Ravi, R.; Guerrero-Preston, R.; Trink, B. Cold plasma selectivity and the possibility of a paradigm shift in cancer therapy. *Br. J. Cancer* **2011**, *105*, 1295–1301. [CrossRef]
35. Zucker, S.N.; Zirnheld, J.; Bagati, A.; DiSanto, T.M.; Des Soye, B.; Wawrzyniak, J.A.; Etemadi, K.; Nikiforov, M.; Berezney, R. Preferential induction of apoptotic cell death in melanoma cells as compared with normal keratinocytes using a non-thermal plasma torch. *Cancer Biol. Ther.* **2012**, *13*, 1299–1306. [CrossRef]
36. Biscop, E.; Lin, A.; Boxem, W.V.; Loenhout, J.V.; Backer, J.; Deben, C.; Dewilde, S.; Smits, E.; Bogaerts, A.A. Influence of Cell Type and Culture Medium on Determining Cancer Selectivity of Cold Atmospheric Plasma Treatment. *Cancers (Basel)* **2019**, *11*, 1287. [CrossRef]
37. Aoudjehane, L.; Podevin, P.; Scatton, O.; Jaffray, P.; Dusanter-Fourt, I.; Feldmann, G.; Massault, P.P.; Grira, L.; Bringuier, A.; Dousset, B.; et al. Interleukin-4 induces human hepatocyte apoptosis through a Fas-independent pathway. *FASEB J.* **2007**, *21*, 1433–1444. [CrossRef]
38. Kurake, N.; Tanaka, H.; Ishikawa, K.; Kondo, T.; Sekine, M.; Nakamura, K.; Kajiyama, H.; Kikkawa, F.; Mizuno, M.; Hori, M. Cell survival of glioblastoma grown in medium containing hydrogen peroxide and/or nitrite, or in plasma-activated medium. *Arch. Biochem. Biophys.* **2016**, *605*, 102–108. [CrossRef]
39. Liedtke, K.R.; Diedrich, S.; Pati, O.; Freund, E.; Flieger, R.; Heidecke, C.D.; Partecke, L.I.; Bekeschus, S. Cold Physical Plasma Selectively Elicits Apoptosis in Murine Pancreatic Cancer Cells In Vitro and In Ovo. *Anticancer Res.* **2018**, *38*, 5655–5663. [CrossRef]
40. Ye, F.; Kaneko, H.; Nagasaka, Y.; Ijima, R.; Nakamura, K.; Nagaya, M.; Takayama, K.; Kajiyama, H.; Senga, T.; Tanaka, H.; et al. Plasma-activated medium suppresses choroidal neovascularization in mice: A new therapeutic concept for age-related macular degeneration. *Sci. Rep.* **2015**, *5*, 7705. [CrossRef]
41. Kaushik, N.K.; Kaushik, N.; Adhikari, M.; Ghimire, B.; Linh, N.N.; Mishra, Y.K.; Lee, S.J.; Choi, E.H. Preventing the Solid Cancer Progression via Release of Anticancer-Cytokines in Co-Culture with Cold Plasma-Stimulated Macrophages. *Cancers (Basel)* **2019**, *11*, 842. [CrossRef] [PubMed]
42. Azzariti, A.; Iacobazzi, R.M.; Di Fonte, R.; Porcelli, L.; Gristina, R.; Favia, P.; Fracassi, F.; Trizio, I.; Silvestris, N.; Guida, G.; et al. Plasma-activated medium triggers cell death and the presentation of immune activating danger signals in melanoma and pancreatic cancer cells. *Sci. Rep.* **2019**, *9*, 4099. [CrossRef] [PubMed]
43. Aoudjehane, L.; Gautheron, J.; Le Goff, W.; Goumard, C.; Gilaizeau, J.; Nget, C.S.; Savier, E.; Atif, M.; Lesnik, P.; Morichon, R.; et al. Novel defatting strategies reduce lipid accumulation in primary human culture models of liver steatosis. *Dis. Model. Mech.* **2020**. [CrossRef] [PubMed]

44. Vaquero, J.; Lobe, C.; Tahraoui, S.; Claperon, A.; Mergey, M.; Merabtene, F.; Wendum, D.; Coulouarn, C.; Housset, C.; Desbois-Mouthon, C.; et al. The IGF2/IR/IGF1R Pathway in Tumor Cells and Myofibroblasts Mediates Resistance to EGFR Inhibition in Cholangiocarcinoma. *Clin. Cancer Res.* **2018**, *24*, 4282–4296. [CrossRef] [PubMed]

11

Selenium-Binding Protein 1 in Human Health and Disease

Mostafa Elhodaky and Alan M. Diamond *

Department of Pathology, University of Illinois at Chicago, Chicago, IL 60612, USA; melhod2@uic.edu
* Correspondence: adiamond@uic.edu

Abstract: Selenium-binding protein 1 (SBP1) is a highly conserved protein that covalently binds selenium. SBP1 may play important roles in several fundamental physiological functions, including protein degradation, intra-Golgi transport, cell differentiation, cellular motility, redox modulation, and the metabolism of sulfur-containing molecules. SBP1 expression is often reduced in many cancer types compared to the corresponding normal tissues and low levels of SBP1 are frequently associated with poor clinical outcome. In this review, the transcriptional regulation of *SBP1*, the different physiological roles reported for SBP1, as well as the implications of SBP1 function in cancer and other diseases are presented.

Keywords: selenium-binding protein 1; SBP1; SELENBP1; hSP56; cancer; disease

---

1. Introduction

Selenium (Se) is a non-metallic, essential trace element for many organisms, including humans. Se has long been recognized for its potential in cancer prevention as evidenced by multiple animal, and human epidemiological studies that have reported an inverse association between Se status and cancer risk [1–8]. Many mechanisms have been suggested for the chemopreventive effect of Se [9–11], including DNA hypomethylation [12], blocked cell cycle progression, enhanced cell death, decreased cell proliferation, increased glutathione peroxidase or thioredoxin reductases activities [13], modulated ER stress response [14], and enhanced DNA repair [15]. Furthermore, Se has been found to play a key role in mammalian development [16] and immune function [17,18]. Low levels of Se may be a contributing factor to several pathologies, including male infertility [19], heart disease [20], inflammation [21,22], and neuromuscular disorders [23]. It is generally recognized that important cellular and organismal functions of Se are likely mediated by the action of selenoproteins constituting the mammalian selenoproteome [24]. While the functions of many selenoproteins are still unknown, they likely have a significant role in human health and disease. Human selenoproteins are generally classified into three categories [11,25]. The first category includes proteins in which Se is cotranslationally incorporated into the elongating peptide as the amino acid selenocysteine in response to an in-frame UGA codon in the corresponding messenger RNA [26]. The human selenoproteome contains 25 genes [25]. The second category consists of proteins in which Se is incorrectly substituted for sulfur in sulfur-containing amino acids due to the similarity in structure between these two elements. The third category is composed of selenium-binding proteins which bind Se by an unknown mechanism. This review will be primarily focused on one member of the latter category, selenium-binding protein 1 (SBP1, SELENBP1, hSP56).

2. SBP1 Discovery

SBP1 was first discovered in mouse liver in 1989 by Bansal et al. using ^{75}Se labelling. Normal 6-week old female BALB/c mice were given a single intraperitoneal injection of ^{75}Se in the form of Na_2SeO_3. After 40 h, animals were euthanized and livers were harvested for preparation of liver cytosols which were then used for a combination of gel filtration, ion-exchange chromatography and SDS-PAGE techniques. This led to identification of four selenium-binding proteins of apparent molecular weights of 12, 14, 24, and 56 kDa [27]. The 56-kDa protein was designated as SBP1, whereas the 24-kDa protein was identified as glutathione peroxidase 1 (GPX1), an enzyme that detoxifies hydroperoxides using reducing equivalents from glutathione [28]. The full-length human *SBP1* cDNA clone was first described by Chang et al. in 1997 and determined to be 1668 base pair (bp) long with an open reading frame encoding 472 amino acids [29]. *SBP1* is abundantly expressed in various human tissues, including liver, lung, prostate, colon, and pancreas, while moderate levels were detected in spleen, heart, and ovary. In contrast, its expression was barely detectable in thymus, testis, and peripheral blood leukocytes [30]. SBP1 is a highly-conserved protein. Flemetakis et al. reported that the predicted amino acid sequence of SBP1 is conserved in both plants and animals, ranging from 77 to 88% in plants, while the identity between the plants and mammalian proteins ranged from 57 to 60% [31]. By comparison, this degree of homology is higher than other conserved proteins, such as HSP60, γ-tubulin, apoptotic cell death 1 protein, and elF4E whose identities of the plant and human proteins are 44, 49, 48, and 52%, respectively [31]. The homology between the mammalian *SBP1* of mice and humans is 86% [31], indicating that the potential fundamental cellular and molecular functions for SBP1 are also conserved across different species. SBP1 is very similar to another selenium-associated protein, selenium liver binding protein (AP-56, SBP2), whose sequence differs by only 14 residues from SBP1 and is encoded by a distinct gene [32]. AP-56 is implicated in the detoxification of acetaminophen in the liver [32]. Although these genes are regulated differently, their similarity may indicate a role for SBP1 in detoxification.

3. The Role of Se in SBP1

The form of Se in SBP1 is currently unknown. Se is stably associated with SBP1, probably through a selenosulfide bond (perselenide), as indicated by the binding of Se to SBP1 being reversed by the addition of a reducing agent during SDS-PAGE [33]. Based on structural and functional studies, it was suggested that one cysteine in SBP1 was the likely binding site for the Se molecule, the cysteine at position 57 [34]. Converting cysteine 57 in SBP1 to a glycine and ectopically expressing that protein in human HCT116 cells that do not express detectable SBP1 levels indicated that the loss of the cysteine reduced the half-life of the protein, induced mitochondrial damage, and attenuated the degree of phosphorylation of signaling proteins such as p53 and GSK3β compared to the native protein expressed at similar levels [35].

The Se in SBP1 may facilitate its interaction with other proteins. SBP1 physically interacts with von Hippel–Lindau protein–interacting deubiquitinating enzyme 1 (VDU1), which plays a role in proteasomal protein degradation [33,36]. This indicates that SBP1, via its interaction with VDU1, may have a role in ubiquitination/deubiquitination-mediated protein degradation and detoxification pathways. When the Se moiety was dissociated from SBP1 by the addition of ß-mercaptoethanol, the interaction with VDU1 was completely blocked, indicating that Se may be essential for the interaction of these two proteins [33]. While the Se moiety is likely required for its interaction with VDU1, the inclusion of Se in SBP1 does not appear to be essential for functioning as methanethiol oxidase (MTO), a recently-discovered novel human SBP1 enzyme activity that metabolizes sulfur-containing molecules [37].

As a non-selenocysteine containing protein, SBP1 is not considered as a part of the "selenium hierarchy" that describes the relative response of selenoproteins to the availability of Se [38]. Initial studies feeding rats varying amounts of Se led to the conclusion that SBP1 levels were not likely dependent upon dietary Se supplementation [39]. However, there may be indirect regulation of SBP1 by Se due to its interaction with GPX1, a member of the selenocysteine-containing selenoproteins. GPX1 is a highly conserved and ubiquitously expressed enzyme that detoxifies hydrogen and lipid peroxides and is implicated in several diseases by human genetics [40]. There is a reciprocal regulatory relationship between SBP1 and GPX1. Ectopically expressing SBP1 in HCT116 human colon cancer cells that do not express endogenous SBP1 resulted in the inhibition of GPX1 enzyme activity without affecting protein levels [28], indicating a likely physical interaction. Consistent with this possibility was data indicating that knocking down *SBP1* in human liver cells resulted in a 4–5 fold increase in GPX activity, also without altering protein levels [41].

Expressing GPX1 in MCF7 human breast cancer cells that do not exhibit detectable GPX1 levels resulted in a decline in both SBP1 mRNA and protein levels [28]. The reciprocal relationship between SBP1 and GPX1 has also been established in mouse colon and duodenum epithelial cells [28], as well as human prostate and liver tissues [41,42]. This raises the possibility that SBP1 can be indirectly downregulated by Se because GPX1 is high on the Se hierarchy, being among the selenoproteins most responsive to Se availability. Support for the indirect regulation of SBP1 by GPX1 comes from experiments showing that increasing Se in the culture media of MCF7 cells caused a dramatic reduction in SBP1 levels only when GPX1 was present and GPX1 levels were increased by the Se supplementation [28].

4. SBP1 Levels Are Reduced in Cancer and Low Levels Are Predictive of Clinical Outcome

One of the striking observations about SBP1 is the diversity of the types of cancers in which SBP1 was found to be reduced compared to normal or benign tissues (reviewed in [43]), including cancers of the thyroid [44], lung [45], stomach [46,47], liver [41], kidney [48], ovary [49–51], breast [52], prostate [53,54], colon [55,56], head and neck [57], and malignant melanoma [58]. In addition to being lower in cancers, the degree of reduction of SBP1 in resected tissues is often predictive of how long a patient will be cancer free and survive their disease [43]. Reduced SBP1 levels have been correlated with poor survival in several types of carcinomas, including colorectal [55,59], gastric [47], nasopharyngeal [57], pulmonary [45], renal [48], and prostate [53] cancers. Recently, a search for genetic variations in selenoprotein genes revealed that a polymorphism in the gene for SBP1, along with variations in the genes of selenocysteine encoding genes, were associated with prostate cancer aggressiveness at diagnosis [60]. The exception to this pattern is ovarian cancer where higher levels of SBP1 were associated with poor survival [50].

In addition to its levels, the distribution of SBP1 between cellular compartments may be relevant to cancer etiology. The associations between prostatic SBP1 levels, tumor grade, and disease recurrence following prostatectomy were investigated using a tissue microarray containing tissue from more than 200 prostate cancer patients who experienced biochemical (PSA) recurrence after prostatectomy and matched control patients whose cancer did not recur [53]. Reduced SBP1 levels were associated with a higher likelihood of prostate cancer recurrence, as has been seen in other cancer types. The subcellular localization of SBP1 was both nuclear and cytoplasmic, with nuclear staining being sporadic (Figure 1). However, a lower nuclear-to-cytoplasmic distribution of SBP1 was associated with a higher tumor grade (Gleason score) [53]. These results indicate that sequestration of SBP1 in a particular cellular compartment may restrict access to relevant substrates or the protein has different functions at these locations.

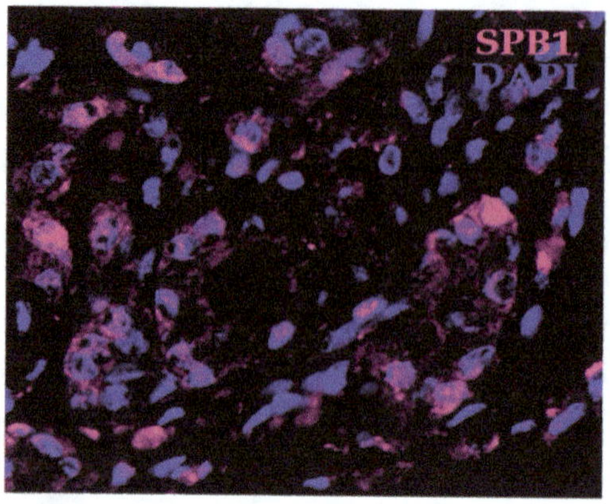

Figure 1. Localization of SBP1 in prostate cancer. Human prostate cancer tissue showing cells that express SBP1 (magenta) mostly in the cytoplasm and several cells that express SBP1 in the nucleus. Nuclei are highlighted with DAPI (blue).

4.1. Is SBP1 a Tumor Suppressor?

The frequent loss of SBP1 in cancer and the association of reduced SBP1 levels with greater mortality could imply that SBP1 is a tumor suppressor. Alternatively, its loss or downregulation may be a consequence of cancer development and progression, and the reduced levels represent a mere "bystander effect". Data supporting the direct role of SBP1 in cancer comes from studies where its levels are altered in cells and consequences relevant to transformation and tumorigenesis are revealed. Over-expressing SBP1 in colon, gastric, and prostate cancer cells have generally yielded results consistent with a tumor suppressor function, including reduced growth in semi-solid media and decreased tumorigenicity in xenograft studies using immune-deficient mice [46,53,54,61,62]. When over-expressed in lung cancer cells, SBP1 reduced proliferation and induced greater apoptosis compared to control cells only when the cells were challenged with H_2O_2 [41]. Some of the phenotypic consequences of over-expressing SBP1 may be due to the downstream activation of the p53 tumor suppressor protein. Over-expression of SBP1 in HCT116 human colon cancer cells resulted in the increased phosphorylation of p53 [53]. In addition to the phosphorylation of p53, SBP1 over-expression in the same cells resulted in the differential expression of 132 proteins, many are associated with energy metabolism and MAPK, Wnt, NF-κB, and Notch signaling [61]. This same study reported that the expression of SBP1 resulted in the reduction of TWIST1, a critical regulator of the epithelial-mesenchymal transition and metastasis.

Consistent with over-expression data, either knocking down *SBP1* or inactivating the gene using CRISPR/Cas9 editing in mouse lung cancer cells and injecting these cells into syngeneic hosts increased the size of tumors obtained compared to controls, although the number of tumors was not increased [63]. Knockout mice that are null for SBP1 exhibit very limited pathology and do not develop tumors [64]. However, examining the ovaries from these animals by gene expression microarrays indicated the increased expression of several genes associated with ovarian carcinogenesis, including *Notch1* and *Fas1* [64]. Less clear is why tumor suppressor genes such as *Apc*, *RB1*, and *Trp53* were also enhanced in the ovaries from these mice. Collectively, studies altering the levels of SBP1 provide substantial evidence that SBP1 serves as a tumor suppressor and its loss or downregulation during cancer development contributes to disease development or progression.

4.2. Is SBP1 Downregulation an Early or Late Event in the Process of Tumorigenesis?

Given the data presented above indicating the frequent downregulation of SBP1 in cancers and its association with poor outcomes, it raises the issue of whether SBP1 loss occurs early in cancer development or late in the process, contributing to cancer progression. This issue was investigated by Zhang et al. who examined SBP1 levels in tissues classified as gastric cancer, precursor lesions, and matched controls of corresponding non-neoplastic epithelial tissues [65]. SBP1 was reduced in most of the gastric cancer tissues compared to its abundant expression in matched non-neoplastic controls and precursor lesions, including tissues obtained from gastric ulcers, gastric polyps, as well as tissues presenting with chronic atrophic gastritis, intestinal metaplasia and dysplasia [65]. SBP1 expression was similar in tissues with different levels of intestinal metaplasia or dysplasia indicating that the reduction of SBP1 levels may be a late event associated with gastric carcinoma progression from normal gastric epithelium or premalignant lesions [65]. These results are consistent with those of Kim et al. who observed much lower levels of SBP1 in colorectal carcinomas compared to matched controls of normal tissues and colon adenomas, supporting the notion that SBP1 loss is a late event during tumorigenesis [59]. In addition, changes in the levels of proteins that occur during the progression of human squamous lung cancer were investigated using isobaric tags for relative and absolute quantitation labeling combined with 2D LC-MS/MS [66]. SBP1 levels were determined by western blotting and immunohistochemistry and shown to be progressively lost during bronchial epithelial cancer progression [66].

In contrast to the data obtained examining gastric, bronchial, and colonic tissues, results have also been reported indicating that the reduction in SBP1 expression may be an early event in the evolution of some tumor types, including ovarian cancer [50] and uterine leiomyoma [67]. Huang et al. identified SBP1 to be the most significantly reduced protein in ovarian cancer cell lines, including DOV13, OVCA429, OVCA882, TOV112D, and SKOV3 using a membrane proteome profiling analysis [50]. However, relatively low levels of SBP1 were also observed in the immortalized human ovarian cell line, HOSE2089, indicating that the reduction of SBP1 may have occurred during the immortalization process [50]. SBP1 expression was also approximately 4-fold lower in leiomyoma samples compared to normal myometrium, as determined by western blotting and immunohistochemistry [67]. However, SBP1 levels were similar in tissues obtained from patients with proliferative secretory and atrophic endometrium in either leiomyoma or normal myometrium. These contrasting results may indicate distinct roles of SBP1 in the development of cancers of different origins.

5. Physiological Roles for SBP1

The impact of SBP1 on normal biological processes and pathologies other than cancer may be due to roles in the modulation of cellular redox homeostasis. The SBP1 amino acid sequence contains two bis (cysteinyl) sequence motifs, Cys-X-X-Cys, at Cys5-X-X-Cys8 and Cys80-X-X-Cys83 shown to be a characteristic feature among several proteins which are involved in modulating the cellular redox state in vivo [68]. In addition, SBP1 may also modulate the redox state of the extracellular environment. Experimental data in support of this comes from a study where the knockdown of *SBP1* in MCF-7 breast cancer and HC116 colon cancer cells by siRNA resulted in increased levels of H_2O_2 and superoxide ion, leading to enhanced apoptosis when cells were exposed to selenite [69]. The authors attributed this effect to the significant increase in extracellular glutathione in the culture media. Changes in either the intracellular or extracellular environment can potentially impact a broad range of biological processes responsive to reactive oxygen in signaling pathways and contribute to the pathology associated with SBP1 dysregulation.

SBP1 has also been implicated in the late stages of intra-Golgi transport. Using an in vitro intra-Golgi cell-free transport assay, both endogenous and recombinant SBP1 (rSBP1) exhibited transport activity in the cell-free assay and the addition of antibodies directed against SBP1 abolished this activity [70]. This data indicates that SBP1 may be regulating vesicular intra-Golgi transport, particularly at the docking or fusions stages [70]. The reported roles for SBP1 are summarized in Figure 2.

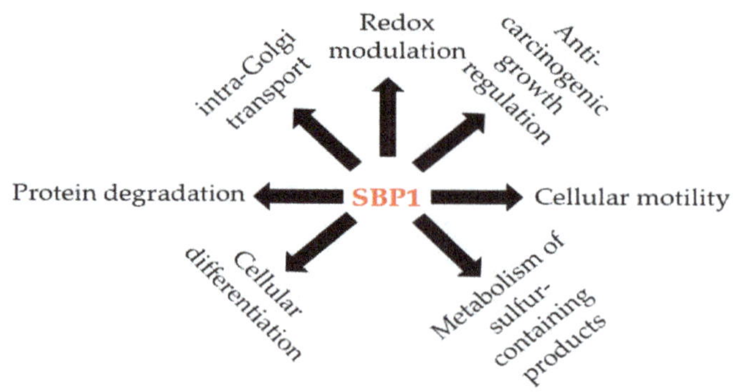

Figure 2. The potential roles of SBP1 in human health and disease. Illustration of the different potential functions reported for SBP1 in the published literature.

Tissue-Specific Roles for SBP1

Several studies have indicated a potential role for SBP1 in neurobiology. SBP1 has been localized at the tips of rapidly extending protrusions in T98G glioblastoma multiforme cells in vitro [71]. Cell protrusive motility, which is tightly associated with actin filament polymerization, is an essential function for multiple cellular processes, including cell proliferation and migration. Monomeric G-actin, but not filamentous F-actin, was shown to be recruited to the SBP1-positive tip, indicating that the recruitment of SBP1 and G-actin at the cell margin precedes actin polymerization [71]. In addition, SBP1 recruitment to the cell margin was observed to precede that of G-actin. The extension of the protrusion will stop when G-actin polymerizes to F-actin at the protruding edges, hence, SBP1 and G-actin disappear from these margins. SBP1 also localized to the growing tips of neurites in SH-SY5Y neuroblastoma cells in vitro [71], possibly indicating a role for SBP1 in neuronal cell outgrowth.

Changes in the levels of SBP1 in neuronal tissues may implicate the protein in several neuropathologies. *SBP1* mRNA has reported to be elevated in the frontal cortex of patients with schizophrenia, indicating a potential specialized role in the pathophysiology of schizophrenia and the central nervous system [72–74]. Genetic data has also implicated SBP1 in the risk of schizophrenia as two single nucleotide polymorphisms in the *SBP1* gene (rs2800953 and rs10788804) have been identified as susceptibility loci for schizophrenia in a family-wide association study [75]. This, and a report of plasma SBP1 protein levels being decreased in patients with recent-onset schizophrenia [76], collectively indicate a potential specialized role for SBP1 in the pathophysiology of this disease. Whether these data indicate a role for SBP1 in the proper functioning of the central nervous system or the potential neuroprotective effect of Se against oxidative and excitatory brain damage [77] remains to be determined.

SBP1 may also be involved with the pathogenesis of glaucoma. Elevated levels of SBP1 have been associated with elevated ocular pressure [78]. It was also identified as a differentially expressed gene in datasets comparing transcripts in glaucoma to normal control tissues, which has been verified in a rat model of acute elevated intraocular pressure [79]. SBP1 was also identified as a novel target antigen in patients with Behçet's disease (BD) with uveitis, where an autoimmune response to retinal antigens is considered to be involved in the pathogenesis of the uveitis in those patients [80,81]. What if any role SBP1 plays in these diseases has not yet been investigated.

6. The Transcriptional Regulation of SBP1

A greater understanding of the biological roles of SBP1 could be gained by examining how its expression is regulated. A subtractive hybridization approach was used to identify transcripts that were more abundant in the relatively fast growing PC-3 human prostate cancer cells compared to slow growing LNCaP cells [30]. The low levels of *SBP1* mRNA in LNCaP cells was shown to be due to the down regulation of *SBP1* transcription as treatment with of androgen-sensitive LNCaP cells with dihydrotestosterone (DHT, active form of androgen) reduced the levels of *SBP1* mRNA in a reversible, concentration-dependent manner [30]. A more complicated picture was revealed by the analysis of the effect of androgen on normal ovarian epithelial cells obtained from the scraping of the ovary surface of patients with benign disease, an immortalized cell line, and ovarian cancer cell lines [50]. Treatment of the primary and immortalized cells with DHT reduced the levels of *SBP1* mRNA while SBP1 levels were increased in four tumor-derived cell lines by DHT treatment. The mechanism accounting for the differential response of these cell lines to DHT has not been resolved.

In addition to androgens, *SBP1* expression is also downregulated by estrogen treatment (17-β estradiol) in estrogen receptor (ER)-positive breast cancer cells, but not in ER-negative cells [52]. The suppression of SBP1 expression by transforming growth factor beta (TGF-β) was also observed using a rhesus monkey renal allograft model to identify molecules involved in the pathogenesis of chronic allograft nephropathy (CAN) [82]. SBP1 was absent or markedly reduced in vascular smooth muscle cells in monkey kidney allografts with CAN. Testing growth factors previously associated with graft rejection, including IFNγ, TNFα, and PDGF, only TGF-β blocked the expression of SBP1 in the normal human vascular smooth muscle cell line, CRL-1999 [82]. It is unlikely that the effects of androgens or estrogens on *SBP1* transcription is a direct consequence of the binding of the corresponding receptor to the *SBP1* promoter as there does not appear to be a consensus binding sequence for the receptor/transcription factor.

The mouse *Sbp1* gene has been identified as a direct target gene of the hypoxia-inducible factor-1α (HIF-1α) transcription factor in primary keratinocyte cell cultures [83]. Scortegagna et al. examined HIF-1α gain of function during multistage murine skin chemical carcinogenesis in K14-HIF-1$\alpha^{Pro402A564G}$ transgenic mice. They concluded that HIF-1α was functioning as a tumor suppressor, most likely by upregulating target genes, including *Sbp1*. Four hypoxia response elements were located within 1400 bp of the transcription start site of the human promoter region of *SBP1*, although the demonstration that these were bona fide response elements was not provided [83]. HIF-1α is a central mediator of the cellular response to environmental stresses, such as hypoxia [84]. It is overexpressed in many types of human cancer [85–87] and its overexpression is associated with treatment failure and increased mortality in some cancers including cancers of the cervix [88,89], breast [90,91], ovary [92], uterus [93], stomach [94], and brain [95]. It is also associated with decreased mortality in other cancers, including those of the head and neck [96] and non-small-cell lung cancer [97]. The consequences of the changes of HIF-1α levels are cancer-type specific and the accompanying molecular alterations, such as SBP1 reduction/loss, can affect the balance between pro- and anti-apoptotic factors. A study by Huang et al. demonstrated that the decreased expression of SBP1 could lead to a higher GPX1 activity and reduced HIF-1α expression in hepatocellular carcinoma, indicating that SBP1 might exert its tumor suppressive function as a regulator of the tumor redox microenvironment [41].

In addition to the putative HIF-1α response elements in the *SBP1* promoter, two potential antioxidant response elements (ARE) with strong homology to the consensus ARE recognition motif are present in promoter region of *SBP1* [28], although the functionality of these sequences as AREs has yet to be established. The presence of functional AREs in the promoter region of *SBP1* may account for the repression of transcription observed when the anti-oxidant selenoprotein GPX1 is ectopically expressed in colon carcinoma cell lines [28], as well as the reciprocal relationship observed in cells and tissues [43]. The factors potentially regulating *SBP1* and some downstream targets are summarized in Figure 3.

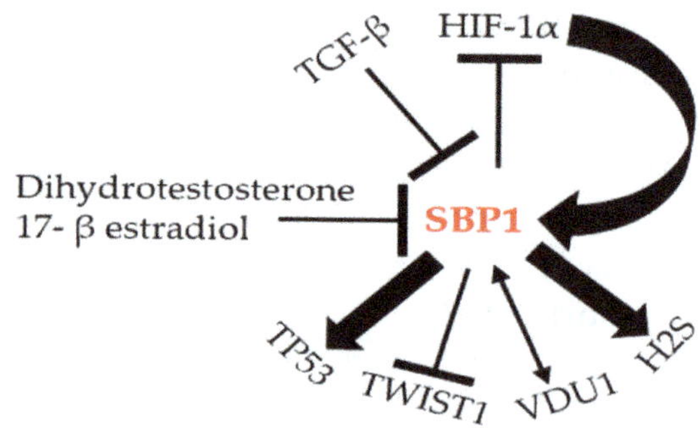

Figure 3. The molecular regulation of SBP1. Illustration of the different proteins that can potentially interact, be regulated by, or regulate SBP1 according to the literature. TGF-β: transforming growth factor beta; HIF-1α: hypoxia-inducible factor-1α; H2S: hydrogen sulfide; VDU1: von Hippel–Lindau protein–interacting deubiquitinating enzyme 1; TWIST1: Twist Family BHLH Transcription Factor 1; TP53: tumor protein p53.

In some cases, epigenetic silencing by promoter methylation may be a mechanism by which the expression of *SBP1* is reduced in human colon cancers. Comparing DNA obtained from colon cancer samples to DNA obtained from matched normal tissue indicated significantly more methylation in the promoter region of samples from the cancers [56]. Hypermethylation of the *SBP1* promoter region was demonstrated in the human colon cell lines SW480, Caco-2, HT-29, and HCT1161 in which the extent of promoter methylation was associated with the degree of SBP1 protein levels. Moreover, treatment of these cells with 5-aza-deoxycytidine, a demethylation agent, decreased promoter methylation and resulted in increased promoter activity and protein levels [56]. In contrast, treatment of three different human colon cancer cell lines, LOVO, SNU-C4, and A549, with 5-aza-deoxycytidine did not result in increased SBP1 expression, nor was there any evidence of genetic loss at the *SBP1* locus [59]. There was also a lack of evidence for either hypermethylation or genetic deletion accounting for the low levels of *SBP1* observed in lung cancers [98]. While there is consistent loss of SBP1 in many cancer types, there may be a multitude of ways in which tumor cells can achieve the reduction in SBP1 expression.

7. SBP1 Is a Methanethiol Oxidase

The enzymatic function of SBP1 was recently revealed by investigators examining the genetic determinants of extraoral halitosis, bad breath [37]. The authors analyzed breaths and body fluids of five affected individuals with extraoral halitosis from three unrelated families using NMR spectroscopy and gas chromatography with a sulfur-specific detector. All patients exhibited elevated levels of methanethiol (MT), dimethylsulfide (DMS), dimethylsufoxide, and dimethylsulfone in breaths and body fluids [37]. The authors postulated that the accumulation of these compounds was due to a defect in a protein which oxidizes MT, leading to its accumulation in affected individuals. Methanethiol oxidases (MTOs) have not previously been reported in humans, but *SBP1* was identified as a candidate gene for extraoral halitosis by searching for human sequences that were similar to the gene encoding an MT-metabolizing protein previously recognized in methylotropic bacteria, the *mtoX* gene. This effort revealed a 26% identity and a 54% sequence similarity between the two genes [37]. Subsequent sequencing of *SBP1* in patients DNAs revealed four different biallelic mutations in the five patients (1039G>T, 481+1G>A, 673G>T, and 985C>T) that were predicted to be pathogenic. Fibroblasts from these patients had significantly reduced SBP1 protein levels and undetectable MTO enzymatic activity, compared to the control cells [37].

MTO converts MT to H_2O_2, formaldehyde, and hydrogen sulfide (H_2S), the latter is a gaseous signaling molecule with distinct functions at different cellular concentrations [99,100]. At low concentrations, H_2S stimulates mitochondrial electron transport in mammalian cells, increasing oxygen consumption [101]. At high concentrations, H_2S is toxic through the inhibition of mitochondrial respiratory-chain complex IV, and consequently reduces oxygen consumption [101]. H_2S has been proposed as a therapy for multiple disorders by suppressing inflammation, affecting apoptotic pathways, increasing anti-oxidant defenses, and vasodilatation [99,102,103]. It is quite conceivable that many of the consequences of SBP1 expression can be due to the effects on H_2S levels as well as the other products of the MTO-mediated reaction, on a broad spectrum of physiological endpoints.

8. Conclusions

Among the selenium-associated proteins, SBP1 is relatively less studied, but is a highly-conserved protein that may be critical for a variety of physiological functions, including cell differentiation, protein degradation, intra-Golgi vesicular transport, cell motility, and redox modulation. The variety of processes where SBP1 has been implicated to have a role is suggestive that there may be cell type-specific functions that are yet to be identified. The only enzymatic function of SBP1 identified to date is MTO activity and it is possible that different levels of both its substrates and products provide differential signals, resulting in distinct intracellular and extracellular environments for the SBP1-expressing cells. With a better understanding of the function of SBP1 in these tissues, its role in diseases such as cancer may be resolved and SBP1 may become a novel therapeutic target for interventions to control it levels and/or activity.

Author Contributions: Both authors contributed to the writing of this manuscript.

References

1. Clark, L.C.; Combs, G.F., Jr.; Turnbull, B.W.; Slate, E.H.; Chalker, D.K.; Chow, J.; Davis, L.S.; Glover, R.A.; Graham, G.F.; Gross, E.G.; et al. Effects of selenium supplementation for cancer prevention in patients with carcinoma of the skin. A randomized controlled trial. Nutritional prevention of cancer study group. *JAMA* **1996**, *276*, 1957–1963. [CrossRef] [PubMed]
2. Clark, L.C.; Dalkin, B.; Krongrad, A.; Combs, G.F., Jr.; Turnbull, B.W.; Slate, E.H.; Witherington, R.; Herlong, J.H.; Janosko, E.; Carpenter, D.; et al. Decreased incidence of prostate cancer with selenium supplementation: Results of a double-blind cancer prevention trial. *Br. J. Urol.* **1998**, *81*, 730–734. [CrossRef] [PubMed]
3. Schrauzer, G.N.; White, D.A.; Schneider, C.J. Cancer mortality correlation studies. Iii. Statistical association with dietary selenium intakes. *Bioinorg. Chem.* **1977**, *7*, 23–34. [CrossRef]
4. Shamberger, R.J.; Frost, D.V. Possible protective effect of selenium against human cancer. *Can. Med. Assoc. J.* **1969**, *100*, 682. [PubMed]
5. Brinkman, M.; Reulen, R.C.; Kellen, E.; Buntinx, F.; Zeegers, M.P. Are men with low selenium levels at increased risk of prostate cancer? *Eur. J. Cancer* **2006**, *42*, 2463–2471. [CrossRef] [PubMed]
6. Fortmann, S.P.; Burda, B.U.; Senger, C.A.; Lin, J.S.; Whitlock, E.P. Vitamin and mineral supplements in the primary prevention of cardiovascular disease and cancer: An updated systematic evidence review for the u.S. Preventive services task force. *Ann. Intern. Med.* **2013**, *159*, 824–834. [CrossRef] [PubMed]
7. Steinbrenner, H.; Speckmann, B.; Sies, H. Toward understanding success and failures in the use of selenium for cancer prevention. *Antioxid. Redox Signal.* **2013**, *19*, 181–191. [CrossRef] [PubMed]
8. Vinceti, M.; Crespi, C.M.; Malagoli, C.; Del Giovane, C.; Krogh, V. Friend or foe? The current epidemiologic evidence on selenium and human cancer risk. *J. Environ. Sci. Health Part C Environ. Carcinog. Ecotoxicol. Rev.* **2013**, *31*, 305–341. [CrossRef] [PubMed]
9. Ip, C. Lessons from basic research in selenium and cancer prevention. *J. Nutr.* **1998**, *128*, 1845–1854. [CrossRef] [PubMed]
10. Klein, E.A. Selenium: Epidemiology and basic science. *J. Urol.* **2004**, *171*, S50–S53. [CrossRef] [PubMed]
11. Behne, D.; Kyriakopoulos, A. Mammalian selenium-containing proteins. *Annu. Rev. Nutr.* **2001**, *21*, 453–473. [CrossRef] [PubMed]
12. Davis, C.D.; Uthus, E.O. Dietary folate and selenium affect dimethylhydrazine-induced aberrant crypt formation, global DNA methylation and one-carbon metabolism in rats. *J. Nutr.* **2003**, *133*, 2907–2914. [CrossRef] [PubMed]

13. Ip, C.; Dong, Y.; Ganther, H. New concepts in selenium chemoprevention. *Cancer Metastasis Rev.* **2002**, *21*, 281–289. [CrossRef] [PubMed]
14. Wu, Y.; Zhang, H.; Dong, Y.; Park, Y.M.; Ip, C. Endoplasmic reticulum stress signal mediators are targets of selenium action. *Cancer Res.* **2005**, *65*, 9073–9079. [CrossRef] [PubMed]
15. Bera, S.; De Rosa, V.; Rachidi, W.; Diamond, A.M. Does a role for selenium in DNA damage repair explain apparent controversies in its use in chemoprevention? *Mutagenesis* **2013**, *28*, 127–134. [CrossRef] [PubMed]
16. Kohrle, J. The deiodinase family: Selenoenzymes regulating thyroid hormone availability and action. *Cell. Mol. Life Sci.* **2000**, *57*, 1853–1863. [CrossRef] [PubMed]
17. Rayman, M.P. Selenium and human health. *Lancet* **2012**, *379*, 1256–1268. [CrossRef]
18. Avery, J.C.; Hoffmann, P.R. Selenium, selenoproteins, and immunity. *Nutrients* **2018**, *10*, 1203. [CrossRef] [PubMed]
19. Turanov, A.A.M.M.; Gladyshev, V.N. Selenium and male reproduction. In *Selenium: Its Molecular Biology and Role in Human Health*, 3rd ed.; Hatfield, D.L.B.M., Gladyshev, V.N., Eds.; Springer: New York, NY, USA, 2012; pp. 409–417.
20. Handy, D.E.L.J. Selenoproteins in cardiovascular redox pathology. In *Selenium: Its Molecular Biology and Role in Human Health*, 3rd ed.; Hatfield, D.L.B.M., Gladyshev, V.N., Eds.; Springer: New York, NY, USA, 2012; pp. 249–259.
21. Kaushal, N.G.U.; Nelson, S.M.; Narayan, V.; Prabhu, K.S. Selenium and inflamation. In *Selenium: Its Molecular Biology and Role in Human Health*, 3rd ed.; Hatfield, D.L.B.M., Gladyshev, V.N., Eds.; Springer: New York, NY, USA, 2012; pp. 443–456.
22. Kudva, A.K.; Shay, A.E.; Prabhu, K.S. Selenium and inflammatory bowel disease. *Am. J. Physiol. Gastrointest. Liver Physiol.* **2015**, *309*, G71–G77. [CrossRef] [PubMed]
23. Moghadaszadeh, B.; Petit, N.; Jaillard, C.; Brockington, M.; Quijano Roy, S.; Merlini, L.; Romero, N.; Estournet, B.; Desguerre, I.; Chaigne, D.; et al. Mutations in sepn1 cause congenital muscular dystrophy with spinal rigidity and restrictive respiratory syndrome. *Nat. Genet.* **2001**, *29*, 17–18. [CrossRef] [PubMed]
24. Labunskyy, V.M.; Hatfield, D.L.; Gladyshev, V.N. Selenoproteins: Molecular pathways and physiological roles. *Physiol. Rev.* **2014**, *94*, 739–777. [CrossRef] [PubMed]
25. Kryukov, G.V.; Castellano, S.; Novoselov, S.V.; Lobanov, A.V.; Zehtab, O.; Guigo, R.; Gladyshev, V.N. Characterization of mammalian selenoproteomes. *Science* **2003**, *300*, 1439–1443. [CrossRef] [PubMed]
26. Hatfield, D.L.; Gladyshev, V.N. How selenium has altered our understanding of the genetic code. *Mol. Cell. Biol.* **2002**, *22*, 3565–3576. [CrossRef] [PubMed]
27. Bansal, M.P.; Oborn, C.J.; Danielson, K.G.; Medina, D. Evidence for two selenium-binding proteins distinct from glutathione peroxidase in mouse liver. *Carcinogenesis* **1989**, *10*, 541–546. [CrossRef] [PubMed]
28. Fang, W.; Goldberg, M.L.; Pohl, N.M.; Bi, X.; Tong, C.; Xiong, B.; Koh, T.J.; Diamond, A.M.; Yang, W. Functional and physical interaction between the selenium-binding protein 1 (sbp1) and the glutathione peroxidase 1 selenoprotein. *Carcinogenesis* **2010**, *31*, 1360–1366. [CrossRef] [PubMed]
29. Chang, P.W.; Tsui, S.K.; Liew, C.; Lee, C.C.; Waye, M.M.; Fung, K.P. Isolation, characterization, and chromosomal mapping of a novel cdna clone encoding human selenium binding protein. *J. Cell. Biochem.* **1997**, *64*, 217–224. [CrossRef]
30. Yang, M.; Sytkowski, A.J. Differential expression and androgen regulation of the human selenium-binding protein gene hsp56 in prostate cancer cells. *Cancer Res.* **1998**, *58*, 3150–3153. [PubMed]
31. Flemetakis, E.; Agalou, A.; Kavroulakis, N.; Dimou, M.; Martsikovskaya, A.; Slater, A.; Spaink, H.P.; Roussis, A.; Katinakis, P. Lotus japonicus gene ljsbp is highly conserved among plants and animals and encodes a homologue to the mammalian selenium-binding proteins. *Mol. Plant Microbe Interact.* **2002**, *15*, 313–322. [CrossRef] [PubMed]
32. Lanfear, J.; Fleming, J.; Walker, M.; Harrison, P. Different patterns of regulation of the genes encoding the closely related 56 kda selenium- and acetaminophen-binding proteins in normal tissues and during carcinogenesis. *Carcinogenesis* **1993**, *14*, 335–340. [CrossRef] [PubMed]
33. Jeong, J.Y.; Wang, Y.; Sytkowski, A.J. Human selenium binding protein-1 (hsp56) interacts with vdu1 in a selenium-dependent manner. *Biochem. Biophys. Res. Commun.* **2009**, *379*, 583–588. [CrossRef] [PubMed]
34. Raucci, R.; Colonna, G.; Guerriero, E.; Capone, F.; Accardo, M.; Castello, G.; Costantini, S. Structural and functional studies of the human selenium binding protein-1 and its involvement in hepatocellular carcinoma. *Biochim. Biophys. Acta* **2011** *1814*, 513–522. [CrossRef] [PubMed]

35. Ying, Q.; Ansong, E.; Diamond, A.M.; Yang, W. A critical role for cysteine 57 in the biological functions of selenium binding protein-1. *Int. J. Mol. Sci.* **2015**, *16*, 27599–27608. [CrossRef] [PubMed]
36. Li, Z.; Na, X.; Wang, D.; Schoen, S.R.; Messing, E.M.; Wu, G. Ubiquitination of a novel deubiquitinating enzyme requires direct binding to von hippel-lindau tumor suppressor protein. *J. Biol. Chem.* **2002**, *277*, 4656–4662. [CrossRef] [PubMed]
37. Pol, A.; Renkema, G.H.; Tangerman, A.; Winkel, E.G.; Engelke, U.F.; de Brouwer, A.P.M.; Lloyd, K.C.; Araiza, R.S.; van den Heuvel, L.; Omran, H.; et al. Mutations in SELENBP1, encoding a novel human methanethiol oxidase, cause extraoral halitosis. *Nat. Genet.* **2018**, *50*, 120–129. [CrossRef] [PubMed]
38. Driscoll, D.M.; Copeland, P.R. Mechanism and regulation of selenoprotein synthesis. *Annu. Rev. Nutr.* **2003**, *23*, 17–40. [CrossRef] [PubMed]
39. Bansal, M.P.; Ip, C.; Medina, D. Levels and 75se-labeling of specific proteins as a consequence of dietary selenium concentration in mice and rats. *Proc. Soc. Exp. Biol. Med.* **1991**, *196*, 147–154. [CrossRef] [PubMed]
40. Lubos, E.; Loscalzo, J.; Handy, D.E. Glutathione peroxidase-1 in health and disease: From molecular mechanisms to therapeutic opportunities. *Antioxid. Redox Signal.* **2011**, *15*, 1957–1997. [CrossRef] [PubMed]
41. Huang, C.; Ding, G.; Gu, C.; Zhou, J.; Kuang, M.; Ji, Y.; He, Y.; Kondo, T.; Fan, J. Decreased selenium-binding protein 1 enhances glutathione peroxidase 1 activity and downregulates hif-1alpha to promote hepatocellular carcinoma invasiveness. *Clin. Cancer Res.* **2012**, *18*, 3042–3053. [CrossRef] [PubMed]
42. Jerome-Morais, A.; Wright, M.E.; Liu, R.; Yang, W.; Jackson, M.I.; Combs, G.F., Jr.; Diamond, A.M. Inverse association between glutathione peroxidase activity and both selenium-binding protein 1 levels and gleason score in human prostate tissue. *Prostate* **2012**, *72*, 1006–1012. [CrossRef] [PubMed]
43. Ansong, E.; Yang, W.; Diamond, A.M. Molecular cross-talk between members of distinct families of selenium containing proteins. *Mol. Nutr. Food Res.* **2014**, *58*, 117–123. [CrossRef] [PubMed]
44. Brown, L.M.; Helmke, S.M.; Hunsucker, S.W.; Netea-Maier, R.T.; Chiang, S.A.; Heinz, D.E.; Shroyer, K.R.; Duncan, M.W.; Haugen, B.R. Quantitative and qualitative differences in protein expression between papillary thyroid carcinoma and normal thyroid tissue. *Mol. Carcinog.* **2006**, *45*, 613–626. [CrossRef] [PubMed]
45. Tan, X.; Liao, L.; Wan, Y.P.; Li, M.X.; Chen, S.H.; Mo, W.J.; Zhao, Q.L.; Huang, L.F.; Zeng, G.Q. Downregulation of selenium-binding protein 1 is associated with poor prognosis in lung squamous cell carcinoma. *World J. Surg. Oncol.* **2016**, *14*, 70. [CrossRef] [PubMed]
46. Zhang, C.; Xu, W.; Pan, W.; Wang, N.; Li, G.; Fan, X.; Xu, X.; Shen, S.; Das, U.N. Selenium-binding protein 1 may decrease gastric cellular proliferation and migration. *Int. J. Oncol.* **2013**, *42*, 1620–1629. [CrossRef] [PubMed]
47. Xia, Y.J.; Ma, Y.Y.; He, X.J.; Wang, H.J.; Ye, Z.Y.; Tao, H.Q. Suppression of selenium-binding protein 1 in gastric cancer is associated with poor survival. *Hum. Pathol.* **2011**, *42*, 1620–1628. [CrossRef] [PubMed]
48. Ha, Y.S.; Lee, G.T.; Kim, Y.H.; Kwon, S.Y.; Choi, S.H.; Kim, T.H.; Kwon, T.G.; Yun, S.J.; Kim, I.Y.; Kim, W.J. Decreased selenium-binding protein 1 mrna expression is associated with poor prognosis in renal cell carcinoma. *World J. Surg. Oncol.* **2014**, *12*, 288. [CrossRef] [PubMed]
49. Zhang, C.; Wang, Y.E.; Zhang, P.; Liu, F.; Sung, C.J.; Steinhoff, M.M.; Quddus, M.R.; Lawrence, W.D. Progressive loss of selenium-binding protein 1 expression correlates with increasing epithelial proliferation and papillary complexity in ovarian serous borderline tumor and low-grade serous carcinoma. *Hum. Pathol.* **2010**, *41*, 255–261. [CrossRef] [PubMed]
50. Huang, K.C.; Park, D.C.; Ng, S.K.; Lee, J.Y.; Ni, X.; Ng, W.C.; Bandera, C.A.; Welch, W.R.; Berkowitz, R.S.; Mok, S.C.; et al. Selenium binding protein 1 in ovarian cancer. *Int. J. Cancer* **2006**, *118*, 2433–2440. [CrossRef] [PubMed]
51. Stammer, K.; Edassery, S.L.; Barua, A.; Bitterman, P.; Bahr, J.M.; Hales, D.B.; Luborsky, J.L. Selenium-binding protein 1 expression in ovaries and ovarian tumors in the laying hen, a spontaneous model of human ovarian cancer. *Gynecol. Oncol.* **2008**, *109*, 115–121. [CrossRef] [PubMed]
52. Zhang, S.; Li, F.; Younes, M.; Liu, H.; Chen, C.; Yao, Q. Reduced selenium-binding protein 1 in breast cancer correlates with poor survival and resistance to the anti-proliferative effects of selenium. *PLoS ONE* **2013**, *8*, e63702. [CrossRef] [PubMed]
53. Ansong, E.; Ying, Q.; Ekoue, D.N.; Deaton, R.; Hall, A.R.; Kajdacsy-Balla, A.; Yang, W.; Gann, P.H.; Diamond, A.M. Evidence that selenium binding protein 1 is a tumor suppressor in prostate cancer. *PLoS ONE* **2015**, *10*, e0127295. [CrossRef] [PubMed]
54. Jeong, J.Y.; Zhou, J.R.; Gao, C.; Feldman, L.; Sytkowski, A.J. Human selenium binding protein-1 (hsp56)

is a negative regulator of hif-1alpha and suppresses the malignant characteristics of prostate cancer cells. *BMB Rep.* **2014**, *47*, 411–416. [CrossRef] [PubMed]

55. Wang, N.; Chen, Y.; Yang, X.; Jiang, Y. Selenium-binding protein 1 is associated with the degree of colorectal cancer differentiation and is regulated by histone modification. *Oncol. Rep.* **2014**, *31*, 2506–2514. [CrossRef] [PubMed]
56. Pohl, N.M.; Tong, C.; Fang, W.; Bi, X.; Li, T.; Yang, W. Transcriptional regulation and biological functions of selenium-binding protein 1 in colorectal cancer in vitro and in nude mouse xenografts. *PLoS ONE* **2009**, *4*, e7774. [CrossRef] [PubMed]
57. Chen, F.; Chen, C.; Qu, Y.; Xiang, H.; Ai, Q.; Yang, F.; Tan, X.; Zhou, Y.; Jiang, G.; Zhang, Z. Selenium-binding protein 1 in head and neck cancer is low-expression and associates with the prognosis of nasopharyngeal carcinoma. *Medicine* **2016**, *95*, e4592. [CrossRef] [PubMed]
58. Schott, M.; de Jel, M.M.; Engelmann, J.C.; Renner, P.; Geissler, E.K.; Bosserhoff, A.K.; Kuphal, S. Selenium-binding protein 1 is down-regulated in malignant melanoma. *Oncotarget* **2018**, *9*, 10445–10456. [CrossRef] [PubMed]
59. Kim, H.; Kang, H.J.; You, K.T.; Kim, S.H.; Lee, K.Y.; Kim, T.I.; Kim, C.; Song, S.Y.; Kim, H.J.; Lee, C.; et al. Suppression of human selenium-binding protein 1 is a late event in colorectal carcinogenesis and is associated with poor survival. *Proteomics* **2006**, *6*, 3466–3476. [CrossRef] [PubMed]
60. Xie, W.; Yang, M.; Chan, J.; Sun, T.; Mucci, L.A.; Penney, K.L.; Lee, G.S.; Kantoff, P.W. Association of genetic variations of selenoprotein genes, plasma selenium levels, and prostate cancer aggressiveness at diagnosis. *Prostate* **2016**, *76*, 691–699. [CrossRef] [PubMed]
61. Ying, Q.; Ansong, E.; Diamond, A.M.; Lu, Z.; Yang, W.; Bie, X. Quantitative proteomic analysis reveals that anti-cancer effects of selenium-binding protein 1 in vivo are associated with metabolic pathways. *PLoS ONE* **2015**, *10*, e0126285. [CrossRef] [PubMed]
62. Gao, P.T.; Ding, G.Y.; Yang, X.; Dong, R.Z.; Hu, B.; Zhu, X.D.; Cai, J.B.; Ji, Y.; Shi, G.M.; Shen, Y.H.; et al. Invasive potential of hepatocellular carcinoma is enhanced by loss of selenium-binding protein 1 and subsequent upregulation of cxcr4. *Am. J. Cancer Res.* **2018**, *8*, 1040–1049. [PubMed]
63. Caswell, D.R.; Chuang, C.H.; Ma, R.K.; Winters, I.P.; Snyder, E.L.; Winslow, M.M. Tumor suppressor activity of SELENBP1, a direct nkx2-1 target, in lung adenocarcinoma. *Mol. Cancer Res.* **2018**. [CrossRef] [PubMed]
64. Tsujimoto, S.; Ishida, T.; Takeda, T.; Ishii, Y.; Onomura, Y.; Tsukimori, K.; Takechi, S.; Yamaguchi, T.; Uchi, H.; Suzuki, S.O.; et al. Selenium-binding protein 1: Its physiological function, dependence on aryl hydrocarbon receptors, and role in wasting syndrome by 2,3,7,8-tetrachlorodibenzo-p-dioxin. *Biochim. Biophys. Acta* **2013**, *1830*, 3616–3624. [CrossRef] [PubMed]
65. Zhang, J.; Zhan, N.; Dong, W.G. Altered expression of selenium-binding protein 1 in gastric carcinoma and precursor lesions. *Med. Oncol.* **2011**, *28*, 951–957. [CrossRef] [PubMed]
66. Zeng, G.Q.; Yi, H.; Zhang, P.F.; Li, X.H.; Hu, R.; Li, M.Y.; Li, C.; Qu, J.Q.; Deng, X.; Xiao, Z.Q. The function and significance of SELENBP1 downregulation in human bronchial epithelial carcinogenic process. *PLoS ONE* **2013**, *8*, e71865. [CrossRef] [PubMed]
67. Zhang, P.; Zhang, C.; Wang, X.; Liu, F.; Sung, C.J.; Quddus, M.R.; Lawrence, W.D. The expression of selenium-binding protein 1 is decreased in uterine leiomyoma. *Diagn. Pathol.* **2010**, *5*, 80. [CrossRef] [PubMed]
68. Hiroshi, I.; Masayuki, I.; Shosuke, K. Early decreases in pulmonary, hepatic and renal glutathione levels in response to cadmium instillation into rat trachea. *J. Appl. Toxicol.* **1991**, *11*, 211–217. [CrossRef]
69. Wang, Y.; Fang, W.; Huang, Y.; Hu, F.; Ying, Q.; Yang, W.; Xiong, B. Reduction of selenium-binding protein 1 sensitizes cancer cells to selenite via elevating extracellular glutathione: A novel mechanism of cancer-specific cytotoxicity of selenite. *Free Radic. Biol. Med.* **2015**, *79*, 186–196. [CrossRef] [PubMed]
70. Porat, A.; Sagiv, Y.; Elazar, Z. A 56-kda selenium-binding protein participates in intra-golgi protein transport. *J. Biol. Chem.* **2000**, *275*, 14457–14465. [CrossRef] [PubMed]
71. Miyaguchi, K. Localization of selenium-binding protein at the tips of rapidly extending protrusions. *Histochem. Cell Biol.* **2004**, *121*, 371–376. [CrossRef] [PubMed]
72. Glatt, S.J.; Everall, I.P.; Kremen, W.S.; Corbeil, J.; Sasik, R.; Khanlou, N.; Han, M.; Liew, C.C.; Tsuang, M.T. Comparative gene expression analysis of blood and brain provides concurrent validation of SELENBP1 up-regulation in schizophrenia. *Proc. Natl. Acad. Sci. USA* **2005**, *102*, 15533–15538. [CrossRef] [PubMed]
73. Kanazawa, T.; Chana, G.; Glatt, S.J.; Mizuno, H.; Masliah, E.; Yoneda, H.; Tsuang, M.T.; Everall, I.P. The utility of SELENBP1 gene expression as a biomarker for major psychotic disorders: Replication in schizophrenia

and extension to bipolar disorder with psychosis. *Am. J. Med. Genet. Part B Neuropsychiatr. Genet.* **2008**, *147B*, 686–689. [CrossRef] [PubMed]

74. Udawela, M.; Money, T.T.; Neo, J.; Seo, M.S.; Scarr, E.; Dean, B.; Everall, I.P. SELENBP1 expression in the prefrontal cortex of subjects with schizophrenia. *Transl. Psychiatry* **2015**, *5*, e615. [CrossRef] [PubMed]
75. Kanazawa, T.; Glatt, S.J.; Faraone, S.V.; Hwu, H.G.; Yoneda, H.; Tsuang, M.T. Family-based association study of SELENBP1 in schizophrenia. *Schizophr. Res.* **2009**, *113*, 268–272. [CrossRef] [PubMed]
76. Chau, E.J.; Mostaid, M.S.; Cropley, V.; McGorry, P.; Pantelis, C.; Bousman, C.A.; Everall, I.P. Downregulation of plasma SELENBP1 protein in patients with recent-onset schizophrenia. *Prog. Neuro-Psychopharmacol. Biol. Psychiatry* **2018**, *85*, 1–6. [CrossRef] [PubMed]
77. Brauer, A.U.; Savaskan, N.E. Molecular actions of selenium in the brain: Neuroprotective mechanisms of an essential trace element. *Rev. Neurosci.* **2004**, *15*, 19–32. [CrossRef] [PubMed]
78. Xue, W.; Du, P.; Lin, S.; Dudley, V.J.; Hernandez, M.R.; Sarthy, V.P. Gene expression changes in retinal muller (glial) cells exposed to elevated pressure. *Curr. Eye Res.* **2011**, *36*, 754–767. [CrossRef] [PubMed]
79. Wang, J.; Qu, D.; An, J.; Yuan, G.; Liu, Y. Integrated microarray analysis provided novel insights to the pathogenesis of glaucoma. *Mol. Med. Rep.* **2017**, *16*, 8735–8746. [CrossRef] [PubMed]
80. Okunuki, Y.; Usui, Y.; Takeuchi, M.; Kezuka, T.; Hattori, T.; Masuko, K.; Nakamura, H.; Yudoh, K.; Usui, M.; Nishioka, K.; et al. Proteomic surveillance of autoimmunity in behcet's disease with uveitis: Selenium binding protein is a novel autoantigen in behcet's disease. *Exp. Eye Res.* **2007**, *84*, 823–831. [CrossRef] [PubMed]
81. Krause, I.; Weinberger, A. Behcet's disease. *Curr. Opin. Rheumatol.* **2008**, *20*, 82–87. [CrossRef] [PubMed]
82. Torrealba, J.R.; Colburn, M.; Golner, S.; Chang, Z.; Scheunemann, T.; Fechner, J.H.; Roenneburg, D.; Hu, H.; Alam, T.; Kim, H.T.; et al. Selenium-binding protein-1 in smooth muscle cells is downregulated in a rhesus monkey model of chronic allograft nephropathy. *Am. J. Transplant.* **2005**, *5*, 58–67. [CrossRef] [PubMed]
83. Scortegagna, M.; Martin, R.J.; Kladney, R.D.; Neumann, R.G.; Arbeit, J.M. Hypoxia-inducible factor-1alpha suppresses squamous carcinogenic progression and epithelial-mesenchymal transition. *Cancer Res.* **2009**, *69*, 2638–2646. [CrossRef] [PubMed]
84. Semenza, G.L. Targeting hif-1 for cancer therapy. *Nat. Rev. Cancer* **2003**, *3*, 721–732. [CrossRef] [PubMed]
85. Zhong, H.; De Marzo, A.M.; Laughner, E.; Lim, M.; Hilton, D.A.; Zagzag, D.; Buechler, P.; Isaacs, W.B.; Semenza, G.L.; Simons, J.W. Overexpression of hypoxia-inducible factor 1alpha in common human cancers and their metastases. *Cancer Res.* **1999**, *59*, 5830–5835. [PubMed]
86. Feldser, D.; Agani, F.; Iyer, N.V.; Pak, B.; Ferreira, G.; Semenza, G.L. Reciprocal positive regulation of hypoxia-inducible factor 1alpha and insulin-like growth factor 2. *Cancer Res.* **1999**, *59*, 3915–3918. [PubMed]
87. Talks, K.L.; Turley, H.; Gatter, K.C.; Maxwell, P.H.; Pugh, C.W.; Ratcliffe, P.J.; Harris, A.L. The expression and distribution of the hypoxia-inducible factors hif-1alpha and hif-2alpha in normal human tissues, cancers, and tumor-associated macrophages. *Am. J. Pathol.* **2000**, *157*, 411–421. [CrossRef]
88. Birner, P.; Schindl, M.; Obermair, A.; Plank, C.; Breitenecker, G.; Oberhuber, G. Overexpression of hypoxia-inducible factor 1alpha is a marker for an unfavorable prognosis in early-stage invasive cervical cancer. *Cancer Res.* **2000**, *60*, 4693–4696. [PubMed]
89. Burri, P.; Djonov, V.; Aebersold, D.M.; Lindel, K.; Studer, U.; Altermatt, H.J.; Mazzucchelli, L.; Greiner, R.H.; Gruber, G. Significant correlation of hypoxia-inducible factor-1alpha with treatment outcome in cervical cancer treated with radical radiotherapy. *Int. J. Radiat. Oncol. Biol. Phys.* **2003**, *56*, 494–501. [CrossRef]
90. Bos, R.; van der Groep, P.; Greijer, A.E.; Shvarts, A.; Meijer, S.; Pinedo, H.M.; Semenza, G.L.; van Diest, P.J.; van der Wall, E. Levels of hypoxia-inducible factor-1alpha independently predict prognosis in patients with lymph node negative breast carcinoma. *Cancer* **2003**, *97*, 1573–1581. [CrossRef] [PubMed]
91. Schindl, M.; Schoppmann, S.F.; Samonigg, H.; Hausmaninger, H.; Kwasny, W.; Gnant, M.; Jakesz, R.; Kubista, E.; Birner, P.; Oberhuber, G.; et al. Overexpression of hypoxia-inducible factor 1alpha is associated with an unfavorable prognosis in lymph node-positive breast cancer. *Clin. Cancer Res.* **2002**, *8*, 1831–1837. [PubMed]
92. Birner, P.; Schindl, M.; Obermair, A.; Breitenecker, G.; Oberhuber, G. Expression of hypoxia-inducible factor 1alpha in epithelial ovarian tumors: Its impact on prognosis and on response to chemotherapy. *Clin. Cancer Res.* **2001**, *7*, 1661–1668. [PubMed]
93. Sivridis, E.; Giatromanolaki, A.; Gatter, K.C.; Harris, A.L.; Koukourakis, M.I.; Tumor and Angiogenesis Research Group. Association of hypoxia-inducible factors 1alpha and 2alpha with activated angiogenic

pathways and prognosis in patients with endometrial carcinoma. *Cancer* **2002**, *95*, 1055–1063. [CrossRef] [PubMed]

94. Takahashi, R.; Tanaka, S.; Hiyama, T.; Ito, M.; Kitadai, Y.; Sumii, M.; Haruma, K.; Chayama, K. Hypoxia-inducible factor-1alpha expression and angiogenesis in gastrointestinal stromal tumor of the stomach. *Oncol. Rep.* **2003**, *10*, 797–802. [PubMed]
95. Birner, P.; Gatterbauer, B.; Oberhuber, G.; Schindl, M.; Rossler, K.; Prodinger, A.; Budka, H.; Hainfellner, J.A. Expression of hypoxia-inducible factor-1 alpha in oligodendrogliomas: Its impact on prognosis and on neoangiogenesis. *Cancer* **2001**, *92*, 165–171. [CrossRef]
96. Beasley, N.J.; Leek, R.; Alam, M.; Turley, H.; Cox, G.J.; Gatter, K.; Millard, P.; Fuggle, S.; Harris, A.L. Hypoxia-inducible factors hif-1alpha and hif-2alpha in head and neck cancer: Relationship to tumor biology and treatment outcome in surgically resected patients. *Cancer Res.* **2002**, *62*, 2493–2497. [PubMed]
97. Volm, M.; Koomagi, R. Hypoxia-inducible factor (hif-1) and its relationship to apoptosis and proliferation in lung cancer. *Anticancer Res.* **2000**, *20*, 1527–1533. [PubMed]
98. Chen, G.; Wang, H.; Miller, C.T.; Thomas, D.G.; Gharib, T.G.; Misek, D.E.; Giordano, T.J.; Orringer, M.B.; Hanash, S.M.; Beer, D.G. Reduced selenium-binding protein 1 expression is associated with poor outcome in lung adenocarcinomas. *J. Pathol.* **2004**, *202*, 321–329. [CrossRef] [PubMed]
99. Barr, L.A.; Calvert, J.W. Discoveries of hydrogen sulfide as a novel cardiovascular therapeutic. *Circ. J.* **2014**, *78*, 2111–2118. [CrossRef] [PubMed]
100. Kohl, J.B.; Mellis, A.T.; Schwarz, G. Homeostatic impact of sulfite and hydrogen sulfide on cysteine catabolism. *Br. J. Pharmacol.* **2018**. [CrossRef] [PubMed]
101. Szabo, C.; Ransy, C.; Modis, K.; Andriamihaja, M.; Murghes, B.; Coletta, C.; Olah, G.; Yanagi, K.; Bouillaud, F. Regulation of mitochondrial bioenergetic function by hydrogen sulfide. Part i. Biochemical and physiological mechanisms. *Br. J. Pharmacol.* **2014**, *171*, 2099–2122. [CrossRef] [PubMed]
102. Bos, E.M.; van Goor, H.; Joles, J.A.; Whiteman, M.; Leuvenink, H.G. Hydrogen sulfide: Physiological properties and therapeutic potential in ischaemia. *Br. J. Pharmacol.* **2015**, *172*, 1479–1493. [CrossRef] [PubMed]
103. Wallace, J.L.; Wang, R. Hydrogen sulfide-based therapeutics: Exploiting a unique but ubiquitous gasotransmitter. *Nat. Rev. Drug Discov.* **2015**, *14*, 329–345. [CrossRef] [PubMed]

12

PET Radiotracers for CNS-Adrenergic Receptors: Developments and Perspectives

Santosh Reddy Alluri [1], Sung Won Kim [2], Nora D. Volkow [2,3,*] and Kun-Eek Kil [1,4,*]

1 University of Missouri Research Reactor, University of Missouri, Columbia, MO 65211-5110, USA; srad3k@missouri.edu
2 Laboratory of Neuroimaging, National Institute on Alcohol Abuse and Alcoholism, National Institutes of Health, Bethesda, MD 20892-1013, USA; kims8@mail.nih.gov
3 National Institute on Drug Abuse, National Institutes of Health, Bethesda, MD 20892-1013, USA
4 Department of Veterinary Medicine and Surgery, University of Missouri, Columbia, MO 65211, USA
* Correspondence: nvolkow@nida.nih.gov (N.D.V.); kilk@missouri.edu (K.-E.K.);

Academic Editor: Krishan Kumar

Abstract: Epinephrine (E) and norepinephrine (NE) play diverse roles in our body's physiology. In addition to their role in the peripheral nervous system (PNS), E/NE systems including their receptors are critical to the central nervous system (CNS) and to mental health. Various antipsychotics, antidepressants, and psychostimulants exert their influence partially through different subtypes of adrenergic receptors (ARs). Despite the potential of pharmacological applications and long history of research related to E/NE systems, research efforts to identify the roles of ARs in the human brain taking advantage of imaging have been limited by the lack of subtype specific ligands for ARs and brain penetrability issues. This review provides an overview of the development of positron emission tomography (PET) radiotracers for in vivo imaging of AR system in the brain.

Keywords: adrenergic receptor; positron emission tomography; radiotracer

1. Introduction

Positron emission tomography (PET) is a noninvasive and highly sensitive in vivo imaging technique that uses small amounts of radiotracers to detect the concentration of relevant biomarkers in tissues such as receptors, enzymes, and transporters. These radiotracers can be used to characterize neurochemical changes in neuropsychiatric diseases and also to measure drug pharmacokinetics and pharmacodynamics directly in the human body including the brain [1,2]. PET technology requires positron-emitting radioisotopes, a radiotracer synthesis unit, a PET scanner, and data acquisition components. Among the PET isotopes, cyclotron produced carbon-11 (C-11, $t_{1/2}$ = 20.34 min), nitrogen-13 (N-13, $t_{1/2}$ = 9.96 min), and fluorine-18 (F-18, $t_{1/2}$ = 109.77 min) are frequently used for PET-neuroimaging. PET imaging is particularly valuable to characterize investigational drugs and their target proteins, providing a valuable tool for clinical neuroscience [3].

PET radiotracers for the central nervous system (CNS) should have proper pharmacokinetic profile in the brain and to achieve this property, they were designed to meet five molecular properties: (a) molecular weight <500 kDa, (b) Log $D_{7.4}$ between ~1 to 3 (lipophilicity factor), (c) number of hydrogen bond donors <5, (d) number of hydrogen bond acceptors <10, and (e) topological polar surface area <90 Å^2. Otherwise, they may either not cross the blood-brain barrier (BBB) or show lack of specific signal due to high nonspecific binding [3–5]. In addition, an ideal PET radiotracer should have, though unachievable, (a) high affinity (preferably subnanomolar range) for its target, (b) high selectivity between subtypes or void on off-targets, (c) high dynamic range in specific binding, (d) appropriate metabolic profile, (e) no adverse toxicology effects, and (f) kinetics suitable for mathematical modelling, which requires fast transfer to BBB and clearance in non-target tissues [3]. In general, a radiotracer with binding potential [ratio of target density (B_{max}) to ligand's affinity (K_d or K_i)] value of at least 10 is expected to provide a reliable specific signal in vivo [6,7]. Furthermore, there are some technical challenges associated with CNS PET radiotracer development, which include: limited synthesis time and/or complex syntheses to prepare a radiotracer, attainment of high molar activity, accurate radiometric metabolite analysis. In addition, the radiotracer ought to ideally address targets that are relevant to brain function and for the diagnosis and therapy of a disease [3,8]. Epinephrine (E) and norepinephrine (NE) were discovered in 1894 and 1907, respectively. They are both neurotransmitters and hormones that belong to the group of catecholamines crucial to the function of the body and brain [9–11]. Neither E nor NE crosses the BBB but they are synthetized in the brain. NE is synthesized in synapse from *L*-phenylalanine in four steps enzymatically through phenylalanine hydroxylase (PAH), tyrosine hydroxylase, dopa decarboxylase (DDC), and dopamine beta-hydroxylase (DBH), respectively. Further, NE is methylated to convert into E with phenylethanolamine-*N*-methyl transferase (PNMT) [12–14]. NE in synaptic cleft is removed either by reuptake via NE transporter (NET) or via metabolism by monoamine oxidase A (MAO-A) or catechol-*O*-methyl transferase (COMT) into various transitional metabolites. Though the noradrenergic neurons are confined to a few relatively small brain areas such as midbrain, pons, locus coeruleus, caudal ventrolateral nucleus, and medulla, they send extensive projections to most brain regions [15]. Table 1 summarizes the brain distribution (reported in mice) and function of various AR subtypes and their involvement in some brain disorders for CNS-ARs.

The effects of NE and E in the CNS and PNS is mediated mainly through two main classes of adrenergic receptors (ARs): alpha-ARs (α-ARs) and beta-ARs (β-ARs) [16]. The ARs were first identified in 1948 and pharmacological and molecular cloning techniques since then have identified various subclasses of ARs [17,18]. α-ARs are divided into α1 and α2 subclasses, wherein, each of these has three subtypes: α1A, α1B, α1D and α2A, α2B, α2C. The three subtypes of β-ARs are β1, β2, and β3 [19]. These receptors in the CNS are G-protein coupled receptors (GPCR) and are implicated in pathophysiology of various diseases, biochemical pathways, and biological functions [18].

Table 1. Brain distribution of AR subtypes and their associated brain disorders.

Receptor		Distribution	Distinct Functions and Associated Disorders	Ref
α1	α1A	High levels in olfactory system, hypothalamic nuclei, and brainstem. Moderate levels in amygdala, cerebral cortex, and cerebellum	Involved in neurotransmission of NE as well as γ-aminobutyric acid (GABA) and NMDA. May mediate effects of anti-depressants in treating depression and obsessive compulsive disorder (OCD)	[18,20–24]
	α1B	Thalamic nuclei, lateral nucleus of amygdala, cerebral cortex, some septal regions, brain stem regions	May play a role in behavioral activation. Associated with addiction, and neurodegenerative disorders (Multiple System Atrophy)	[18,20,21,24–27]
	α1D	Olfactory bulb, cerebral cortex, hippocampus, reticular thalamic nuclei, and amygdala	Mediates changes in locomotor behaviors. Associated with stress.	[18,20,23,28,29]
α2	α2A	Locus coeruleus, midbrain, hypothalamus, amygdala, cerebral cortex, and brain stem	Mediate functions of most of the α2-agonists used in sedation, antinociception, and behavioral actions. Associated with ADHD, anxiety	[18,23,30–35]
	α2B	Thalamus, hypothalamus, cerebellar Purkinje layer	Mediate antinociceptive action of nitrous oxide	[18,30,31]
	α2C	Hippocampus, striatum, olfactory tubercle, medulla, and basal ganglia	Involved in the neuronal release of NE as well as dopamine and serotonin. Potential therapeutic targets in depression & schizophrenia	[18,30,31,36–39]
β	β1, β2, β3	Homologous distribution. Expression was found (mostly β1 and β2) in frontal cortex, striatum, thalamus, putamen, amygdala, cerebellum, cerebral cortex and hippocampus.	Essential to motor learning, emotional memory storage and regulation of neuronal regeneration. Associated with mood disorders, aging, Alzheimer's disease, Parkinson's disease.	[16,18,40–48]

Given its biological significance, the adrenergic system has emerged as an important target for PET studies. Although ARs play major roles in the brain, most PET studies of ARs have focused on cardiac imaging [49,50] and PET studies of CNS-ARs are very limited. The other components of adrenergic system such as NET and MAO-A were studied using PET. Various C-11 and F-18 radiotracers of NET-selective anti-depressants (e.g., reboxetine) were examined using PET to monitor the function of noradrenergic system in CNS. Radiotracers, for example, (*S,S*)-[^{11}C]*O*-methyl-reboxetine ([^{11}C]MRB) and [^{18}F]FMeNER-D_2, were shown to exhibit desirable in vivo properties and their regional distribution in the brain is consistent with known distribution of NET in preclinical/clinical settings [51–54]. These radiotracers have been employed to monitor NET availability in different related diseases, including obesity, major depressive disorder, and Parkinson's disease. Likewise, radiotracers, for instance, [^{11}C]Harmine demonstrated clinical success for in vivo brain imaging of MAO-A, respectively [55–57]. [^{11}C]Harmine has been applied in several-PET neuroimaging studies to study the role of MAO-A in different pathological conditions, including nicotine/alcohol dependence, and Alzheimer's disease.

However, the metabolic functions of MAO-A do not necessarily reflect the activities of adrenergic system as they also metabolize other neurotransmitters, such as, dopamine and serotonin (5-HT). Therefore, the in vivo activities of adrenergic neurons, thus far, were exclusively examined by PET imaging based on NET. Since the activities of NET reflect only on presynaptic systems of adrenergic neurons, novel PET radiotracers that can observe the features of postsynaptic adrenergic system are still required. PET-neuroimaging of AR subtypes combined with NET can scrutinize the unique implications of adrenergic system in various pathophysiological conditions of the brain. Subtype specific PET radiotracers for CNS-ARs have the potential to help clarify the roles of ARs in brain pathophysiology and provide suggestions towards the diagnosis and treatment for diseases such as depression, attention deficit hyperactivity disorder (ADHD), substance use disorders, schizophrenia, and neurodegenerative diseases that involve ARs. This review, based on reports published through 2019, summarizes the development of PET radioligands for CNS-ARs in animal models and human subjects and presents suggestions for further development for CNS-AR radiotracers.

2. α1-AR PET Radiotracers

Three highly homologous subunits of α-1 ARs, α1A, α1B, and α1D, have been shown to have different amino acid sequence, pharmacological properties, and tissue distributions [58–60]. A detailed review of α1-AR pharmacology is given by Michael and Perez [58]. Binding of NE/E to any of the α1-AR subtypes is stimulatory and activates $G_{q/11}$-signalling pathway, which involves phospholipase C activation, generation of secondary messengers, inositol triphosphate and diacyl glycerol and intracellular calcium mobilization. In PNS, as well as in the brain's vascular system it results in smooth muscle contraction and vasoconstriction. While the signaling effects of α1-ARs in the cardiovascular system are well studied [61,62], the role of α1-ARs in CNS is complex and not completely understood. The Bmax values of α-1 ARs were measured from saturation assays using [^{3}H]prazosin (a selective α-1 blocker) with tissue homogenates from rats and the observed binding capacities (fmol/mg tissue) of prazosin in cortex, hippocampus, and cerebellum were 14.49 ± 0.38, 11.03 ± 0.39, and 7.72 ± 0.11, respectively [23,63]. The α1-ARs are postsynaptic receptors and can also modulate release of NE. In the human brain, α1-AR subtypes are localized in amygdala, cerebellum, thalamus, hippocampus, and to some extent in striatum [20,22,64].

The anti-depressant effects of noradrenergic enhancing drugs as well as their effects on anxiety and stress reactivity points to their relevance of α1A, α1D to these behaviors [21,28,65]. Furthermore, α1A-ARs regulate GABAergic and NMDAergic neurons [20]. A decrease in α1A-AR mRNA expression was observed in prefrontal cortex of subjects with dementia [66,67]. The α1B-ARs has also been shown to be crucial to brain function and disease [18]. For example, α1B-knockout (KO) mice study revealed that α1B-AR modulates behavior, showing increased reaction to novel situations [24,27]. In addition, the locomotor and rewarding effects of psychostimulants and opiates were decreased in α1B-KO mice, highlighting their role in the pharmacological effects of these drugs [24]. On the other hand, studies using the α1B-overexpression model suggest their involvement in neurodegenerative diseases [25].

Several α1-AR agonists and antagonists (α1-blockers) are available in the market as drugs to treat various heart and brain disorders [68,69]. Pharmacology of most of these drugs is complicated by the fact that they have strong affinities for other receptor systems, such as serotonin and dopamine receptors. The need to develop α1-AR selective/α1-AR subtype specific drugs is demanding. Undoubtedly, PET radiotracers selective for α1-AR are valuable to assess α1-ARs contribution to brain function and disease. In the late 1980s, prazosin, used for the treatment of hypertension, was labelled with carbon-11 to image α1-ARs with PET [49]. Following this, [^{11}C]prazosin analogous, [^{11}C]bunazosin and [^{11}C]GB67 (Figure 1A) were developed as PET radiotracers to image α1-ARs in the cardiovascular system [49,70]. These tracers were shown to have limited BBB permeability and were deemed to be not suitable for PET-neuroimaging. Efforts to develop PET radiotracers to image α1-ARs in the CNS was mainly based on antipsychotic drugs such as clozapine, sertindole, olanzapine, and risperidone that have mixed binding affinities for D_2, $5HT_{2A}$ receptors and α1-ARs in the nanomolar range. Their affinity for α1-ARs has been shown to contribute to antipsychotic efficacy uncovering their role in psychoses [71,72].

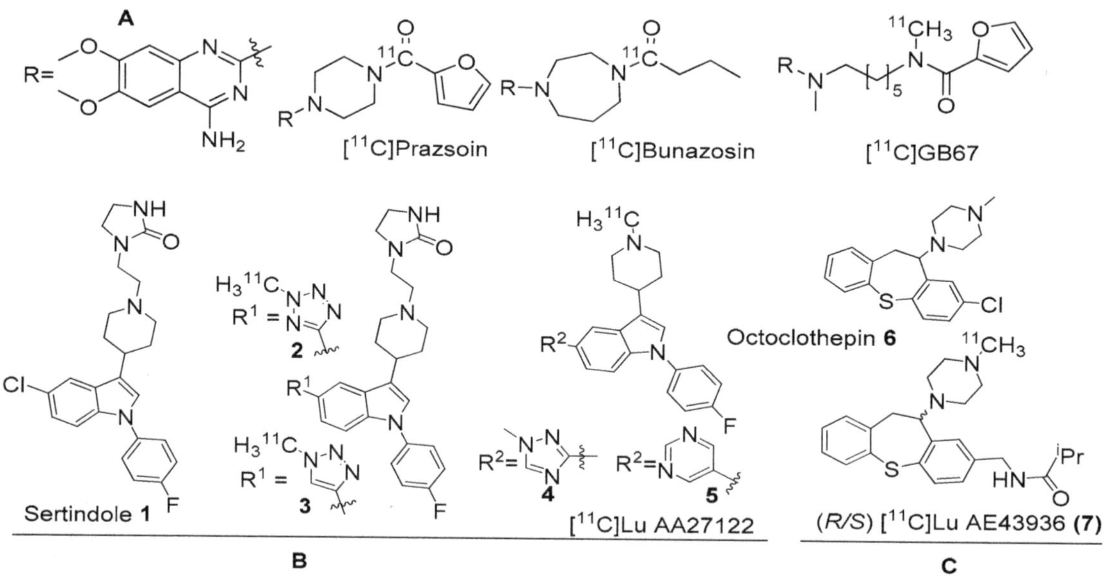

Figure 1. (**A**) Earlier PET radiotracers, [^{11}C]Prazosin, [^{11}C]Bunazosin, and [^{11}C]GB67 for cardiac α1-AR imaging. (**B**) Antagonist PET radiotracers based on sertindole. (**C**) Antagonist PET radiotracers based on octoclothepin for brain α1-AR imaging.

Two C-11 labelled analogs of the atypical antipsychotic drug sertindole were first reported by Balle et al. In the early 2000s (Figure 1B) [73,74]. Several other analogs with good affinities (K_i < 10 nM) for α1-ARs were subsequently reported by the same group. Two analogs, in which chlorine in sertindole (**1**) is replaced by a 2-methyl-tetrazol-5-yl (**2**) and a 1-methyl-1,2,3-triazol-4-yl (**3**), were labelled with C-11 [73,74]. The in vitro affinities (K_i) of **1**, **2** and **3** for α1-ARs are 1.4, 1.8 and 9.5 nM, respectively. Both [^{11}C]**2** and [^{11}C]**3** were prepared using ^{11}C-methylation with [^{11}C]methyl triflate from their corresponding *N*-desmethyl precursors. The molar activity of [^{11}C]**2** and [^{11}C]**3** was reported at 70 GBq/µmol and 15 GBq/µmol, respectively. Their brain distribution examined with PET in Cynomolgus monkeys showed that brain uptake of [^{11}C]**2** and [^{11}C]**3** was slow and low, with [^{11}C]**3** showing somewhat higher brain uptake than [^{11}C]**2**. Their brain distribution was homogenous and specific binding to α1-ARs could not be demonstrated. It was also concluded that these two radiotracers were not suitable to image α1-ARs in brain owing to rapid metabolism, substantial distribution to other organs, and substrates for active efflux mechanism.

In the early 2010s, further optimization of structure-activity relationship (SAR) studies led to the identification of two more sertindole analogs, **4** and **5** (Lu AA27122), with higher α1-AR selectivity over D_2 receptors (Figure 1B). Compared to the in vitro affinity for α1A-AR subtype (K_i = 0.16, 0.52 nM for **4** and **5**), the affinity for the α1B and α1D subtypes is 4 to 15 times less potent (Table 2). The $LogD_{7.4}$ values for **4** (2.7) and **5** (1.9) were in the optimal range for in vivo brain imaging [75–77]. Both [^{11}C]**4** and [^{11}C]**5** were prepared in a similar manner like above with >370 GBq/μmol molar activity for non-human primate studies [75]. Interestingly, while [^{11}C]**4** showed very poor brain uptake, [^{11}C]**5** had suitable brain uptake (4.6% ID/cc at 36 min). However, its binding was not blocked with a pharmacological dose of prazosin pretreatment, indicating lack of α1-AR specificity.

Table 2. In vitro affinities of compounds **1** to **7** for α1-ARs, D_2 and $5HT_{2C}$ receptors [73,75,76].

Compound	Receptor K_i (nM)				
	α1A	α1B	α1D	D_2	$5HT_{2C}$
1	0.37	0.33	0.66	0.45	0.55
2	0.23	1.1	2.0	140	330
3	3.0	6.0	8.6	310	1500
4	0.16	6.4	15	220	-
5	0.52	1.9	2.5	120	-
6	0.37	0.33	0.66	0.45	0.51
(*R*)-**7**	0.43	0.27	0.64	31	8.0
(*S*)-**7**	0.16	0.20	0.21	4.5	93

At the same time, another C-11 labelled radiotracer, [^{11}C]**7** ([^{11}C]Lu AE43936, Figure 1C) for brain α1-ARs was developed and evaluated by Risgaard et al. [76]. This radiotracer was based on the antipsychotic octoclothepin (**6**, Figure 1C), which belongs to the tricylic dibenzotheiepin group and has inverse agonist effects at dopamine, serotonin, and α1 receptor sites [78]. Two enantiomers of **7** (*R*/*S*) were radiolabelled on the basis of their varying selectivity and specificity for α1-AR subtypes (Table 2) and imaged with PET in female Danish Landrace pigs. The baseline PET imaging results indicated that neither of the radiolabelled isomers entered the pig's brain. Pretreatment with cyclosporin A (CsA) [79] increased the brain uptake of (*R*)-**7** in α1-AR rich cortex, thalamus (above 2 SUV), suggesting that (*R*)-**7** was a substrate for active efflux transporters. Further cell studies specified that (*R*)-**7** is a substrate for p-glycoprotein (Pgp).

So far, none of the reported radiotracers showed promising results for in vivo brain imaging of α1-ARs for they were limited by poor BBB penetration, being substrates of Pgp or lack of binding specificity. Therefore, novel α1-AR radiotracers that overcome brain permeability and display good affinity and subtype-selectivity are required to evaluate the role of α1-AR subtypes in brain pathophysiology. Several α1-AR subtype specific (high affinity for one subtype over the other) and nonspecific compounds have been reported over the years [26,29,80,81]. Either direct radiolabeling (if possible) or chemical modification and then radiolabeling of the most specific compounds could be an optimal approach for developing new α1-subtype specific radiotracer, considering the aforementioned CNS-PET radiotracer criteria.

3. α2-AR Subtype and Nonspecific PET Radiotracers

Unlike α1-ARs, α2-ARs decrease adenyl cyclase activity in association with G_i heterotrimeric G-protein and hence are inhibitory. They mediate many NE effects including cognition and readiness for action [11,30]. The brain distribution of the three subtypes, α2A, α2B, and α2C, was characterized by autoradiography and immunohistochemistry techniques. Among the three subtypes, α2A-ARs are the most abundant in the brain and localized in locus coeruleus, midbrain, hippocampus, hypothalamus, amygdala, cerebral cortex and brain stem. The α2B-ARs are located in thalamus and hypothalamus and α2C-ARs in cortex, hippocampus, olfactory tubercle and basal ganglia [51–53]. In the mouse brain, ~90% of α2-ARs are α2A-ARs and ~10% are α2C-ARs [30–32,82]. Notably, binding experiments using [^{3}H]2-methoxyidazoxan (a selective α-2 AR antagonist) with postmortem human brain detected 100% of α2A-ARs population in the hippocampus, cerebellum, and brainstem (B_{max} = 34–90 fmol/mg protein). In addition to this, α2A-AR (B_{max} = 53 fmol/mg of protein) and α2B/C-AR (B_{max} = 8 fmol/mg of protein) were detected in the frontal cortex [30]. An extensive array of agonists and antagonists for α2-ARs have been developed. The main limitation of these ligands is lack of subtype selectivity for α2-ARs and off-target binding to other receptors [83,84]. α2A-ARs are mostly presynaptic and agonists inhibit NE release from the terminals and are used to treat hypertension, drug withdrawal, and ADHD whereas antagonists increase NE release and are used as antidepressants. Development of α2-AR subtype selective PET tracers would facilitate medication development and help gain further understanding of their role in brain diseases.

During the 1980s, two research groups identified two potent α2-AR selective antagonists via radioligand binding assays. One WY-26703 belongs to the benzoquinolizine class, and the other MK-492 belongs to the benzo[b]furo-quinolizine class [85,86]. Based on these templates, Bylund's group developed two PET tracers: [^{11}C]WY-26703 (**8**) in 1992 and [^{11}C]MK-912 (**9**) in 1998 (Figure 2) [87,88]. Both radiotracers were prepared from their respective *N*-desmethyl precursors via ^{11}C-methylation with 30.71–34.41 GBq/μmol molar activity. The in vitro binding assays and ex vivo biodistribution studies (tissue dissection followed by γ-counting) in rodents indicated that both radiotracers crossed the BBB and **9** showed higher affinity and specific binding to α2-ARs than **8**. However, PET studies of **8** and **9** in Rhesus monkeys showed fast washout from brain and nonspecific binding; thus it was concluded that they were not appropriate for PET imaging of α2-ARs in brain.

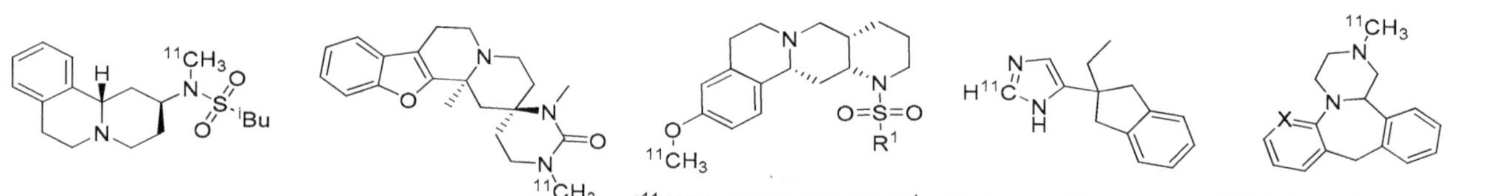

[^{11}C]WY-26703, **8** [^{11}C]MK-912, **9** [^{11}C]RS-15385-197, **10** (R^1 = Me) [^{11}C]RS-79948-197, **11** (R^1 = Et) **12** [^{11}C]mianserin, **13** (X = CH) [^{11}C]mitrazepine, **14** (X = N)

Figure 2. Various classes of α2-ARs antagonist radiotracers.

In 1997, Pike's group developed [^{11}C]RS-15385-197 (**10**) and [^{11}C]79948-197 (**11**) as PET α2-ARs ligands (Figure 2) [89]. These radiotracers were prepared from their respective *O*-desmethyl precursors through the ^{11}C-methylation method with 61 ± 17 GBq/μmol (**10**) and 64 ± 3 GBq/μmol molar activity (**11**). Biodistribution, brain uptake, and metabolic profile studies were done in male Sprague-Dawley rats. They observed specific signals in brain (mainly cerebellum) at 30–90 min (70–95% radioactivity of parent radioligand), which was analogous to their results with [^{3}H]**10**. Nonspecific binding in brain was **11** > **10**, which mostly likely reflected their differential metabolism (**11** > **10**). Thus, they chose **10** to quantify α2-ARs in the human brain using PET [90]. Studies in two volunteers with **10** revealed a low brain uptake index (BUI) due to high affinity to human plasma proteins. Consequently, **10** was not studied further.

In 2002, Crouzel's group chose atipamezole, an α2-AR selective antagonist, to develop [^{11}C]atipamezole, **12** (Figure 2) [91]. The radiotracer was prepared through an unique approach using 2-ethyl-2-oxoacetylindane, [^{11}C]formaldehyde ([^{11}C]HCHO) in the presence of zinc oxide and ammonium hydroxide (similar to Debus-Radziszewski imidazole synthesis) with an overall yield of 1.5%. However, no PET studies were reported with **12**.

Furthermore, in 2002, Smith's group developed two tetracyclic based anti-depressant radiotracers, mianserin (**13**) and mitrazepine (**14**), that have potent antagonist properties at α2-ARs and also at serotonin receptors ($5HT_{2A}$, $5HT_{2C}$) and labelled them with C-11 to prepare **13** and **14** (Figure 2) [92,93]. The radiotracers **13** and **14** were prepared from their respective *N*-desmethyl precursors via ^{11}C-methylation with ~40 GBq/μmol and 5–7 GBq/μmol molar activity, respectively. PET studies in female pigs with **13** showed limited binding potential in brain whereas **14** showed more favorable properties including slow metabolism, fast brain uptake and sufficient target-to-background ratio for pharmacokinetic parameters estimation.

Radiotracer **14** had higher binding in the frontal cortex, thalamus, and basal ganglia where pretreatment with unlabeled mitrazepine revealed that its binding was reversible, whereas, in the cerebellum and olfactory tubercle, it was not. Notably, using the α2-AR subtype KO mouse model they validated the receptor selectivity of **14**. In 2004 and 2009, this group conducted a clinical trial with volunteers using **14** to study its distribution, metabolism and pharmacokinetics [94,95]. The results revealed that **14** can serve as a PET radiotracer to image α2-ARs in the brain, though identification of its metabolites and its nonselective binding are limitations.

Two years later, Leysen's group developed a reversible, potent and selective α2-AR antagonist, viz. R107474 (**15**, Figure 3) [96]. They prepared [^{11}C]**15** through Pictet-Spengler condensation method using [^{11}C]HCHO and the respective secondary amine with 24–28 GBq/μmol molar activity at the end of bombardment (EOB). They carried out ex vivo autoradiography to measure in vivo α2A-ARs and α2C-ARs occupancy of **15** in rats. Biodistribution studies showed rapid uptake of **15** into brain and other tissues with the brain showing the highest uptake other than liver and kidneys. In the brain the highest uptake of **15** was in the septum (3.54 ± 0.52 ID/g) and entorhinal cortex (1.57 ± 0.50 ID/g) whereas the lowest was in the cerebellum, a region with very low density of α2-ARs. However, the potential of **15** was not investigated further.

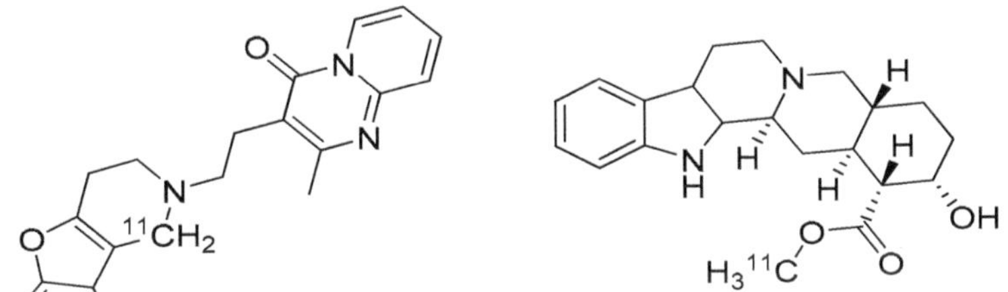
[^{11}C]R107474, **15**   [^{11}C]yohimbine, **16**

Figure 3. Anti-depressive & antihypertensive based α2-AR PET radiotracers.

In 2006, Jacobsen's group developed C-11 labelled yohimbine (**16**, Figure 3) [97], an antihypertensive agent. Yohimbine has potent antagonist properties at α2-ARs, but also interacts with α1 and 5-hydroxy tryptamine 1A receptors (5-HT_{1A}). The radiotracer **16** was prepared through ^{11}C-methylation of yohimbinic acid using C-11 methyl iodide ([^{11}C]CH_3I) and obtained with 40 GBq/μmol molar activity.

PET studies were performed in pigs to obtain whole-body and dosimetry recordings and for dynamic brain imaging. Interestingly, no radioactive metabolites of **16** were reported in pig plasma and binding of **16** was observed in α2-AR-rich regions where it was displaceable by co-injection of pharmacological doses of yohimbine or selective α2-AR antagonist (Figure 4). Later, **16** was used to image α2-ARs in the human brain (n = 6) using PET [98]. Highest binding of **16** was observed in cortex and hippocampus and the lowest in corpus callosum, which was used as a reference region to estimate the average total distribution (V_T) in other brain regions. The radiotracer **16** seems to be a suitable radiotracer to image α2-ARs but has similar issues as of **14,** which need to be addressed.

The concentration of α2-subtype receptors in the brain is low (5–90 fmol/mg range) increasing the challenge for their detection by PET [31]. Therefore, α2- subtype specific PET tracers (with subnanomolar affinities and >30-fold selectivity) still need to be developed for the quantification of α2-subtype receptors and to assess their role in brain diseases. A few research groups have developed α2-subtype specific PET radiotracers, but success has been limited.

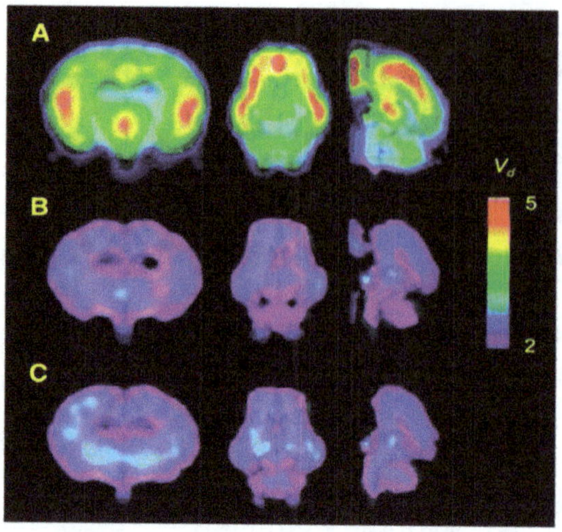

Figure 4. Parametric maps of **16** in living porcine brain. (**A**) Baseline study using **16** showed regional differences in its distribution. (**B**) Blocking experiment (yohimbine at 0.07 mg/kg) reduced the scale of distribution volume (V_d) to ~2 mL g^{-1} in all the α2-AR bound regions. (**C**) Increased dose of yohimbine (1.6 mg/kg) had no further significant effect in comparison to the low dose (n = 3) Maps are superimposed on the MR image. Adapted from JNM publication by Jacobsen S, Pedersen, K.; Smith, D.F.; Jensen, S.B.; Munk, O.L.; Cumming P [97]. Permission obtained from SNMMI.

3.1. *α2A-Specific PET Radiotracers*

Kumar's group in 2010 developed [^{11}C]MPTQ (**17**, Figure 5) for the quantification of α2A-ARs in vivo [35]. Compound **17** was shown to have blocking effects on α2A-ARs in vivo in brain and has stronger affinities for α2A-AR (K_i = 1.6 nM) than α2C-AR (K_i = 4.5 nM) and 5-HTT (serotonin transporter, K_i = 16 nM) [99]. They anticipated no binding of **17** to α2B and α2C-ARs since the densities of these receptors are lower than α2A-ARs. In addition, the 10-fold higher affinity of **17** α2A-ARs over 5-HTT is advantageous for α2A-ARs as both have similar B_{max} values. The radiosynthesis of **17** was accomplished through ^{11}C-methylation of its respective *N*-desmethyl precursor with 74–88.8 GBq/μmol molar activity at the end of synthesis (EOS). PET studies in baboons with **17** showed that it penetrated the BBB and accumulated in α2A-AR-rich brain areas. They ruled out binding of **17** to 5-HTT due to its low uptake in the hippocampus, temporal cortex, and occipital cortex, which are the brain regions with the highest binding of 5-HTT radiotracers. No further studies were reported using **17**.

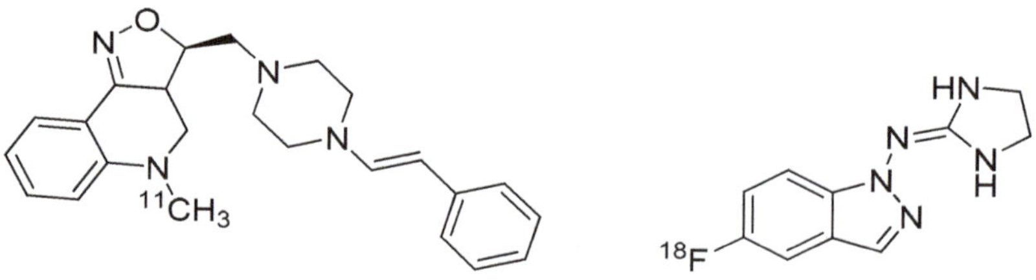

[^{11}C]MPTQ, **17** 6-[^{18}F]fluoromarsanidine, **18**

Figure 5. α2A-antagonist (**17**) and agonist (**18**) PET radiotracers.

In search of a selective agonist to α2-ARs, Lehmann's group identified 1-[(imidazolidin-2-yl) imino]indazole (marsanidine) [100] and later developed an α2A subtype specific ligand by introducing fluorine to marsanidine [33]. The reported binding affinity (K_d) of 6-fluoromarsanidine for α2A (33 nM) is higher than for α2B (72 nM) and α2C (600 nM). Solin et al., in 2019, prepared 6-[^{18}F]fluoromarsanidine (**18**, Figure 5) through electrophilic ^{18}F-radiofluorination using [^{18}F]selectfluor bis(triflate) and a corresponding precursor with 3–26 GBq/μmol molar activity at the EOS [34]. In vivo PET was performed in rats and α2A-KO mice, but the radiotracer was not continued further because of its rapid metabolism and high nonspecific uptake in rat and mouse brain.

3.2. α2C-Specific PET Radiotracers

Animal models, such as the forced swimming test (FST) and the prepulse inhibition (PPI) are used to screen for anti-depressants and anti-psychotics, respectively. The use of α2C-KO and α2C-overexpression (α2C-OE) mouse models in FST and PPI paradigms suggested that α2C-specific compounds may have therapeutic benefits for depression and schizophrenia [32,38]. In 2007, Orion pharma from Finland identified an acridine-based compound, JP-1302 [38], and a research group from Japan identified a methyl benzofuran based compound, MBF [101], as selective α2C antagonists. Both these ligands have high affinities for α2C (JP-1302 K_i = 28 nM, MBF K_i = 20 nM) than for α2A (JP-1302 K_i = 3500 nM, MBF K_i = 17,000 nM) and α2B (JP-1302 K_i = 1500 nM, MBF K_i = 750 nM). Based on these findings, Zhang's group, in 2010, synthesized [^{11}C]JP-1302 (**19**) and [^{11}C]MBF (**20**)(Figure 6) as PET probes to evaluate their BBB penetration and α2C selective binding in the brain [37]. The radiotracers **19** (molar activity 95 ± 24 GBq/μmol) and **20** (molar activity 62 ± 15 GBq/μmol) were prepared using ^{11}C-methylation from *N*-desmethyl and *O*-desmethyl precursors, respectively. PET studies were conducted in WT and Pgp, breast cancer resistance protein (BCRP) KO mice using both radiotracers.

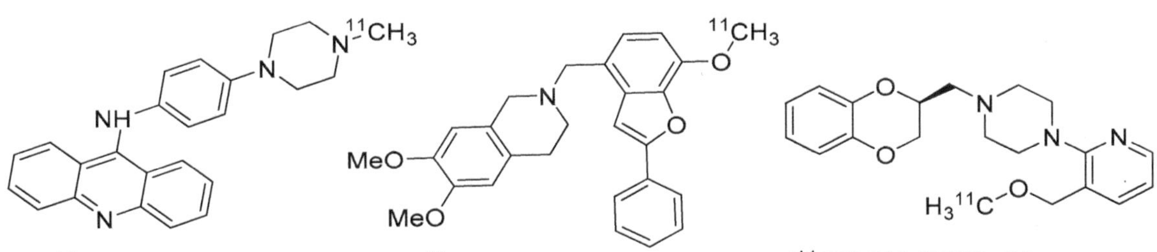

[^{11}C]JP-1302, **19** [^{11}C]MBF, **20** [^{11}C]ORM-13070, **21**

Figure 6. PET radiotracers for α2C-ARs.

This combined KO model is useful to evaluate whether brain penetration of PET probes is sensitive to Pgp and BCRP. After injection of the radiotracers, their levels in the brain were low in WT mice whereas they were higher in Pgp and BCRP KO mice. The regional binding of these radiotracers did not correspond with the regional brain distribution of α2C, so it was concluded that they were inadequate to evaluate α2C-ARs in brain with PET.

In 2014, researchers from Turku PET center and Orion Pharma reported the radiosynthesis of [^{11}C]ORM13070 (**21**, Figure 6) with molar activity 690 ± 340 GBq/μmol and its evaluation in rats and in α2A and α2AC KO mice with PET [36,102]. The binding affinities of **21** for α2C (3.8 nM) is higher than for α2A (109 nM) and α2B (23 nM).

The in vivo PET and ex vivo autoradiography of **21** in rat indicated that its brain distribution corresponds to the regional distribution of α2C in brain, with highest levels in striatum and olfactory tubercle. Pretreatment with atipamezole, a α2-sutype nonselective antagonist blocked the binding of **21** into these regions. Furthermore, by using α2A and α2AC KO model mice, they demonstrated α2C specificity of **21**. The brain uptake of **21** in α2A-KO and WT mice was similar whereas, negligible uptake occurred in α2AC KO (Figure 7, left). They represented time-activity curves for striatum and cerebellar cortex of three mice types (Figure 7, right) and the radioactivity ratios at 5–15 min for α2A, α2AC KO mice, and WT mice were 1.51–1.51, 1.06–1.09 and 1.51–1.57, respectively.

Accordingly, **21** was studied in healthy men to estimate its metabolism, pharmacokinetics, whole-body distribution and radiation dosimetry [39]. Good results were obtained in rodent and human PET studies with **21**, except for its fast washout from brain. Better pharmacokinetics, higher affinity, and specificity can potentially be enhanced by structural modifications to **21**. Given that the α2A-ARs are widely distributed in brain in contrast to α2C-ARs, a candidate with subnanomolar affinity for α2C-ARs (>50-fold affinity than α2A-ARs) is needed for a PET radiotracer. As α2C-ARs are of interest as therapeutic targets in brain diseases, the α2C-specifc PET radiotracers would facilitate their development as medications and help in investigations of α2C-ARs in the human brain.

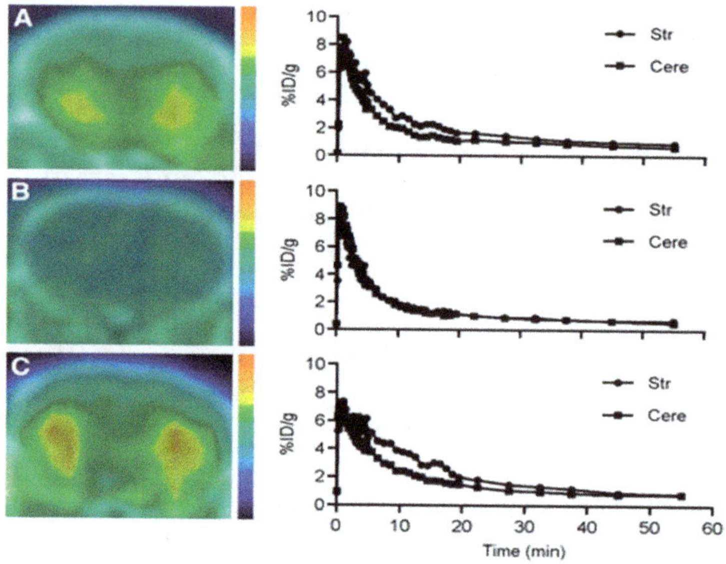

Figure 7. PET/CT images and time-activity curves of **21** for striatum and cerebellar cortex of (**A**) α2A KO (**B**) α2AC KO and (**C**) WT mice. Brain uptake of **21** in α2AC KO is negligible and is similar in α2A KO and WT mice with 7.8–8.1% ID/g at 1 min and 1.2% ID/g at 30 min after **21** injection. The striatum to cerebellar cortex radioactivity ratios (at 5–15 min) for α2AC KO mice did not differ and for α2A KO and WT mice are alike. Adapted from JNM publication by Arponen E.; Helin, S.; Marjamäki, P.; Grönroos, T.; Holm, P.; Löyttyniemi, E.; Någren, K.; Scheinin, M.; Haaparanta-Solin, M.; Sallinen, J.; [36]. Permission obtained from SNMMI.

4. β-ARs and Nonselective PET Radiotracers

β-ARs are associated with G_s-heterotrimeric G-protein and mediate intracellular signaling through adenyl cyclase activation and cyclic adenosine monophosphate (cAMP) production. β-ARs are classified into β1, β2, and β3 subtypes, in which, the former two have been much more explored [42,46]. Quite a lot of selective and nonselective β-AR agonists and antagonists (blockers) are available as drugs in the market to treat various cardiac and pulmonary disorders. In the brain, β-ARs are localized in the frontal cortex, striatum, thalamus, putamen, amygdala, cerebellum and hippocampus [48]. The density of β-ARs in brain is sensitive to brain pathophysiology. Notably, the density of β-ARs decrease with age [40]. Light microscopic autoradiography using [^{3}H]dihydroaloprenolol (a selective β-blocker) with rat brain sections has shown a wide distribution of β-ARs in forebrain and cerebellum regions (B_{max} = 23 fmol/mg tissue) [103]. Similarly, B_{max} value of 18 fmol/mg protein was reported in pre-frontal cortex of subjects with Parkinson's disease [48,104]. By altering the Ca^{2+} levels through *N*-methyl-*D*-aspartate (NMDA) receptors in hippocampus, β-ARs modulate synaptic plasticity, including that needed for memory [44,45]. The blockade of β-ARs is associated with a small increased risk for Alzheimer's and Parkinson's disease [43,105]. In addition, abnormal function and densities of β-ARs have been reported in mood disorders and schizophrenia [41,47,106].

Several radioligands, mostly based on β-blockers, were validated for imaging of β-ARs in the heart [50]. The majority of β-blockers possess a hydroxyl propylamine moiety in their structures that is vital for binding to β-ARs and this moiety was maintained in most of these radioligands. PET radiotracers have succeeded in imaging and quantifying myocardial and pulmonary β-ARs in human [107,108], whereas, PET radiotracers for cerebral β-ARs have been more challenging. The clinical PET radiotracers for cardiac β-ARs have negative Log P values (<-2), which is not suitable for imaging the brain. Several lipophilic and high to moderate affinity β-AR nonselective antagonists were explored as PET radiotracers to image β-ARs in the brain.

During the 1980s, propranolol, a β-blocker drug was labelled with C-11 (**22**, Figure 8) but was unsuitable as a PET ligand for β-ARs because of high nonspecific binding in vivo [109,110]. Subsequently, Berridge's group described the synthesis of two isomers (*R*/*S*) of [^{18}F]fluorocarazolol

(**23**, Figure 8) through reductive amination using [^{18}F]fluoroacetone and desisopropylcarazolol with 18.5–37 GBq/μmol molar activity [111,112]. The radiotracer **23** has subnanomolar K_i values for β-ARs (β1 0.4 nM, β2 0.1 nM) and Log $P_{7.4}$ value of 2.19. The same group used *S*-**23** for PET imaging of the pig heart and lungs to validate the β-AR biding. In 1997, Waarde et al., employed *S*-**23** to image β-ARs in the human brain and obtained positive results [113]. They observed specific binding (blocked with pindolol) of *S*-**23** in β-AR rich areas, striatum and various cortical areas. However, the radiotracer was discontinued for further human studies as fluorocarazolol was positive for the Ames test i.e., mutagenic [114].

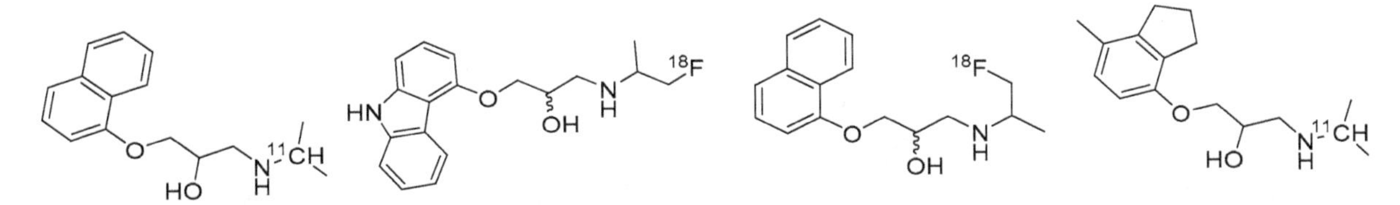

[^{11}C]propranolol **22** [^{18}F]fluorocarazolol **23** [^{18}F]fluoropropranolol **24** [^{11}C]ICI 118551 **25**

Figure 8. Early PET radiotracers for cerebral β-ARs.

Two research groups conducted biodistribution studies in rats using [^{18}F]fluoropropranolol (**24**) and [^{11}C]ICI 118,551 (**25**) (Figure 8), which failed because of their nonspecific binding [115,116]. In 2001, Fazio's group described two isomers (*R/S*) of C-11 labelled bisprolol (β1 K_i 1.6 nM, β2 K_i 100 nM and Log $P_{7.4} = -0.2$) (**26**, Figure 9) to image β1-ARs in the brain [117]. The radiosynthesis of **26** was accomplished via reductive amination using [^{11}C]acetone and desisopropyl bisprolol precursor with 129.5 ± 37 GBq/μmol molar activity at the EOS. They observed little specific uptake of **26** in β1-AR rich regions in the rat's brain and also high nonspecific uptake in the pituitary (1.8 ± 0.3 ID at 30 min), a region with high β2-ARs levels. No further studies were reported using **26** to image β-ARs.

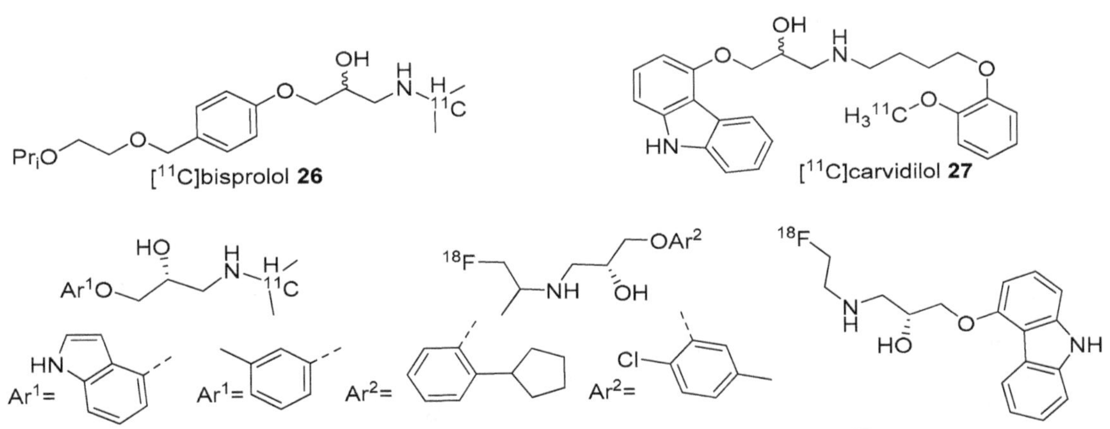

[^{11}C]pindolol **28** [^{11}C]toliprolol **29** [^{18}F]fluorobupranolol **30** [^{18}F]fluoropenbutalol **31** [^{18}F]fluoroethylcarazolol **32**

Figure 9. Radiotracers based on various β-AR blockers.

In 2002, Elsinga's group reported five different potent and lipophilic β-AR antagonists (carvedilol, pindolol, toliprolol, bupranolol, and penbutolol) as PET probes to image β-ARs in rat brain [118]. C-11 labelled carvedilol (**27**, Figure 9; molar activity 12.97–25.9 GBq/μmol) was prepared through ^{11}C-methylation using [^{11}C]CH_3I and its respective *O*-desmethyl precursor, whereas, [^{11}C]pindolol (**28**, molar activity 25.9–37 GBq/μmol) and [^{11}C]toliprolol (**29**, molar activity 22.2–25.9 GBq/μmol) were prepared via reductive amination using [^{11}C]acetone and the respective desisopropyl precursors. The F-18 tracers of bupranolol (**30**, molar activity 11.1–18.5 GBq/μmol) and penbutolol (**31**, 22.2–99.9 GBq/μmol) were also prepared by means of reductive amination but using [^{18}F]fluoroacetone and the respective des-fluoro-isopropyl precursors.

The five radiotracers had strong affinities (subnanomolar K_d) for β1 and β2-ARs. Although these radiotracers had sufficient affinity and lipophilicity for in vivo imaging, none showed good brain uptake. This group also evaluated S-[^{18}F]fluoroethylcarazolol (**32**, β1 K_i = 0.5 nM, β2 K_i = 0.4 nM and Log $P_{7.4}$ = 1.94) for in vivo imaging of β-ARs in rat brain [119]. The radiotracer **32** (Figure 9) was prepared via an epoxide ring-opening using [^{18}F]fluoroethylamine and the corresponding epoxide with >10 GBq/μmol molar activity. The radiotracer accumulated in brain with uptake reflecting cerebral β-ARs binding. However, no further PET imaging studies were reported using **32** probably because of its analogous nature to **23** which was shown to be positive Ames test [114,120].

In 2008, Elsinga's and Vasdev's groups chose exaprolol (β-AR K_d = 9–9.5 nM) and developed *S*-[^{11}C]exaprolol (**33**) and *S*-[^{18}F]fluoroexaprolol (**34**), respectively, to image β-ARs with PET (Figure 10) [120,121]. Radiotracer **33** was prepared via reductive amination using [^{11}C]acetone and desisopropylexaprolol precursor with >10 GBq/μmol molar activity and the radiotracer **34** was prepared through a nucleophilic substitution reaction using [^{18}F]fluoride and a corresponding tosylate precursor followed by reductive hydrolysis, with 34.29 GBq/μmol molar activity. Regardless of good binding and kinetic properties, both these radiotracers showed high nonspecific uptake in the brain and were found to be inadequate for PET imaging of β-ARs.

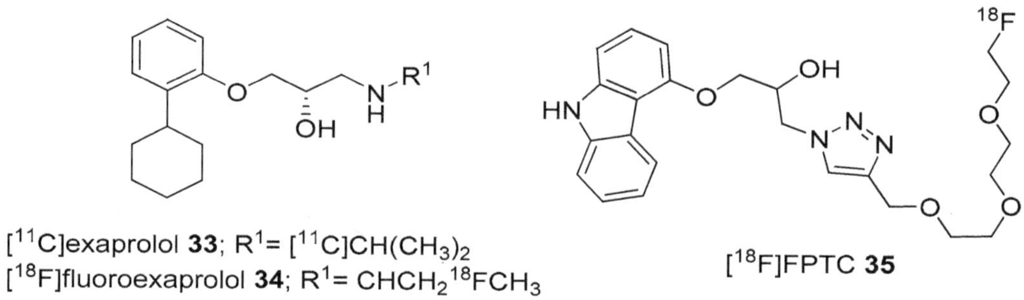

Figure 10. Another set of latest β-AR PET radiotracers.

Again in 2014, Elsinga's group developed [^{18}F]FPTC (**35**, Figure 10) for PET imaging of β-ARs in brain [122]. The radiotracer **35** is a derivative of carazolol, wherein, isopropylamine group of carazolol was replaced by a PEGylated triazole group. It was prepared through Huisgen's 1,3-dipolar cycloaddition (click reaction) using F-18 labelled PEGylated alkyne and the corresponding azide with >120 GBq/μmol molar activity. Although **35** was shown to have appropriate Log$P_{7.4}$ (2.48) and specific binding in in vitro assays, it could not visualize β-ARs in the brain, lung or heart using micro-PET.

Thus, the development of PET radiotracers for neuroimaging of β-ARs remains a challenge and as of now, there are no β-AR subtype specific PET radiotracers. Such radiotracers are important to expand our understanding of the role of β-ARs in aging and memory formation and also to assess their function in behavioral disorders. Future research, as suggested by Elsinga and Waarde [48], should consider modifying the imaging agents used for myocardial β-ARs rather than radiolabeling existing β-blocker drugs. Alterations should optimize Log $P_{7.4}$ (2-3), high affinity and selectivity to β-ARs and no substrate affinity for Pgp.

5. Conclusions

Over the past four decades, significant efforts have been made to develop CNS-ARs PET ligands for brain imaging. Despite these efforts, very few PET radiotracers are available to selectively image AR subtypes in the brain. The development of specific radiotracers is hindered mainly by the low receptor densities of each AR subclass within the brain, which requires further optimization processes for highly potent and BBB permeable ligands. Though challenging, AR subtype specific agonist/antagonist PET radiotracers are needed to ascertain AR's role in brain pathophysiology and for medication development.

References

1. Scott, J.A. Positron Emission Tomography: Basic Science and Clinical Practice. *Am. J. Roentgenol.* **2004**, *182*, 418. [CrossRef]
2. Shukla, A.; Kumar, U. Positron emission tomography: An overview. *J. Med. Phys.* **2006**, *31*, 13–21. [CrossRef] [PubMed]
3. McCluskey, S.P.; Plisson, C.; Rabiner, E.A.; Howes, O. Advances in CNS PET: The state-of-the-art for new imaging targets for pathophysiology and drug development. *Eur. J. Nucl. Med. Mol. Imaging* **2020**, *47*, 451–489. [CrossRef]
4. Rankovic, Z. CNS Drug Design: Balancing Physicochemical Properties for Optimal Brain Exposure. *J. Med. Chem.* **2015**, *58*, 2584–2608. [CrossRef] [PubMed]
5. Adenot, M.; Lahana, R. Blood-Brain Barrier Permeation Models: Discriminating between Potential CNS and Non-CNS Drugs Including P-Glycoprotein Substrates. *J. Chem. Inf. Comput. Sci.* **2004**, *44*, 239–248. [CrossRef]
6. Agdeppa, E.D.; Spilker, M.E. A review of imaging agent development. *AAPS J.* **2009**, *11*, 286–299. [CrossRef]
7. Kumar, J.S.; Mann, J. PET Tracers for Serotonin Receptors and Their Applications. *Cent. Nerv. Syst. Agents Med. Chem.* **2014**, *14*, 96–112. [CrossRef]
8. Dunphy, M.P.S.; Lewis, J.S. Radiopharmaceuticals in preclinical and clinical development for monitoring of therapy with PET. *J. Nucl. Med.* **2009**, *50*, 106–122. [CrossRef]
9. Sneader, W. The discovery and synthesis of epinephrine. *Drug News Perspect.* **2001**, *14*, 491–494. [CrossRef]
10. Arthur, G. Epinephrine: A short history. *Lancet Respir. Med.* **2015**, *3*, 350–351. [CrossRef]
11. Schmidt, K.T.; Weinshenker, D. Adrenaline rush: The role of adrenergic receptors in stimulant-induced behaviors. *Mol. Pharmacol.* **2014**, *85*, 640–650. [CrossRef] [PubMed]
12. Eisenhofer, G.; Kopin, I.J.; Goldstein, D.S. Catecholamine metabolism: A contemporary view with implications for physiology and medicine. *Pharmacol. Rev.* **2004**, *56*, 331–349. [CrossRef] [PubMed]
13. Kirshner, N. Biosynthesis of adrenaline and noradrenaline. *Pharmacol. Rev.* **1959**, *11*, 350–357. [PubMed]
14. Flatmark, T. Catecholamine biosynthesis and physiological regulation in neuroendocrine cells. *Acta Physiol. Scand.* **2000**, *168*, 1–17. [CrossRef] [PubMed]
15. Ranjbar-Slamloo, Y.; Fazlali, Z. Dopamine and Noradrenaline in the Brain; Overlapping or Dissociate Functions? *Front. Mol. Neurosci.* **2020**, *12*, 1–8. [CrossRef]
16. Strosberg, A.D. Structure, function, and regulation of adrenergic receptors. *Protein Sci.* **1993**, *2*, 1198–1209. [CrossRef]
17. Ahlquist, R.P. A study of the adrenotropic receptors. *Am. J. Physiol.* **1948**, *153*, 586–600. [CrossRef]
18. Philipp, M.; Hein, L. Adrenergic receptor knockout mice: Distinct functions of 9 receptor subtypes. *Pharmacol. Ther.* **2004**, *101*, 65–74. [CrossRef]
19. Paul, J.; Bylund, B.; Lefkowitz, J.; Eikenburg, C.; Ruffolo, R.; Langer, Z.; Minneman, P. International Union of Pharmacology X. Recommendation for Nomenclature of adrenoreceptors: Consensus update. *Am. Soc. Pharmacol. Exp. Ther.* **1995**, *47*, 267–270.
20. Day, H.E.W.; Campeau, S.; Watson, S.J.; Akil, H. Distribution of α(1a)-, α(1b)- and α(1d)-adrenergic receptor mRNA in the rat brain and spinal cord. *J. Chem. Neuroanat.* **1997**, *13*, 115–139. [CrossRef]
21. Doze, V.A.; Handel, E.M.; Jensen, K.A.; Darsie, B.; Luger, E.J.; Haselton, J.R.; Talbot, J.N.; Rorabaugh, B.R. α1A- and α1B-adrenergic receptors differentially modulate antidepressant-like behavior in the mouse. *Brain Res.* **2009**, *1285*, 148–157. [CrossRef] [PubMed]
22. Leslie, A. Characterization of a1-Adrenergic Receptor Subtypes in Rat Brain: A Reevaluation of [3H] WB41 04 and [3H] Prazosin Binding. *Pharmacol. Exet. Am. Chem. Sciety Pharmacol. Experiemntal Ther.* **1986**, *29*, 321–330.
23. Reader, T.A.; Brière, R.; Grondin, L. Alpha-1 and alpha-2 adrenoceptor binding in cerebral cortex: Competition studies with [3H]prazosin and [3H]idazoxan. *J. Neural Transm.* **1987**, *68*, 79–95. [CrossRef] [PubMed]
24. Drouin, C.; Darracq, L.; Trovero, F.; Blanc, G.; Glowinski, J.; Cotecchia, S.; Tassin, J.P. α1b-Adrenergic Receptors Control Locomotor and Rewarding Effects of Psychostimulants and Opiates. *J. Neurosci.* **2002**, *22*, 2873–2884. [CrossRef]
25. Zuscik, M.J.; Sands, S.; Ross, S.A.; Waugh, D.J.J.; Gaivin, R.J.; Morilak, D.; Perez, D.M. Overexpression of the α(1B)-adrenergic receptor causes apoptotic neurodegeneration: Multiple system atrophy. *Nat. Med.* **2000**, *6*, 1388–1394. [CrossRef]

26. Hayashi, R.; Ohmori, E.; Isogaya, M.; Moriwaki, M.; Kumagai, H. Design and synthesis of selective α1B adrenoceptor antagonists. *Bioorg. Med. Chem. Lett.* **2006**, *16*, 4045–4047. [CrossRef]
27. Spreng, M.; Cotecchia, S.; Schenk, F. A behavioral study of alpha-1b adrenergic receptor knockout mice: Increased reaction to novelty and selectively reduced learning capacities. *Neurobiol. Learn. Mem.* **2001**, *75*, 214–229. [CrossRef]
28. Sadalge, A.; Coughlin, L.; Fu, H.; Wang, B.; Valladares, O.; Valentino, R.; Blendy, J.A. A1D Adrenoceptor Signaling Is Required for Stimulus Induced Locomotor Activity. *Mol. Psychiatry* **2003**, *8*, 664–672. [CrossRef]
29. Buckner, S.A.; Milicic, I.; Daza, A.; Lynch, J.J.; Kolasa, T.; Nakane, M.; Sullivan, J.P.; Brioni, J.D. A-315456: A selective α1D-adrenoceptor antagonist with minimal dopamine D2 and 5-HT1A receptor affinity. *Eur. J. Pharmacol.* **2001**, *433*, 123–127. [CrossRef]
30. Saunders, C.; Limbird, L.E. Localization and trafficking of α2-adrenergic receptor subtypes in cells and tissues. *Pharmacol. Ther.* **1999**, *84*, 193–205. [CrossRef]
31. Sastre, M.; García-Sevilla, J.A. α 2-Adrenoceptor Subtypes Identified by [3H]RX821002 Binding in the Human Brain: The Agonist Guanoxabenz Does Not Discriminate Different Forms of the Predominant α2A Subtype. *J. Neurochem.* **1994**, *63*, 1077–1085. [CrossRef] [PubMed]
32. Gilsbach, R.; Hein, L. Are the pharmacology and physiology of α 2adrenoceptors determined by α 2-heteroreceptors and autoreceptors respectively? *Br. J. Pharmacol.* **2012**, *165*, 90–102. [CrossRef] [PubMed]
33. Wasilewska, A.; Sączewski, F.; Hudson, A.L.; Ferdousi, M.; Scheinin, M.; Laurila, J.M.; Rybczyńska, A.; Boblewski, K.; Lehmann, A. Fluorinated analogues of marsanidine, a highly α2-AR/imidazoline I1 binding site-selective hypotensive agent. Synthesis and biological activities. *Eur. J. Med. Chem.* **2014**, *87*, 386–397. [CrossRef] [PubMed]
34. Krzyczmonik, A.; Keller, T.; López-Picón, F.R.; Forsback, S.; Kirjavainen, A.K.; Takkinen, J.S.; Wasilewska, A.; Scheinin, M.; Haaparanta-Solin, M.; Sączewski, F.; et al. Radiosynthesis and Preclinical Evaluation of an α2A-Adrenoceptor Tracer Candidate, 6-[18F]Fluoro-marsanidine. *Mol. Imaging Biol.* **2019**, *21*, 879–887. [CrossRef] [PubMed]
35. Prabhakaran, J.; Majo, V.J.; Milak, M.S.; Mali, P.; Savenkova, L.; Mann, J.J.; Parsey, R.V.; Kumar, J.S.D. Synthesis and in vivo evaluation of [11C]MPTQ: A potential PET tracer for alpha2A-adrenergic receptors. *Bioorg. Med. Chem. Lett.* **2010**, *20*, 3654–3657. [CrossRef]
36. Arponen, E.; Helin, S.; Marjamäki, P.; Grönroos, T.; Holm, P.; Löyttyniemi, E.; Någren, K.; Scheinin, M.; Haaparanta-Solin, M.; Sallinen, J.; et al. A PET tracer for brain α2C adrenoceptors, 11C-ORM-13070: Radiosynthesis and preclinical evaluation in rats and knockout mice. *J. Nucl. Med.* **2014**, *55*, 1171–1177. [CrossRef]
37. Kawamura, K.; Akiyama, M.; Yui, J.; Yamasaki, T.; Hatori, A.; Kumata, K.; Wakizaka, H.; Takei, M.; Nengaki, N.; Yanamoto, K.; et al. In vivo evaluation of limiting brain penetration of probes for α2C-adrenoceptor using small-animal positron emission tomography. *ACS Chem. Neurosci.* **2010**, *1*, 520–528. [CrossRef]
38. Sallinen, J.; Höglund, I.; Engström, M.; Lehtimäki, J.; Virtanen, R.; Sirviö, J.; Wurster, S.; Savola, J.M.; Haapalinna, A. Pharmacological characterization and CNS effects of a novel highly selective α2C-adrenoceptor antagonist JP-1302. *Br. J. Pharmacol.* **2007**, *150*, 391–402. [CrossRef]
39. Luoto, P.; Suilamo, S.; Oikonen, V.; Arponen, E.; Helin, S.; Herttuainen, J.; Hietamäki, J.; Holopainen, A.; Kailajärvi, M.; Peltonen, J.M.; et al. 11C-ORM-13070, a novel PET ligand for brain α2C-adrenoceptors: Radiometabolism, plasma pharmacokinetics, whole-body distribution and radiation dosimetry in healthy men. *Eur. J. Nucl. Med. Mol. Imaging* **2014**, *41*, 1947–1956. [CrossRef]
40. Sscarpace, P.J.; Abrass, I.B. Alpha- and beta-adrenergic receptor function in the brain during senescence. *Neurobiol. Aging* **1988**, *9*, 53–58. [CrossRef]
41. Pandey, S.C.; Ren, X.; Sagen, J.; Pandey, G.N. β-Adrenergic receptor subtypes in stress-induced behavioral depression. *Pharmacol. Biochem. Behav.* **1995**, *51*, 339–344. [CrossRef]
42. Wallukat, G. The β-adrenergic receptors. *Herz* **2002**, *27*, 683–690. [CrossRef] [PubMed]
43. Lu'O'Ng, K.V.Q.; Nguyen, L.T.H. The role of beta-adrenergic receptor blockers in Alzheimer's disease: Potential genetic and cellular signaling mechanisms. *Am. J. Alzheimers. Dis. Demen.* **2013**, *28*, 427–439. [CrossRef] [PubMed]
44. O'Dell, T.J.; Connor, S.A.; Guglietta, R.; Nguyen, P.V. β-Adrenergic receptor signaling and modulation of long-term potentiation in the mammalian hippocampus. *Learn. Mem.* **2015**, *22*, 461–471. [CrossRef]

45. Gelinas, J.; Nguyen, P. Neuromodulation of Hippocampal Synaptic Plasticity, Learning, and Memory by Noradrenaline. *Cent. Nerv. Syst. Agents Med. Chem.* **2008**, *7*, 17–33. [CrossRef]
46. Wachter, S.B.; Gilbert, E.M. Beta-adrenergic receptors, from their discovery and characterization through their manipulation to beneficial clinical application. *Cardiology* **2012**, *122*, 104–112. [CrossRef]
47. Joyce, J.N.; Lexow, N.; Kim, S.J.; Artymyshyn, R.; Senzon, S.; Lawerence, D.; Cassanova, M.F.; Kleinman, J.E.; Bird, E.D.; Winokur, A. Distribution of beta-adrenergic receptor subtypes in human post-mortem brain: Alterations in limbic regions of schizophrenics. *Synapse* **1992**, *10*, 228–246. [CrossRef]
48. Waarde, A.; Vaalburg, W.; Doze, P.; Bosker, F.; Elsinga, P. PET Imaging of Beta-Adrenoceptors in Human Brain: A Realistic Goal or a Mirage? *Curr. Pharm. Des.* **2005**, *10*, 1519–1536. [CrossRef]
49. Pike, V.W.; Law, M.P.; Osman, S.; Davenport, R.J.; Rimoldi, O.; Giardinà, D.; Camici, P.G. Selection, design and evaluation of new radioligands for PET studies of cardiac adrenoceptors. *Pharm. Acta Helv.* **2000**, *74*, 191–200. [CrossRef]
50. Chen, X.; Werner, R.A.; Javadi, M.S.; Maya, Y.; Decker, M.; Lapa, C.; Herrmann, K.; Higuchi, T. Radionuclide imaging of neurohormonal system of the heart. *Theranostics* **2015**, *5*, 545–558. [CrossRef]
51. Logan, J.; Wang, G.J.; Telang, F.; Fowler, J.S.; Alexoff, D.; Zabroski, J.; Jayne, M.; Hubbard, B.; King, P.; Carter, P.; et al. Imaging the norepinephrine transporter in humans with (S,S)-[11C]O-methyl reboxetine and PET: Problems and progress. *Nucl. Med. Biol.* **2007**, *34*, 667–679. [CrossRef] [PubMed]
52. Chen, X.; Kudo, T.; Lapa, C.; Buck, A.; Higuchi, T. Recent advances in radiotracers targeting norepinephrine transporter: Structural development and radiolabeling improvements. *J. Neural Transm.* **2020**, *127*, 851–873. [CrossRef] [PubMed]
53. Zeng, F.; Mun, J.; Jarkas, N.; Stehouwer, J.S.; Voll, R.J.; Tamagnan, G.D.; Howell, L.; Votaw, J.R.; Kilts, C.D.; Nemeroff, C.B.; et al. Synthesis, Radiosynthesis, and Biological Evaluation of Carbon-11 and Fluorine-18 Labeled Reboxetine Analogs: Potential Positron Emission Tomography Radioligands for in Vivo Imaging of the Norepinephrine Transporter. *J. Med. Chem.* **2009**, *52*, 62–73. [CrossRef] [PubMed]
54. Moriguchi, S.; Kimura, Y.; Ichise, M.; Arakawa, R.; Takano, H.; Seki, C.; Ikoma, Y.; Takahata, K.; Nagashima, T.; Yamada, M.; et al. PET quantification of the norepinephrine transporter in human brain with (S,S)-18F-FMeNER-D2. *J. Nucl. Med.* **2017**, *58*, 1140–1145. [CrossRef]
55. Narayanaswami, V.; Drake, L.R.; Brooks, A.F.; Meyer, J.H.; Houle, S.; Kilbourn, M.R.; Scott, P.J.H.; Vasdev, N. Classics in Neuroimaging: Development of PET Tracers for Imaging Monoamine Oxidases. *ACS Chem. Neurosci.* **2019**, *10*, 1867–1871. [CrossRef]
56. Fowler, J.S.; Logan, J.; Shumay, E.; Alia-Klein, N.; Wang, G.J.; Volkow, N.D. Monoamine oxidase: Radiotracer chemistry and human studies. *J. Label. Compd. Radiopharm.* **2015**, *58*, 51–64. [CrossRef]
57. Narayanaswami, V.; Dahl, K.; Bernard-Gauthier, V.; Josephson, L.; Cumming, P.; Vasdev, N. Emerging PET Radiotracers and Targets for Imaging of Neuroinflammation in Neurodegenerative Diseases: Outlook Beyond TSPO. *Mol. Imaging* **2018**, *17*, 1–25. [CrossRef]
58. Piascik, M.T.; Perez, D.M. α1-Adrenergic receptors: New insights and directions. *J. Pharmacol. Exp. Ther.* **2001**, *298*, 403–410.
59. Graham, R.M.; Perez, D.M.; Hwa, J.; Piascik, M.T. α1 -Adrenergic Receptor Subtypes. *Circ. Res.* **1996**, *78*, 737–749. [CrossRef]
60. Chen, Z.J.; Minneman, K.P. Recent progress in α1-adrenergic receptor research. *Acta Pharmacol. Sin.* **2005**, *26*, 1281–1287. [CrossRef]
61. O'Connell, T.D.; Jensen, B.C.; Baker, A.J.; Simpson, P.C. Cardiac alpha1-adrenergic receptors: Novel aspects of expression, signaling mechanisms, physiologic function, and clinical importance. *Pharmacol. Rev.* **2014**, *66*, 308–333. [CrossRef] [PubMed]
62. Jensen, B.C.; O'Connell, T.D.; Simpson, P.C. Alpha-1-adrenergic receptors in heart failure: The adaptive arm of the cardiac response to chronic catecholamine stimulation. *J. Cardiovasc. Pharmacol.* **2014**, *63*, 291–301. [CrossRef] [PubMed]
63. Morrow, A.L.; Creese, I. Characterization of Alpha-1-Adrenergic Receptor Subtypes in Rat-Brain—A Reevaluation of [H-3] Wb4104 and [H-3] Prazosin Binding. *Mol. Pharmacol.* **1986**, *29*, 321–330. [PubMed]
64. Romero-grimaldi, C.; Moreno-lo, B. Age-Dependent Effect of Nitric Oxide on Subventricular Zone and Olfactory Bulb. *J. Comp. Neurol.* **2008**, *346*, 339–346. [CrossRef] [PubMed]
65. Campeau, S.; Nyhuis, T.J.; Kryskow, E.M.; Masini, C.V.; Babb, J.A.; Sasse, S.K.; Greenwood, B.N.; Fleshner, M.;

Day, H.E.W. Stress rapidly increases alpha 1d adrenergic receptor mRNA in the rat dentate gyrus. *Brain Res.* **2010**, *1323*, 109–118. [CrossRef]

66. Szot, P.; White, S.S.; Greenup, J.L.; Leverenz, J.B.; Peskind, E.R.; Raskind, M.A. Changes in Adrenoreceptors in The Prefrontal Cortex Of Subjects With Dementia: Evidence Of Compensatory Changes. *Neuroscience* **2007**, *146*, 471–480. [CrossRef]
67. Perez, D.M.; Doze, V.A. Cardiac and neuroprotection regulated by alpha1-AR subtypes. *J. Recept Signal. Transduct Res.* **2011**, *31*, 98–110. [CrossRef]
68. Sica, D. Alpha-1 adrenergic Blockers: Current Usage Considerations. *J. Clin. Hypertens.* **2005**, *7*, 757–762. [CrossRef]
69. Miriam, H.; Hein, L. α1-Adrenozeptor-Antagonisten. Bei BPS und Hypertonie. *Pharm. Unserer Zeit* **2008**, *37*, 290–295. [CrossRef]
70. Law, M.P.; Osman, S.; Pike, V.W.; Davenport, R.J.; Cunningham, V.J.; Rimoldi, O.; Rhodes, C.G.; Giardinà, D.; Camici, P.G. Evaluation of [11C]GB67, a novel radioligand for imaging myocardial (α1-adrenoceptors with positron emission tomography. *Eur. J. Nucl. Med.* **2000**, *27*, 7–17. [CrossRef]
71. Nyberg, S.; Eriksson, B.; Oxenstierna, G.; Halldin, C.; Farde, L. Suggested minimal effective dose of risperidone based on PET-measured D2 and 5-HT(2A) receptor occupancy in schizophrenic patients. *Am. J. Psychiatry* **1999**, *156*, 869–875. [CrossRef] [PubMed]
72. Nyberg, S.; Olsson, H.; Nilsson, U.; Maehlum, E.; Halldin, C.; Farde, L. Low striatal and extra-striatal D2 receptor occupancy during treatment with the atypical antipsychotic sertindole. *Psychopharmacology (Berl.)* **2002**, *162*, 37–41. [CrossRef]
73. Balle, T.; Perregaard, J.; Ramirez, M.T.; Larsen, A.K.; Søby, K.K.; Liljefors, T.; Andersen, K. Synthesis and structure-affinity relationship investigations of 5-heteroaryl-substituted analogues of the antipsychotic sertindole. A new class of highly selective α1 adrenoceptor antagonists. *J. Med. Chem.* **2003**, *46*, 265–283. [CrossRef] [PubMed]
74. Balle, T.; Halldin, C.; Andersen, L.; Alifrangis, L.H.; Badolo, L.; Jensen, K.G.; Chou, Y.W.; Andersen, K.; Perregaard, J.; Farde, L. New α1-adrenoceptor antagonists derived from the antipsychotic sertindole—Carbon-11 labelling and pet examination of brain uptake in the cynomolgus monkey. *Nucl. Med. Biol.* **2004**, *31*, 327–336. [CrossRef] [PubMed]
75. Airaksinen, A.J.; Finnema, S.J.; Balle, T.; Varnäs, K.; Bang-Andersen, B.; Gulyás, B.; Farde, L.; Halldin, C. Radiosynthesis and evaluation of new α1-adrenoceptor antagonists as PET radioligands for brain imaging. *Nucl. Med. Biol.* **2013**, *40*, 747–754. [CrossRef]
76. Risgaard, R.; Ettrup, A.; Balle, T.; Dyssegaard, A.; Hansen, H.D.; Lehel, S.; Madsen, J.; Pedersen, H.; Püschl, A.; Badolo, L.; et al. Radiolabelling and PET brain imaging of the α1-adrenoceptor antagonist Lu AE43936. *Nucl. Med. Biol.* **2013**, *40*, 135–140. [CrossRef]
77. Jorgensen, M.; Jorgensen, P.N.; Christoffersen, C.T.; Jensen, K.G.; Balle, T.; Bang-Andersen, B. Discovery of novel α1-adrenoceptor ligands based on the antipsychotic sertindole suitable for labeling as PET ligands. *Bioorg. Med. Chem.* **2013**, *21*, 196–204. [CrossRef]
78. Bøgesø, K.P.; Arnt, J.; Hyttel, J.; Pedersen, H.; Liljefors, T. Octoclothepin Enantiomers. A Reinvestigation of Their Biochemical and Pharmacological Activity in Relation to a New Receptor-Interaction Model for Dopamine D-2 Receptor Antagonists. *J. Med. Chem.* **1991**, *34*, 2023–2030. [CrossRef]
79. Liow, J.S.; Lu, S.; McCarron, J.A.; Hong, J.; Musachio, J.L.; Pike, V.W.; Innis, R.B.; Zoghbi, S.S. Effect of a P-Glycoprotein Inhibitor, Cyclosporin A, on the Disposition in Rodent Brain and Blood of the 5-HT1A Receptor Radioligand, [11C](R)-(—)-RWAY. *Synapse* **2007**, *61*, 96–105. [CrossRef]
80. Roberts, L.R.; Bryans, J.; Conlon, K.; McMurray, G.; Stobie, A.; Whitlock, G.A. Novel 2-imidazoles as potent, selective and CNS penetrant α1A adrenoceptor partial agonists. *Bioorg. Med. Chem. Lett.* **2008**, *18*, 6437–6440. [CrossRef]
81. Whitlock, G.A.; Brennan, P.E.; Roberts, L.R.; Stobie, A. Potent and selective α1A adrenoceptor partial agonists-Novel imidazole frameworks. *Bioorg. Med. Chem. Lett.* **2009**, *19*, 3118–3121. [CrossRef] [PubMed]
82. Bücheler, M.M.; Hadamek, K.; Hein, L. Two α2-adrenergic receptor subtypes, α2A and α2C, inhibit transmitter release in the brain of gene-targeted mice. *Neuroscience* **2002**, *109*, 819–826. [CrossRef]
83. Nguyen, V.; Tiemann, D.; Park, E.; Salehi, A. Alpha-2 Agonists. *Anesthesiol. Clin.* **2017**, *35*, 233–245. [CrossRef] [PubMed]

84. Khan, Z.P.; Ferguson, C.N.; Jones, R.M. Alpha-2 and imidazoline receptor agonists. Their pharmacology and therapeutic role. *Anaesthesia* **1999** *54*, 146–165. [CrossRef]

85. Paciorek, P.M.; Pierce, V.; Shepperson, N.B.; Waterfall, J.F. An investigation into the selectivity of a novel series of benzoquinolizines for α2-adrenoceptors in vivo. *Br. J. Pharmacol.* **1984**, *82*, 127–134. [CrossRef]

86. Pettibone, D.J.; Flagg, S.D.; Totarol, J.A.; Clineschmidt, B.V.; Huff, J.R.; Young, S.D.; Chen, R. [3H]L-657, 743 (MK-912): A new, high affinity, selective radioligand for brain α-2 adrenoceptors. *Life Sci.* **1989**, *44*, 459–467. [CrossRef]

87. Pleus, R.C.; Shiue, C.Y.; Shiue, G.G.; Rysavy, J.A.; Huang, H.; Cornish, K.G.; Sunderland, J.J.; Bylund, D.B. Synthesis and biodistribution of the alpha 2-adrenergic receptor antagonist (11C)WY26703. Use as a radioligand for positron emission tomography. *Receptor* **1992**, *2*, 241–252.

88. Shiue, C.Y.; Pleus, R.C.; Shiue, G.G.; Rysavy, J.A.; Sunderland, J.J.; Cornish, K.G.; Young, S.D.; Bylund, D.B. Synthesis and biological evaluation of [11C]MK-912 as an α2- adrenergic receptor radioligand for PET studies. *Nucl. Med. Biol.* **1998**, *25*, 127–133. [CrossRef]

89. BK, F.D.; Terrazzino, S.; Tavitian, B.; Hinnen, F.; Vaufrey, F.; Crouzel, C. XIIth international symposium on radiopharmaceutical chemistry: Abstracts and programme. *J. Label. Compd. Radiopharm.* **1997**, *40*, 1–72. [CrossRef]

90. Hume, S.P.; Hirani, E.; Opacka-Juffry, J.; Osman, S.; Myers, R.; Gunn, R.N.; McCarron, J.A.; Clark, R.D.; Melichar, J.; Nutt, D.J.; et al. Evaluation of [O-methyl-11C]RS.15385-197 as a positron emission tomography radioligand for central α2-adrenoceptors. *Eur. J. Nucl. Med.* **2000**, *27*, 475–484. [CrossRef]

91. Roeda, D.; Sipil, H.T.; Bramoull, Y.; Enas, J.D.; Vaufrey, F.; Doll, F.; Crouzel, C. Synthesis of [11C]atipamezole, a potential PET ligand for the α2-adrenergic receptor in the brain. *J. Label. Compd. Radiopharm.* **2002**, *45*, 37–47. [CrossRef]

92. Marthi, K.; Bender, D.; Watanabe, H.; Smith, D.F. PET evaluation of a tetracyclic, atypical antidepressant, [N-methyl-11C]mianserin, in the living porcine brain. *Nucl. Med. Biol.* **2002**, *29*, 317–319. [CrossRef]

93. Marthi, K.; Bender, D.; Gjedde, A.; Smith, D.F. [11C]Mirtazapine for PET neuroimaging: Radiosynthesis and initial evaluation in the living porcine brain. *Eur. Neuropsychopharmacol.* **2002**, *12*, 427–432. [CrossRef]

94. Marthi, K.; Jakobsen, S.; Bender, D.; Hansen, S.B.; Smith, S.B.; Hermansen, F.; Rosenberg, R.; Smith, D.F. [N-methyl-11C]Mirtazapine for positron emission tomography neuroimaging of antidepressant actions in humans. *Psychopharmacology (Berl.)* **2004**, *174*, 260–265. [CrossRef] [PubMed]

95. Smith, D.F.; Stork, B.S.; Wegener, G.; Ashkanian, M.; Jakobsen, S.; Bender, D.; Audrain, H.; Vase, K.H.; Hansen, S.B.; Videbech, P.; et al. [11C]mirtazapine binding in depressed antidepressant nonresponders studied by PET neuroimaging. *Psychopharmacology (Berl.)* **2009**, *206*, 133–140. [CrossRef] [PubMed]

96. Van der Mey, M.; Windhorst, A.D.; Klok, R.P.; Herscheid, J.D.M.; Kennis, L.E.; Bischoff, F.; Bakker, M.; Langlois, X.; Heylen, L.; Jurzak, M.; et al. Synthesis and biodistribution of [11C]R107474, a new radiolabeled α2-adrenoceptor antagonist. *Bioorg. Med. Chem.* **2006**, *14*, 4526–4534. [CrossRef]

97. Jakobsen, S.; Pedersen, K.; Smith, D.F.; Jensen, S.B.; Munk, O.L.; Cumming, P. Detection of a 2 -Adrenergic Receptors in Brain of Living Pig with 11 C-Yohimbine. *J. Nucl. Med.* **2006**, *47*, 2008–2015.

98. Nahimi, A.; Jakobsen, S.; Munk, O.L.; Vang, K.; Phan, J.A.; Rodell, A.; Gjedde, A. Mapping α2 adrenoceptors of the human brain with11C-yohimbine. *J. Nucl. Med.* **2015**, *56*, 392–398. [CrossRef]

99. Andrés, J.I.; Alcázar, J.; Alonso, J.M.; Alvarez, R.M.; Bakker, M.H.; Biesmans, I.; Cid, J.M.; De Lucas, A.I.; Fernández, J.; Font, L.M.; et al. Discovery of a new series of centrally active tricyclic isoxazoles combining serotonin (5-HT) reuptake inhibition with α2- adrenoceptor blocking activity. *J. Med. Chem.* **2005**, *48*, 2054–2071. [CrossRef]

100. Sa̧czewski, F.; Kornicka, A.; Rybczyńska, A.; Hudson, A.L.; Shu, S.M.; Gdaniec, M.; Boblewski, K.; Lehmann, A. 1-[(imidazolidin-2-yl)imino]indazole. Highly α2/I 1 selective agonist: Synthesis, X-ray structure, and biological activity. *J. Med. Chem.* **2008**, *51*, 3599–3608. [CrossRef]

101. Hagihara, K.; Kashima, H.; Iida, K.; Enokizono, J.; Uchida, S.I.; Nonaka, H.; Kurokawa, M.; Shimada, J. Novel 4-(6,7-dimethoxy-1,2,3,4-tetrahydroisoquinolin-2-yl)methylbenzofuran derivatives as selective α2C-adrenergic receptor antagonists. *Bioorg. Med. Chem. Lett.* **2007**, *17*, 1616–1621. [CrossRef] [PubMed]

102. Finnema, S.J.; Hughes, Z.A.; Haaparanta-Solin, M.; Stepanov, V.; Nakao, R.; Varnäs, K.; Varrone, A.; Arponen, E.; Marjamäki, P.; Pohjanoksa, K.; et al. Amphetamine decreases α2C-adrenoceptor binding of [11C]ORM-13070: A PET study in the primate brain. *Int. J. Neuropsychopharmacol.* **2015**, *18*, 1–10. [CrossRef] [PubMed]

103. Palacios, J.M.; Kuhar, M.J. Beta adrenergic receptor localization in rat brain by light microscopic autoradiography. *Neurochem. Int.* **1982**, *4*, 473–490. [CrossRef]
104. Cash, R.; Ruberg, M.; Raisman, R.; Agid, Y. Adrenergic receptors in Parkinson's disease. *Brain Res.* **1984**, *322*, 269–275. [CrossRef]
105. Hopfner, F.; Höglinger, G.U.; Kuhlenbäumer, G.; Pottegård, A.; Wod, M.; Christensen, K.; Tanner, C.M.; Deuschl, G. β-adrenoreceptors and the risk of Parkinson's disease. *Lancet Neurol.* **2020**, *19*, 247–254. [CrossRef]
106. Klimek, V.; Rajkowska, G.; Luker, S.N.; Dilley, G.; Meltzer, H.Y.; Overholser, J.C.; Stockmeier, C.A.; Ordway, G.A. Brain noradrenergic receptors in major depression and schizophrenia. *Neuropsychopharmacology* **1999**, *21*, 69–81. [CrossRef]
107. Ueki, J.; Rhodes, C.G.; Hughes, J.M.; De Silva, R.; Lefroy, D.C.; Ind, P.W.; Qing, F.; Brady, F.; Luthra, S.K.; Steel, C.J. In vivo quantification of pulmonary B-adrenoceptor density in humans with (*S*)-[11C]CGP-12177 and PET. *Am. Physiol. Soc.* **1993**, *75*, 559–565. [CrossRef] [PubMed]
108. Elsinga, P.H.; Doze, P.; Van Waarde, A.; Pieterman, R.M.; Blanksma, P.K.; Willemsen, A.T.M.; Vaalburg, W. Imaging of β-adrenoceptors in the human thorax using (*S*)-[11C]CGP12388 and positron emission tomography. *Eur. J. Pharmacol.* **2001**, *433*, 173–176. [CrossRef]
109. Berger, G.; Maziere, M.; Prenant, C.; Sastre, J.; Syrota, A.; Comar, D. Synthesis of 11 C propranolol. *J. Radioanal. Chem.* **1982**, *74*, 301–306. [CrossRef]
110. Antoni, G.; Ulin, J.; Långström, B. Synthesis of the 11C-labelled β-adrenergic receptor ligands atenolol, metoprolol and propranolol. *Int. J. Radiat. Appl. Instrum. Part A* **1989**, *40*, 561–564. [CrossRef]
111. Berridge, M.S.; Nelson, A.D.; Zheng, L.; Leisure, G.P.; Miraldi, F. Specific beta-adrenergic receptor binding of carazolol measured with PET. *J. Nucl. Med.* **1994**, *35*, 1665–1676.
112. Zheng, L.; Berridge, M.S.; Ernsberger, P. Synthesis, Binding Properties, and 18F Labeling of Fluorocarazolol, a High-Affinity β-Adrenergic Receptor Antagonist. *J. Med. Chem.* **1994**, *37*, 3219–3230. [CrossRef] [PubMed]
113. Doze, P.; Van Waarde, A.; Elsinga, P.H.; Van-Loenen Weemaes, A.M.A.; Willemsen, A.T.M.; Vaalburg, W. Validation of S-1′-[18F]fluorocarazolol for in vivo imaging and quantification of cerebral β-adrenoceptors. *Eur. J. Pharmacol.* **1998**, *353*, 215–226. [CrossRef]
114. Doze, P.; Elsinga, P.H.; De Vries, E.F.J.; Van Waarde, A.; Vaalburg, W. Mutagenic activity of a fluorinated analog of the beta-adrenoceptor ligand carazolol in the Ames test. *Nucl. Med. Biol.* **2000**, *27*, 315–319. [CrossRef]
115. Tewson, T.J.; Stekhova, S.; Kinsey, B.; Chen, L.; Wiens, L.; Barber, R. Synthesis and biodistribution of R- and S-isomers of [18F]- fluoropropranolol, a lipophilic ligand for the β-adrenergic receptor. *Nucl. Med. Biol.* **1999**, *26*, 891–896. [CrossRef]
116. Moresco, R.M.; Matarrese, M.; Soloviev, D.; Simonelli, P.; Rigamonti, M.; Gobbo, C.; Todde, S.; Carpinelli, A.; Galli Kienle, M.; Fazio, F. Synthesis and in vivo evaluation of [11C]ICI 118551 as a putative subtype selective β2-adrenergic radioligand. *Int. J. Pharm.* **2000**, *204*, 101–109. [CrossRef]
117. Soloviev, D.V.; Matarrese, M.; Moresco, R.M.; Todde, S.; Bonasera, T.A.; Sudati, F.; Simonelli, P.; Magni, F.; Colombo, D.; Carpinelli, A.; et al. Asymmetric synthesis and preliminary evaluation of (*R*)- and (*S*)-[11C]bisoprolol, a putative β1-selective adrenoceptor radioligand. *Neurochem. Int.* **2001**, *38*, 169–180. [CrossRef]
118. Doze, P.; Elsinga, P.H.; Maas, B.; Van Waarde, A.; Wegman, T.; Vaalburg, W. Synthesis and evaluation of radiolabeled antagonists for imaging of β-adrenoceptors in the brain with PET. *Neurochem. Int.* **2002**, *40*, 145–155. [CrossRef]
119. Doze, P.; Van Waarde, A.; Tewson, T.J.; Vaalburg, W.; Elsinga, P.H. Synthesis and evaluation of (*S*)-[18F]-fluoroethylcarazolol for in vivo β-adrenoceptor imaging in the brain. *Neurochem. Int.* **2002**, *41*, 17–27. [CrossRef]
120. van Waarde, A.; Doorduin, J.; de Jong, J.R.; Dierckx, R.A.; Elsinga, P.H. Synthesis and preliminary evaluation of (*S*)-[11C]-exaprolol, a novel β-adrenoceptor ligand for PET. *Neurochem. Int.* **2008**, *52*, 729–733. [CrossRef]
121. Stephenson, K.A.; van Oosten, E.M.; Wilson, A.A.; Meyer, J.H.; Houle, S.; Vasdev, N. Synthesis and preliminary evaluation of [18F]-fluoro-(2S)-Exaprolol for imaging cerebral β-adrenergic receptors with PET. *Neurochem. Int.* **2008**, *53*, 173–179. [CrossRef] [PubMed]
122. Mirfeizi, L.; Rybczynska, A.A.; van Waarde, A.; Campbell-Verduyn, L.; Feringa, B.L.; Dierckx, R.A.J.O.; Elsinga, P.H. [18F]-(fluoromethoxy)ethoxy)methyl)-1H-1,2,3-triazol-1-yl)propan-2-ol ([18F FPTC) a novel PET-ligand for cerebral beta-adrenoceptors. *Nucl. Med. Biol.* **2014**, *41*, 203–209. [CrossRef] [PubMed]

13

Pyrazoles as Key Scaffolds for the Development of Fluorine-18-Labeled Radiotracers for Positron Emission Tomography (PET)

Pedro M. O. Gomes, Artur M. S. Silva and Vera L. M. Silva *

LAQV-REQUIMTE, Department of Chemistry, University of Aveiro, 3810-193 Aveiro, Portugal; pm.gomes@ua.pt (P.M.O.G.); artur.silva@ua.pt (A.M.S.S.)

* Correspondence: verasilva@ua.pt

Academic Editor: Krishan Kumar

Abstract: The need for increasingly personalized medicine solutions (precision medicine) and quality medical treatments, has led to a growing demand and research for image-guided therapeutic solutions. Positron emission tomography (PET) is a powerful imaging technique that can be established using complementary imaging systems and selective imaging agents—chemical probes or radiotracers—which are drugs labeled with a radionuclide, also called radiopharmaceuticals. PET has two complementary purposes: selective imaging for diagnosis and monitoring of disease progression and response to treatment. The development of selective imaging agents is a growing research area, with a high number of diverse drugs, labeled with different radionuclides, being reported nowadays. This review article is focused on the use of pyrazoles as suitable scaffolds for the development of ^{18}F-labeled radiotracers for PET imaging. A brief introduction to PET and pyrazoles, as key scaffolds in medicinal chemistry, is presented, followed by a description of the most important [^{18}F]pyrazole-derived radiotracers (PET tracers) that have been developed in the last 20 years for selective PET imaging, grouped according to their specific targets.

Keywords: positron emission tomography (PET); pyrazoles; fluorine-18; radionuclides; PET probes; imaging pharmaceuticals

---

1. Introduction

Positron emission tomography (PET) is a nuclear medicine functional imaging technique that uses gamma rays (formed as a result of the annihilation of the emitted positrons) to provide three-dimensional images that give information about the functioning of a person's specific organs. PET is based on the detection of tiny amounts (picomolar) of a biological substance labeled with a short-lived positron-emitting radionuclide (PET tracer) without disturbing the biological system and has the advantage of being a noninvasive, functional and highly sensitive technique which provides a great wealth of information [1]. The PET tracers are drugs or biomolecules labeled with radionuclides such as ^{11}C, ^{13}N, ^{15}O, ^{18}F, ^{64}Cu, ^{68}Ga, ^{89}Zr and ^{124}I. Since radionuclides can replace the stable analogues, the PET probes have the same chemical structure as the drugs and biomolecules without altering their biological activity. The choice of the PET radionuclide must follow some criteria: (i) physical and chemical characteristics, (ii) availability and (iii) timescale of the biological process in the study. For different biological processes, some radionuclides are better than others. If the biological process in the study gives results hours or days after the injection of PET probe, ^{64}Cu, ^{89}Zr or ^{124}I can be used, because these three radionuclides have a long half-life time (12.8 h, 78.4 h and 4.17 days, respectively). On the contrary, radionuclides as ^{11}C or ^{18}F are used for labeling small organic compounds for faster biological processes [1]. To avoid unnecessary radiation, it is important to choose a radionuclide with a half-life that enable the reaction of the radionuclide with the carrier molecule and matches the timescale of the biological process in the study. ^{18}F is the ideal radionuclide for routine PET imaging, because it has a short half-life (109.8 min) but enough to allow all the process of synthesis, transport and imaging. Furthermore, it is a 97% positron-emitter, and the low positron energy of ^{18}F leads to a high resolution of PET imaging [1,2].

In the last three decades, the interest in PET has been growing, and nowadays, this technique is used in several areas of medicine, such as oncology [3], cardiology [4], neurology [5] and also in drug development and evaluation [6]. Besides the aforementioned advantages of PET, there are also some limitations; pregnant women should not undergo in PET imaging; the radioactivity of PET tracers limits the number of times one patient can undergo PET scans and is a very expensive treatment [7]. Moreover, the potential of PET strongly depends on the availability of suitable PET radiotracers. For instance, 2-[^{18}F]fluoro-2-deoxyglucose ([^{18}F]FDG) is one of the most used radiotracers for the clinical diagnosis and evaluation of cancer. However, it has inherent drawbacks, namely its high accumulation in inflamed and infected tissues giving false-positive results and its low uptake in tumors that grow slowly, which can lead to false-negative results [8]. Finally, the development of new PET-imaging probes is not trivial, and radiochemistry is a major limiting factor for this field. Hence, the research and development of new PET tracers is a challenging issue of major importance within the scientific community.

Following our interest in the synthesis and biological evaluation of pyrazole-type compounds envisaging their use in medicine [9–14] and considering their huge potential for application in PET field, herein we present an overview of pyrazole-derived PET radiotracers developed in the last 20 years. Pyrazoles labeled with ^{18}F radionuclide will be the focus of this review article, given the aforementioned advantages of this radionuclide for routine PET imaging.

2. Pyrazoles

This family of compounds is characterized by a simple heteroaromatic five-membered ring containing three carbon and two nitrogen atoms in adjacent positions [15]. The occurrence of the pyrazole core in nature is rare, probably due to the difficulty of living organisms to make a N-N bound [16]. Until now, there are only approximately 20 natural compounds with a pyrazole core on their structures [17]. Although scarce in nature, pyrazole (1*H*-pyrazole (**1**), Figure 1) and its reduced derivatives (pyrazolines **2–4**, Figure 1) are considered privileged structures in medicinal chemistry. Pyrazole scaffold is present in several synthetic drugs, being celecoxib (Celebrex®), sildenafil (Viagra®), rimonabant, fomepizole, penthiopyrad and sulfaphenazole the most notorious [15].

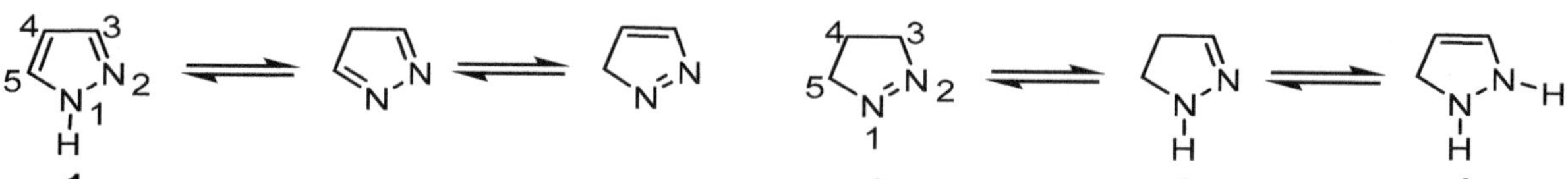

Figure 1. Chemical structures and numbering of pyrazole (**1**) and dihydropyrazole (pyrazoline) tautomers **2–4** [18].

Pyrazole derivatives act on diverse and relevant biological targets, which make them attractive for the development of PET tracers, and possess a wide range of pharmaceutical activities. Abdel-Maksoud et al. have demonstrated antitumoral activity of several compounds with a pyrazole and sulfonamide moieties [19]; antibacterial and antifungal activity of pyrazole was demonstrated by Chowdary et al. [20]. Pyrazoles also showed good activity as monoamine oxidase inhibitors, antidepressant and anticonvulsant agents [21], as BRAF inhibitors [22] and DNA gyrase inhibitors [23] and present antileishmanial, anti-inflammatory, analgesic, antidiabetic and cannabinoid activity; cyclin-dependent kinase and tissue-nonspecific alkaline phosphatase inhibitory activity and moderate antihepatotoxic activity, among others [9,11,24–29]. In 2013, Prabhu et. al. reported the antioxidant activity of pyrazole [30]. They demonstrated that pyrazole (1,2-diazole) can be used to prevent nephrotoxicity caused by cisplatin, a drug used to treat several cancers. Cisplatin provokes renal damage because of its toxicity to proximal tubule cells and can reduce glomerular filtration, resulting in renal failure. One of the reasons of nephrotoxicity induced by cisplatin is the decreasing concentration of glutathione (GSH). Pyrazole prevents nephrotoxicity induced by cisplatin by counteracting this effect, increasing the concentration of this enzyme [30]. Recently, Silva et al. reported the antioxidant activity of around three hundred pyrazoles [18].

2.1. *Pyrazoles as Probes for PET Imaging*

The labeling of pyrazole-type compounds with ^{18}F for PET imaging is a research issue that has been growing significantly, as evidenced by the number of papers and citations in the last years, according to our search on Web of Science using the keywords (pyrazole) and (positron emission tomography) and (^{18}F) (Figure 2). In this section are described the most important [^{18}F]-labeled pyrazoles developed for use as PET radiotracers. The compounds are presented according to their specific targets, which are indicated by alphabetical order and not by their relevance in the PET field. Whenever possible, the most promising applications of these compounds in this field are discussed.

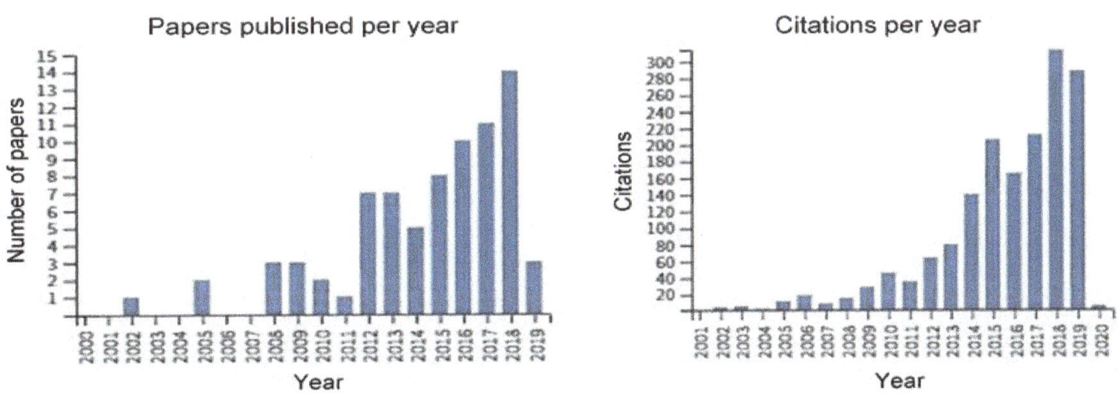

Figure 2. Number of papers published and citations per year found using the keywords "pyrazoles" and "positron emission tomography" and "^{18}F" in Web of Science in the period 2000–2020.

2.1.1. Adenosine Receptors Ligands

Adenosine, an endogenous-signaling substance, is a purine ribonucleoside composed of adenine (purine base) and ribose (sugar molecule), which is produced in response to metabolic stress and cell damage. It induces several physiopathological effects, regulating the central nervous, cardiovascular, peripheral, and immune systems due to the rapid generation of adenosine from cellular metabolism and the widespread distribution of its receptor subtypes in almost all organs and tissues [31]. There are four types of adenosine receptors: A_1, A_{2A}, A_{2B} and A_3. A_{2A}R are abundant in dopamine-rich regions of the brain, being the striatum the region with a higher concentration of A_{2A}R [31]. In preclinical studies, A_{2A}R antagonists showed potential benefits in the treatment of some neurodegenerative diseases like Alzheimer's disease (AD) and Parkinson's disease (PD), neuroinflammation, ischemia, spinal cord injury, drug addiction and other conditions [31]. Khanapur et al. developed a pyrazolo[4,3-*e*]-1,2,4-triazolo[1,5-*c*]pyrimidine labeled with carbon-11, [^{11}C]SCH442416 (**5**) and its [^{18}F]fluoroethyl and [^{18}F]fluoropropyl derivatives ([^{18}F]FESCH (**6**) and [^{18}F]FPSCH (**7**), respectively) (Figure 3), and both radioligands showed a distribution in the rat brain corresponding to the regional A_{2A}R densities, as evidenced by in vitro autoradiography (ARG) experiments and binding assays [32]. These two tracers showed a similar ratio specific/nonspecific binding, using the striatum as the specific binding and cerebellum as the nonspecific binding (4.6 at 25 and 37 min after injection, respectively) and reversible binding in rat brains, although their kinetics were slightly different [32]. Recently, the same authors studied the full kinetics of radioligands **6** and **7** in rat brains. On the basis of the Akaike information criterion, they have found that 1TCM was the most appropriate model for describing [^{18}F]FPSCH kinetics, whereas 2TCM was the most suitable model for [^{18}F]FESCH kinetics. Using dynamic PET imaging, under baseline and full blocking conditions, they proved that **6** is the most suitable PET radioligand for quantifying $A_{2A}R$ receptor expression in the rat brain. However, before starting the clinical use of **6**, it will be necessary to reevaluate the brain uptake in humans due to possible interspecies differences in tracer kinetics and metabolisms [33].

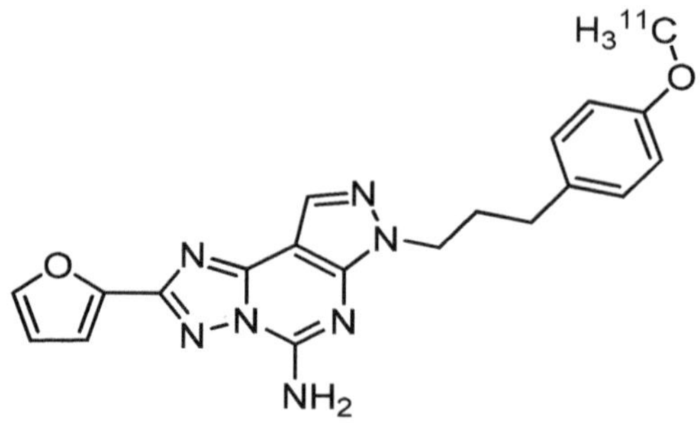

[^{11}C]SCH442416

5

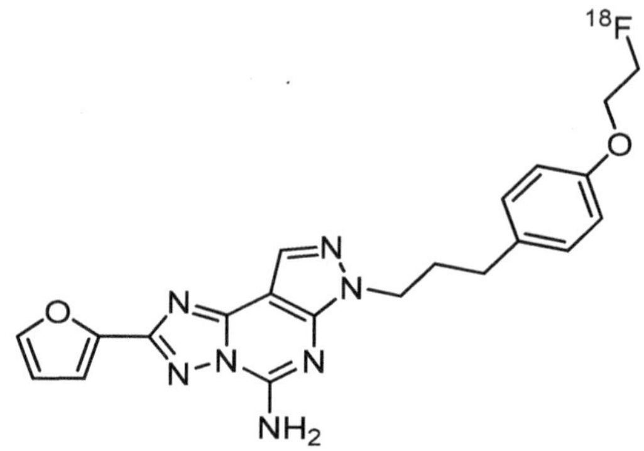

[^{18}F]FESCH

6

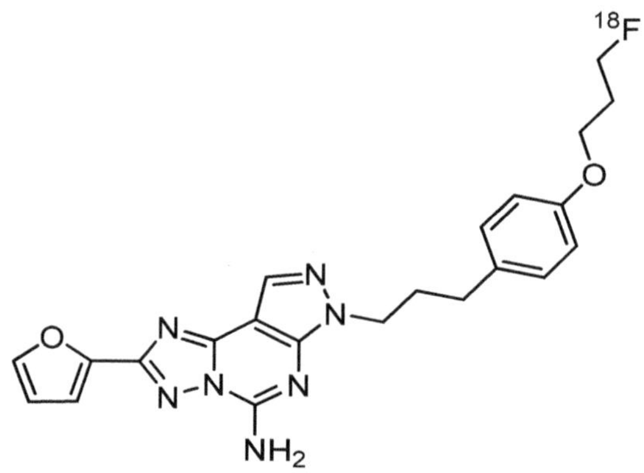

[^{18}F]FPSCH

7

Figure 3. Adenosine receptor ($A_{2A}R$) radioantagonists **5**–**7** for PET imaging [32,33].

2.1.2. Cannabinoid Receptors Ligands

Products derived from *Cannabis sativa* are some of the oldest and widely used drugs in the world. These products are known as natural cannabinoids, but several synthetic cannabinoids have been developed as well. Cannabinoids have been used as analgesics for more than 100 years [34]. Additionally, they have been used as antiemetic agents to prevent chemotherapy-induced nausea and vomiting, because they can bind to opiate receptors in the forebrain, blocking the vomiting center in the medulla [35]. In 1998, Williams and Kirkham have demonstrated that anandamide, an endogenous cannabinoid, provokes hyperphagia in satiated rats [36]. Cannabinoid-type compounds bind to cannabinoid receptors, which can be divided in two groups—cannabinoid receptor type 1 (CB_1), predominantly found in the brain, and the peripheral cannabinoid receptor type 2 (CB_2), mainly expressed in immune tissues, and both are G-protein-coupled membrane receptors [37].

The imaging of the CB_1 receptor is of great importance for studying its role in neuropsychiatric disorders, including depression, and in obesity, drug or alcohol addiction, and is an active target for in vivo imaging development [38]. The first selective CB_1 receptor antagonist was [*N*-(piperidin-1-yl)-5-(4-chlorophenyl)-1-(2,4-dichlorophenyl)-4-methyl-1*H*-pyrazole-3-carboxamide] SR141716 (**8**), known as rimonabant (Figure 4) [39]. This compound was approved in Europe, in 2006, to treat obesity by reducing the patient's appetite. Two years later, the European Medicines Agency (EMA) withdrew rimonabant from sale due to its evident secondary effects. Some studies demonstrated that SR141716 induced anxiety, depression, agitation, eating disorders, irritability, aggression and insomnia. Rimonabant was not approved in the USA by the Food and Drug Administration (FDA) [40]. However, some analogs of SR141716 (**8**) have been labeled with radionuclides for PET imaging. [^{18}F]SR144385 (**9**) and [^{18}F]SR147963 (**10**) [37,41], [^{18}F]NIDA-42033 (**11**) and its related ester derivative (**12**) [42], [^{18}F]O-1302 (**13**) [43] and [^{18}F]AM5144 (**14**) [44] are some examples of PET tracers labeled with ^{18}F (Figure 4), while [^{123}I]AM251 (**15**) and [^{123}I]AM281 (**16**) [44] are two examples of PET tracers labeled with ^{123}I (Figure 5).

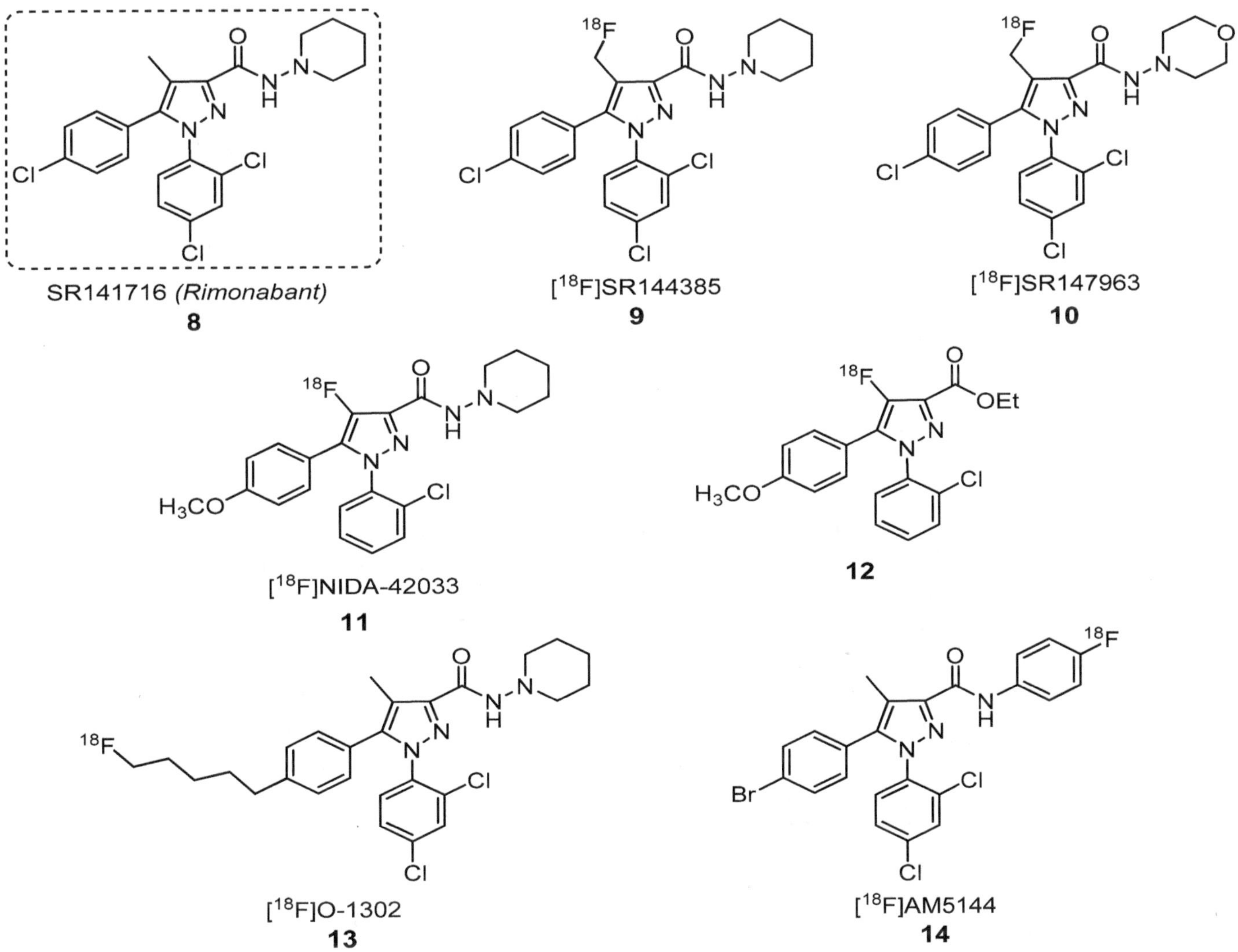

Figure 4. Structure of rimonabant (**8**) and structurally related [^{18}F]pyrazole PET tracers **9–14** [37,39,41–44].

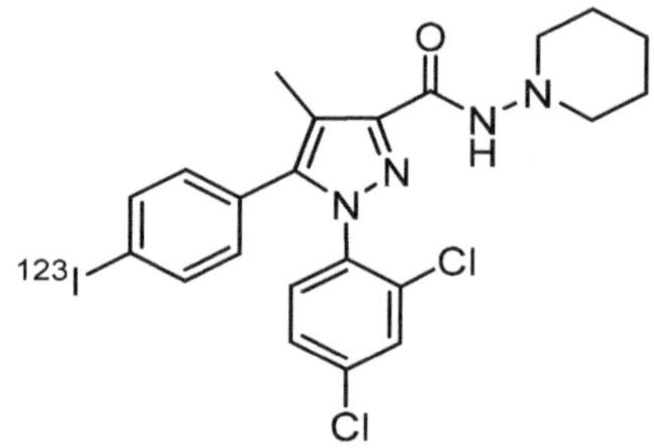

[^{123}I]AM251
15

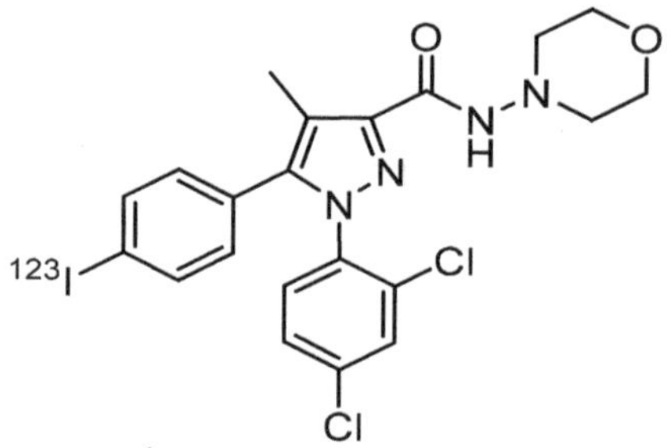

[^{123}I]AM281
16

Figure 5. Pyrazole-derived PET tracers **15** and **16** labeled with ^{123}I [44].

Studies were performed to evaluate the specificity of cannabinoids [^{18}F]SR144385 (**9**) and [^{18}F]SR147963 (**10**) (Figure 4) for CB_1 receptors [37]. After 15 min of injection in male CD-1 mice (25–30 g), compound **10** showed a higher brain uptake compared to compound **9** (5.70% ID/g and 3.06% ID/g, respectively). The hippocampus was the brain region that exhibited the highest uptake of both tracers, followed by the striatum, cerebellum, frontal cortex, cortex, olfactory tubercles and hypothalamus. Both the brain stem and thalamus showed low uptakes of the tracers, and the thalamus showed the fastest decrease of %ID/g. These results are in accordance with the knowledge of CB_1 receptors' brain density in rats, which was found to be lower in the thalamus region. For evaluation of the target to nontarget ratio, the thalamus was used as indicator of nonspecific binding. Compounds **9** and **10** showed differences in the post-injection time they reached the maximum target to nontarget ratio (90 min for compound **9** with a ratio of 2.50 and 60 min for compound **10** with a ratio of 1.69) [37]. In vivo selectivity and specificity studies of [^{18}F]SR144385 (**9**) showed that significant blocking of this tracer uptake was achieved when a 1-mg/kg dose of the structurally similar blocking agent SR141716 (**8**) was given 30 min prior to the radiotracer. Likewise, the uptake of [^{18}F]SR147963 (**10**) at either 30 or 60 min post-injection was also blocked by a 1-mg/kg dose of SR141716 (**8**) given 30 min before the radiotracer.

In 2005, Li et al. synthetized the radioactive pyrazole [^{18}F]AM5144 (**14**) (Figure 4) as a PET radioligand candidate for cannabinoid CB_1 receptors. Using baboons, they demonstrated that the highest radioactivity concentration of compound **14** was found on the cerebellum, and the lowest concentration was found in the thalamus. They concluded that there was a poor brain uptake of **14** and of other related [^{18}F]pyrazoles because of their high lipophilicity, although this property is not the key factor in brain uptake. This study proved that there is no close relationship between the clogP value and brain uptake, indicating that there are other uptake key factors [44]. Despite the high in vitro-binding affinity and moderate lipophilicity of [^{18}F]O-1302 (**13**) (Figure 4), it is not suitable for imaging the CB_1 receptor in the brain due to poor brain entry and high levels of nonspecific binding [43]. Although radiotracer uptake in the brain is often considered a function of the log P that peaks between a log P of 2 and 3, the investigation of the factors that affect brain uptake beyond lipophilicity is crucial to a better comprehension of this process. Some studies highlighted that there may be large species differences in brain penetration for a given PET radiotracer; for example, the brain uptake of [^{123}I]AM251 (**15**) (Figure 5) is very different comparing mice and monkeys, being higher for mice [44,45].

Chang et al. observed that [^{18}F]DBPR211 (**17**) (Figure 6) was distributed in the brain, liver, heart, thigh muscle and kidney when intravenously injected in mice. In the brain, it was found in a very low percentage (less than 1%) over 90-min scans. This result is evidence of its action as a peripherally restricted CB_1 antagonist [46]. Taking into account these observations, this radiotracer can be seen as a promising tool to study metabolic processes associated with peripheral CB_1 receptors.

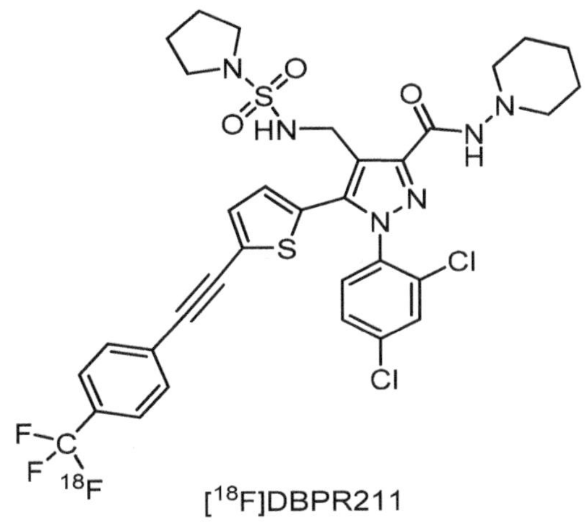

[18F]DBPR211
17

Figure 6. [^{18}F]pyrazole-derived peripheral CB_1 antagonist **17** [46].

2.1.3. Cyclooxygenase Inhibitors

Cyclooxygenase-2 (COX-2) is an enzyme with high-level expressions at sites of inflammation and cancer and is also a promising target for neuroinflammation imaging [47,48]. The development of agents capable of monitoring COX-2 levels is highly desirable for cancer prevention and therapy. To achieve this goal, Uddin et al. synthetized several indomethacin and celecoxib derivatives and evaluated their IC_{50} values for the inhibition of COX-2 in vivo and in intact cells [49]. Indomethacin derivatives were effective COX-2 inhibitors in intact cells (0.09–0.26 µmol/L), but the synthesis of the respective radiotracer has some drawbacks, because the *p*-chlorobenzoyl group is not stable in the conditions of radiochemical synthesis. Among celecoxib derivatives, the more effective COX-2 inhibitor was compound **18** with an IC_{50} value of 0.16 µmol/L. After the synthesis of ^{18}F-**18** (Figure 7), in vivo biodistribution was studied in the inflamed and contralateral footpad of male Sprague Dawley rats. The major advantage of this inflammation model is the possibility to image the inflamed footpad in comparison with the noninflamed contralateral footpad. Compound **18** had a higher accumulation in the inflamed footpad in comparison with the noninflamed. The selective binding between **18** and COX-2 was proved with an assay using celecoxib to block COX-2 before the injection of **18.** To confirm the COX-2 specificity of **18**, COX-2-null mice were injected with carrageenan to promote inflammation. COX-2-null feet demonstrated a 1.08 ± 0.09 ratio of inflamed/noninflamed feet. On other hand, the wild-type mice group, used as the control, had an uptake ratio of 1.48 ± 0.04. The ability of **18** to target COX-2 in human tumor xenografts was also demonstrated using 1483 HNSCC cells and HCT116 cells injected in the left and right hip of female nude mice. In the COX-2-null HCT116 tumor cells, the uptake of **18** was minimal, while, in the 1483 HNSCC cells, a significative uptake of the radiotracer was observed. Once again, to prove that the difference in the uptake of **18** was related with the expression of COX-2, mice bearing 1483 xenografts were pretreated with celecoxib to block the active site of COX-2. There was a significative lower uptake of **18** for mice pretreated with celecoxib when compared with the control group [49].

Lebedev et al. developed a new, high-affinity ^{18}F-COX-2 inhibitor **19** (Figure 7) that is radiolabeled directly on a heteroaromatic ring with the purpose to increase biodistribution and metabolic stability [50]. In vitro studies demonstrated a clear correlation between COX-2 expression and uptake of this radiotracer. Moreover, pharmacokinetic studies in healthy mice revealed no bone retention or defluorination within 2 h of injection, significant blood clearance, since the molecule is excreted from blood within an hour mainly through the hepatobiliary excretion pathway, crossing of blood-brain barrier (BBB) and no significant metabolites in major organs. Although these properties make this probe ideal for PET imaging, some aspects related to radiochemical synthesis severely limit the application of this compound as a probe. In fact, the use of $Et_4NF^{+}4HF$ has limited the specific activity to 3 Ci/mmol, and the current decay-corrected radiochemical yield of 2%, although enough for preclinical studies and the production of a single patient dose, need further improvement to achieve the successful use of this compound as a PET tracer.

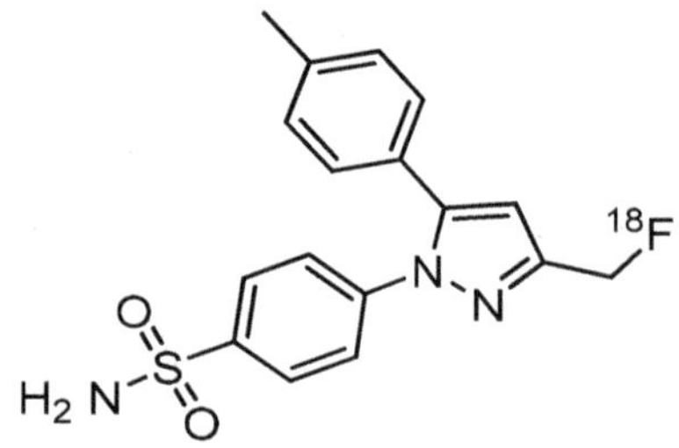

18

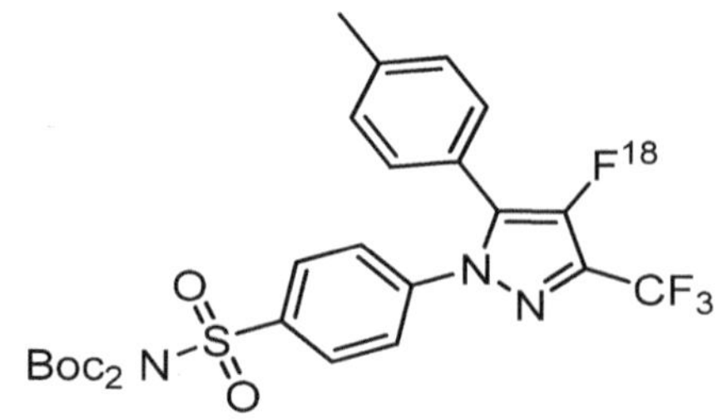

19

Figure 7. [^{18}F]-labeled COX-2 inhibitors **18** and **19** [49,50].

Aiming to develop selective probes for the two COX enzyme subtypes, COX-1 and COX-2, McCharty et al. have prepared [^{18}F]SC63217 (**20**) and [^{18}F]SC58125 (**21**) (Figure 8), starting from the corresponding nonradioactive COX-1 and COX-2 selective inhibitors, SC63217 and SC58125, respectively [51]. Both compounds are structurally similar, presenting only a different substituent on only one aromatic ring. In vitro binding studies of both compounds, using J774 macrophages, revealed that compound **20** is a potential probe for COX-2, while **21** was not a good marker of COX-1 due to high nonspecific binding. In vivo studies showed that, for each tracer, rat biodistribution was well-matched with the known distribution of these enzymes [51].

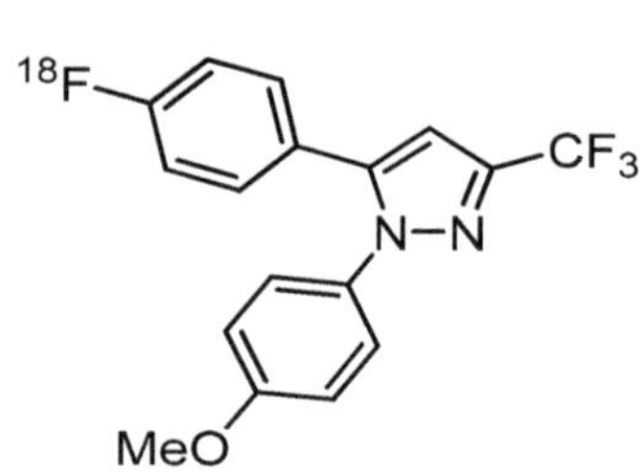

[^{18}F]SC63217
20

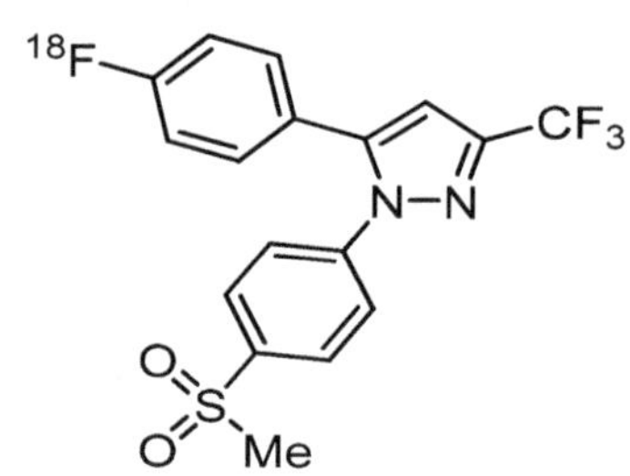

[^{18}F]SC58125
21

Figure 8. [^{18}F]-labeled pyrazoles as probes for COX-1 **20** and COX-2 **21** [51].

2.1.4. Dopamine Receptors Ligands

The subfamily of D_2-like dopamine receptors includes the D_2-, D_3- and D_4-receptor subtypes and mediates the action of dopamine in the brain by the inhibition of adenylate cyclase activity. While the distribution of D_2- and D_3- receptors is well-known, there are still some uncertainties regarding D_4-receptor (D_4R) expression. If D_4R selective radioligands are available, PET can be suited to gain deeper knowledge into the distribution and pathophysiological role of D_4R in humans.

In 2008, the pyrazolo[1,5-*a*]pyridine derivatives, FAUC 113 (**22**) and FAUC 213 (**23**) (Figure 9), bearing a (4-chlorophenyl)piperazinylmethyl moiety in the 3 and 2 positions of the pyrazolo[1,5-*a*]pyridine core, were synthetized. After an evaluation of their binding affinities for D_4-like dopamine receptors, **22** and **23** were chosen as lead compounds for the development of [^{18}F]-labeled PET tracers. A novel compound with a fluoroethoxyphenyl substituent in the *para*-position of the phenylpiperazinyl moiety showed the highest specificity to the D_4 receptor. Due to these results, the next step was radiochemical synthesis to prepare the same labeled derivative, [^{18}F]FAUC F41 (**24**) (Figure 9). Using coronal rat brains, in vivo AGR studies were performed to evaluate the specific binding of **24** to D_4R. An increased uptake of this compound was detected in the hippocampus, hypothalamus, cortex, medial habenular nucleus and central medial thalamic nucleus. The observed binding pattern was mainly consistent with the known D_4R distribution in the rat brains. The log P value for this compound was found to be 2.9, which may indicate adequate BBB penetration. Moreover, this ligand revealed high stability in human serum, even after long-term incubation for up to 90 min [52]. These results demonstrate that [^{18}F]FAUC F41 (**24**) represents a potential radioligand for studying the D_4R in vivo by PET imaging.

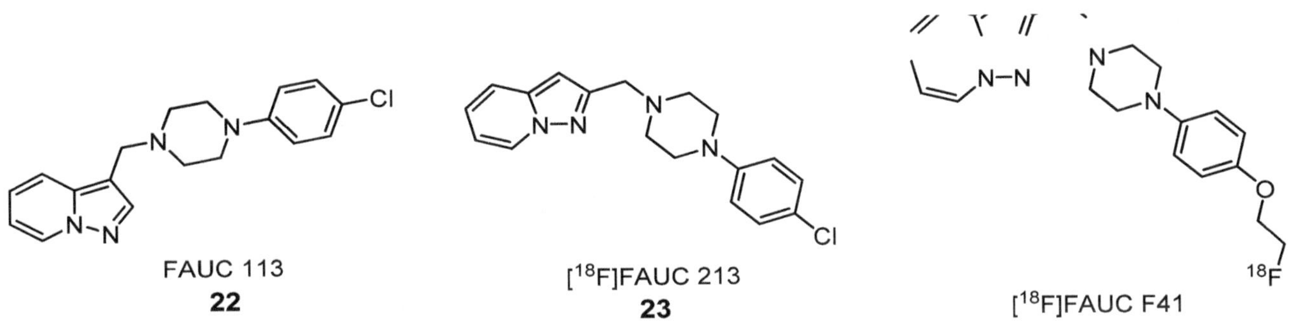

Figure 9. [^{18}F]-labeled high-affinity dopamine receptor (D_4R) tracers **22–24** [52].

With the aim to develop a radiotracer with high selectivity and favorable lipophilicity for imaging of the D_3-receptor in the brain, Stößel et al. have synthetized compound **26** as the radioactive [^{18}F]-labeled analogue of the D_3 ligand FAUC 329 (**25**) (Figure 10) [53]. In vitro AGR studies showed that **26** successfully visualized D_3-rich brain regions, including the islands of Calleja. However, in vivo PET imaging revealed that it does not significantly accumulate in the CNS structures of rat brains, probably due to a low BBB penetration. Instead, a significant uptake occurred in the brain ventricular system, due to a significant penetration of this compound in the blood-liquor barrier and, more noticeable, in the pituitary gland, outside the BBB [53]. The results of PET studies also suggest that the main mode of action of FAUC 329, in vivo, could be due to binding to the dopamine receptors in the pituitary gland.

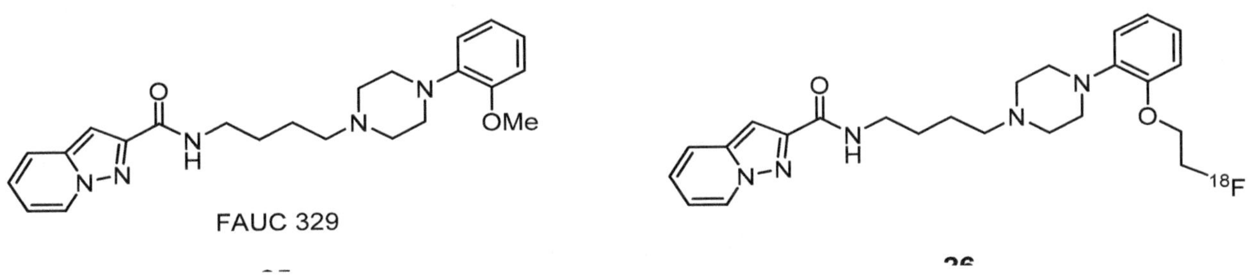

Figure 10. Radiotracer **26** derived from the dopamine D_3 receptor ligand FAUC 329 (**25**) [53].

2.1.5. Glucocorticoid Receptor Ligands

In 1998, Hoyte et al. reported a series of aryl-pyrazolo steroids similar to the potent glucocorticoid cortivazol **27** and evaluated the affinity of these compounds for glucocorticoid receptors (GRs). Among them, the fluoro analog **28,** which showed good binding and was a very potent glucocorticoid, was labeled with ^{18}F to be used as a glucocorticoid receptor-mediated imaging agent for PET (Figure 11) [54].

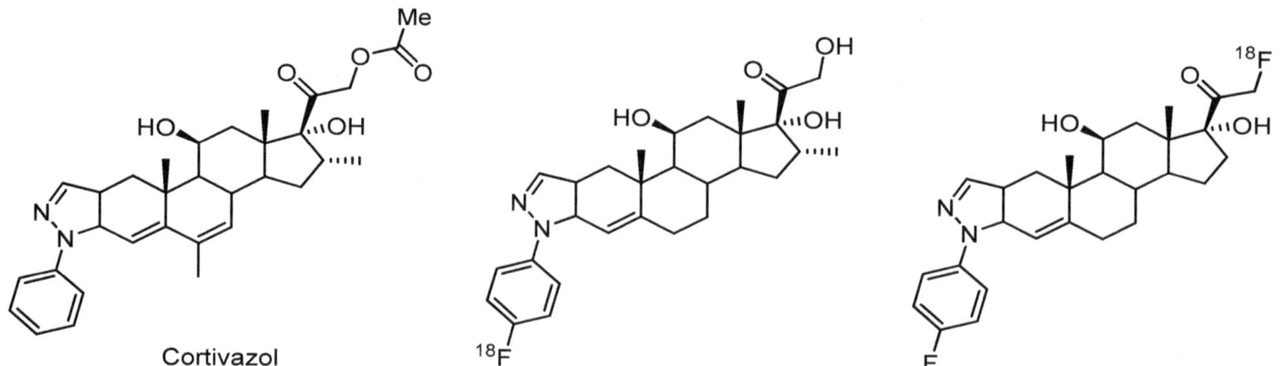

Cortivazol
27

28

29

Figure 11. Cortivazol (**27**) and related [^{18}F]arylpyrazolo steroids **28**–**29** as potential glucocorticoid receptor ligands for PET imaging [54,55].

Later, Würst et al. used the 2′-(4-fluorophenyl)-21-[^{18}F]fluoro-20-oxo-11β,17α-dihydroxypregn-4-eno[3,2-*c*]pyrazole (**29**) (Figure 11) as a ligand for studying brain GRs. Biodistribution and radiopharmacological studies with male Wistar rats revealed promising brain uptakes and low in vivo radiodefluorinations in comparison with other PET radioligands for brain GRs [55].

2.1.6. Insulin-Like Growth Factor-1 Receptor Ligands

Insulin-like growth factor-1 receptor (IGF-1R) is a potential therapeutic target, because it is overexpressed in many cancers, AD, traumatic brain injury, amyotrophic lateral sclerosis (ALS), Friedreich ataxia and aging. In 2013, Majo et al. synthetized and evaluated in vitro [^{18}F]BMS-754807 (**30**) (Figure 12), a potent and reversible small molecule inhibitor of the IGF-1R/IR kinases' family, currently in phase II clinical trials. ARG studies using surgically removed and pathologically identified grade IV glioblastoma, breast cancer and pancreatic tumors demonstrate that **30** binds to IGF-1R. The selectivity over other kinases, the presence of metabolically stable fluorine in the 2-substituted pyridine ring, which is amenable for radiolabeling by nucleophilic displacement with [^{18}F]fluoride and a calculated lipophilicity (clogP) of 3.5, make this ligand a potential PET-imaging agent for in vivo monitoring of IGF-1R [56].

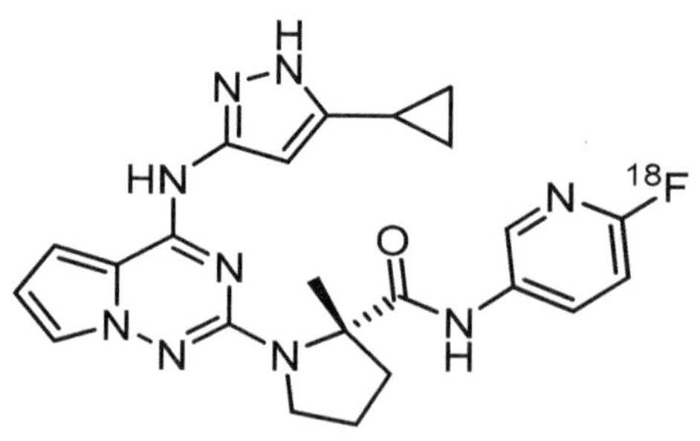

[^{18}F]BMS-754807
30

Figure 12. Potential PET radiotracer **30** for IGF-IR imaging [56].

2.1.7. Phosphodiester-10A Enzyme Inhibitors

Phosphodiester-10A (PDE10A) is an enzyme that hydrolyzes adenosine and/or guanosine 3′,5′-cyclic monophosphates (cAMP and cGMP, respectively). In the medium spiny neurons of the striatum, PDE10A messenger RNA and the corresponding protein are highly abundant. PDE10A inhibitors are a potential target for the diagnosis of schizophrenia, Huntington's disease, PD, obsessive-compulsive disorder and addiction.

In 2010, Tu et al. made a first attempt to visualize PDE10A using a ^{11}C-radiolabeled PDE10A inhibitor named papaverine (**31**) (Figure 13). In vitro ^{11}C-papaverine showed selective PDE10A binding, but in vivo failed because of rapid washout of the tracer [57]. To overcome this problem, Celen et al. synthetized a specific and selective radioligand for PDE10A, the ^{18}F-quinoline-labeled [^{18}F]JNJ-41510417 (**32**) (Figure 13). They used rats and PDE10A knockout mice to show that **32** binds specifically and reversibly to PDE10A in the striatum, presenting high accumulation therein. This brain region was the only to show an increase of tracer concentration after the injection (1.6 SUV after 2 min vs. 2.6 SUV after 60 min). Other brain regions, the hippocampus, cortex and cerebellum showed a washout of the radiotracer. These results are in accordance with the distribution of PDE10A. Despite the [^{18}F]JNJ-41510417 (**32**) good target specificity and signal-to-noise characteristics, slow brain kinetics due to its high potency is a limitation [58].

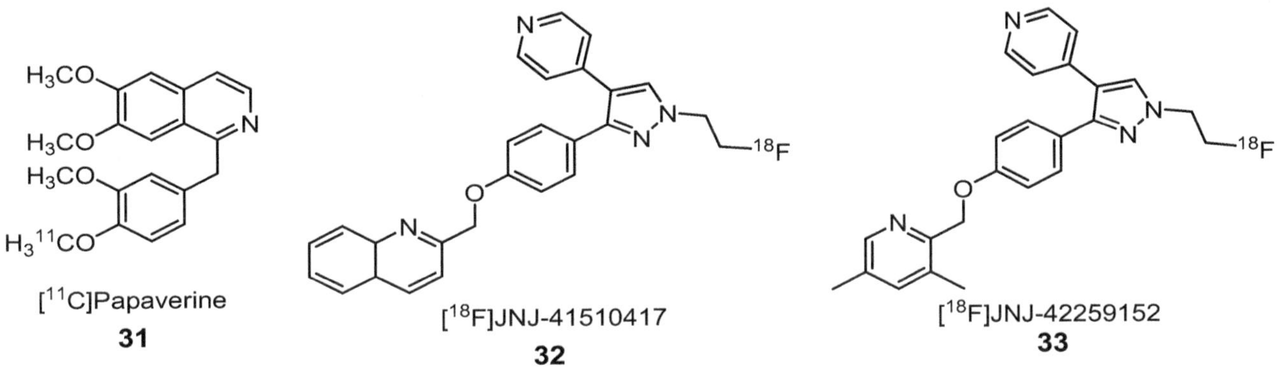

Figure 13. Radiotracers **31–33** for phosphodiester-10A (PDE10A) visualization in the brain by PET imaging [57–62].

Then, Laere et al., in collaboration with Janssen Pharmaceuticals, synthetized and studied the human biodistribution of another radioligand [^{18}F]JNJ-42259152 (**33**) [2-(4-(1-(2[^{18}F]fluoroethyl)-4-(4-pyridinyl)-1*H*-pyrazol-3-yl)phenoxy)methyl)-3,5-dimethylpyridine] (Figure 13), which belongs to a series of structurally related analogues of MP10 in which the 2-quinolinyl heterocycle was replaced with substituted 2-pyridinyl moieties, resulting in a slightly lower potency compared to [^{18}F]JNJ-41510417 (**32**) [59,60]. Six healthy male Caucasians (23–69 years; 3 younger than 40 years and 3 older than 60 years) have been volunteers in the study managed by Laere. Compound **33** showed a rapid uptake in the striatum, a few minutes after the injection, with a high clearance rate consistent with specific binding in this target region. The results of this pilot study are in accordance with the distribution of PDE10A in the human brain and show a promising kinetics and biodistribution of [^{18}F]JNJ-42259152 (**33**) [60].

Laere et al. have demonstrated that PDE10A activity in the brain can be reliably quantified using [^{18}F]JNJ-42259152 (**33**) [61]. A relatively fast kinetics for the striatal region was observed, followed by a subsequent moderately fast washout. The regional in vivo distribution of this radiotracer was in agreement with the known distribution of PDE10A, being found predominantly in the putamen followed by the caudate nucleus, ventral striatum and substantia nigra. Compared with the activity in the striatum, the cortical and cerebellar activity were more than 10-fold lower. Later, Ooms et al. have investigated the effect of alterations in cAMP levels on [^{18}F]JNJ-42259152 binding to PDE10A in the striatum homogenates. Increased affinity of this radiotracer for PDE10A was observed in the presence of cAMP, which seems to have an important role in the allosteric regulation of PDE10A [62].

Stepanov et al. described the synthesis of two [^{18}F]-labeled PET radioligands to target PDE10A, the [^{18}F]FM-T-773-d$_2$ (**34**) and [^{18}F]FE-T-773-d$_4$ (**35**) (Figure 14), and their in vivo evaluation in nonhuman primates [63]. High brain uptake was measured for both radioligands and a fast washout. Specific binding reached the maximum after 30 min for [^{18}F]FM-T-773-d$_2$ (**34**) and after 45 min for

[^{18}F]FE-T-773-d_4 (**35**). On account of brain uptake specific binding and kinetics, [^{18}F]FM-T-773-d_2 (**34**) was considered the more promising PET radioligand for further clinical evaluation.

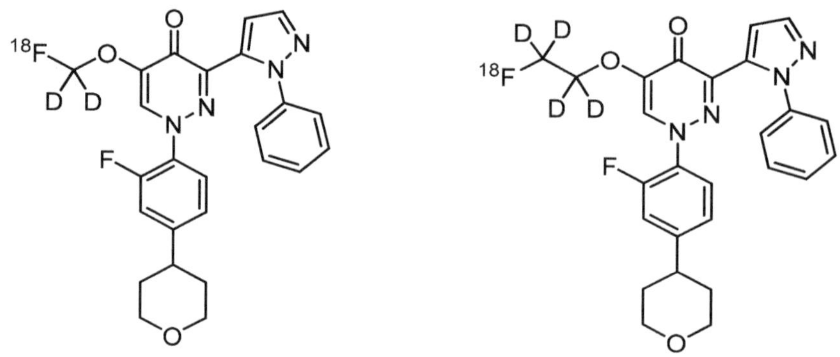

[^{18}F]FM-T-773-d_2
34

[^{18}F]FE-T-773-d_4
35

Figure 14. PET radiotracers **34** and **35** for in vivo phosphodiester-10A (PDE10A) evaluation in nonhuman primates' brains [63].

2.1.8. Translocator Protein Receptor Ligands

The translocator protein (TSPO) receptor is an 18 kDa protein organized around five large transmembrane α-helices and located on the mitochondrial outer membrane [2]. This protein has a key role in the regulation of several cellular processes: steroid biosynthesis, cholesterol metabolism, apoptosis and cellular metabolism [64]. TSPO is highly expressed in organs involved in steroid synthesis as adrenal glands, testis, ovaries and pituitary glands [65]. In the central nervous system (CNS) and liver, TSPO expression is modest. However, in the case of acute or neurodegenerative pathologies associated with microglia or astrocytes, levels of TSPO in the brain are upregulated. The upregulation of this protein is directly correlated with the degree of neuronal damage. For these reasons, TSPO is considered a very promising target for the early imaging of neuroinflammation [66] and a possible indirect marker of neuronal loss progression, multiple sclerosis and AD [66–68] and has high relevance in neuroscience. The expression of this protein is also elevated in several cancers: colon, breast, glioma, prostate, colorectal, liver and ovary cancer, relating TSPO with disease progression and survival [2,64,65,69]. These evidences increased the interest in TSPO and led to the development of several radiolabeled ligands for the evaluation of the expression of this protein and detection of some of the aforementioned diseases by PET imaging.

Since the discovery of the first nonbenzodiazepine ligand for TSPO, the isoquinoline carboxamide PK11195 (**36**) [70–72], several families of compounds were evaluated as TSPO ligands—among them, [^{11}C]DPA-713 (**37**), [^{18}F]DPA-714 (**38**), [^{18}F]DPA (**39**), [^{18}F]VUIIS1008 (**40**) and [^{18}F]DPA-716 (or [^{18}F]PBR146) (**41**), which are pyrazolo[1,5-*a*]pyrimidine acetamides (Figure 15) [72,73].

Chauveau et al. compared compound **38** with **36** and **37** using a rat model of acute neuroinflammation. (*R,S*)-α-amino-3-hydroxy-5-methyl-4-isoxazolopropionic acid (AMPA) was used to provoke neuroinflammation. Compounds **37** and **38** were specifically localized in the neuroinflammatory site with a similar signal-to-noise ratio in vitro. However, the fluorine-labeled tracer **38** achieved a higher bioavailability in the brain, higher uptake and higher binding potential than the other radiotracers. In the reference zone (contralateral area), a lower uptake of **37** and **38** were found when compared with **36**. These results showed that **37** and **38** have lower nonspecific bindings than **36** [74].

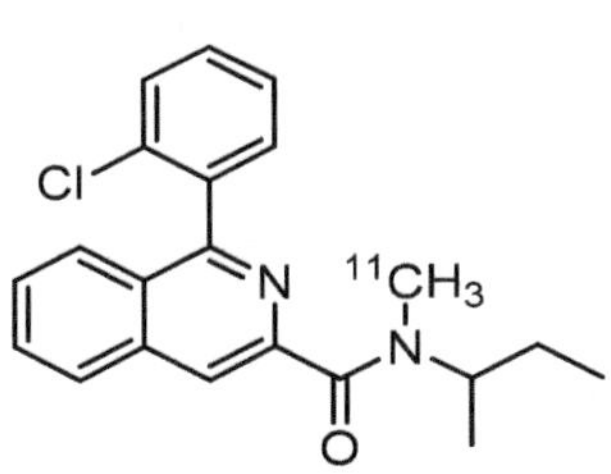

[^{11}C]PK11195
36

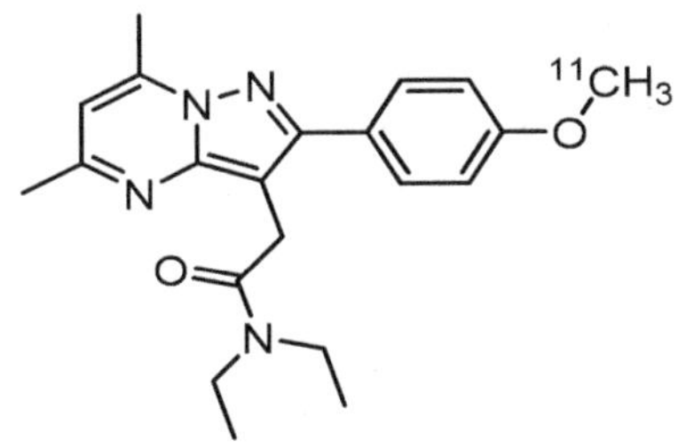

[^{11}C]DPA-713
37

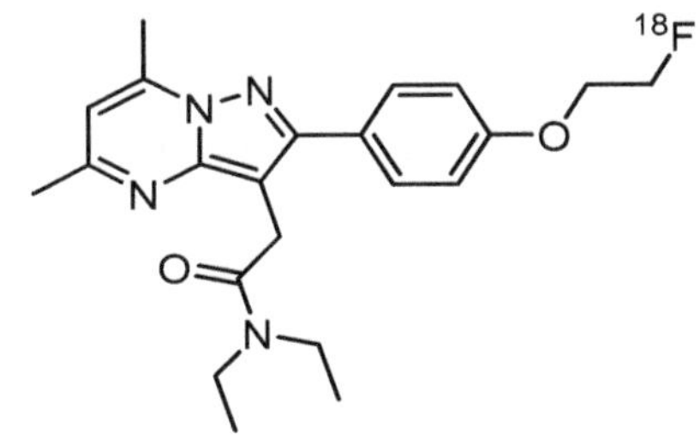

[^{18}F]DPA-714
38

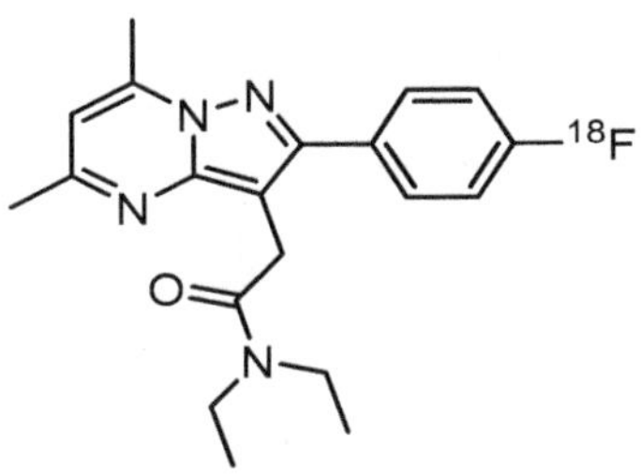

[^{18}F]F-DPA
39

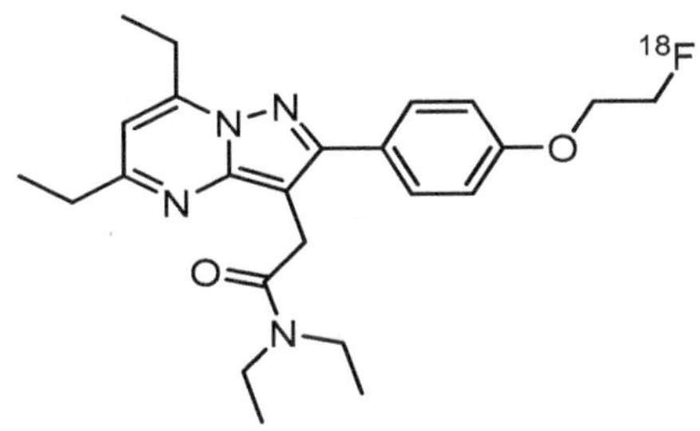

[^{18}F]VUIIS1008
40

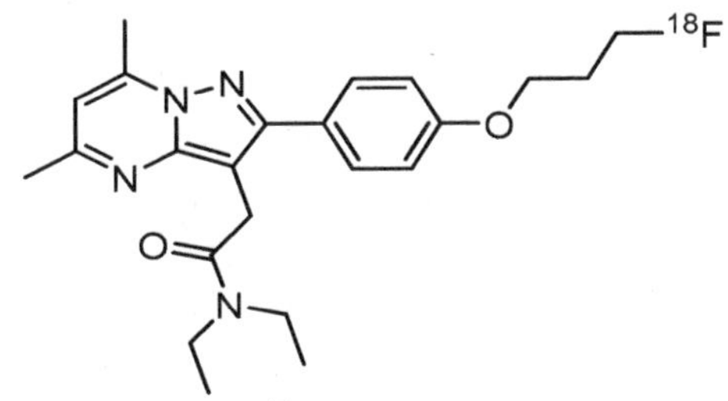

[^{18}F]DPA-716
(or [^{18}F]PBR146)
41

Figure 15. [^{11}C]PK11195 (**36**) and pyrazolopyrimidine-derived radiotracers **37**–**41** for translocator protein (TSPO) PET imaging [72–82].

Compound **38** was also used to monitor the TSPO levels after the injection of some antibiotic like minocycline. This drug inhibits the activation of microglial cells [75]. Furthermore, the radiotracer **38** was used on studies of rodent models of excitotoxicity, herpes encephalitis [76], astrocytic activation, excitotoxically lesioned nonhuman primate brains, abdominal aortic aneurysm [77], rheumatoid arthritis [78,79] and neuroinflammatory changes in the brain after morphine exposure [65,67]. It demonstrated a good uptake in the primate brain and an eight-fold higher uptake in the lesioned striatum of a quinolinic acid-lesioned rat model of activated microglia. Both **37** and **38** showed better imaging properties than **36** in the striatum of lesioned rats. A study using a rat model of herpes simplex encephalitis (HSE) suggested that **38**, as an agonist of TSPO, is potentially suitable for visualizing mild neuroinflammation [76].

Kuszpit et al. demonstrated that [^{18}F]DPA-714 (**38**) is a sensitive tool for the detection of neuroinflammation, induced by Zika virus (ZIKV) infection, using a mice model of ZIKV neurological disease. Moreover, the evaluation of therapeutics being developed for the treatment of the disease is also possible by [^{18}F]DPA-714 (**38**) imaging [80].

In 2017, Keller et al. compared the activity of **38** with its analogue [^{18}F]F-DPA (**39**) (Figure 15), which presents the radionuclide directly linked to the phenyl ring. This study showed that compound **39** is metabolically more stable than its analogue **38** in rats' brains, being regarded as a promising TSPO radiotracer, because it shows a higher ratio between specific and nonspecific binding [81]. Later, in 2018, the same author described the potential of [^{18}F]F-DPA **39** to visualize activated microglia at an early stage of AD pathology. The in vivo PET imaging and ex vivo brain AGR data indicated and increased uptake of this radiotracer **39** with age in the brains of transgenic animals (APP/PS1-21 mouse models of AD) in comparison with wild-type animals [68].

In 2012, Tang et al. used glioma-bearing rats to study the feasibility of using [^{18}F]DPA-714 (**38**) for the visualization of TSPO expressing in brain tumors. This PET tracer showed to be highly specific to TSPO in glioma cell line homogenates. In vivo studies showed a higher uptake of **38** in tumor tissues than in other brain regions, suggesting that this compound could be used as a novel predictive cancer imaging tool [82]. In 2013, the same author carried out the synthesis and structure-activity relationship study of pyrazolopyrimidine-derived radioligands, presenting different substituents, namely at the 5, 6 and 7 positions, in order to find the more robust PET ligand. The best result was achieved with compound [^{18}F]VUIIS1008 (**40**) (Figure 15), which showed a negligible binding in normal brains but a much higher binding in tumor tissues [64]. This result demonstrated that this radiotracer is a promising PET ligand for TSPO in tumors.

In 2014, Médran-Navarrete et al. evaluated a new ^{18}F-labeled analogue of [^{18}F]DPA-714 (**38**), the [^{18}F]DPA-C5yne (**42**) (Figure 16), as a TSPO radioligand. In vitro studies revealed that **42** was stable in plasma at 37 °C for at least 90 min. AGR studies, using slices of AMPA-lesioned rat brains, showed a high specificity of binding and selectivity for TSPO, highlighting the potential of **42** as a radiotracer for TSPO [83]. One year later, Damont et al. synthetized a series of novel pyrazolo[1,5-*a*]pyrimidines and evaluated, in vitro, their affinity, lipophilicity and metabolism. Based on the results obtained, two of the synthetized compounds were chosen for ^{18}F-radiolabeling affording ligands [^{18}F]DPA-C5yne (**42**) and (**43**) an analogue of [^{18}F]DPA-714 (**38**), where the oxygen atom was replaced by a methylene group (Figure 16). Neuroinflammation PET images, using anesthetized Wistar rats seven days after AMPA-induced brain lesions in the right striatum, showed that both radiotracers **42** and **43** have a high in vivo-specific binding for TSPO. Compound **43** presented an ipsilateral-to-contralateral ratio of 3.57 ± 0.48 comparable to **38** (3.71 ± 0.39), and **42** showed an ipsilateral-to-contralateral ratio of 4.62 ± 0.44. These results suggest that both **42** and **43** are appropriate for neuroinflammation imaging [72].

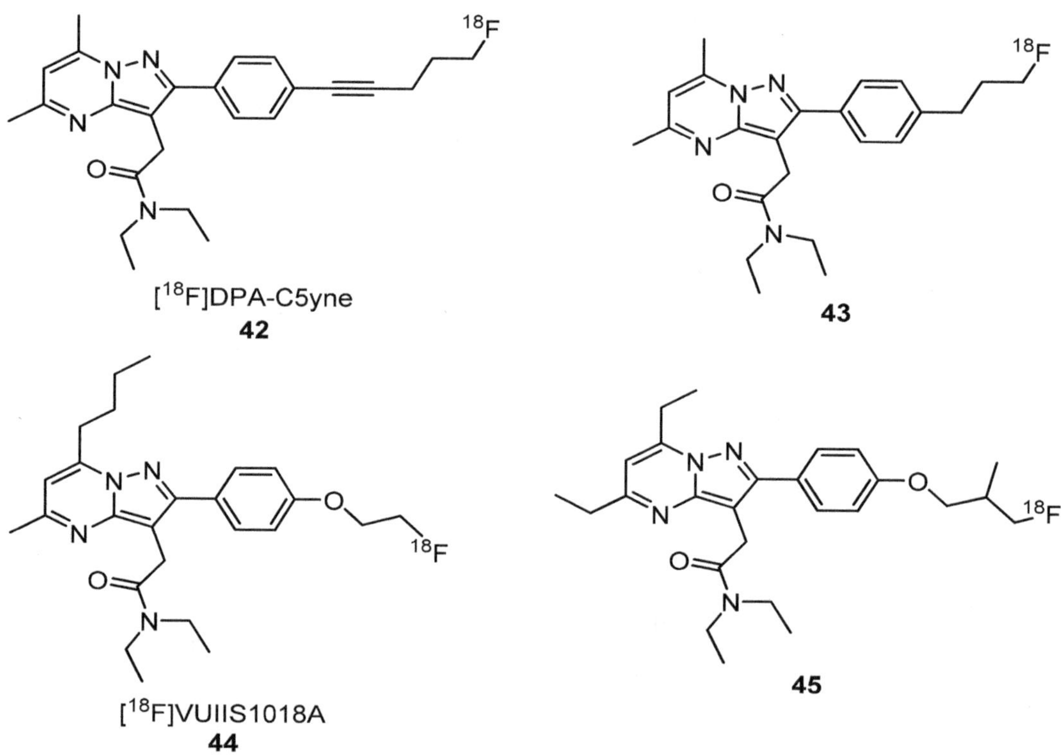

Figure 16. Pyrazolopyrimidine-derived radiotracers **42**–**45** for TSPO PET imaging [83–87].

Recently, Tang et al. synthetized a new TSPO PET tracer [^{18}F]VUIIS1018A (**44**), an analogue of [^{18}F]DPA-714 (**38**) where the 7-methyl group of the pyrazolopyrimidine ring was replaced by a *n*-butyl group (Figure 16), and evaluated its behavior in a preclinical model of neuroinflammation. These authors concluded that this structural modification increased the lipophilicity of **44** compared with **38** (3.7 vs. 2.4, respectively). After 60 min of injection of **44**, more than 85% of this probe was intact, indicating that it is very stable in the brain. It is noteworthy that, for **38**, just 50% of the probe was intact after 60 min of injection. In vivo blocking experiments and in vitro AGR assays confirmed a high binding specificity of **44** for TSPO, showing that it can be a promising TSPO PET tracer [84]. Tang et al.

developed a preclinical evaluation to image glioma. In this work, **44** exhibited a lower accumulation in healthy brains, what was regarded as an advantage to distinguish lower-grade gliomas. Compared with [^{18}F]DPA-714 (**38**) and [^{18}F]VUIIS1008 (**40**), **44** had an improved tumor-to-background ratio, a higher specific-to-nonspecific binding ratio and a higher tumor-binding potential. These results showed that **44** is a promising candidate to detect tumors with modest TSPO expression [85].

A series of novel 2-phenylpyrazolo[1,5-a]pyrimidin-3-ylacetamides were synthesized, and their in vitro binding affinities for TSPO and lipophilicity (log $P_{7.5}$) were evaluated using [^{18}F]DPA-714 (**38**) as the control. Based on the results of these assays, the tosylated precursor was selected for radiofluorination, affording **45** (Figure 16). Using LPS induced neuroinflammation rat models, a dynamic micro-PET study was performed and demonstrated a higher uptake of **45** in the ipsilateral region and a higher ratio of target-to-background than **38**. These results suggest that **45** can be a promising PET probe candidate for TSPO imaging [86].

In 2018, Verweij et al. measured the cellular response in patients after an acute coronary syndrome by PET imaging using [^{18}F]DPA-714 (**38**) as a probe. TSPO receptor is highly expressed in myeloid cells. Using a PET tracer with a high affinity for the TSPO receptor as **38** was possible to determine the hematopoietic activity. In the acute phase, the treatment with **38** revealed a higher uptake in the bone marrow and the spleen. Three months after, the bone marrow uptake decreased to levels comparable to the healthy control. On the other hand, the spleen uptake remained elevated [87].

3. Conclusions

Considering that ^{18}F is the most suitable radionuclide for routine PET imaging and that pyrazoles are a key motif in medicinal chemistry and drug design, we made a compilation of [^{18}F]pyrazole-derived imaging probes that have been developed and evaluated in the last 20 years. Regarding the examples presented herein, it is evident that pyrazoles are important scaffolds for the development of radiotracers for the diagnosis of several pathologies. In fact, pyrazoles interact with remarkable targets, namely with adenosine receptors, cannabinoid receptors, cyclooxygenase enzymes, dopamine receptors, glucocorticoid receptor, insulin-like growth factor-1 receptor, phosphodiester-10A enzyme and the translocator protein receptor. Among the probes presented herein, most are cannabinoid ligands and dopamine ligands, with a huge potential for brain imaging and TSPO ligands, namely pyrazolopyrimidine-derived radiotracers, that have shown important applications for the imaging of neuroinflammation and cancer.

The successful use of the described pyrazoles-imaging probes in clinics may help to increase the understanding of several diseases such as AD, PD, Huntington's disease, atherosclerosis, neuropsychiatric disorders, neuroinflammation, cardiovascular diseases and cancer, among others, and to identify ways to improve therapy. In this sense, the pyrazoles described herein can be regarded as potential theragnostic agents and as important templates for the development of novel radiotracers with improved properties for PET imaging.

Author Contributions: V.L.M.S. and P.M.O.G. idealized the manuscript. P.M.O.G. did the bibliographic research and prepared the original draft. V.L.M.S. and A.M.S.S. supervised the manuscript preparation, revised it and did the necessary corrections. All authors have read and agreed to the published version of the manuscript.

References

1. Li, Z.; Conti, P.S. Radiopharmaceutical chemistry for positron emission tomography. *Adv. Drug Deliv. Rev.* **2010**, *62*, 1031–1051. [CrossRef] [PubMed]
2. Damont, A.; Roeda, D.; Dollé, F. The potential of carbon-11 and fluorine-18 chemistry: Illustration through the development of positron emission tomography radioligands targeting the translocator protein 18 kDa. *J. Label. Compd. Radiopharm.* **2013**, *56*, 96–104. [CrossRef] [PubMed]
3. Coleman, R.E. Clinical PET in oncology. *Clin. Positron Imaging* **1998** *1*, 15–30. [CrossRef]

4. Anderson, C.J.; Bulte, J.W.M.; Chen, K.; Chen, X.; Khaw, B.-A.; Shokeen, M.; Wooley, K.L.; VanBrocklin, H.F. Design of targeted cardiovascular molecular imaging probes. *J. Nucl. Med.* **2010**, *51*, 3S–17S. [CrossRef]
5. Xiong, K.L.; Yang, Q.W.; Gong, S.G.; Zhang, W.G. The role of positron emission tomography imaging of β-amyloid in patients with Alzheimer's disease. *Nucl. Med. Commun.* **2010**, *31*, 4–11. [CrossRef]
6. Murphy, P.S.; McCarthy, T.J.; Dzik-Jurasz, A.S.K. The role of clinical imaging in oncological drug development. *Br. J. Radiol.* **2008**, *81*, 685–692. [CrossRef]
7. Cazzato, R.L.; Garnon, J.; Shaygi, B.; Koch, G.; Tsoumakidou, G.; Caudrelier, J.; Addeo, P.; Bachellier, P.; Namer, I.J.; Gangi, A. PET/CT-guided interventions: Indications, advantages, disadvantages and the state of the art. *Minim. Invasive Ther. Allied Technol.* **2018**, *27*, 27–32. [CrossRef]
8. Wood, K.A.; Hoskin, P.J.; Saunders, M.I. Positron emission tomography in oncology: A review. *Clin. Oncol.* **2007**, *19*, 237–255. [CrossRef]
9. Silva, V.L.M.; Silva, A.M.S.; Pinto, D.C.G.A.; Jagerovic, N.; Callado, L.F.; Cavaleiro, J.A.S.; Elguero, J. Synthesis and pharmacological evaluation of chlorinated *N*-alkyl-3- and -5-(2-hydroxyphenyl)pyrazoles as CB_1 cannabinoid ligands. *Monatsh. Chem.* **2007**, *138*, 797–811. [CrossRef]
10. Silva, V.L.M.; Silva, A.M.S.; Pinto, D.C.G.A.; Cavaleiro, J.A.S.; Elguero, J. Synthesis of (*E*)- and (*Z*)-3(5)-(2-hydroxyphenyl)-4-styrylpyrazoles. *Monatsh. Chem.* **2009**, *140*, 87–95. [CrossRef]
11. Silva, V.L.M.; Silva, A.M.S.; Pinto, D.C.G.A.; Rodríguez, P.; Gómez, M.; Jagerovic, N.; Callado, L.F.; Cavaleiro, J.A.S.; Elguero, J.; Fernández-Ruiz, J. Synthesis and pharmacological evaluation of new (*E*)- and (*Z*)-3-aryl-4-styryl-1*H*-pyrazoles as potential cannabinoid ligands. *Arkivoc* **2010**, 226–247. [CrossRef]
12. Marques, J.; Silva, V.L.M.; Silva, A.M.S.; Marques, M.P.M.; Braga, S.S. Ru(II) trithiacyclononane 3-(2-hydroxyphenyl)-5-(4-methoxystyryl)pyrazole, a complex with facile synthesis and high cytotoxicity against PC-3 and MDA-MB-231 cells. *Complex Metals* **2014**, *1*, 7–12. [CrossRef]
13. Soengas, R.G.; Silva, V.L.M.; Ide, D.; Kato, A.; Cardoso, S.M.; Almeida Paz, F.A.; Silva, A.M.S. Synthesis of 3-(2-nitrovinyl)-4*H*-chromones: Useful scaffolds for the construction of biologically relevant 3-(pyrazol-5-yl)chromones. *Tetrahedron* **2016**, *72*, 3198–3203. [CrossRef]
14. Carreira, A.R.F.; Pereira, D.M.; Andrade, P.B.; Valentão, P.; Silva, A.M.S.; Braga, S.S.; Silva, V.L.M. Novel styrylpyrazole-glucosides and their unexpected dioxolo-bridged doppelgangers: Synthesis and cytotoxicity. *New J. Chem.* **2019**, *43*, 8299–8310. [CrossRef]
15. Abrigach, F.; Touzani, R. Pyrazole derivatives with NCN junction and their biological activity: A review. *Med. Chem.* **2016**, *6*, 292–298. [CrossRef]
16. Suri, M.; Jousseaume, T.; Neumann, J.J.; Glorius, F. An efficient copper-catalyzed formation of highly substituted pyrazoles using molecular oxygen as the oxidant. *Green Chem.* **2012**, *14*, 2193–2196. [CrossRef]
17. Kumar, V.; Kaur, K.; Gupta, G.K.; Sharma, A.K. Pyrazole containing natural products: Synthetic preview and biological significance. *Eur. J. Med. Chem.* **2013**, *69*, 735–753. [CrossRef]
18. Silva, V.L.M.; Elguero, J.; Silva, A.M.S. Current progress on antioxidants incorporating the pyrazole core. *Eur. J. Med. Chem.* **2018**, *15*, 394–429. [CrossRef]
19. Abdel-Maksoud, M.S.; El-Gamal, M.I.; Gamal El-Din, M.M.; Oh, C.H. Design, synthesis, in vitro anticancer evaluation, kinase inhibitory effects, and pharmacokinetic profile of new 1,3,4-triarylpyrazole derivatives possessing terminal sulfonamide moiety. *J. Enz. Inhib. Med. Chem.* **2019**, *34*, 97–109. [CrossRef]
20. Chowdary, B.N.; Umashankara, M.; Dinesh, B.; Girish, K.; Baba, A.R. Development of 5-(aryl)-3-phenyl-1*H*-pyrazole derivatives as potent antimicrobial compounds. *Asian J. Chem.* **2019**, *31*, 45–50. [CrossRef]
21. Secci, D.; Bolasco, A.; Chimenti, P.; Carradori, S. The state of the art of pyrazole derivatives as monoamine oxidase inhibitors and antidepressant/anticonvulsant agents. *Curr. Med. Chem.* **2011**, *18*, 5114–5144. [CrossRef] [PubMed]
22. Liu, J.J.; Zhang, H.; Sun, J.; Wang, Z.C.; Yang, Y.S.; Li, D.D.; Zhang, F.; Gong, H.B.; Zhu, H.L. Synthesis, biological evaluation of novel 4,5-dihydro-2*H*-pyrazole 2-hydroxyphenyl derivatives as BRAF inhibitors. *Bioorg. Med. Chem.* **2012**, *20*, 6089–6096. [CrossRef] [PubMed]
23. Tanitame, A.; Oyamada, Y.; Ofuji, K.; Fujimoto, M.; Iwai, N.; Hiyama, Y.; Suzuki, K.; Ito, H.; Terauchi, H.; Kawasaki, M.; et al. Synthesis and antibacterial activity of a novel series of potent DNA gyrase inhibitors. Pyrazole derivatives. *J. Med. Chem.* **2004**, *47*, 3693–3696. [CrossRef] [PubMed]
24. Ansari, A.; Ali, A.; Asif, M.; Shamsuzzaman, S. Review: Biologically active pyrazole derivatives. *New J. Chem.* **2016**, *41*, 16–41. [CrossRef]

25. Liu, J.-J.; Zhao, M.-Y.; Zhang, X.; Zhao, X.; Zhu, H.-L. Pyrazole derivatives as antitumor, anti-inflammatory and antibacterial agents. *Mini Rev. Med. Chem.* **2013**, *13*, 1957–1966. [CrossRef]
26. Küçükgüzel, S.G.; Senkardes, S. Recent advances in bioactive pyrazoles. *Eur. J. Med. Chem.* **2015**, *97*, 786–815. [CrossRef]
27. Santos, C.M.M.; Silva, V.L.M.; Silva, A.M.S. Synthesis of chromone-related pyrazole compounds. *Molecules* **2017**, *22*, 1665. [CrossRef]
28. Faria, J.V.; Vegi, P.F.; Miguita, A.G.C.; dos Santos, M.S.; Boechat, N.; Bernardino, A.M.R. Recently reported biological activities of pyrazole compounds. *Bioorg. Med. Chem.* **2017**, *25*, 5891–5903. [CrossRef]
29. Perez-Fernandez, R.; Goya, P.; Elguero, J. A review of recent progress (2002–2012) on the biological activities of pyrazoles. *Arkivoc* **2014**, 233–293. [CrossRef]
30. Prabhu, V.V.; Kannan, N.; Guruvayoorappan, C. 1,2-Diazole prevents cisplatin-induced nephrotoxicity in experimental rats. *Pharmacol. Reports* **2013**, *65*, 980–990. [CrossRef]
31. Borea, P.A.; Gessi, S.; Merighi, S.; Vincenzi, F.; Varani, K. Pharmacology of adenosine receptors: The state of the art. *Physiol. Rev.* **2018**, *98*, 1591–1625. [CrossRef] [PubMed]
32. Khanapur, S.; Paul, S.; Shah, A.; Vatakuti, S.; Koole, M.J.B.; Zijlma, R.; Dierckx, R.A.J.O.; Luurtsema, G.; Garg, P.; van Waarde, A.; et al. Development of [^{18}F]-labelled pyrazolo[4,3-*e*]-1,2,4-triazolo[1,5-*c*]pyrimidine (SCH442416) analogs for the imaging of cerebral adenosine A_2A receptors with positron emission tomography. *J. Med. Chem.* **2014**, *57*, 6765–6780. [CrossRef] [PubMed]
33. Khanapur, S.; van Waarde, A.; Dierckx, R.A.J.O.; Elsinga, P.H.; Koole, M.J.B. Preclinical evaluation and quantification of ^{18}F-fluoroethyl and ^{18}F-fluoropropyl analogs of SCH442416 as radioligands for PET imaging of the adenosine A_2A receptor in rat brain. *J. Nucl. Med.* **2017**, *58*, 466–472. [CrossRef] [PubMed]
34. Li, J.; Daughters, R.S.; Bullis, C.; Bengiamin, R.; Stucky, M.W.; Brennan, J.; Simone, D.A. The cannabinoid receptor agonist WIN 55,212-2 mesylate blocks the development of hyperalgesia produced by capsaicin in rats. *Pain* **1999**, *81*, 25–33. [CrossRef]
35. Gonzalez-Rosales, F.; Walsh, D. Intractable nausea and vomiting due to gastrointestinal mucosal metastases relieved by tetrahydrocannabinol (Dronabinol). *J. Pain Symptom Manag.* **1997**, *14*, 311–314. [CrossRef]
36. Williams, C.M.; Kirkham, T.C. Anandamide induces overeating: Mediation by central cannabinoid (CB_1) receptors. *Psychopharmacology* **1999**, *143*, 315–317. [CrossRef]
37. Mathews, W.B.; Scheffel, U.; Finley, P.; Ravert, H.T.; Frank, R.A.; Rinaldi-Carmona, M.; Barth, F.; Dannals, R.F. Biodistribution of [^{18}F]SR144385 and [^{18}F]SR147963: Selective radioligands for positron emission tomographic studies of brain cannabinoid receptors. *Nucl. Med. Biol.* **2000**, *27*, 757–762. [CrossRef]
38. Horti, A.G.; Fan, H.; Kuwabara, H.; Hilton, J.; Ravert, H.T.; Holt, D.P.; Alexander, M.; Kumar, A.; Rahmim, A.; Scheffel, U.; et al. ^{11}C-JHU75528: A radiotracer for PET imaging of CB_1 cannabinoid receptors. *J. Nucl. Med.* **2006**, *47*, 1689–1696.
39. Rinaldi-Carmona, M.; Barth, F.; Héaulme, M.; Shire, D.; Calandra, B.; Congy, C.; Martinez, S.; Maruani, J.; Néliat, G.; Caput, D.; et al. SR141716A, a potent and selective antagonist of the brain cannabinoid receptor. *FEBS Lett.* **1994**, *350*, 240–244. [CrossRef]
40. Moreira, F.A.; Crippa, J.A.S. The psychiatric side-effects of rimonabant. *Braz. J. Psychiatry* **2009**, *31*, 145–153. [CrossRef]
41. Mathews, W.B.; Ravert, H.T.; Musachio, J.L.; Frank, R.A.; Rinaldi-Carmona, M.; Barth, F.; Dannals, R.F. Synthesis of [^{18}F]SR144385: A selective radioligand for positron emission tomography studies of brain cannabinoid receptors. *J. Label. Compd. Radiopharm.* **1999**, *42*, 589–596. [CrossRef]
42. Katoch-Rouse, R.; Horti, A.G. Synthesis of *N*-(piperidin-1-yl)-5-(4-methoxyphenyl)-1-(2-chlorophenyl)-4-[^{18}F]fluoro-1*H*-pyrazole-3-carboxamide by nucleophilic [^{18}F] fluorination: A PET radiotracer for studying CB_1 cannabinoid receptors. *J. Label. Compd. Radiopharm.* **2003**, *46*, 93–98. [CrossRef]
43. Nojiri, Y.; Ishiwata, K.; Qinggeletu; Tobiishi, S.; Sasada, T.; Yamamoto, F.; Mukai, T.; Maeda, M. Radiosynthesis and biodistribution in mice of a ^{18}F-labelled analog of O-1302 for use in cerebral CB_1 cannabinoid receptor imaging. *Biol. Pharm. Bull.* **2008**, *31*, 1274–1278. [CrossRef] [PubMed]
44. Li, Z.; Gifford, A.; Liu, Q.; Thotapally, R.; Ding, Y.-S.; Makriyannis, A.; Gatley, S.J. Candidate PET radioligands for cannabinoid CB_1 receptors: [^{18}F]AM5144 and related pyrazole compounds. *Nucl. Med. Biol.* **2005**, *32*, 361–366. [CrossRef]
45. Gatley, S.J.; Lan, R.; Volkow, N.D.; Pappas, N.; King, P.; Wong, C.T.; Gifford, A.N.; Pyatt, B.; Dewey, S.L.;

Makriyannis, A. Imaging the brain marijuana receptor: Development of a radioligand that binds to cannabinoid CB1 receptors in vivo. *J. Neurochem.* **1998**, *70*, 417–423. [CrossRef]
46. Chang, C.-P.; Huang, H.-L.; Huang, J.-K.; Hung, M.-S.; Wu, C.-H.; Song, J.-S.; Lee, C.-J.; Yub, C.-S.; Shia, K.-S. Fluorine-18 isotope labeling for positron emission tomography imaging. Direct evidence for DBPR211 as a peripherally restricted CB_1 inverse agonist. *Bioorg. Med. Chem.* **2019**, *27*, 216–223. [CrossRef]
47. Taketo, M.M. Cyclooxygenase-2 inhibitors in tumorigenesis (Part II). *J. Natl. Can. Inst.* **1998**, *90*, 1529–1536. [CrossRef]
48. Minghetti, L. Cyclooxygenase-2 (COX-2) in inflammatory and degenerative brain diseases. *J. Neuropath. Exp. Neur.* **2004**, *63*, 901–910. [CrossRef]
49. Uddin, M.J.; Crews, B.C.; Ghebreselasie, K.; Huda, I.; Kingsley, P.J.; Ansari, M.S.; Tantawy, M.N.; Reese, J.J.; Marnett, L.J. Fluorinated COX-2 inhibitors as agents in PET imaging of inflammation and cancer. *Cancer Prev. Res.* **2011**, *4*, 1536–1545. [CrossRef]
50. Lebedev, A.; Jiao, J.; Lee, J.; Yang, F.; Allison, N.; Herschman, H.; Sadeghi, S. Radiochemistry on electrodes: Synthesis of an ^{18}F-labelled and in vivo stable COX-2 inhibitor. *PLoS ONE* **2017**, *12*, e0176606. [CrossRef]
51. McCarthy, T.J.; Sheriff, A.U.; Graneto, M.J.; Talley, J.J.; Welch, M.J. Radiosynthesis, in vitro validation, and in vivo evaluation of ^{18}F-labeled COX-1 and COX-2 inhibitors. *J. Nucl. Med.* **2002**, *43*, 117–124. [PubMed]
52. Prante, O.; Tietze, R.; Hocke, C.; Löber, S.; Hübner, H.; Kuwert, T.; Gmeiner, P. Synthesis, radiofluorination, and in vitro evaluation of pyrazolo[1,5-*a*]pyridine-based dopamine D_4-receptor ligands: Discovery of an inverse agonist radioligand for PET. *J. Med. Chem.* **2008**, *51*, 1800–1810. [CrossRef] [PubMed]
53. Stößel, A.; Box, R.; Purkayastha, N.; Hübner, H.; Hocke, C.; Prante, O.; Gmeiner, P. Development of molecular tools based on the dopamine D_3 receptor ligand FAUC 329 showing inhibiting effects on drug and food maintained behavior. *Bioorg. Med. Chem.* **2017**, *25*, 3491–3499. [CrossRef]
54. Hoyte, R.M.; Labaree, D.C.; Fede, J.-M.; Harris, C.; Hochberg, R.B. Iodinated and fluorinated steroid 2′-aryl-[3,2-*c*] pyrazoles as potential glucocorticoid receptor imaging agents. *Steroids* **1998**, *63*, 595–602. [CrossRef]
55. Würst, F.; Kniess, T.; Kretzschmar, M.; Bergmann, R. Synthesis and radiopharmacological evaluation of 2′-(4-fluorophenyl)-21-[^{18}F]fluoro-20-oxo-11β,17α-dihydroxypregn-4-eno[3,2-c]pyrazole as potential glucocorticoid receptor ligand for positron emission tomography (PET). *Bioorg. Med. Chem. Lett.* **2005**, *15*, 1303–1306. [CrossRef] [PubMed]
56. Majo, V.J.; Arango, V.; Simpson, N.R.; Prabhakaran, J.; Kassir, S.A.; Underwood, M.D.; Bakalian, M.; Canoll, P.; Mann, J.J.; Dileep Kumar, J.S. Synthesis and in vitro evaluation of [^{18}F]BMS-754807: A potential PET ligand for IGF-1R. *Bioorg. Med. Chem. Lett.* **2013**, *23*, 4191–4194. [CrossRef]
57. Tu, Z.; Xu, J.; Jones, L.A.; Li, S.; Mach, R.H. Carbon-11 labelled papaverine as a PET tracer for imaging PDE10A: Radiosynthesis, in vitro and in vivo evaluation. *Nucl. Med. Biol.* **2010**, *37*, 509–516. [CrossRef]
58. Celen, S.; Koole, M.; De Angelis, M.; Sannen, I.; Chitneni, S.K.; Alcazar, J.; Dedeurwaerdere, S.; Moechars, D.; Schmidt, M.; Verbruggen, A.; et al. Preclinical evaluation of ^{18}F-JNJ41510417 as a radioligand for PET imaging of phosphodiesterase-10A in the brain. *J. Nucl. Med.* **2010**, *51*, 1584–1591. [CrossRef]
59. Andres, J.-I.; De Angelis, M.; Alcazar, J.; Iturrino, L.; Langlois, X.; Dedeurwaerdere, S.; Lenaerts, I.; Vanhoof, G.; Celen, S.; Bormans, G. Synthesis, in vivo occupancy, and radiolabeling of potent phosphodiesterase subtype-10 inhibitors as candidates for positron emission tomography imaging. *J. Med. Chem.* **2011**, *54*, 5820–5835. [CrossRef]
60. Laere, K.V.; Ahmad, R.U.; Hudyana, H.; Celen, S.; Dubois, K.; Schmidt, M.E.; Bormans, G.; Koole, M. Human biodistribution and dosimetry of ^{18}F-JNJ42259152, a radioligand for phosphodiesterase 10A imaging. *Eur. J. Nucl. Med. Mol. Imaging* **2013**, *40*, 254–261. [CrossRef]
61. Laere, K.V.; Ahmad, R.U.; Hudyana, H.; Dubois, K.; Schmidt, M.E.; Celen, S.; Bormans, G.; Koole, M. Quantification of ^{18}F-JNJ-42259152, a novel phosphodiesterase 10A PET tracer: Kinetic modelling and test-retest study in human brain. *J. Nucl. Med.* **2013**, *54*, 1285–1293. [CrossRef] [PubMed]
62. Ooms, M.; Altili, B.; Celen, S.; Koole, M.; Verbruggen, A.; Laere, K.V.; Bormans, G. [^{18}F]JNJ-42259152 binding to phosphodiesterase 10A, a key regulator of medium spiny neuron excitability, is altered in the presence of cyclic AMP. *J. Neurochem.* **2016**, *139*, 897–906. [CrossRef] [PubMed]
63. Stepanov, V.; Takano, A.; Nakao, R.; Amini, N.; Miura, S.; Kimura, H.; Taniguchi, T.; Halldin, C. Development of two fluorine-18 labeled PET radioligands targeting PDE10A and in vivo PET evaluation in nonhuman primates. *Nucl. Med Biol.* **2018**, *57*, 12–19. [CrossRef] [PubMed]

64. Tang, D.; McKinley, E.T.; Hight, M.R.; Uddin, M.I.; Harp, J.M.; Fu, A.; Nickels, M.L.; Buck, J.R.; Manning, H.C. Synthesis and structure-activity relationships of 5,6,7-substituted pyrazolopyrimidines: Discovery of a novel TSPO PET ligand for cancer imaging. *J. Med. Chem.* **2013**, *56*, 3429–3433. [CrossRef]
65. Zheng, J.; Winkeler, A.; Peyronneau, M.A.; Dollé, F.; Boisgard, R. Evaluation of PET imaging performance of the TSPO radioligand [^{18}F]DPA-714 in mouse and rat models of cancer and inflammation. *Mol. Imaging Biol.* **2016**, *18*, 127–134. [CrossRef]
66. Hagens, M.H.J.; Golla, S.V.; Wijburg, M.T.; Yaqub, M.; Heijtel, D.; Steenwijk, M.D.; Schober, P.; Brevé, J.J.P.; Schuit, R.C.; Reekie, T.A.; et al. In vivo assessment of neuroinflammation in progressive multiple sclerosis: A proof of concept study with [^{18}F]DPA714 PET. *J. Neuroinflammation* **2018**, *15*, 314–324. [CrossRef]
67. Lavisse, S.; Inoue, K.; Jan, C.; Peyronneau, M.A.; Petit, F.; Goutal, S.; Dauguet, J.; Guillermier, M.; Dollé, F.; Rbah-Vidal, L.; et al. [^{18}F]DPA-714 PET imaging of translocator protein TSPO (18 kDa) in the normal and excitotoxically-lesioned nonhuman primate brain. *Eur. J. Nucl. Med. Mol. Imaging* **2015**, *42*, 478–494. [CrossRef]
68. Keller, T.; López-Picón, F.R.; Krzyczmonik, A.; Forsback, S.; Kirjavainen, A.K.; Takkinen, J.S.; Alzghool, O.; Rajander, J.; Teperi, S.; Cacheux, F.; et al. [^{18}F]F-DPA for the detection of activated microglia in a mouse model of Alzheimer's disease. *Nucl. Med. Biol.* **2018**, *67*, 1–9. [CrossRef]
69. Gungor, H.; Saleem, A.; Babar, S.; Dina, R.; El-Bahrawy, M.A.; Curry, E.; Rama, N.; Chen, M.; Pickford, E.; Agarwal, R.; et al. Dose-finding quantitative ^{18}F-FDG PET imaging study with the oral Pan-AKT inhibitor GSK2141795 in patients with gynecologic malignancies. *J. Nucl. Med.* **2015**, *56*, 1828–1835. [CrossRef]
70. Inoue, O.; Yamasaki, T.; Hashimoto, K.; Kojima, M. Evaluation of ^{3}H-PK11195 as a radioligand for the in vivo study of peripheral benzodiazepine receptor. *Kaku Igaku.* **1985**, *22*, 1385–1389.
71. Camsonne, R.; Moulin, M.A.; Crouzel, C.; Syrota, A.; Maziere, M.; Comar, D. Carbon-11 labelling of PK11195 and visualization of benzodiazepine peripheral receptors using positron emission tomography. *J. Pharmacol.* **1986**, *17*, 383.
72. Damont, A.; Médran-Navarrete, V.; Cacheux, F.; Kuhnast, B.; Pottier, G.; Bernards, N.; Marquet, F.; Puech, F.; Boisgard, R.; Dollé, F. Novel pyrazolo[1,5-*a*]pyrimidines as translocator protein 18 kDa (TSPO) ligands: Synthesis, in vitro biological evaluation, [^{18}F]-labeling, and in vivo neuroinflammation PET images. *J. Med. Chem.* **2015**, *58*, 7449–7464. [CrossRef] [PubMed]
73. Fookes, C.J.R.; Pham, T.Q.; Mattner, F.; Greguric, I.; Loc'h, C.; Liu, X.; Berghofer, P.; Shepherd, R.; Gregoire, M.-C.; Katsifis, A. Synthesis and biological evaluation of substituted [^{18}F]imidazo[1,2-*a*]pyridines and [^{18}F]pyrazolo[1,5-*a*]pyrimidines for the study of the peripheral benzodiazepine receptor using positron emission tomography. *J. Med. Chem.* **2008**, *51*, 3700–3712. [CrossRef] [PubMed]
74. Chauveau, F.; Camp, N.V.; Dollé, F.; Kuhnast, B.; Hinnen, F.; Damont, A.; Boutin, H.; James, M.; Kassiou, M.; Tavitian, B. Comparative evaluation of the translocator protein radioligands ^{11}C-DPA-713, ^{18}F-DPA-714, and ^{11}C-PK11195 in a rat model of acute neuroinflammation. *J. Nucl. Med.* **2009**, *50*, 468–476. [CrossRef] [PubMed]
75. Martín, A.; Boisgard, R.; Kassiou, M.; Dollé, F.; Tavitian, B. Reduced PBR/TSPO expression after minocycline treatment in a rat model of focal cerebral ischemia: A PET study using [^{18}F]DPA-714. *Mol. Imaging Biol.* **2011**, *13*, 10–15. [CrossRef]
76. Doorduin, J.; Klein, H.C.; Dierckx, R.A.; James, M.; Kassiou, M.; de Vries, E.F.J. [^{11}C]-DPA-713 and [^{18}F]-DPA-714 as new PET tracers for TSPO: A comparison with [^{11}C]-(R)-PK11195 in a rat model of herpes encephalitis. *Mol. Imaging Biol.* **2009**, *11*, 386–398. [CrossRef]
77. Sarda-Mantel, L.; Alsac, J.M.; Boisgard, R.; Hervatin, F.; Montravers, F.; Tavitian, B.; Michel, J.B.; Le Guludec, D. Comparison of ^{18}F-fluoro-deoxy-glucose, ^{18}F-fluoro-methyl-choline, and ^{18}F-DPA714 for positron-emission tomography imaging of leukocyte accumulation in the aortic wall of experimental abdominal aneurysms. *J. Vasc. Surg.* **2012**, *56*, 765–773. [CrossRef]
78. Pottier, G.; Bernards, N.; Dollé, F.; Boisgard, R. [^{18}F]DPA-714 as a biomarker for positron emission tomography imaging of rheumatoid arthritis in an animal model. *Arthritis Res. Ther.* **2014**, *16*, R69. [CrossRef]
79. Gent, Y.Y.J.; Weijers, K.; Molthoff, C.F.M.; Windhorst, A.D.; Huisman, M.C.; Kassiou, M.; Jansen, G.; Lammertsma, A.A.; van der Laken, C.J. Promising potential of new generation translocator protein tracers providing enhanced contrast of arthritis. *Arthritis Res. Ther.* **2014**, *16*, R70. [CrossRef]
80. Kuszpit, K.; Hollidge, B.S.; Zeng, X.; Stafford, R.G.; Daye, S.; Zhang, X.; Basuli, F.; Golden, J.W.; Swenson, R.E.;

Smith, D.R.; et al. [^{18}F]DPA-714 PET imaging reveals global neuroinflammation in Zika Virus-infected mice. *Mol. Imaging Biol.* **2018**, *20*, 275–283. [CrossRef]
81. Keller, T.; Krzyczmonik, A.; Forsback, S.; Picón, F.R.L.; Kirjavainen, A.K.; Takkinen, J.; Rajander, J.; Cacheux, F.; Damont, A.; Dollé, F.; et al. Radiosynthesis and preclinical evaluation of [^{18}F]F-DPA, a novel pyrazolo[1,5-*a*]pyrimidine acetamide TSPO radioligand, in healthy Sprague Dawley rats. *Mol. Imaging Biol.* **2017**, *19*, 736–745. [CrossRef] [PubMed]
82. Tang, D.; Hight, M.R.; McKinley, E.T.; Fu, A.; Buck, J.R.; Smith, R.A.; Tantawy, M.N.; Peterson, T.E.; Colvin, D.C.; Ansari, M.S.; et al. Quantitative preclinical imaging of TSPO expression in glioma using *N,N*-diethyl-2-(2-(4-(2-^{18}F-fluoroethoxy)phenyl)-5,7-dimethylpyrazolo[1,5-*a*]pyrimidin-3-yl)acetamide. *J. Nucl. Med.* **2012**, *53*, 287–294. [CrossRef] [PubMed]
83. Médran-Navarrete, V.; Bernards, N.; Kuhnast, B.; Damont, A.; Pottier, G.; Peyronneau, M.A.; Kassiou, M.; Marguet, F.; Puech, F.; Boisgard, R.; et al. [^{18}F]DPA-C5yne, a novel fluorine-18-labelled analogue of DPA-714: Radiosynthesis and preliminary evaluation as a radiotracer for imaging neuroinflammation with PET. *J. Label Compd. Radiopharm.* **2014**, *57*, 410–418. [CrossRef] [PubMed]
84. Tang, D.; Fujinaga, M.; Hatori, A.; Zhang, Y.; Yamasaki, T.; Xie, L.; Mori, W.; Kumata, K.; Liu, J.; Manning, H.C.; et al. Evaluation of the novel TSPO radiotracer 2-(7-butyl-2-(4-(2-([^{18}F]fluoroethoxy)phenyl)-5-methylpyrazolo[1,5-*a*]pyrimidin-3-yl)-*N,N*-diethylacetamide in a preclinical model of neuroinflammation. *Eur. J. Med. Chem.* **2018**, *150*, 1–8. [CrossRef] [PubMed]
85. Tang, D.; Li, J.; Nickels, M.L.; Huang, G.; Cohen, A.S.; Manning, H.C. Preclinical evaluation of a novel TSPO PET ligand 2-(7-butyl-2-(4-(2-[^{18}F]fluoroethoxy)phenyl)-5-methylpyrazolo[1,5-*a*]pyrimidin-3-yl)-*N,N*-diethylacetamide (^{18}F-VUIIS1018A) to image glioma. *Mol. Imaging Biol.* **2019**, *21*, 113–121. [CrossRef] [PubMed]
86. Kwon, Y.D.; Kang, S.; Park, H.; Cheong, I.K.; Chang, K.A.; Lee, S.Y.; Jung, J.H.; Lee, B.C.; Lim, S.T.; Kim, H.K. Novel potential pyrazolopyrimidine based translocator protein ligands for the evaluation of neuroinflammation with PET. *Eur. J. Med. Chem.* **2018**, *159*, 292–306. [CrossRef]
87. Verweij, S.L.; Stiekema, L.C.A.; Delewi, R.; Zheng, K.H.; Moens, S.J.B.; Kroon, J.; Stroes, C.I.; Versloot, M.; Piek, J.J.; Verberne, H.J.; et al. Prolonged hematopoietic and myeloid cellular response in patients after an acute coronary syndrome measured with ^{18}F-DPA-714 PET/CT. *Eur. J. Nucl. Med. Mol. Imaging* **2018**, *45*, 1956–1963. [CrossRef]

Permissions

All chapters in this book were first published by MDPI; hereby published with permission under the Creative Commons Attribution License or equivalent. Every chapter published in this book has been scrutinized by our experts. Their significance has been extensively debated. The topics covered herein carry significant findings which will fuel the growth of the discipline. They may even be implemented as practical applications or may be referred to as a beginning point for another development.

The contributors of this book come from diverse backgrounds, making this book a truly international effort. This book will bring forth new frontiers with its revolutionizing research information and detailed analysis of the nascent developments around the world.

We would like to thank all the contributing authors for lending their expertise to make the book truly unique. They have played a crucial role in the development of this book. Without their invaluable contributions this book wouldn't have been possible. They have made vital efforts to compile up to date information on the varied aspects of this subject to make this book a valuable addition to the collection of many professionals and students.

This book was conceptualized with the vision of imparting up-to-date information and advanced data in this field. To ensure the same, a matchless editorial board was set up. Every individual on the board went through rigorous rounds of assessment to prove their worth. After which they invested a large part of their time researching and compiling the most relevant data for our readers.

The editorial board has been involved in producing this book since its inception. They have spent rigorous hours researching and exploring the diverse topics which have resulted in the successful publishing of this book. They have passed on their knowledge of decades through this book. To expedite this challenging task, the publisher supported the team at every step. A small team of assistant editors was also appointed to further simplify the editing procedure and attain best results for the readers.

Apart from the editorial board, the designing team has also invested a significant amount of their time in understanding the subject and creating the most relevant covers. They scrutinized every image to scout for the most suitable representation of the subject and create an appropriate cover for the book.

The publishing team has been an ardent support to the editorial, designing and production team. Their endless efforts to recruit the best for this project, has resulted in the accomplishment of this book. They are a veteran in the field of academics and their pool of knowledge is as vast as their experience in printing. Their expertise and guidance has proved useful at every step. Their uncompromising quality standards have made this book an exceptional effort. Their encouragement from time to time has been an inspiration for everyone.

The publisher and the editorial board hope that this book will prove to be a valuable piece of knowledge for researchers, students, practitioners and scholars across the globe.

List of Contributors

Chih-Yuan Wang
National Taiwan University College of Medicine, Taipei 10051, Taiwan
Department of Internal Medicine, National Taiwan University Hospital, Taipei 10002, Taiwan

Shyang-Rong Shih
National Taiwan University College of Medicine, Taipei 10051, Taiwan
Department of Internal Medicine, National Taiwan University Hospital, Taipei 10002, Taiwan
Center of Anti-Aging and Health Consultation, National Taiwan University Hospital, Taipei 10002, Taiwan

Yung-Lien Hsiao
Department of Internal Medicine, National Taiwan University Hospital, Taipei 10002, Taiwan

I-Shiow Jan
Department of Laboratory Medicine, National Taiwan University Hospital, Taipei 10002, Taiwan

Kuen-Yuan Chen
Department of Surgery, National Taiwan University Hospital, Taipei 10002, Taiwan

Tien-Chun Chang
National Taiwan University College of Medicine, Taipei 10051, Taiwan
Center of Anti-Aging and Health Consultation, National Taiwan University Hospital, Taipei 10002, Taiwan
Far Eastern Polyclinic, Taipei 10043, Taiwan

Argon Chen
Institute of Industrial Engineering, National Taiwan University, Taipei 10617, Taiwan

Sungbin Park, Heejoo Kim, Hwee Won Ji, Hyeon Woo Kim, Sung Hwan Yun and Sun Jung Kim
Department of Life Science, Dongguk University-Seoul, Goyang 10326, Korea

Parvesh Singh
School of Chemistry and Physics, University of Kwa-Zulu Natal (UKZN), Westville Campus, Durban 4000, South Africa

Richard J. Lobb
Tumour Microenvironment Laboratory, QIMR Berghofer Medical Research Institute, Herston, QLD 4006, Australia

Gregory M. Jacobson and Ray T. Cursons
Department of Biological Sciences, University ofWaikato, Hamilton 3216, New Zealand

Michael B. Jameson
Oncology Department, Waikato Hospital, Hamilton 3204, New Zealand
Waikato Clinical Campus, Faculty of Medical and Health Sciences, University of Auckland, Hamilton 3204, New Zealand

John T. Lafin
Department of Urology, University of Texas Southwestern Medical Center, Dallas, TX 75235, USA

Ehab H. Sarsour, Amanda L. Kalen, Brett A. Wagner, Garry R. Buettner and Prabhat C. Goswami
The University of Iowa Free Radical and Radiation Biology Program, Department of Radiation Oncology, University of Iowa, Iowa City, IA 52242, USA

Verónica Alcolea, Daniel Plano, Juan Antonio Palop and Carmen Sanmartín
Department of Pharmaceutical Technology and Chemistry, School of Pharmacy and Nutrition, University of Navarra, Irunlarrea 1, E-31008 Pamplona, Spain
Instituto de Investigación Sanitaria de Navarra (IdiSNA), Irunlarrea 3, E-31008 Pamplona, Spain

Deepkamal N. Karelia, Manoj K. Pandey, Shantu Amin and Arun K. Sharma
Department of Pharmacology, Penn State Cancer Institute, CH72, Penn State College of Medicine, 500 University Drive, Hershey, PA 17033, USA
Department of Biomedical Sciences, Cooper Medical School of Rowan University, Camden, NJ 08103, USA

Eun Ha Choi
Plasma Bioscience Research Center, Kwangwoon University, Seoul 01897, Korea

Wan-Yu Chuang
AmCad BioMed Corporation, Taipei 10547, Taiwan

Eric Benoist
UPS, CNRS, SPCMIB (Laboratoire de Synthèse et Physico-Chimie deMolécules d'Intérêt Biologique)—UMR 5068, Université de Toulouse, F-31062 Toulouse, France

Romain Eychenne
UPS, CNRS, SPCMIB (Laboratoire de Synthèse et Physico-Chimie deMolécules d'Intérêt Biologique)—UMR 5068, Université de Toulouse, F-31062 Toulouse, France
Groupement d'Intérêt Public ARRONAX, 1 Rue Aronnax, F-44817 Saint Herblain, France
CNRS, CRCINA (Centre de Recherche en Cancérologie et Immunologie Nantes—Angers)—UMR 1232, ERL 6001, Inserm, Université de Nantes, F-44000 Nantes, France

Mickael Bourgeois
Groupement d'Intérêt Public ARRONAX, 1 Rue Aronnax, F-44817 Saint Herblain, France
CNRS, CRCINA (Centre de Recherche en Cancérologie et Immunologie Nantes—Angers)—UMR 1232, ERL 6001, Inserm, Université de Nantes, F-44000 Nantes, France

Christelle Bouvry
Comprehensive Cancer Center Eugène Marquis, Rennes, F-35000, France
CNRS, ISCR (Institut des Sciences Chimiques de Rennes)—UMR 6226, Univ Rennes, F-35000 Rennes, France

Pascal Loyer
INRAE, Institut NUMECAN (Nutrition, Métabolismes et Cancer)—UMR_A 1341, UMR_S 1241, Inserm, Univ Rennes, F-35000 Rennes, France

Nicolas Lepareur
Comprehensive Cancer Center Eugène Marquis, Rennes, F-35000, France
INRAE, Institut NUMECAN (Nutrition, Métabolismes et Cancer)—UMR_A 1341, UMR_S 1241, Inserm, Univ Rennes, F-35000 Rennes, France

Bing-Ze Lin and Min-Ying Lin
Department of Biomedical Imaging and Radiological Sciences, National Yang-Ming University, No. 155, Sec. 2, Linong St. Beitou District, Taipei 11221, Taiwan

Shen-Ying Wan
Department of Biomedical Imaging and Radiological Sciences, National Yang-Ming University, No. 155, Sec. 2, Linong St. Beitou District, Taipei 11221, Taiwan
Department of Nuclear Medicine, Far Eastern Memorial Hospital, New Taipei City 22000, Taiwan

Chih-Hsien Chang
Department of Biomedical Imaging and Radiological Sciences, National Yang-Ming University, No. 155, Sec. 2, Linong St. Beitou District, Taipei 11221, Taiwan
Isotope Application Division, Institute of Nuclear Energy Research, Taoyuan 32546, Taiwan

Ting-Wen Chen
Institute of Bioinformatics and Systems Biology, National Chiao Tung University, Hsinchu 30068, Taiwan
Department of Biological Science and Technology, National Chiao Tung University, Hsinchu 30068, Taiwan
Center For Intelligent Drug Systems and Smart Bio-devices (IDS2B), National Chiao Tung University, Hsinchu 30068, Taiwan

Yi-Jang Lee
Department of Biomedical Imaging and Radiological Sciences, National Yang-Ming University, No. 155, Sec. 2, Linong St. Beitou District, Taipei 11221, Taiwan
Cancer Progression Research Center, National Yang-Ming University, Taipei 11221, Taiwan

Muh-Hwa Yang
Cancer Progression Research Center, National Yang-Ming University, Taipei 11221, Taiwan
Institute of Clinical Medicine, National Yang-Ming University, Taipei 11221, Taiwan
Division of Medical Oncology, Department of Oncology, Taipei Veteran General Hospital, Taipei 11217, Taiwan

Eline Biscop, Wilma Van Boxem and Annemie Bogaerts
PLASMANT Research Group, Department of Chemistry, University of Antwerp, 2610 Antwerp, Belgium

Abraham Lin
PLASMANT Research Group, Department of Chemistry, University of Antwerp, 2610 Antwerp, Belgium
Center for Oncological Research, University of Antwerp, 2610 Antwerp, Belgium

Jinthe Van Loenhout, Christophe Deben and Evelien Smits
Center for Oncological Research, University of Antwerp, 2610 Antwerp, Belgium

Joey De Backer and Sylvia Dewilde
Department of Biomedical Sciences, University of Antwerp, 2610 Antwerp, Belgium

Miguel Mateu-Sanz, Juan Tornín, Anna Khlyustova and Cristina Canal
Biomaterials, Biomechanics and Tissue Engineering Group, Department Materials Science and Metallurgy, Technical University of Catalonia (UPC), Escola d'Enginyeria Barcelona Est (EEBE), c/Eduard Maristany 14, 08019 Barcelona, Spain
Barcelona Research Center in Multiscale Science and Engineering, UPC, 08019 Barcelona, Spain
Research Centre for Biomedical Engineering (CREB), UPC, 08019 Barcelona, Spain

Maria-Pau Ginebra
Biomaterials, Biomechanics and Tissue Engineering Group, Department Materials Science and Metallurgy, Technical University of Catalonia (UPC), Escola d'Enginyeria Barcelona Est (EEBE), c/Eduard Maristany 14, 08019 Barcelona, Spain
Barcelona Research Center in Multiscale Science and Engineering, UPC, 08019 Barcelona, Spain
Research Centre for Biomedical Engineering (CREB), UPC, 08019 Barcelona, Spain
Institute for Bioengineering of Catalonia (IBEC), Barcelona Institute of Science and Technology (BIST), c/Baldiri i Reixach 10-12, 08028 Barcelona, Spain

Bénédicte Brulin and Pierre Layrolle
Inserm, UMR 1238, PHY-OS, Laboratory of Bone Sarcomas and Remodeling of Calcified Tissues, Faculty of Medicine, University of Nantes, 44035 Nantes, France

Marie Vallette, Ander Arbelaiz, Fatiha Merabtene, Jérémy Augustin and Laura Fouassier
Institut National de la Santé et de la Recherche Médicale (Inserm), Centre de Recherche Saint-Antoine, CRSA, Sorbonne Université, 75012 Paris, France

Florian Judée, Thierry Dufour and Henri Decauchy
LPP (Laboratoire de Physique des Plasmas, UMR 7648), Sorbonne Université, Centre National de la Recherche Scientifique (CNRS), Ecole Polytechnique, 75005 Paris, France

Javier Vaquero
Institut National de la Santé et de la Recherche Médicale (Inserm), Centre de Recherche Saint-Antoine, CRSA, Sorbonne Université, 75012 Paris, France
LPP (Laboratoire de Physique des Plasmas, UMR 7648), Sorbonne Université, Centre National de la Recherche Scientifique (CNRS), Ecole Polytechnique, 75005 Paris, France
TGF-β and Cancer Group, Oncobell Program, Bellvitge Biomedical Research Institute (IDIBELL), 08908 Barcelona, Spain
Oncology Program, CIBEREHD, National Biomedical Research Institute on Liver and Gastrointestinal Diseases, Instituto de Salud Carlos III, 28029 Madrid, Spain

Ester Gonzalez-Sanchez
Institut National de la Santé et de la Recherche Médicale (Inserm), Centre de Recherche Saint-Antoine, CRSA, Sorbonne Université, 75012 Paris, France
TGF-β and Cancer Group, Oncobell Program, Bellvitge Biomedical Research Institute (IDIBELL), 08908 Barcelona, Spain
Oncology Program, CIBEREHD, National Biomedical Research Institute on Liver and Gastrointestinal Diseases, Instituto de Salud Carlos III, 28029 Madrid, Spain

Lynda Aoudjehane
Institut National de la Santé et de la Recherche Médicale (Inserm), Centre de Recherche Saint-Antoine, CRSA, Sorbonne Université, 75012 Paris, France
Inserm, Institute of Cardiometabolism and Nutrition (ICAN), Sorbonne Université, 75013 Paris, France

Olivier Scatton
Institut National de la Santé et de la Recherche Médicale (Inserm), Centre de Recherche Saint-Antoine, CRSA, Sorbonne Université, 75012 Paris, France
Inserm, Institute of Cardiometabolism and Nutrition (ICAN), Sorbonne Université, 75013 Paris, France
Department of Hepatobiliary Surgery and Liver Transplantation, Pitié-Salpêtrière Hospital, Assistance Publique-Hôpitaux de Paris (AP-HP), 75013 Paris, France

Chantal Housset
Institut National de la Santé et de la Recherche Médicale (Inserm), Centre de Recherche Saint-Antoine, CRSA, Sorbonne Université, 75012 Paris, France
Inserm, Institute of Cardiometabolism and Nutrition (ICAN), Sorbonne Université, 75013 Paris, France
Department of Hepatology, Reference Center for Inflammatory Biliary Diseases and Autoimmune Hepatitis (Centre de Référence Maladies Rares (CRMR), Maladies Inflammatoires des Voies Biliaires et Hépatites Auto-Immunes (MIVB-H), AP-HP, 75012 Paris, France

Mostafa Elhodaky and Alan M. Diamond
Department of Pathology, University of Illinois at Chicago, Chicago, IL 60612, USA

Santosh Reddy Alluri
University of Missouri Research Reactor, University of Missouri, Columbia, MO 65211-5110, USA

Sung Won Kim
Laboratory of Neuroimaging, National Institute on Alcohol Abuse and Alcoholism, National Institutes of Health, Bethesda, MD 20892-1013, USA

Nora D. Volkow
Laboratory of Neuroimaging, National Institute on Alcohol Abuse and Alcoholism, National Institutes of Health, Bethesda, MD 20892-1013, USA
National Institute on Drug Abuse, National Institutes of Health, Bethesda, MD 20892-1013, USA

Kun-Eek Kil
University of Missouri Research Reactor, University of Missouri, Columbia, MO 65211-5110, USA
Department of Veterinary Medicine and Surgery, University of Missouri, Columbia, MO 65211, USA

Pedro M. O. Gomes, Artur M. S. Silva and Vera L. M. Silva
LAQV-REQUIMTE, Department of Chemistry, University of Aveiro, 3810-193 Aveiro, Portugal

Index

A

Adjuvant, 38-39, 88, 141

Alanine Aminotransferase, 162, 174

Amino Acid, 61, 63, 66, 71, 98, 181-182, 185, 197

Angiogenesis, 26, 54, 63, 193-194

Anticancer Agents, 35, 54, 61, 157

Apoptosis, 13-14, 20, 22, 27-28, 30, 32, 35-36, 46-47, 51, 53-54, 58-60, 63, 66, 68, 71, 85, 88, 92, 110, 113, 124-125, 129, 139-143, 151-152, 154, 156, 158, 160, 163-166, 168-171, 175-176, 179, 184-185, 194, 224

B

Biliary Tree, 160-161

Bioluminescent Imaging, 104, 106, 108

Bone Cancer, 142, 146, 157

Brain Cancer, 129-130, 132-133, 138

Breast Cancer, 13-14, 20-21, 23-24, 36, 47, 50, 82, 102, 124-125, 139-140, 178, 183, 185, 187, 191, 193, 203

C

Cancer Cells, 13-15, 20, 24, 27-28, 32, 36-38, 40-41, 46-47, 52, 56, 110, 124-126, 129, 131-134, 137, 139-141, 143, 151-152, 156-158, 169, 171-172, 177-179, 183-187, 190, 192

Cancerous Cells, 128-129, 131-134, 138

Cell Culture Medium, 128-134, 136-138, 143, 150-151

Cell Cycle, 13, 43, 51, 53, 60, 63, 68, 110, 113, 143, 160-161, 165-167, 169-172, 176, 181

Cell Death, 14, 20, 31, 36, 39, 43, 46, 51, 53, 57-58, 60-61, 63, 124, 126, 129, 134-135, 140-141, 143, 146, 148, 151-152, 154, 156-161, 164-165, 171, 177, 179, 181-182

Cell Proliferation, 14, 21, 54, 59-60, 66, 71, 110-111, 124-125, 141, 152, 161, 171, 181, 186

Chemotherapy, 13, 23, 26-27, 29-35, 38, 49-50, 52, 85, 90, 105, 128, 142, 152, 159, 161, 193

Cholangiocarcinoma, 72-73, 92, 160-163, 165, 177-178, 180

Cold Atmospheric Plasma, 13-14, 24, 128, 139-140, 142, 155-163, 165, 169, 173-174, 177-179

Colorectal Cancer, 35, 67, 105, 115, 124-125, 158, 173, 192

Cytology, 1, 7, 12

Cytotoxic Effects, 26, 53, 129-130, 138, 142-144, 146, 151-152, 155

Cytotoxicity, 13, 26-27, 32-33, 37, 43, 45, 47, 53, 65, 130-131, 138, 140, 142-143, 146, 158, 192, 228

D

Dielectric Barrier Discharge, 21, 128, 136, 139, 141, 158

Dna Damage, 26-27, 30-33, 37, 106, 117, 126, 142, 146, 148, 152, 154, 156-157, 159, 164-167, 169, 171-172, 176, 179, 190

Drug Efflux, 13-14

E

Endoplasmic Reticulum, 26-28, 36, 115, 171, 179, 190

Epinephrine, 135-136, 195, 207

F

Fetal Bovine Serum, 21, 48, 64, 66, 119, 135, 152, 173

Fibroblasts, 36, 38-39, 41, 48, 51, 130, 133, 138, 158, 161, 169-170, 172, 188

Follicular Neoplasm, 1, 4, 6, 8

G

Gemcitabine, 139, 161-166, 169-171, 173, 175, 177-178

Genome-wide Expression, 13, 16, 20

Glioblastoma, 14, 24, 72, 124, 130-132, 134-135, 139, 143, 159, 170, 172, 178-179, 186

Glutathione, 26-29, 33-34, 36-39, 43-52, 134, 172, 181-182, 185, 190-192

Growth Hormone, 70-73, 91

H

Head And Neck Cancer, 35, 38, 51, 105-106, 112, 117-118, 123, 126, 135, 139, 141, 159, 192, 194

Healthy Cells, 58, 129, 134-135, 143, 146, 151, 172

Hepatocytes, 161, 165-167, 169-173, 175, 177

Hyperplasia, 1-2, 4, 6-7, 9

Hypopharyngeal Cancer, 104-105, 108, 118, 122

I

Intraperitoneal Injection, 162, 171, 173, 181

Isoselenourea, 53-54, 56, 62, 66

L

Lactate Dehydrogenase, 162-163, 174

Lipid Peroxidation, 38-39, 42-43, 45-47, 50-51

Lymphoma, 35-36, 73, 157, 159

M

Macrophage, 160, 169, 178

Melanocytes, 53, 131, 135-136

Metastasis, 24, 36, 53-54, 59-60, 63, 67-68, 92, 110, 124-125, 178, 184, 190

Methylseleninic Acid, 26-28, 34, 36, 38-40, 48-51

Methylselenol, 27, 32, 39, 42-47, 50, 69

Mitogen-activated Protein Kinase, 54, 66, 179

Mononuclear Blood Cells, 26, 31

Morphometry, 1-2, 7, 12

N
Necrosis, 32, 58, 88, 152, 169
Neurotransmitters, 70, 197
Nuclear-cytoplasmic Ratio, 2

O
Oncology, 26, 35, 38, 91, 93, 100, 103-104, 126, 139, 158, 160-161, 171, 178, 227-228
Optical Emission Spectroscopy, 150, 153
Organotypic Cultures, 142, 144, 146, 149, 152-153, 155
Osteosarcoma, 124, 142, 155-159
Ovarian Cancer, 14, 24, 32, 35, 46, 50, 105, 123, 129, 133, 140, 178, 183, 185, 187, 191
Oxidative Stress, 28, 36, 63, 130, 134, 140-141, 143, 151, 159, 165, 170-171, 179

P
Paclitaxel, 13, 23-24, 39, 47, 50
Papillary Thyroid Cancer, 1-2, 4-6, 12
Penicillin, 21, 33, 64, 119, 135, 152, 173
Peptide Hormone, 70-71
Phosphorylation, 14, 28, 53, 59-61, 63, 123, 134, 160, 165-167, 169, 171, 182, 184
Plasma Membrane, 14, 20
Plasma-activated Ringer's Saline, 142, 144-145, 153
Prognosis, 7, 12-14, 20, 53, 67-68, 105, 111, 124-125, 142, 161, 191-194

R
Radiation Sensitivity, 38, 45, 49
Radiation Therapy, 23, 38-39, 118, 126
Radiolabeling, 70, 76, 78-79, 81-82, 86, 93-94, 97-98, 122, 199, 206, 209, 226
Radionuclide Therapy, 70, 85, 87, 94, 97, 99-103, 122
Radiopharmaceuticals, 70, 75, 77, 79, 82-83, 85, 90, 93-94, 96, 100-102, 105, 122, 207, 213
Radiotherapy, 26-27, 31, 35, 50-51, 70, 90, 95, 99-101, 103, 105, 118, 123, 125-126, 128, 142, 193
Reactive Oxygen Species, 13-14, 21, 24, 32, 46, 50, 140-142, 144-145, 153, 158

S
Selenium, 26, 28, 30, 34-39, 41-42, 44, 46-47, 49-51, 53-54, 56, 62-63, 67-68, 181-182, 189-194
Signaling Pathways, 54, 66, 70-72, 104-105, 115, 164, 166, 171-172, 185
Solid Tumor, 123, 142
Somatostatin, 70-75, 78-85, 87-103, 105, 122
Streptomycin, 21, 33, 64, 135, 152, 173

T
Therapeutic Chemical, 13
Thyroid Nodules, 1-2, 7, 11-12
Tocopherol, 38, 42-43, 45-46
Tumor Microenvironment, 160-161, 172
Tumor Tissue, 39, 135

V
Vemurafenib, 53-54, 67

www.ingramcontent.com/pod-product-compliance
Lightning Source LLC
LaVergne TN
LVHW061513220926
848485LV00018B/1027